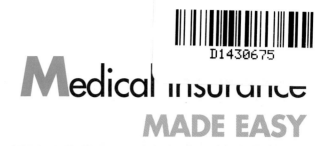

Medical Insurance
MADE EASY

Understanding the Claim Cycle

Medical Insurance
MADE EASY

Understanding the Claim Cycle

JILL L. BROWN, RN, CPC, CPC-H, MPA

Program Coordinator
Medical Billing and Coding Specialist Program
Americare School of Nursing and Health Professions
Fern Park, Florida;
Former Captain
United States Air Force;
Former Instructor
Medical Assisting Program
Central Florida College (formerly Career Training Institute)
Orlando, Florida

SECOND EDITION

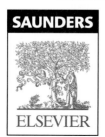

SAUNDERS

ELSEVIER

SAUNDERS
ELSEVIER

11830 Westline Industrial Drive
St. Louis, Missouri 63146

MEDICAL INSURANCE MADE EASY: UNDERSTANDING
THE CLAIM CYCLE, SECOND EDITION

ISBN-13: 978-0-7216-0556-2
ISBN-10: 0-7216-0556-7

Notice

Knowledge and best practice in this field are constantly changing. As new research and experience broaden our knowledge, changes in practice, treatment, and drug therapy may become necessary or appropriate. Readers are advised to check the most current information provided (i) on procedures featured or (ii) by the manufacturer of each product to be administered, to verify the recommended dose or formula, the method and duration of administration, and contraindications. It is the responsibility of the practitioner, relying on his or her own experience and knowledge of the patient, to make diagnoses, to determine dosages and the best treatment for each individual patient, and to take all appropriate safety precautions. To the fullest extent of the law, neither the Publisher nor the Author assumes any liability for any injury and/or damage to persons or property arising out of or related to any use of the material contained in this book.

The Publisher

ISBN-13: 978-0-7216-0556-2
ISBN-10: 0-7216-0556-7

Publishing Director: Andrew M. Allen
Senior Acquisitions Editor: Susan Cole
Developmental Editor: Beth LoGiudice
Publishing Services Manager: Patricia Tannian
Project Manager: Kristine Feeherty
Design Direction: Andrea Lutes

Printed in the United States of America

Last digit is the print number: 9 8 7 6 5 4 3 2 1

To my family

My children, **Jeremiah** and **Jason**
My mother, **Vivian**

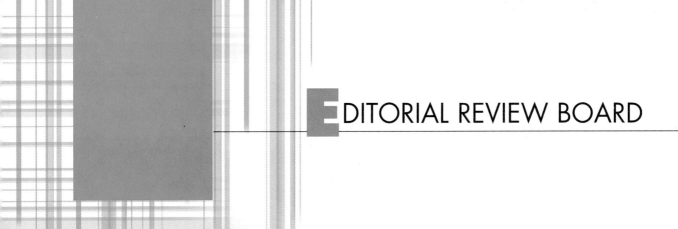

EDITORIAL REVIEW BOARD

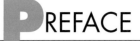

PREFACE

Why Learn About Medical Insurance?

Although the practice of medicine dates back to the earliest civilizations, medical insurance is a relative newcomer, invented only during the past century. Over the course of the last 45 years, laws regulating health care have become increasingly complex as both government and private medical insurance plans have tried to control rapidly growing costs.

In the medical office, clinical employees are primarily responsible for production (the process of delivering medical care), and business office employees are primarily responsible for collections (the process of collecting payment). However, both clinical employees and business office employees play a significant role in the reimbursement process. Clinical employees are held accountable for collecting physician-supplied information for the bottom half of the medical claim form, and the physicians are held accountable for meeting clinical documentation requirements. Business office employees are held accountable for collecting patient-supplied information for the top half of the medical claim form and for filing medical claims and collecting all payments due.

Delivering medical care is expensive. The business expenses—rent, telephone, electricity, furniture,

equipment, supplies, malpractice insurance, salaries, and employee benefits—are paid from the revenue (money) that is collected. A medical business cannot survive unless correct payment is collected for every service delivered.

In the average medical office today, a large portion of the payments is collected from medical insurance companies, and only small portions are collected from individual patients. Collecting payment from medical insurance plans can be very time consuming, and the rules that must be followed often change every year. One tiny piece of missing information or one missed step in the documentation process can result in a payment of 30% or less of the amount rightfully earned by the physician, and occasionally the payment is zero. Therefore it is imperative that every employee learns about medical insurance and that all employees learn to work together as a cohesive reimbursement team.

Note: Increasingly, nonphysician providers, such as physician's assistants (PAs) and nurse practitioners (NPs), also provide medical care. Unless an exception is noted in the text, items that apply to physicians also apply to nonphysician providers.

Text Objectives

Those completing this text will be able to demonstrate how to file clean claims using payor-specific rules and determine whether or not the correct reimbursement has been collected from specific payors. In the process, readers will gain an appreciation for each piece of clinical documentation and billing information, no matter how small and insignificant it may seem, and they will gain an appreciation for the importance of every employee position in a medical office.

Chapter 1, *Learning to Speak the Language,* explains how to interpret the language that is unique to medical offices.

Chapter 2, *You're Part of a Team,* demonstrates the role each employee plays in collecting the information required to file a medical claim.

Chapter 3, *How the Medical Claim Cycle Works,* introduces and gives an overview of the claim-filing process. It explains the lifecycle of a clean claim and illustrates the forms used to gather the required information. The topics introduced in Chapter 3 are covered in more detail throughout the remaining chapters.

Chapter 4, *CMS-1500 Claim Form,* illustrates the requirements for each field on the CMS-1500 medical insurance claim form used by physicians and other outpatient providers. The claim form is taught using the perspective of the payor's expectations, and this chapter includes many practical billing tips.

Chapter 5, *Basic Principles of Diagnosis Coding;* Chapter 6, *Basic Principles for Evaluation and Management (E/M) Services;* and Chapter 7, *Basic Principles of Procedure Coding,* offer a basic understanding of how medical coding is used to bill for the services delivered and explain how medical documentation and coding influence reimbursement. ICD-9-CM, CPT-4, and HCPCS codes are covered in these chapters. Also included is coverage on ICD-10, CPT-5, the Correct Coding Initiative, 1995 and 1997 documentation guidelines, and the ideas that have been proposed for new guidelines. These coding chapters cover basic coding in more detail than many competing textbooks.

Chapter 8, *Private Indemnity and Managed Care Medical Plans,* and Chapter 9, *Other Insurance Plans with Medical Coverage and Disability Plans,* define basic differences and similarities between the types of private medical plans (including private managed care plans) and other private plans with medical coverage one may encounter while working in a physician's office.

Chapter 10, *Medicare,* and Chapter 11, *Other Government Medical Plans,* define differences and similarities among the various government medical plans (including government managed care plans) one may encounter while working in a physician's office.

Chapter 12, *Hospital/Facility Billing Rules,* defines the prospective payment systems used by Medicare to pay physicians (RBRVS), inpatient hospital charges (DRG), outpatient hospital charges (APC), and other facility charges. It then illustrates the requirements for each field on the UB-92 medical insurance claim form used by hospitals and facilities. The claim form is taught using the perspective of the payor's expectations, and this chapter includes many practical billing tips. This chapter covers the UB-92 claim form in more detail than many competing textbooks.

Chapter 13, *Reimbursement Success,* teaches how to evaluate each payment received and determine whether additional actions are warranted. It also includes a selection of the actual reason codes used by payors to explain reimbursement decisions.

Chapter 14, *Developing Critical Thinking Skills: Analyzing Problems and Making Decisions,* teaches critical thinking skills, suggesting how to analyze a variety of potential problems and make decisions. Also included is the timetable for the implementation of key provisions of the Health Insurance Portability and Accountability Act of 1996 (HIPAA).

Text Features

Learning Objectives found at the beginning of each chapter offer students an overview of the chapter and help them measure their progress. They also assist the instructor in preparing lecture material.

Objectives   After completing this chapter, you should be able to:

- Relate three or more responsibilities of business office personnel
- Briefly explain how each business office employee influences medical reimbursement
- Discuss legal aspects for each business office position
- Relate three or more of the responsibilities of the clinical staff
- Briefly explain clinical staff responsibilities for documentation and how it influences reimbursement
- Discuss legal aspects for each clinical staff position

Key Terms, also found at the beginning of each chapter, are found in bold print throughout the text and are defined at the beginning of the chapter, in the text, and in the glossary found in the back of the book. Many of the key terms are important in subsequent chapters, and the glossary makes it easy to locate definitions quickly.

Key Terms

ancillary medical providers professionals with a limited license to practice medicine, and medical therapists who perform billable services.

billing manager the supervisor in charge of medical billing and collections; may or may not include medical coding.

business office personnel employees in the medical business office: office manager, billing manager, schedulers, receptionists, billers, collections employees, medical records employees, and professional medical coders.

certified coding professional someone who has met the educational and experience prerequisites and who has passed a medical coding certification test administered by a professional coding organization.

collections employee an employee with responsibility for collecting payments from insurance companies and patients.

credentialing the process of verifying credentials to establish that a person has not misrepresented accomplishments, that licensure remains current, and that the person has not been excluded from participation in federal medical plans.

custodian of records the employee who is legally responsible for the care and handling of medical records for the medical practice.

DC doctor of chiropractic medicine; schooling focuses on medical health in relation to spinal alignment; fully licensed to practice chiropractic medicine.

DO doctor of osteopathy; similar to an MD, but schooling

Stop and Review Exercises are located at intervals throughout each chapter to allow students to master each chapter one section at a time. Most Stop and Review sections have 10 exercises. They are presented in a variety of formats, including true/false, multiple choice, mix and match, fill in the blank, and short answer.

STOP & REVIEW

Please answer the following questions:

1. When patients arrive for an appointment, they should check in by signing their name on a community sign-in sheet.

    ____True   ____False

2. If the scheduler entered all the registration information into the computer at the time the appointment was scheduled, a new patient does not need to fill out a patient registration form on the day of the appointment.

    ____True   ____False

3. Circle the correct answer. The patient history form is designed to:
    A. Report the patient's past medical history
    B. Report past medical history for blood relatives
    C. Report the patient's social history
    D. Report the social history for those who live with the patient
    E. All of the above

4. The interim history form may be used if a complete history is on file for an established patient. It reports changes since the patient's last visit.

    ____True   ____False

5. The patient may not list just a P.O. box address on the registration form. The physical address where the patient lives must also be listed in case an ambulance should need to be dispatched in the future.

    ____True   ____False

6. There is only one correct way to design a form for a medical office.

    ____True   ____False

Match the circumstance in column A with the form in column B:

COLUMN A

7. Medicare service listed as noncovered
8. Treatment with significant risks
9. Provider opted out of Medicare
10. Service possibly not medically necessary by Medicare's definitions

COLUMN B

A. Waiver of Medicare Part B Entitlement
B. ABN of Medicare Medical Necessity
C. Consent to Treatment
D. ABN of Non covered Medicare Part B Services

Use the birthday rule to determine whose plan is the primary payor:

Mother's birthday is October 10; father's birthday is October 2.

_____

Mother's birthday is September 6; father's birthday is May 18.

_____

Mother's birthday is February 9; father's birthday is December 29.

Clinical Application Exercises occur periodically throughout the text to provide students with practical application of discussed concepts.

Clinical Application Exercise

Thomas is a 14-year-old boy with a history of cerebral palsy, spastic diplegia with quadriparesis, since infancy. He normally ambulates short distances and uses a wheelchair the remainder of the time. Thomas lost his balance and fell 10 days ago while walking at home and injured his right foot. Home treatment for a sprain has proven ineffective, and he is now unable to ambulate at all. An x-ray of the foot shows a closed fracture of the fourth metatarsal and a loss of bone density in the right foot. Because of Thomas's unusual gait and the presence of osteoporosis from disuse, a decision is made to apply a cast.

Code the diagnoses for this visit.

1. _____   3. _____

2. _____   4. _____

"Sidebars" are set off from the core subject matter and contain additional important information to augment the text discussion.

policyholder for the second plan. When the patient is the insured for both the primary and the secondary plans, this field is left blank.

> When a husband and a wife both have family policies issued by their respective employers, special rules apply. When the husband is the patient, his policy is always primary. When the wife is the patient, her policy is always primary. In both instances, the spouse's plan is secondary.

Examples illustrate the correct use of guidelines and concepts presented in text discussion.

specificity, as well as the presence or absence of significant comorbidities, greatly influence the statistical value of medical research.

For example: A new wound management system is the subject of a study. Unfortunately, most of the medical claims submitted list only the diagnosis for the wound and only the procedure for the new treatment. Medical researchers and insurance actuaries are unable to determine how other variables, such as comorbidities (e.g., diabetes, heart disease, kidney disease) and other procedures (e.g., whirlpool treatments or wound debridement), might have influenced the study's findings.

Insurance companies use the results of medical research to determine the cost effectiveness of one treatment over another. When variables are tracked

Chapter Reviews that consist of a summary review followed by review exercises are found at the end of each chapter. Most Chapter Review sections contain 20 exercises. Like the Stop and Review exercises, they are presented in a variety of formats.

Chapter Review

In the United States, ICD-9-CM is the codebook currently used for diagnosis coding. ICD-9-CM stands for "International Classification of Diseases, Ninth Revision, Clinical Modification."

Volume 1 contains the tabular list and is followed by supplements for V-codes, E-codes, and five informational appendices. The information in the tabular list is divided into chapters, sections, categories, subcategories, and subclassifications. Symbols and abbreviations also are used to convey information.

Volume 2 contains the alphabetical index of diseases (the diagnosis code index), the hypertension table, the neoplasm table, a table of drugs and chemicals, and an alphabetical index to the causes of external injuries and poisoning (the E-code index).

Answer the following questions:

1. Is it possible to code accurately from the alphabetical index alone? Why or why not?

2. Which is the correct standard code order?
   A. Primary diagnosis, secondary conditions, anything else that influences treatment
   B. The order in which codes are listed in the patient's medical record
   C. Principal diagnosis, primary diagnosis, secondary diagnoses
   D. The order in which codes are listed on the SuperBill

Appendix A contains a full set of the 1997 documentation guideline examination tables. **Appendix B** contains a directory of state insurance departments and other resources. **Appendix C** contains billing information for a fictional medical office and 10 realistic case studies. The case studies range in difficulty from easy to complex, and they may be used with the coding chapters (Chapters 5, 6, and 7) for additional coding practice. The fee schedule may be used with Chapter 3 and Chapter 13 for additional reimbursement practice. **Appendix D** contains the *Quick Guide to HIPAA for the Physician's Office* for reference when studying HIPAA guidelines.

Supplements

STUDENT PRACTICE CD-ROM

Ten case studies from the fictional Lake Eola Family Practice Associates, featured in Appendix C, are presented on a free CD-ROM bound in the back of this textbook to give students practical experience in completing CMS-1500 claim forms for a variety of payors. The case studies range in difficulty from easy to complex. Students will gain a greater understanding of how to complete the claim form by gathering information from the patient files presented. This software will give students a real-world, hands-on approach, helping them to gain the knowledge and experience needed for working in the medical office.

Students learn to set up a medical practice from scratch, including setting up the office and each physician in the fictional Lake Eola Family Practice Associates (featured in Appendix C). Students then register each new patient presented in Appendix C as the patient checks in for his or her appointment, check out the patient at the conclusion of his or her appointment, print claims (on plain paper), check the claims for accuracy (copy a CMS-1500 form onto transparency film and place it over each "plain-paper claim"), post both patient and insurance payments, and post write-offs to give a realistic medical office experience without leaving school.

A demonstration version of AltaPoint practice management software is available for download on the Evolve site for extra practice.

INSTRUCTOR'S RESOURCE MANUAL WITH CD-ROM

This comprehensive instructor resource presented on CD-ROM contains a variety of features for each chapter. In addition to introductions, learning objectives, key terms with definitions, and answers to Stop and Review and Chapter Review sections, this resource will also include:

- ☐ Class activities
- ☐ PowerPoint slides
- ☐ Additional learning references
- ☐ Additional learning tools with answers

A computerized test bank is also included on this CD-ROM, containing more than 1000 test questions with answers. Test questions are organized by chapter and presented in a variety of formats, including true/false, multiple choice, fill in the blank, and short answer. Rationales are provided for many of the answers.

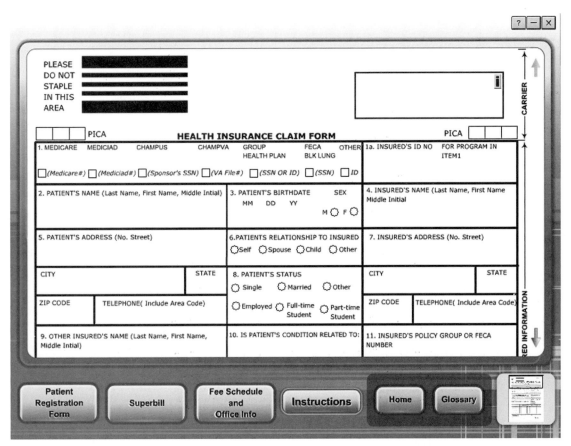

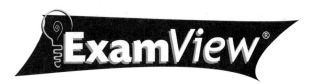

ACKNOWLEDGMENTS

My grateful thanks to the many wonderful people who participated in the creation, production, and marketing of this book:

I thank the entire staff at Elsevier for their dedication, perseverance, and patience as I wrote this text during an exceptionally difficult period of my life and missed deadline after deadline. I especially thank Susan Cole, Senior Acquisitions Editor for Health Professions; Beth LoGiudice, Developmental Editor; and Kristine Feeherty, Project Manager, for their endless patience and skillful guidance.

I thank my students, friends, and colleagues who offered inspiration, encouragement, verification of facts, and practical suggestions.

Finally, I thank all of the education professionals who took time out of their busy schedules to review this text and offer professional opinions and suggestions.

Jill L. Brown

CONTENTS

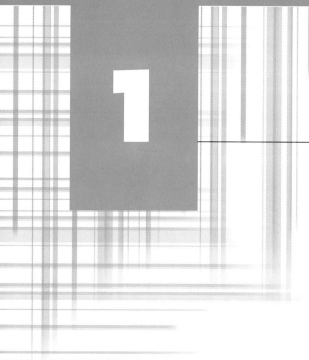

1

LEARNING TO SPEAK THE LANGUAGE

Objectives After completing this chapter, you should be able to:

- Determine the meaning of medical words and phrases frequently encountered in a medical office
- Recite basic information about human anatomy and physiology
- Use root words, prefixes, and suffixes to obtain clues to the meanings of many medical words
- Demonstrate abbreviations frequently used in medical offices and clinics
- Distinguish among signs, symptoms, and significant findings
- Recognize terms used in medical prescriptions
- Recognize units of measure used in medical offices and clinics

Key Terms

circulatory system uses the heart, blood, and blood vessels in a complex delivery system for the body. The heart pumps the blood and keeps it flowing through the blood vessels. Arteries carry blood away from the heart and veins carry blood back to the heart.

combining vowel a vowel inserted to link word parts together to make them easier to read.

constitutional signs and symptoms includes vital signs and an assessment of a person's general well being.

digestive system processes food to provide nutrients to the body and processes solid waste that is expelled by the body.

endocrine system uses ductless glands to produce hormones. Hormones regulate many body functions.

eponym a word, such as a medical diagnosis or procedure, that is named after a person or a place.

genitourinary system the reproductive and urinary systems. The male and female reproductive systems work together to create a baby. The urinary system processes and expels liquid waste from the body.

immune system uses the lymphatic system and the spleen to fight infection and regulate immune responses. Also regulates the amount of fluid in and around body cells.

integumentary system consists of skin, hair, nails, sebaceous glands, and sweat glands. It is the body's largest organ system and the first line of defense against infection.

musculoskeletal system muscles and bones provide the framework that gives the body shape, form, and movement.

nervous system the electronic computer system for the body. It gathers, stores, and interprets information, and it initiates responses. It includes the central nervous system, the peripheral nervous system, and the autonomic nervous system.

prefix a word part attached at the beginning of a word to add to or alter the meaning of the word.

prescription an order for a drug, treatment, or device, written or given by a properly licensed professional.

respiratory system uses breathing to bring oxygen into the body and to expel carbon dioxide from the body.

root word the word part that gives the basic meaning of the word.

sign a change from normal noted or observed by the examiner.

significant finding a change from normal (a sign or a symptom) or a significant normal finding that narrows the options and leads to a diagnosis.

suffix a word part attached at the end of a word that adds to or alters the meaning of the word.

symptom a change or suspected change from normal noted or observed by the patient.

vital signs a minimum of 3 of 10 possible examination items identified by the American Medical Association considered critical to assess body function.

Introduction

Taking the time to learn the meanings of common medical words is very important for every medical office employee. The physicians, your co-workers, and the patients must have confidence that you understand what they are saying.

The easiest way to learn the meaning of medical words is to learn how to break them into smaller parts. In this chapter, you will learn how to interpret medical words using basic word parts that give clues to the meaning of each word. *If you have already completed a medical terminology course or an anatomy and physiology course, you will find this chapter to be a good review.* If you wish to take a medical terminology or an anatomy and physiology course later, you will find this chapter to be a valuable introduction for those courses.

Word Parts

Most medical words are developed by combining root words that describe the structure and function of the body. A **root word** gives the basic meaning of the word. A word must have at least one root to be considered a word, and a word with one root can stand alone as a complete word. Medical words often have more than one root word.

In addition, medical words often contain prefixes and suffixes. A **prefix** is a word part that is attached to the beginning of a word. A **suffix** is a word part that is attached at the end of a word. Prefixes and suffixes have specific meanings that either add to or alter the meaning of the root word, but they do not contain root words, and they are seldom used alone. When a prefix is listed alone, a hyphen is attached at the end of the prefix to indicate that something should come after (e.g., epi-). When a suffix is listed alone, a hyphen is attached at the beginning of the suffix to indicate that something should come before (e.g., -ic).

When you separate a word into various word parts, a slash (/) is used to show where the divisions occur. The word epi/gastr/ic has a prefix, a root word, and a suffix. The prefix *epi-* means "above"; the root word *gastr* means "stomach"; the suffix *-ic* means "pertaining to." Therefore *epigastric* means "pertaining to above the stomach."

Combining vowels make words easier to read. Whereas *o* is the most commonly used combining vowel, it is not the only combining vowel: *a* and *i* are also used. A combining vowel is always inserted to link root words together and is sometimes inserted to link root words to suffixes. The only time a combining vowel is dropped is when a suffix begins with a vowel. It is not dropped if a root word begins with a vowel. The word *hemat/o/logy* has a root word, a combining vowel, and a suffix. *Hemat* is the root word and means "blood"; *o* is the combining vowel; *-logy* is the suffix and means "study of." Therefore *hematology* means "the study of blood."

When a medical term is named after a person or a place and does not have a combination of word parts that give clues to the meaning of the word, the term is called an **eponym.** Many diseases and conditions are named for the person who discovered them. Eponyms are always capitalized.

To help you learn to use combining vowels correctly, the root words listed in word part tables throughout this chapter will be listed with combining vowels. By learning the most common root words, prefixes, and suffixes and how they are combined, you will be able to determine the meanings of most medical words. Many of the word part tables also list a few select eponyms and common abbreviations.

STOP & REVIEW Use the root words, prefixes, and suffixes from Table 1-1 and follow the directions to complete the exercises. Rewrite each word using slashes to separate the word parts, and then write the meaning.

1. abdominal

_____

2. abdominoplasty

_____

3. endocardiac

_____

Write medical terms by combining word parts, and then write the meaning.

4. cardi/o + my/o + -pathy

_____

5. bi- + later/o + -al

_____

6. hist/o + -logy

_____

7. tachy- + cardi/o + -ia

_____

Write a term to match the meanings.

8. A condition in which the heart is slow

_____

9. Pertaining to one side

_____

10. Inflammation around the heart

_____

Musculoskeletal System

The **musculoskeletal system** (Figure 1-1) provides the framework that gives the human body shape, form, and movement. It is made up of bones, joints, muscles, and connective tissue. The skeleton consists of bones and gives the basic shape to the body. The places where the bones come together are called joints. Some joints allow movement, and muscles provide the movement. The bones, joints, and muscles are held in place by connective tissue such as tendons and ligaments. There are many types of bones, muscles, and joints. Each type has a specific function and purpose.

The hard, rigid exterior of a bone gives strength to the skeleton and protects the important, soft interior of the bone, called marrow. New blood cells develop and mature in the marrow.

Skeletal muscles give the body form, and they work with nerves and joints to give the body movement. Skeletal muscles contract and relax in response to the signals sent by the central nervous system (voluntary movement). Smooth muscles are present in many of the organ systems (digestive, respiratory, circulatory, lymphatic, and genitourinary), and they contract and relax in response to signals sent by the parasympathetic nervous system (involuntary movement).

Joints can either be fixed, with no movement (as in the skull), or they can allow movement. Some are hinged joints, allowing movement in two directions (as in knees, elbows, fingers, and toes), and others are ball-in-socket joints, allowing rotation and movement in many directions (as in shoulders and hips).

TABLE 1-1
Word Parts

Root Words Root—Meaning	Prefixes Prefix—Meaning	Suffixes Suffix—Meaning
abdomin/o—abdomen	**bi-**—two	**-ac, -al, -ic**—pertaining to
cardi/o—heart	**brady-**—slow	**-itis**—inflammation
hist/o—tissue	**end-, endo-**—inside	**-ia**—condition
immun/o—immune	**peri-**—around	**-logy**—study, science
later/o—side	**tachy-**—fast	**-pathy**—disease
my/o—muscle	**uni-**—one	**-plasty**—surgical repair

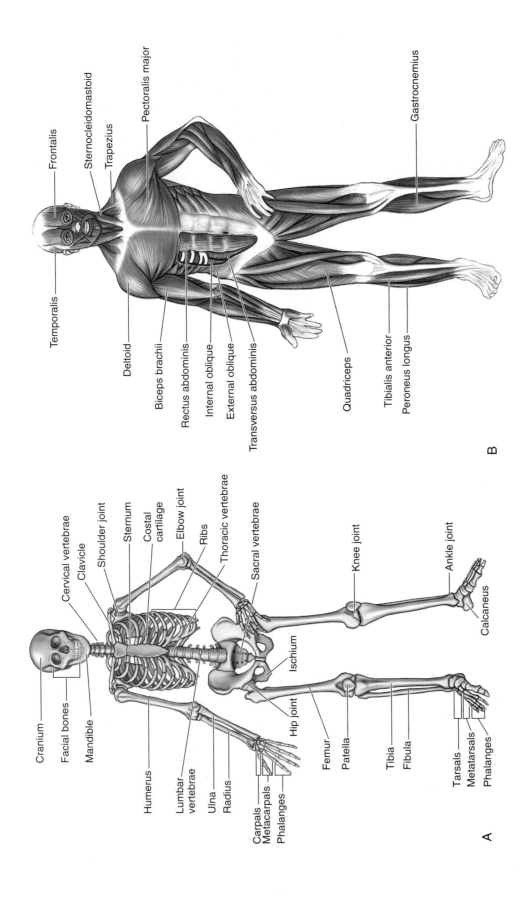

FIGURE 1-1

The musculoskeletal system. **A**, skeleton; **B**, muscles. (Modified from from Herlihy B and Maebius N: The Human Body in Health and Illness. Philadelphia, WB Saunders, 2000, pp. 111, 150.)

STOP & REVIEW

Complete the following statements:

1. _____ give the body shape. They have a hard exterior and a soft interior.

2. _____ give the body form and work with _____ and nerves to give the body movement.

3. _____ holds the rest of the musculoskeletal system in place.

Use Table 1-2 to define the following:

4. Chondromalacia _____

5. Arthrodesis _____

6. Spondylolisthesis _____

7. Myasthenia _____

8. Lyme disease _____

9. RA _____

10. DTR _____

TABLE 1-2
Word Parts for Musculoskeletal System Terminology

Root Words

Root—Meaning	Root—Meaning	Root—Meaning
acetabulo/o—acetabulum (hip socket)	**infer/o**—inferior, situated below	**phylang/o**—phalanges (bones in fingers and toes)
ankyl/o—crooked, bent, or stiff joint	**kinesi/o**—movement	**plant/o**—sole (bottom) of the foot
arthr/o, articul/o—joint, articulation (joint movement)	**kyph/o**—humpback (outward curve in upper back)	**proxim/o**—proximal, near
burs/o—bursa (provides lubrication for joints)	**later/o**—side	**radi/o**—radius (one of lower arm bones) or radiant energy (x-rays)
calc/o, calci/o—calcium	**ligament/o**—ligament (connective tissue binding bones to bones)	**rhabdomy/o**—skeletal muscle connected to bones
carp/o—carpals (wrist bones)	**lord/o**—swayback (inward curve of the lower back)	**rheumat/o**—watery flow (usually in joints)
cephal/o—head	**lumb/o**—lower back, loins	**scapul/o**—scapula (shoulder bone)
cervic/o—neck	**mandibul/o**—mandible (lower jaw)	**scoli/o**—crooked, bent (back curves sideways)
chir/o—hand	**maxill/o**—maxilla (upper jaw)	**spondyl/o**—vertebral (conditions)
chondr/o—cartilage	**medi/o**—medial, middle	**stern/o**—sternum (breast bone)
clavicul/o—clavicle (collar bone)	**metacarp/o**—metacarpals (hand bones)	**synov/o**—synovial membrane (lining in movable joints)
coccyg/o—coccyx (tailbone)	**metatars/o**—metatarsals (foot bones)	**tars/o**—tarsals (ankle bones)
cost/o—ribs	**my/o, myos/o**—muscles	**ten/o, tendin/o**—tendons (connective tissue binding muscles to bones)
crani/o—cranium (skull bones)	**myel/o**—bone marrow, spinal cord	**thorac/o**—thorax, chest
dactyl/o—digit (fingers and toes)	**onc/o**—tumor	**tibi/o**—tibia (shin bone in lower leg)
dors/o—dorsal (back)	**orth/o**—straight	**uln/o**—ulna (one of lower arm bones)
fasci/o—fascia (forms sheaths enveloping muscles)	**oste/o**—bone	**vertebr/o**—vertebral (structure)
femor/o—femur (thigh bone)	**patell/a, patell/o**—patella (kneecap)	
fibr/o—fibrous connective tissue	**path/o**—disease	
fibul/o, perone/o—fibula (one of two bones in lower leg)	**ped/o**—foot, child	
humer/o—humerus (upper arm bone)	**pelv/i**—pelvis (hip bone)	
ili/o—ilium (upper part of the pelvic bone)		

Prefixes

Prefix—Meaning	Prefix—Meaning	Prefix—Meaning
a-, an-—no, not, without	**dys-**—bad, painful, difficul	**multi-**—many
ab-—away from	**hemi-**—half	**poly-**—many, much
ad-—toward	**infra-**—situated below	**pre-**—before
anti-—against	**inter-**—between	**retro-**—backward, behind
contra-—against, not, opposite	**intra-**—within	**super-, supra-**—above, excess
dorsi-—back	**meta-**—change, next	**syn-**—joined, together

Continued.

TABLE 1-2
Word Parts for Musculoskeletal System Terminology—cont'd

Suffixes		
Suffix—Meaning	Suffix—Meaning	Suffix—Meaning
-ac, -al, -ic, -eal—pertaining to	**-listhesis**—slipping	**-plegia**—paralysis (loss of ability to move body parts)
-ad—toward	**-malacia—softening**	**-porosis**—pore, passage
-algia, -dynia—pain	**-oma**—tumor, mass, swelling	**-schisis**—split
-asthenia—weakness, lack of strength	**-osis**—abnormal condition, disease, abnormal increase	**-scopy**—viewing, examining
-clasia—break	**-paresis**—less than total paralysis	**-stenosis**—narrowing
-desis—to bind, tie together, fuse	**-physis**—to grow	**-trophy**—development, nourishment
-ectomy—surgical removal, excision		**-y**—state, condition
-ema, -ia, -iasis—condition		

Eponyms
Eponym—Meaning
Bence Jones protein—a protein found almost exclusively in the urine of a patient with multiple myeloma.
Ewing's sarcoma—a malignant bone tumor most often found in children and teenagers; pain and swelling are common. It is treated with radiation therapy and chemotherapy.
Lyme disease—a disease carried by a tick; recurrent symptoms include weakness, muscle pain, joint pain, impairment of nerves, and impairment of heart. It is treated with antibiotics.

Abbreviations		
Abbreviation—Meaning	Abbreviation—Meaning	Abbreviation—Meaning
BK—below knee	**IM**—intramuscular injection	**ROM**—range of motion
Ca—calcium	**lab**—laboratory	**SLE**—systemic lupus erythematosus
CTS—carpal tunnel syndrome	**LS**—lumbosacral	**SLR**—straight-leg raising
C1-C7—cervical vertebrae 1-7	**L1-L5**—lumbar vertebrae 1-5	**TMJ**—temporomandibular joint
DJD—degenerative joint disease	**ortho**—orthopedic, orthopaedic	**T1-T12**—thoracic vertebrae 1-12
DTR—deep tendon reflexes	**RA**—rheumatoid arthritis	**x-ray**—a diagnostic test to investigate the integrity of body structures
EMG—electromyelogram	**RF**—rheumatoid factor	

STOP & REVIEW

Complete the following:

1. Skin has _____ layers.

2. This layer of skin contains the blood vessels and nerve fibers. _____

3. This layer of skin is composed of fat cells. _____
   _____

4. Why does the skin have oil glands? _____
   _____

Use Table 1-3 to define the following:

5. Bactericidal _____

6. Subcutaneous _____

7. Dermatitis _____

8. Mohs' surgery _____

9. I & D _____

10. Subq _____

TABLE 1-3
Word Parts for Integumentary System Terminology

Root Words		
Root—Meaning	Root—Meaning	Root—Meaning
adip/o, lip/o, steat/o—fat	**hidr/o**—sweat	**pil/o, trich/o**—hair, hair follicle
albin/o—white	**ichthy/o**—fish, scaly, dry	**py/o**—pus
axill/o—armpit	**kerat/o**—hard horny tissue, cornea	**rhytid/o**—wrinkle
bacter/i—bacteria	**leuk/o**—white	**seb/o**—sebum (oily secretion from sebaceous glands in skin)
caus/o—burn, burning	**melan/o**—black	**seps/o, sept/o**—infection, septum
cry/o—cold	**myc/o**—fungus (yeast, molds, mushrooms)	**squam/o**—scalelike
cutane/o, derm/o, dermat/o—skin	**necr/o**—dead or death	**therm/o**—heat
diaphor/o—profuse sweating	**onych/o, ungu/o**—nail	**xanth/o**—yellow
erythem/o, erythmat/o—redness	**phyt/o**—plant	**xer/o**—dry
heli/o—sun		

TABLE 1-3
Word Parts for Integumentary System Terminology—cont'd

Prefixes

Prefix—Meaning	Prefix—Meaning	Prefix—Meaning
dia-—through **hyper-**—above, excessive, more than normal	**hypo-**—below, deficient, less than **in-**—in, into, not	**meso-**—middle **sub-**—under

Suffixes

Suffix—Meaning	Suffix—Meaning	Suffix—Meaning
-ac, -al, -ic—pertaining to **-algesia**—sensitivity to pain **-algia**—pain **-cidal**—killing **-derma**—skin	**-edema**—swelling **-itis**—inflammation **-oma**—tumor, mass, swelling **-osis**—abnormal condition,	**-ous**—pertaining to, characterized by **-pathy**—disease disease, abnormal increase **-plasia, -plasm**—formation, growth

Eponyms
Eponym—Meaning

acne vulgaris—a condition caused by a buildup of oil and keratin in the skin. *Vulgaris* means ordinary. Sometimes pores become partially or completely blocked, which can lead to infection. Severe cases are treated with antibiotics and drying agents.

Mohs' surgery—microscopically controlled surgery in which thin layers of a malignant growth are removed and examined under a microscope.

Abbreviations

Abbreviation—Meaning	Abbreviation—Meaning	Abbreviation—Meaning
Bx, bx—biopsy **Derm**—Dermatology **DLE**—discoid lupus erythematosus **EAHF**—eczema, asthma, and hay fever	**I & D**—incise and drain **LE**—lupus erythematosus **Subq, subq**—subcutaneous	**TENS**—transcutaneous electrical **UV**—ultraviolet nerve stimulation

Integumentary System

The **integumentary system** (Figure 1-2) contains skin, hair, nails, sweat glands, oil glands, a blood supply, a lymph supply, a nerve supply, and a layer of fat. Skin is the largest organ of the body, and the first line of defense against infection. Skin has three layers.

The thin outer layer is called the epidermis. The epidermis is composed of dead cells that form a tough protective coating on the outside and living cells on the inside. As the dead cells are worn away, the living cells multiply and replace them. Nails are part of the epidermis. The middle layer, called the dermis, is the thickest layer. Many consider it to be true skin. The dermis contains hair roots, sweat glands, oil glands (called sebaceous glands), the blood supply, the lymph supply, hair muscles, and the nerve supply. Each is held in place by connective tissue. The innermost layer, called the subcutaneous layer, is composed entirely of fat cells. These fatty substances make skin waterproof.

Skin is a sensory organ. It allows you to tell the difference between touch, temperature, pain, pressure, and itching. It also helps regulate body temperature. When the body is hot, the sweat glands produce perspiration and the blood vessels dilate (get bigger) to get rid of heat. When the body is cold, the blood vessels constrict (get smaller) to retain heat. The sebaceous glands produce an oily substance to keep skin supple. There are no sebaceous glands on the palms of the hands or the soles of the feet.

Respiratory System

Respiration is the process by which oxygen reaches body cells. It is used for metabolism, and is the process by which carbon dioxide, a waste product from metabolism, is expelled from the body. We inhale (breathe in) oxygen and exhale (breathe out) carbon dioxide. The **respiratory system** (Figure 1-3) works closely with the circulatory system.

Air containing oxygen is drawn in through the nose or mouth where it is warmed, filtered, and moistened before it travels through the trachea (windpipe) to

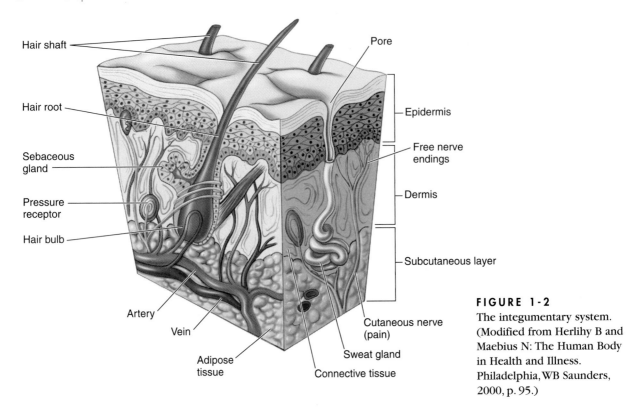

Hair shaft

Hair root

Sebaceous gland

Pressure receptor

Hair bulb

Artery

Vein

Adipose tissue

Connective tissue

Sweat gland

Cutaneous nerve (pain)

Pore

Epidermis

Free nerve endings

Dermis

Subcutaneous layer

FIGURE 1-2
The integumentary system. (Modified from Herlihy B and Maebius N: The Human Body in Health and Illness. Philadelphia, WB Saunders, 2000, p. 95.)

reach the branching tubes called bronchi that deliver it to the lungs. In the lungs, each bronchus branches further into bronchioles. Bronchioles end with small air sacs called alveoli.

The pulmonary artery leads from the right side of the heart and delivers blood full of carbon dioxide to the alveoli in the lungs, where the carbon dioxide is removed and oxygen is picked up. The pulmonary veins deliver the blood full of oxygen back to the left side of the heart for distribution to the rest of the body. The pulmonary circulatory system is the only circulatory system in which arteries carry blood full of carbon dioxide, and the veins carry blood full of oxygen.

In the systemic circulatory system, arteries carry blood full of oxygen to individual cells in the body where the oxygen is used for metabolism. Metabolism is the process by which cells are nourished and energy is produced. Carbon dioxide is a waste product of metabolism that is removed by respiration. Blood full of carbon dioxide is carried back to the heart through veins and is then pumped back to the lungs through the pulmonary artery, and the cycle starts over again.

The ability to speak is also dependent on the respiratory system. The larynx, or voice box, forms the Adam's apple and is larger in men. The larynx is a small pouch in front of the trachea (windpipe), and it contains the vocal cords. Sound is produced when air is drawn into the larynx and passes over the vocal cords. Muscles in the larynx determine when to draw air into the larynx, and they determine the shape of the larynx to produce the desired sound.

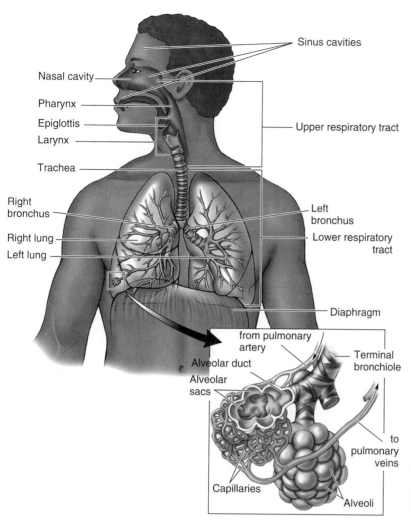

FIGURE 1-3
The respiratory system. (Modified from Herlihy B and Maebius N: The Human Body in Health and Illness. Philadelphia, WB Saunders, 2000, p. 363.)

STOP & REVIEW

Complete the following statements:

1. The medical name for the windpipe is the _____.

2. The air sacs where the oxygen is absorbed and the carbon dioxide is released are called _____.

3. The medical name for the voice box is the _____.

Use Table 1-4 to define the following:

4. Orthopnea _____

5. Pneumonia _____

6. Sinusitis _____

7. Spirometry _____

8. URI _____

9. SOB _____

10. COPD _____

TABLE 1-4
Word Parts for Respiratory System Terminology

Root Words

Root—Meaning	Root—Meaning	Root—Meaning
acid/o—acid	**coni/o**—dust	**phas/o**—speech
adenoid/o—adenoids (lymph tissue in the nose and throat)	**cyan/o**—blue	**phon/o**—voice
alkal/o—alkaline, basic	**epiglott/o**—epiglottis (lidlike cartilage that covers the larynx)	**plas/o**—formation, development
alveol/o—alveolus, alveoli (air sacs in lungs)	**fibr/o**—fiber, fibrous	**pleg/o**—paralysis
anthrac/o, —coal	**gen/o**—origin, beginning	**pleur/o**—pleura (membrane surrounding each lung)
bronch/o, bronchi/o—bronchus, bronchi (tubes leading into lungs; branch from lower end of windpipe)	**laryng/o**—larynx (voice box)	**pneum/o, pneumon/o**—air, lungs
	lob/o—lobe of the lung	**pulm/o, pulmon/o**—lungs
	nas/o—nose	**rhin/o**—nose
bronchiol/o—bronchiole (smaller tubes leading from bronchi to alveoli)	**or/o**—mouth	**sinus/o**—sinus, cavity
	orth/o—straight, upright	**spir/o**—breathing
	ox/o—oxygen	**tel/o**—complete
capn/o—carbon dioxide	**palat/o**—palate (roof of mouth)	**thorac/o**—chest
	pector/o—chest	**tonsill/o**—tonsils
	pharyng/o—pharynx, throat	**trache/o**—trachea, windpipe

Prefixes

Prefix—Meaning	Prefix—Meaning	Prefix—Meaning
a; an-—no, not, without	**dys-**—bad, painful, difficult	**ex-**—out, without, away from
bi-—two	**epi-**—above, upon	**in-**—in, inside, negative

Suffixes

Suffix—Meaning	Suffix—Meaning	Suffix—Meaning
-algia—pain	**-itis**—inflammation	**-plagia**—formation, development
-capnia—carbon dioxide	**-metry**—the process of measuring	**-plegia**—paralysis
-centesis—surgical puncture	**-ole**—little, small	**-pnea**—breathing
-ectasia, -ectasis—stretching, dilation	**-osmia**—smell	**-ptosis**—prolapse
-ectomy—surgical removal, excision	**-osis**—abnormal condition, disease, abnormal increase	**-ptysis**—splitting
-ema, -ia, -iasis—condition	**-pathy**—disease	**-sphyxia**—pulse
-genesis, -genic, -genous—origin, beginning, produced by	**-phasia**—speech	**-thorax**—pleural cavity, chest

Abbreviations

Abbreviation—Meaning	Abbreviation—Meaning	Abbreviation—Meaning
AFB—acid fast bacillus (organism that causes tuberculosis)	**CXR**—chest x-ray	**RDS**—respiratory distress syndrome
ARDS—adult respiratory distress syndrome	**DPT**—diphtheria, pertussis, tetanus immunization	**RLL**—right lower lobe (of lung)
	FVC—forced vital capacity	**RUL**—right upper lobe (of lung)
bronch—bronchoscopy	**LLL**—left lower lobe (of lung)	**SIDS**—sudden infant death syndrome
COPD—chronic obstructive pulmonary disease (emphysema)	**LUL**—left upper lobe (of lung)	**SOB**—shortness of breath
CPR—cardiopulmonory resuscitation	**PFT**—pulmonary function test	**TB**—tuberculosis
CTA—clear to auscultation (by listening)	**PPD**—purified protein derivative (used in test for tuberculosis)	**URI**—upper respiratory (tract) infection

Digestive System

The **digestive system** (Figure 1-4) breaks down food into chemical components the body can use for nourishment. It consists of the digestive tract and various associated organs, and it works closely with the circulatory and lymphatic systems.

The digestive tract is also called the gastrointestinal tract and the alimentary canal. It is basically a tube through which food passes and extends from the mouth to the anus. The upper portion of the digestive tract processes food and makes the nourishment available to the body. The lower portion of the digestive tract removes excess liquid from any remaining food and expels solid waste products.

Digestive glands release substances that break down food into usable components. Digestive glands include the salivary glands in the mouth, the gastric glands in the stomach, the liver, the gallbladder, the pancreas, and the intestinal glands.

The circulatory and lymphatic systems pick up nutrients from the upper digestive tract and deliver

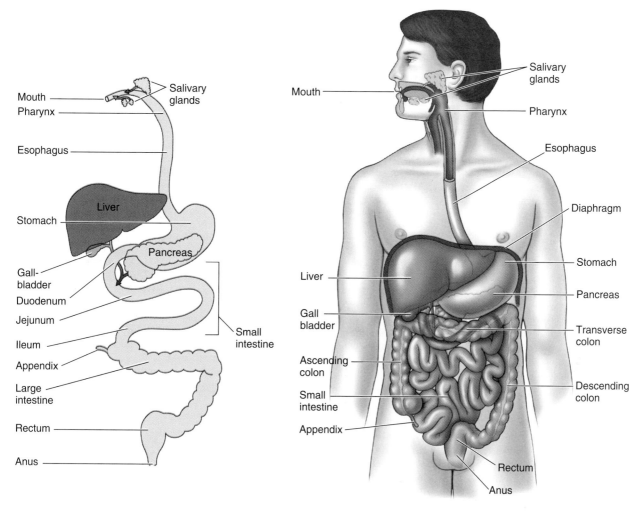

FIGURE 1-4
The digestive system. (Modified from Herlihy B and Maebius N: The Human Body in Health and Illness. Philadelphia, WB Saunders, 2000, p. 389.)

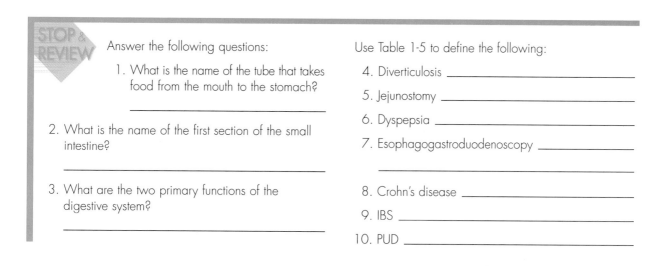

STOP & REVIEW

Answer the following questions:

1. What is the name of the tube that takes food from the mouth to the stomach?

   _____

2. What is the name of the first section of the small intestine?

   _____

3. What are the two primary functions of the digestive system?

   _____

Use Table 1-5 to define the following:

4. Diverticulosis _____

5. Jejunostomy _____

6. Dyspepsia _____

7. Esophagogastroduodenoscopy _____

   _____

8. Crohn's disease _____

9. IBS _____

10. PUD _____

TABLE 1-5
Word Parts for Digestive System Terminology

Root Words

Root—Meaning	Root—Meaning	Root—Meaning
amyl/o—starch	**enter/o**—intestines; usually small intestines	**palat/o**—palate (roof of mouth)
an/o—anus	**esophag/o**—esophagus (the food tube leading from the mouth to the stomach)	**pancreat/o**—pancreas (organ that produces insulin and digestive enzymes)
append/o, appendic/o—appendix		
bil/i, chol/e—bile, gall		
bilirubin/o—bilirubin (the orange-yellow bile pigment)	**faci/o**—face	**peritone/o**—peritoneum (a membrane that lines the walls of the abdominal and pelvic cavities)
bucc/o—cheek	**fruct/o**—fruit	
cec/o—cecum (where large intestine and small intestine meet)	**gastr/o**—stomach	
	gingiv/o—gums	**pex/o**—surgical fixation
celi/o—belly, abdomen	**gloss/o, lingu/o**—tongue	**pharyng/o**—throat
cheil/o—lip	**gluc/o, glyc/o**—sugar	**proct/o, rect/o**—anus and rectum (the end of the digestive tract)
cholecyst/o—gallbladder	**ile/o**—ileum (the third segment of the small intestine; leads into the large intestine)	
choledoch/o—common bile duct		**prote/o**—protein
col/o, colon/o—colon, large intestine		**pylor/o**—pylorus (the lower part of the stomach), pyloric sphincter (the muscle that controls the flow of food from the stomach into the small intestine)
	jejun/o—jejunum (the second segment of the small intestine)	
cyst/o—bladder, sac		
dent/i—tooth, teeth	**labi/o**—lip	
dips/o—thirst	**lact/o**—milk	
diverticul/o—diverticulum (an abnormal out-pouching, usually of the colon)	**lapar/o**—abdomen	**sial/o, sialaden/o**—saliva, salivary glands
	lip/o, steat/o—fat	
	lith/o—stone	**sigmoid/o**—sigmoid colon (the lower end of the colon)
duoden/o—duodenum (the first segment of the small intestine; leads from the stomach)	**mandibul/o**—mandible (lower jaw)	**stomat/o**—mouth
	odont/o—tooth	**vag/o**—vagus nerve (a branch of this nerve controls gastric secretions)
	or/o—mouth	

Prefixes

Prefix—Meaning	Prefix—Meaning	Prefix—Meaning
aniso-—unequal	**hyper-**—excessive, above	**par-, para-**—near, beside, abnormal
dys-—bad, painful, difficult	**hypo-**—deficient, below	**peri-**—around, during
eu-—normal, well, good	**iso-**—equal, same	**post-**—after, behind
hetero-—different	**mal-**—bad, poor	**pre-**—before
homo-—same	**mega-, megalo-**—large	**sub-**—below, under

Suffixes

Suffix—Meaning	Suffix—Meaning	Suffix—Meaning
-ac, -al, -ic—pertaining to	**-iasis**—abnormal condition	**-rrhagia, -rrhage**—bursting forth of blood, excessive bleeding
-algia—pain	**-lysis**—destruction, breakdown, separation	
-ase—enzyme (digestive enzymes help break down food)		**-rrhaphy**—surgical repair, suture
	-megaly—large	**-rrhea**—flow, discharge
-cele—hernia	**-ose**—sugar	**-scopy**—to view or examine
-centesis—puncture of a cavity to remove fluid	**-osis**—abnormal condition, disease, abnormal increase	**-spasm**—sudden involuntary muscle cramp
-chezia—defecation, elimination of wastes	**-ous**—pertaining to, characterized by	**-stasis**—stopping, controlling
	-pepsia—digestion	**-stenosis**—tightening, stricture, narrowing
-clysis—irrigation, washing out	**-pexy**—surgical fixation	**-stomy**—a new permanent opening
-ectasis, -ectasia—stretching, dilation, dilatation	**-phagia**—eating, swallowing	**-tomy**—cutting into (incision)
	-prandial—meal	**-tresia**—opening
-ectomy—surgical removal (excision)	**-ptosis**—prolapse, fall, sag	**-tripsy**—crushing, destroying (e.g., gallstones)
-emesis—vomiting	**-ptysis**—spitting	
-itis—inflammation		

Eponyms
Eponym—Meaning

Crohn's disease—chronic inflammation of the intestinal tract. Symptoms include diarrhea, cramping, and fever.

TABLE 1-5
Word Parts for Digestive System Terminology—cont'd

Abbreviations		
Abbreviation—Meaning	Abbreviation—Meaning	Abbreviation—Meaning
alk phos, ALP—alkaline phosphatase (liver function test)	**GB**—gallbladder	**NPO**—nulla per os (nothing by mouth)
BE, BaE—barium enema (lower-GI x-ray using contrast medium)	**GI**—gastrointestinal	**PUD**—peptic ulcer disease
BM—bowel movement	**IBS**—irritable bowel syndrome	**TPN**—total parenteral nutrition (a concentrated IV solution with complete nutrition given through an IV line into a large vein or into the heart)
EGD—esophagogastroduodenoscopy	**IVC**—intravenous cholangiogram (x-ray of the bile ducts using IV contrast material)	
ERCP—endoscopic retrograde cholangiopancreatography (x-ray of pancreatic and bile ducts using contrast medium)	**LFT**—liver function tests	**UGI**—upper gastrointestinal (x-rays of the esophagus, stomach, and small intestine using swallowed contrast material)
GA—gastric analysis	**NG tube**—nasogastric tube (tube inserted through nose and passed into stomach; for food, medication, or to remove stomach contents)	

them to body cells. They pick up waste products from body cells and deliver them to the lower digestive tract where they are expelled from the body.

The digestive process begins in the mouth. Teeth are used to chop food, and salivary glands produce saliva to make it easier to swallow chopped food. Saliva contains water, mucus, and salts to keep the mouth wet and to lubricate food, as well as an enzyme that works to break down starches.

The tongue also plays a role in the digestive system. The tongue manipulates food to bring it into position to be chewed and swallowed, and it contains sensory nerves called taste buds.

Swallowing pushes food from the back of the throat into the esophagus. The esophagus is a muscular tube that propels food in one direction into the stomach; it has no other function. In the stomach, food is mixed with acids and digestive enzymes produced by the gastric glands. When the food is semiliquid, it passes out of the stomach into the first portion of the small intestine, the duodenum.

The liver produces bile salts and acids, which are stored in the gallbladder until they are needed for digestion. The gallbladder releases the bile salts and acids into the duodenum to process fat. The pancreas also releases digestive enzymes into the duodenum to process carbohydrates, fats, and protein.

The liquid food then travels to the jejunum, the middle section of the small intestine, and then the ileum, the last section of the small intestine. In these sections, intestinal glands release enzymes to complete the digestion of the food, and the nutrients are picked up by the circulatory system and, to a lesser degree, the lymphatic system for delivery to the body. The next stop for the digestive system is the liver, where the blood is filtered and most harmful substances are either removed or rendered harmless (a process called detoxification). The liver also produces hemoglobin, which is a component of red blood cells that transports oxygen to the cells.

Any remaining liquid food is passed out of the small intestine into the large intestine through a juncture called the cecum. The appendix is a small sac located near the cecum. The appendix is generally considered to have no function, but it contains a small amount of lymph tissue, so it might serve to prevent infection. As food travels through the large intestine, most of the remaining water is removed by the circulatory system and, to a lesser degree, the lymph system, and other waste products are passed into the large intestine, or colon.

The large intestine has three sections. The first section is the ascending colon and is located on the right side of the abdomen. The second section is the transverse colon and it flows from right to left across the upper abdomen. The last section is the descending colon. It is located on the left side of the abdomen and it ends in the anus. The lowest portion of the descending colon, just before it exits the body, is called the rectum. Solid waste called feces is held in the rectum until defecation expels it from the body through the anus.

Genitourinary System

In both men and women, the urinary and reproductive systems are located very close to each other, and problems that affect one system can sometimes affect both. For that reason, they are usually studied together as the **genitourinary system** (Figure 1-5).

The urinary system removes liquid waste from the body. It consists of:

- ❑ Two kidneys
- ❑ Two tubes called ureters, one leading from each kidney to the bladder
- ❑ The bladder, where urine is collected until it is expelled
- ❑ The urethra, a tube leading from the bladder to the urinary or urethral meatus
- ❑ The urinary or urethral meatus, where urine is expelled from the body

The kidneys filter blood. Their main purpose is to eliminate liquid waste products. In addition, a hormone released by the kidneys regulates the production and release of red blood cells in the bone marrow. The adrenal glands sit on top of each kidney and produce hormones. One hormone regulates blood pressure and another regulates the blood levels of sodium and potassium (chemicals called electrolytes). The kidneys respond to hormones produced by the adrenal glands to control the electrolytes in the blood and the acid-base balance in the body. This, in turn, helps control blood pressure.

Excess liquid in the digestive system and liquid waste products in body cells, including urea, a waste product from protein metabolism, are picked up by the circulatory system and transported to the kidneys, where blood is filtered. The kidneys convert water and liquid waste products into urine, and the urine moves through small tubes called ureters to the bladder for storage.

The urinary bladder can store more than a pint of urine. The bladder is made of involuntary smooth muscle that expands and contracts according to the amount of urine present. As the bladder fills, nerve endings send signals to the brain so a decision can be made to empty the bladder. A somewhat larger tube, called a urethra, carries urine from the bladder out of the body. A voluntary sphincter muscle at the base of the bladder opens and closes to regulate the flow of urine into the urethra. The point where the urethra exits the body is called the urinary or urethral meatus.

The female reproductive system is situated between the urinary bladder and the rectum. It consists of two ovaries, two fallopian tubes, a uterus, a vagina, and external genitalia.

Eggs are produced and released by ovaries. Typically, one egg is produced each month. The released egg travels down a fallopian tube, where fertilization can occur, to the uterus. If the egg is not fertilized, the egg, together with the lining of the uterus that had been prepared to nourish a fertilized egg, moves out of the uterus, through the vagina, and is expelled from the body. This discharge is called a menstrual flow or period.

The cervix, often called the neck of the uterus, is a round muscle that connects the uterus to the vagina. When the cervix is closed, the contents of the uterus stay in the uterus. When the cervix is open, the uterine contents may move into the vagina.

There are external skin folds outside of the vagina that roll together, like lips, to make it difficult for contaminants to enter the vagina. These external folds, or genitalia, are called the vulva. The urinary or urethral meatus is located near the top wall of the vagina, either just inside the vagina or just outside the vagina in the vulva.

When an egg is fertilized by a sperm cell, usually in the fallopian tube, conception occurs, and the woman is now pregnant. Unless there are complications, an unborn baby goes through several stages of growth over a 40-week period, preparing for birth.

The fertilized egg, now called a zygote, begins to grow, travels to the uterus, and attaches itself to the inner wall of the uterus. This takes about 2 weeks. Once implanted in the uterus, the zygote is called an *embryo*. By the ninth week after conception, the placenta and umbilical cord have formed, and the embryo, now called a fetus, is cushioned in a fluid-filled amniotic sac. The unborn baby matures in the uterus as a fetus for another 31 weeks until the cervix of the uterus dilates, and the fetus moves through the vagina in a process called a vaginal birth or vaginal delivery.

When complications prevent a vaginal delivery, an incision is made through the abdominal wall, the bladder is moved to the side, and an incision is made through the uterus to deliver the baby. This is called a cesarian, or C-section, birth or delivery.

When a baby is born alive more than 2 weeks early, the process is called a premature birth. When the cervix opens and an unborn baby that weighs less than 500 g is involuntarily expelled from the woman's body, the process is called a miscarriage or spontaneous abortion. If an unborn baby that weighs 500 g or more dies before birth, the vaginal or C-section delivery is called a stillbirth. A voluntary

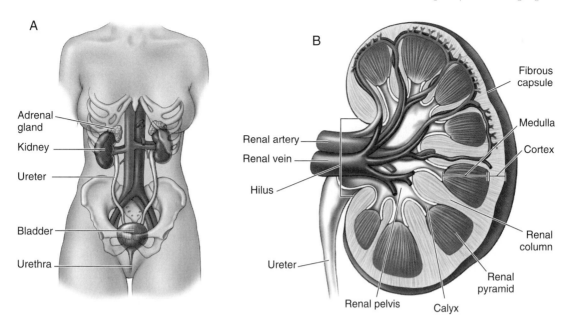

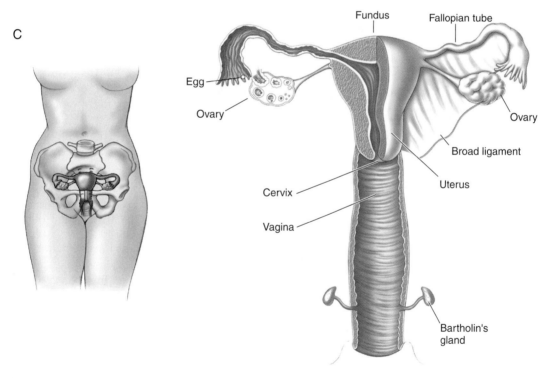

FIGURE 1-5
The genitourinary system. **A,** urinary system; **B,** kidney; **C,** female reproductive system.   *Continued.*

D

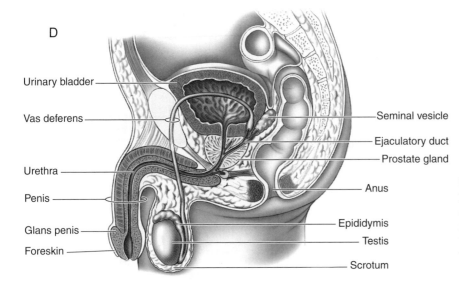

Urinary bladder

Vas deferens

Urethra

Penis

Glans penis

Foreskin

Seminal vesicle

Ejaculatory duct

Prostate gland

Anus

Epididymis

Testis

Scrotum

FIGURE 1-5, cont'd
D, male reproductive system.
(Modified from Herlihy B and
Maebius N: The Human Body in
Health and Illness. Philadelphia,
WB Saunders, 2000, pp. 421,
453, 459.)

interruption or termination of pregnancy, at any stage of pregnancy, is called a voluntary abortion.

The male reproductive system is located below the bladder and in front of the rectum. It consists of the testicles, the scrotum, the epididymis, the vas deferens, the seminal vesicles, the prostate gland, and the penis.

The testicles are located in the scrotum, a pouch outside the main body cavity, behind the penis and before the anus. Sperm produced in the testicles are sent into a long coiled tube, also located in the scrotum, called the epididymis, where they are stored and they mature. Millions of sperm are released at one time.

Shortly before the sperm are ejected from the body, they travel from the epididymis through another long tube called the vas deferens into the seminal vesicles located just behind the bladder. The seminal vesicles add fluid to the sperm and then send it into tubes that pass through the prostate gland, where more fluid is added before the sperm are emptied into the urethra. The prostate gland is located under the bladder and it surrounds the upper urethra. The fluid containing the sperm is now called semen. Erectile tissue makes the penis firm before the sperm are ejected from the urethra. The male urinary or urethral meatus is located at the tip of the penis.

If the male penis is inside the female vagina when the semen is ejected, the sperm travel up the vagina, pass through the cervix into the uterus, and travel up the uterus and into the fallopian tubes in search of an egg to fertilize. In artificial insemination, semen is ejected into a sterile cup, and sterile instruments are used to transfer the semen from the cup into the uterus.

STOP & REVIEW

Complete the following sentences:

1. The kidneys _____ blood to remove liquid waste products.

2. _____, a waste product from protein metabolism, is expelled in urine.

3. From the time a human embryo is implanted in the wall of the uterus until about 9 weeks after conception, the unborn baby is called

_____ .

4. The reproductive fluid containing sperm that is dumped into the male urethra is called

_____ .

Use Table 1-6 to define the following:

5. Oliguria _____

6 Primigravida _____

7. Lithotripsy _____

8. Marshall-Marchetti-Krantz operation _____

_____

9. STD _____

10. UTI _____

TABLE 1-6
Word Parts for Genitourinary System Terminology

Root Words

Root—Meaning	Root—Meaning	Root—Meaning
albumin/o—albumin (a protein found in blood and body tissues)	**genit/o**—genitals (organs of reproduction)	**par/o**—bearing of offspring
amni/o—amnion (inner membrane around developing fetus in pregnancy)	**glomerul/o**—glomerulus (tiny blood vessels in the cortex of the kidney)	**perine/o**—the perineum (in females, the area between the anus and the vagina)
andr/o—male	**glycos/o**—sweet, sugar	**phor/o**—to bear
azot/o—nitrogen (an element released	**gon/o**—seed, genitals, reproduction	**prostat/o**—prostate (a male genital gland that surrounds the lowest portion of the bladder and the urethra)
bacteri/o—bacteria	**gynec/o**—woman, female	
balan/o—glans penis (the sensitive tip of in urine, feces, and sweat) the penis)	**hydr/o**—water, fluid (the genital organ where a developing fetus grows)	**py/o**—pus
cali/o, calic/o—calix, calx (a collecting region in the renal pelvis of the kidney)	**hyster/o, uter/o**—uterus, womb	**pyel/o**—renal pelvis (the part of the kidney where collecting takes place)
	ket/o, keton/o—ketones (a substance produced during fat metabolism in the liver and excreted through the kidneys)	**ren/o**—kidney
cervic/o—neck, neck of uterus		**salping/o**—fallopian tubes, oviducts, uterine tubes
chori/o, chorion/o—chorion (the outer membrane surrounding a developing fetus in pregnancy)	**lact/o**—milk	**semin/i, semin/o**—semen, seed
	lapar/o—abdominal wall	**sperm/o, spermat/o**—sperm, spermatozoa
colp/o—vagina	**lith/o**—stone (as in kidney stone or gallstone)	
cry/o—cold		**terat/o**—monster
crypt/o—hidden	**mamm/o, mast/o**—breast	**test/o**—testis, testicle (male gonads or genitals)
culd/o—cul-de-sac (pouch of peritoneum between the rectum and the uterus)	**meat/o**—meatus (the external opening of the urethra; where urine exits the body)	**top/o**—place
	men/o—month, menses, menstruation	**trigon/o**—trigone (triangular area in the bladder marked by the two ureters and the urethra)
cyst/o—urinary bladder	**metr/o, metri/o**—measure, uterine tissue	
dipl/o—double		**ur/o, urin/o**—urea, urine
dips/o—thirst	**my/o**—muscle	**ureter/o**—ureter (tubes between
epididym/o—epididymis (tube for sperm located on top of each testis in a male)	**myom/o**—muscle tumor	**urethra/o**—urethra (tube between kidneys and bladder) bladder and meatus)
	nat/i—birth	
	nephr/o—kidney	
episi/o—vulva (external genitalia in a female)	**noct/i**—night	**vas/o**—vessel, duct, vas deferens
	o/o, ov/o, ovul/o—egg	**vesic/o**—urinary bladder
fet/o—fetus (the developing unborn baby during pregnancy)	**olig/o**—scanty, small	**zo/o**—animal life (tube between epididymis and urethra in a male)
galact/o—milk	**oophor/o, ovari/o**—ovary (genital organ that produces eggs in a woman)	

Prefixes

Prefix—Meaning	Prefix—Meaning	Prefix—Meaning
ante-, pre-—before, forward	**in-**—in	**post-**—after, behind
bi-—two	**intra-**—within	**pre-**—before
dys-—painful	**multi-**—many	**primi-**—first
ecto-—situated outside	**neo-**—new	**pseudo-**—false
endo-—within	**nulli-**—none	**retro-**—backward
extra-—outside	**peri-**—around, during	**supra-**—above

Suffixes

Suffix—Meaning	Suffix—Meaning	Suffix—Meaning
-ac, -al, -ic—pertaining to	**-parous**—to bear, bring forth (also used as a noun, para, followed by a number to indicate the number of live births for a woman)	**-rrhexis**—rupture
-arche—beginning		**-salpinx**—fallopian tube, oviduct, uterine tube
-cyesis—pregnancy		**-tocia**—labor, birth
-gravida—pregnancy (sometimes used as a noun followed by a number to indicate the number of pregnancies for a woman)	**-poietin**—a substance that forms	**-tripsy**—to crush (used with kidney stones)
	-rrhagia—profuse bleeding	**-urea**—urination, urine condition
	-rrhaphy—suture or repair	**-version**—act of turning

Eponyms
Eponym—Meaning

Down syndrome—a chromosomal abnormality that features mental retardation and many physical defects. Also called *mongolism*.
Marshall-Marchetti-Krantz operation—a surgical operation to repair damage to the bladder and the urethra. In women, may also include repair of the vagina.
Wilms' tumor—a malignant tumor of the kidney that occurs in childhood.

Continued.

TABLE 1-6
Word Parts for Genitourinary System Terminology—cont'd

	Abbreviations	
Abbreviation—Meaning	Abbreviation—Meaning	Abbreviation—Meaning
AB—abortion (may be spontaneous, as in miscarriage, or may be induced)	**DUB**—dysfunctional uterine bleeding	**Multip, multip**—multipara, multiparous (not the first pregnancy)
ADH—antidiuretic hormone	**EDC**—estimated date of confinement (due date for a pregnant woman)	**OB**—obstetrics (management of pregnancy and delivery)
AFP—alpha-fetoprotein (high levels in amniotic fluid or pregnant woman's blood indicate risk of neurological birth defect in infant)	**ERT**—estrogen replacement therapy	**OCP**—oral contraceptive pill (birth control pill)
	ESRD—end-stage renal disease	**Pap smear**—Papanicolaou smear (test for cervical or vaginal cancer)
ARF—acute renal failure	**ESWL**—extracorporeal shock wave lithotripsy (shock waves are used to crush kidney stones)	
BPH—benign prostatic hypertrophy (benign enlarged prostate in a man)		**PID**—pelvic inflammatory disease
BUN—blood urea nitrogen (a measure of kidney function)	**FHT**—fetal heart tone (the heartbeat of an unborn baby)	**PKU**—phenylketonuria (a birth defect in which a digestive enzyme is lacking; the resulting buildup of phenylalanine is poisonous to the brain)
CAPD—continuous ambulatory peritoneal dialysis (special fluid is placed in abdomen and then removed hours later to eliminate wastes from blood when kidneys do not function)	**FSH**—follicle stimulating hormone (causes eggs and sperm to mature)	
	GC—gonococcus (the organism that causes gonorrhea)	**PMS**—premenstrual syndrome
	GFR—glomerular filtration rate (a measure of kidney function)	**Primip**—primipara, primiparous (first pregnancy)
	GU—genitourinary in a man)	**PSA**—prostate specific antigen (an elevated level indicates prostate cancer)
Cath, cath—catheter, catheterization	**GYN**—gynecology	
CIS—carcinoma in situ (cancer that is localized in one place; it has not spread)	**HCG**—human chorionic gonadotropin (a hormone produced by the placenta; presence in blood indicates pregnancy)	**RPR**—rapid plasma reagin (test for syphilis)
Cl—chloride (an electrolyte excreted through the kidney)	**HD**—hemodialysis (blood is filtered through a machine to remove waste products when the kidney does not function)	**STD**—sexually transmitted disease
CPD—cephalopelvic disproportion (when an unborn baby's head is too large to fit through the mother's pelvis)		**TAH**—total abdominal hysterectomy (removal of uterus through abdominal incision)
	HSG—hysterosalpingography (a test to show if the fallopian tubes are open enough for an egg to pass from the ovary to the uterus)	**TAH-BSO**—total abdominal hysterectomy and bilateral salpingo-oophorectomy (removal of uterus, both tubes, and both ovaries through abdominal incision)
CRF—chronic renal failure		
Cx—cervix (the muscle that controls the entrance from the vagina into the uterus)	**IUD**—intrauterine device (contraceptive; to prevent pregnancy)	**TRUS**—transrectal ultrasound (evaluates prostate)
Cysto, cysto—cystoscopic examination (a look at the inside of the urinary bladder through a lighted instrument)	**IVP**—intravenous pyelogram (an x-ray of kidney function using IV contrast material)	**TUR/TURP**—transurethral resection of the prostate (removal of the prostate or part of the prostate
C-section—cesarean section (delivery of baby through an abdominal incision)	**KUB**—an x-ray of the kidneys, ureters, and bladder	**UA**—urinalysis
		UTI—urinary tract infection
D & C—dilatation and curettage (the process of dilating a woman's cervix and scraping out the lining and any contents of the uterus)	**LMP**—last menstrual period (used to calculate due date in a pregnant woman)	**VD**—venereal disease (sexually transmitted disease)
		VDRL—Venereal Disease Research Lab
		VIP—voluntary interruption of pregnancy (a blood test for venereal diseases)

Endocrine System

The **endocrine system** (Figure 1-6) is a system of ductless glands that produce hormones. The hormones are released directly into the bloodstream. Hormones are chemical substances that regulate many body functions. For example, one regulates the growth of bones, another blood pressure, another blood sugar. Others regulate the reproductive system, and still others control metabolism and the amounts of various chemicals in the body. A hormone produced in one part of the body may regulate functions in the same part of the body or in other, distant parts of the body.

The pituitary and pineal glands are located in the brain. The pituitary gland is often called the master gland because it receives information from the brain and sends directions to other endocrine glands, thereby coordinating the response of the entire body. The thyroid and parathyroid are located in the neck, in front of the trachea, near the voice box. The thymus is located in the upper chest and may extend up into the neck. The adrenal glands are located in the abdomen, on top of the kidneys. The pancreas is located in the abdomen, on the left side, under the liver, near the stomach. Only part of the pancreas, called the islets of Langerhans, has an endocrine function. (The rest of the pancreas uses ducts to deliver digestive enzymes into the duodenum.) The male testicles are located in the scrotum, just outside of the pelvis, and female ovaries are located in the pelvis.

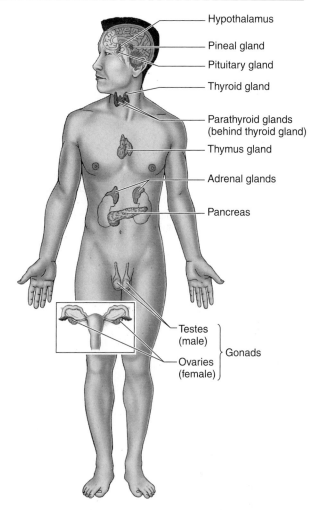

Hypothalamus
Pineal gland
Pituitary gland
Thyroid gland
Parathyroid glands (behind thyroid gland)
Thymus gland
Adrenal glands
Pancreas
Testes (male)
Ovaries (female)
Gonads

FIGURE 1-6
The endocrine system. (Modified from Herlihy B and Maebius N: The Human Body in Health and Illness. Philadelphia, WB Saunders, 2000, p. 239.)

STOP & REVIEW

Answer the following:

1. What gland contains the islets of Langerhans?

   _____

2. What endocrine gland is located on top of the kidneys?

   _____

3. Name an endocrine gland that only men have.

   _____

4. What physical feature distinguishes endocrine glands from other glands?

   _____

Use Table 1-7 to define the following:

5. Somatotropic _____

6. Lactose _____

7. Gonadotropin _____

8. Graves' disease _____

   _____

9. BMR _____

10. GTT _____

TABLE 1-7
Word Parts for Endocrine System Terminology

Root Words

Root—Meaning	Root—Meaning	Root—Meaning
aden/o—gland	**home/o**—sameness, constant	**pancreat/o**—pancreas (an endocrine
adren/o, adrenal/o—adrenal	**hormon/o**—hormone (substance	gland behind the stomach)
glands	produced by an endocrine gland that	**parathyroid/o**—parathyroid gland
adrenalin/o—adrenaline, also called	regulates the function of an organ)	(four small endocrine glands behind
epinephrine (increases heart rate	**insulin/o**—insulin (lowers blood sugar)	the thyroid gland)
and blood pressure)	**iod/o**—iodine (an essential trace	**phys/o**—growing
andr/o—male or masculine	element; 80% of the iodine in the	**pituitar/o**—pituitary (endocrine
calc/o—calcium	body is found in the thyroid gland)	gland at the base of the brain)
cortic/o—cortex (outer region)	**kal/i**—potassium (an electrolyte—a	**somat/o**—body
crin/o—secrete	mineral salt found in blood and tissues	**ster/o**—solid structure
dips/o—thirst	and needed for proper functioning)	**thyr/o, thyroid/o**—thyroid gland
estr/o—female	**lact/o**—milk	(endocrine gland in the neck)
gigant/o—large	**mamm/o, mast/o**—breast	**toc/o**—childbirth
glyc/o—sugar	**myx/o**—mucous	**toxic/o**—poison
gonad/o—gonad, sex gland (ovaries	**natr/o**—sodium (an electrolyte)	**trop/o**—to stimulate
and testes)		**ur/o**—urine

Prefixes

Prefix—Meaning	Prefix—Meaning	Prefix—Meaning
anti-—against	**oxy-**—rapid, sharp, acid	**tetra-**—four
eu-—good, normal	**pan-**—all	**trans-**—across
exo-—outside, outward	**pro-**—before, for	**tri-**—three

Suffixes

Suffix—Meaning	Suffix—Meaning	Suffix—Meaning
-agon—assemble, gather together	**-plasia**—formation, development	**-tropin**—that which stimulates
-in, -ine—a substance	**-poietin**—a substance that forms	(to turn or act upon)
-ose—sugar	**-tropic**—stimulate	**-uria**—urea, urine condition
-physis—growth		

Eponyms

Eponym—Meaning

Addison's disease—a life-threatening disease caused by partial or complete failure of the adrenal gland.
Cushing's syndrome—a disorder resulting from too much ACTH made by the pituitary gland, usually a side effect from long-term steroid use. Symptoms include obesity, moon face, hump back, high blood sugar, and low potassium.
Graves' disease—hyperthyroidism, usually with an enlarged thyroid. Symptoms include bulging eyes, weight loss, nervousness, and tremors.

Abbreviations

Abbreviation—Meaning	Abbreviation—Meaning	Abbreviation—Meaning
ACTH—adrenocorticotropic hormone (produced by the pituitary gland; stimulates the adrenal cortex)	**GTT**—glucose tolerance test (measures blood sugar levels over several hours in response to a known amount of sugar intake)	**PTH**—parathyroid hormone, parathormone (produced by the parathyroid gland; increases blood calcium)
ADH—antidiuretic hormone (produced by the pituitary gland; increases reabsorption of water by the kidney)	**HGH**—human growth hormone	**RAIU**—radioactive iodine uptake (measures thyroid function)
BMR—basal metabolic rate (measures the amount of energy needed to maintain body function; an indicator of thyroid function)	**ICSH**—interstitial cell-stimulating hormone	**RIA**—radio-immunoassay (measures hormone levels in plasma)
	IDDM—insulin-dependent diabetes mellitus	**SIADH**—syndrome of inappropriate ADH (symptoms include weight gain despite loss of appetite)
DI—diabetes insipidus (insufficient secretion of ADH)	**K, K$^+$**—potassium	**STH**—somatotropic hormone (produced by the pituitary; also called *growth hormone*)
DM—diabetes mellitus (lack of or insufficient insulin secretion from pancreas)	**LH**—puteinizing hormone (produced by the pituitary; stimulates ovulation in women and stimulates testosterone secretion in men)	**T$_3$**—triioothyronine (produced by the thyroid gland; increases metabolism in cells)
FBS—fasting blood sugar	**MSH**—melanocyte-stimulating hormone (produced by the pituitary; high levels increase pigmentation of the skin)	**T$_4$**—thyroxine (produced by the thyroid gland; increases metabolism in cells)
FSH—follicle stimulating hormone (produced by pituitary; stimulates hormone secretion and egg or sperm production)	**17-OH**—17-hydroxy-corticosteroids (any of the hormones produced by the adrenal glands)	**TFT**—thyroid function test
GH—growth hormone (produced by the pituitary; stimulates growth of bones and tissue)	**PRL**—prolactin (produced by the pituitary gland; promotes milk secretion)	**TSH**—thyroid stimulating hormone (produced by the pituitary gland; promotes thyroid function)

Circulatory System

The **circulatory system** (Figure 1-7) is a delivery service for the rest of the body. It includes the heart, the blood, and a network of blood vessels called arteries and veins. The smallest blood vessels are called capillaries.

The circulatory system delivers oxygen and waste products for the respiratory system. It delivers nutrients and waste products for the digestive system. It delivers hormones for the endocrine system. It delivers fluids and waste products for the urinary system.

Bones manufacture red blood cells in the musculoskeletal system. Blood cells are carried through the body by an intricate network of blood vessels in the circulatory system. Blood can only flow in one direction in a blood vessel. There is a systemic circulatory system that goes to the whole body and a pulmonary circulatory system that just goes to the lungs. The same blood flows through both systems and the heart ties the two together.

The heart is the pump that keeps blood flowing through the body. The right side of the heart maintains the pulmonary circulatory system. It receives blood from the whole body and sends it to the lungs to get rid of carbon dioxide and pick up oxygen. The left side of the heart maintains the systemic circulatory system. It receives blood back from the lungs and sends it out to the rest of the body.

The blood vessels that carry blood from the heart to the body cells are called arteries. In the systemic circulatory system, the blood in the arteries is loaded with good things (oxygen, food, hormones, etc.) sent from many body systems to be delivered to the body cells. The blood vessels that carry blood from the body cells back to the heart are called veins. In the systemic circulatory system, the veins carry waste products from the body cells for disposal through the appropriate body systems.

The pulmonary circulatory system does things in reverse. The pulmonary artery carries the waste products to be expelled through the lungs and the pulmonary veins carry oxygen from the lungs to be delivered to the rest of the body. Blood that is low in oxygen is blue and blood that is high in oxygen is red.

STOP & REVIEW

Answer or complete the following:

1. The _____ side of the heart sends blood to the lungs.
2. The _____ side of the heart sends blood to the entire body, except the lungs.
3. _____ arteries carry blood laden with oxygen and nutrients for the entire body.
4. The _____ artery carries blood low in oxygen and laden with carbon dioxide waste products.

Use Table 1-8 to define the following:

5. Cyanosis _____
6. Cholesterolemia _____
7. Hemoglobin _____
8. Tetralogy of Fallot _____
_____
9. CABG _____
10. CHF _____

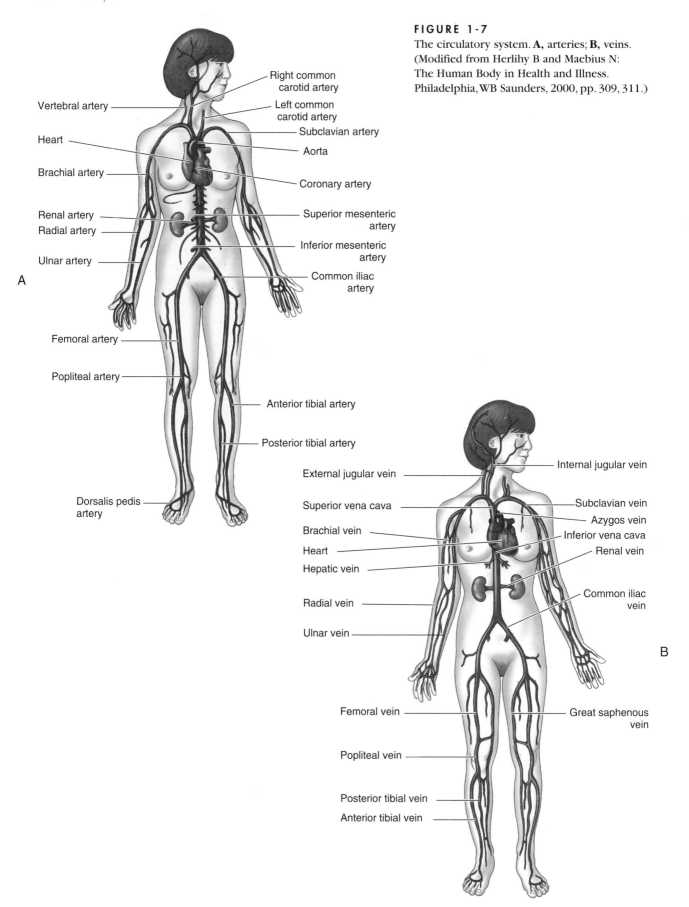

FIGURE 1-7
The circulatory system. **A,** arteries; **B,** veins.
(Modified from Herlihy B and Maebius N:
The Human Body in Health and Illness.
Philadelphia, WB Saunders, 2000, pp. 309, 311.)

A

Right common carotid artery
Vertebral artery
Left common carotid artery
Heart
Subclavian artery
Aorta
Brachial artery
Coronary artery
Renal artery
Superior mesenteric artery
Radial artery
Inferior mesenteric artery
Ulnar artery
Common iliac artery
Femoral artery
Popliteal artery
Anterior tibial artery
Posterior tibial artery
Dorsalis pedis artery

B

External jugular vein
Internal jugular vein
Superior vena cava
Subclavian vein
Azygos vein
Brachial vein
Inferior vena cava
Heart
Renal vein
Hepatic vein
Radial vein
Common iliac vein
Ulnar vein
Femoral vein
Great saphenous vein
Popliteal vein
Posterior tibial vein
Anterior tibial vein

TABLE 1-8
Word Parts for Circulatory System Terminology

Root Words

Root—Meaning	Root—Meaning	Root—Meaning
aer/o—air	**coron/o**—heart (pumps blood throughout the body)	**neutr/o**—neutral (neither acid nor base)
agglutin/o—clumping, sticking together	**cyan/o**—blue (blood low in oxygen is blue)	**ox/o**—oxygen
angi/o, vas/o—vessel (blood vessels	**cyt/o**—cell	**pericardi/o**—pericardial (around the heart)
aort/o—aorta (the largest artery in the body)	**ech/o, son/o**—sound	**phag/o**—to eat, swallow
arter/o, arteri/o—artery (the large blood vessels that carry blood away from the heart to the rest of the body)	**eosin/o**—red, rosy, dawn	**phil/o**—attraction
	erythr/o—red	**phleb/o, ven/o**—vein (a blood vessel that carries blood from the body to the heart)
arteriol/o—arteriole (a smaller branch of an artery)	**fibrin/o**—fibrin (a protein in blood clots)	**poikil/o**—irregular, varied
ather/o—a yellowish fatty plaque that can build up in blood vessels and narrow or block the space available for blood flow	**granul/o**—granules (important for wound healing)	**rhythm/o**—rhythm
	hem/a, hem/o, hemat/o—blood	**scler/o**—hard, hardening
	hemoglobin/o—hemoglobin (a protein in red blood cells that allows them to carry oxygen)	**scop/o**—to view or examine
atri/o—atrium (an upper chamber in the heart)		**sept/o**—septum, partition (such as found in the heart and nose)
bas/o—base (alkaline; the opposite of acid)	**is/o**—same, equal include both arteries and veins)	**sider/o**—iron
brachi/o—arm	**kary/o, nucle/o**—nucleus (control center of a cell or group of cells)	**spher/o**—round, globe
cancer/o, carcin/o—cancer (an abnormal growth, or tumor, that harms the body)	**leuk/o**—white	**sphygm/o**—pulse, pulse pressure
	lys/o—destruction, dissolving	**steth/o**—chest
cardi/o—heart	**macr/o, megal/o**—large, enlarged	**thromb/o**—thrombus (blood clot)
cholesterol/o—cholesterol (found in animal fat; in humans it plays a role in the endocrine, circulatory, and nervous systems. High amounts are linked to plaque buildup in blood vessels.)	**mediastin/o**—mediastinum (area between spine and breastbone; contains all chest organs except lungs)	**valv/o, valvul/o**—valve (allows fluid to flow in one direction and controls the flow of fluid)
	melan/o—black	**vas/o, vascul/o**—vessel (a small tube that carries fluid)
	micr/o—small	**ventricle/o**—ventricle (lower heart chamber)
chrom/o—color	**mon/o**—one, single	**venul/o**—venule (small blood vessels that join together to form veins)
coagul/o—coagulation (turning a liquid into a solid, as in a blood clot)	**morph/o**—shape, form	**xanth/o**—yellow
	myel/o—bone marrow	

Prefixes

Prefix—Meaning	Prefix—Meaning	Prefix—Meaning
a-—no, not, without	**hyper-**—excessive, more than normal	**poly-**—many
anti-—against	**peri-**—around	**trans-**—across
bi-—two		**tri-**—three
de-—down, from, reversing		

Suffixes

Suffix—Meaning	Suffix—Meaning	Suffix—Meaning
-apheresis—removal, carry away	**-lysis**—destruction (as in surgical destruction)	**-philia**—attraction for or an increase in cell numbers
-blast—immature, embryonic	**-lytic**—capable of destroying (as in a condition)	**-phobia**—abnormal fear
-cyte—cell	**-meter**—instrument used to measure	**-phoresis**—carrying, transmission
-cytosis—abnormal condition of cells (i.e., increased number of cells)	**-metry**—process of measuring	**-poiesis**—production, formation
-ectomy—removal, excision	**-oid**—like, resembling, derived from	**-scope**—instrument used to view or examine
-edema—swelling	**-oma**—tumor, swelling	**-scopy**—viewing, examining
-emia—blood, blood condition	**-opia**—vision	**-stasis**—stop, control
-globin—a specific protein (combines	**-osis**—abnormal condition	**-stenosis**—narrowing, stricture
-globulin—a broad category of proteins with iron in the blood)	**-ous**—pertaining to, characterized by	**-tome**—cutting instrument
-ium—membrane	**-penia**—deficiency, decreased	**-y**—state or condition
-lysin—a substance that dissolves or destroys	**-phage**—eat, swallow	

Continued.

TABLE 1-8
Word Parts for Circulatory System Terminology—cont'd

Eponyms
Eponym—Meaning

Raynaud's phenomenon—short episodes of pallor and numbness of the fingers and toes due to temporary constriction of the arterioles in the skin.

tetralogy of Fallot—a congenital heart defect involving four distinct defects.

Abbreviations		
Abbreviation—Meaning	Abbreviation—Meaning	Abbreviation—Meaning
ABO—blood groups, blood types	**BP**—blood pressure (measures the stress placed on walls of the veins and arteries by the pumping action of the heart)	**ECG, EKG**—electrocardiogram (a measurement of the electrical activity in the heart)
AF—atrial fibrillation (the upper heart chambers beat too rapidly and unevenly; ineffective heartbeat)	**CABG**—coronary artery bypass graft (surgery to replace blocked arteries in the heart)	**ECHO**—echocardiogram (sound waves are used to study the structure and motion of the heart)
AHF—antihemophilic factor (a blood clotting factor)	**CAD**—coronary artery disease (any abnormal condition that affects the arteries of the heart)	**ETT**—exercise tolerance test (also called a *stress test*)
AI—aortic insufficiency, aortic regurgitation (the reverse flow of blood from the aorta back into the left ventricle of the heart)	**Cath, cath**—catheterization (putting a tube into a body cavity or organ; cardiac catheterization is used to visualize and/or treat heart problems)	**hct**—hematocrit (a measure of the number of red cells found in blood)
ALL, CLL—acute or chronic lymphocytic leukemia (a cancer of the blood-forming tissues; ALL is seen mainly in children, CLL in adults)	**CBC**—complete blood count	**hgb**—hemoglobin (a protein in blood that carries oxygen to the cells)
AML, CML—acute or chronic myelocytic leukemia (a cancer of blood-forming tissues; AML is seen in all ages, CML in adults)	**CHF**—congestive heart failure (circulatory congestion caused by heart disorders)	**MI**—myocardial infarction (heart attack)
AS—aortic stenosis (defect of the aortic valve in the heart; the flow of blood into the aorta is blocked)	**CPK**—creatinine phosphokinase (released into bloodstream following injury to heart or skeletal muscles)	**PAC**—premature atrial contraction (premature beat from upper heart chamber)
ASD—atrial septal defect (a hole in the wall between the upper heart chambers)	**CPR**—cardiopulmonary resuscitation (a life-saving measure; artificial respiration and heart massage are used to restart the heart and lungs)	**PT**—prothrombin time (a test for blood clotting defects)
ASHD—arteriosclerotic heart disease (hardening of the arteries due to calcium deposits; decreased blood flow, especially to the brain and legs)	**DIC**—disseminated intravascular coagulation (a severe disorder in which disease or injury triggers clotting in blood vessels)	**PTT**—partial prothrombin time (a test for blood clotting defects)
AV, A-V—atrioventricular (pertaining to the upper and lower heart chambers or the function and structures between them)	**DOE**—dyspnea on exertion (shortness of breath or difficulty breathing)	**PVC**—premature ventricular contraction (premature beat from lower heart chamber)
BMT—bone marrow transplant	**DVT**—deep vein thrombosis (a blood clot in a deep vein; the condition may be life-threatening)	**RBC**—red blood cell, red blood count
		VSD—ventricular septal defect (a hole in the wall between the lower heart chambers)
		VT—ventricular tachycardia (lower heart chamber beats too fast)
		WBC—white blood cell, white blood count

Immune System

The **immune system** defends the body against an invasion by bacteria, viruses, cancer cells, and other abnormal growths or foreign bodies. It also helps regulate and maintain the fluid environment in and around body cells. It includes the lymphatic vascular system (Figure 1-8), lymphatic glands and tissue, and white blood cells. The thymus and spleen are lymphatic organs, and tonsils and adenoids are lymphatic tissue.

Lymph vessels are similar to blood vessels, but they have more valves to keep blood out of the lymph network, and they have filters called lymph nodes. The heart only pumps blood; it does not pump lymph. The movement of body parts helps keep lymph flowing through the lymphatic system. Lymph fluid is collected throughout the body by the lymphatic network and eventually drains into the blood vessel network. Much of the fluid collected by the lymph system is the fluid found between body cells.

The thymus is the primary central gland of the lymphatic system. It produces a hormone that is critical to lymph function. The spleen is the largest organ in the lymphatic system. It removes and destroys worn-out red blood cells and fights infection. When the bone marrow is impaired, the spleen can produce red blood cells. The spleen is not an essential organ; other parts of the lymphatic system take over if the spleen is removed. The tonsils and adenoids fight infection in the upper respiratory system.

Cancer usually spreads from one part of the body to another through the lymphatic system and the circulatory system. Therefore when cancer cells are found in the lymph nodes, it is an indication that the cancer may have already spread to another part of the body.

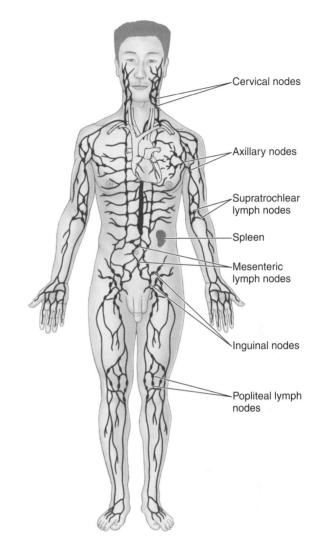

Cervical nodes

Axillary nodes

Supratrochlear lymph nodes

Spleen

Mesenteric lymph nodes

Inguinal nodes

Popliteal lymph nodes

FIGURE 1-8

The lymphatic system. (Modified from Herlihy B and Maebius N: The Human Body in Health and Illness. Philadelphia, WB Saunders, 2000, p. 337.)

STOP & REVIEW

Answer or complete the following:
1. Name the filter found in lymphatic vessels.

_____

2. Where does lymph eventually drain?

_____

3. What organ has the most control over the lymphatic system?

_____

4. What is the largest organ in the lymphatic system?

_____

Use Table 1-9 to define the following:

5. Lymphedema _____

6. Tonsillectomy _____

7. Papilloma _____

8. Hodgkin's disease _____

_____

9. T & A _____

10. ca _____

TABLE 1-9
Word Parts for Immune System Terminology

Root Words

Root—Meaning	Root—Meaning	Root—Meaning
aden/o—gland	**immun/o**—protection	**plas/o**—formation
adenoid/o—adenoids	**lymph/o**—lymph (a watery fluid that circulates through the body using lymph vessels)	**ple/o**—many, more
albin/o, leuk/o—white		**polyp/o**—polyp (a small tumorlike growth on the surface of a mucous membrane)
alveol/o—a small saclike structure	**lymphaden/o**—lymph node (gland)	
angi/o, vas/o—vessel (tube that carries fluid)	**lymphangi/o**—lymph vessel	**radi/o**—rays, x-rays
	lymphat/o—lymphatics	**sarc/o**—flesh, connective tissue
cac/o; mal/o—bad	**medull/o**—soft inner part	**scirrh/o**—hard
cancer/o, carcin/o—cancer (an abnormal growth or tumor that harms the body)	**melan/o**—black	**splen/o**—spleen (an organ located above the stomach on the left side of the body; part of the lymphatic system)
	muc/o—mucous	
	mut/o—genetic change	
cauter/o—burn, heat	**mutagen/o**—causing genetic change	
chem/o, pharmac/o—chemical, drug, medication	**myc/o**—fungus (includes yeasts and molds)	**thym/o**—thymus (located in the neck, under the thyroid, it is the primary gland of the lymphatic system)
cry/o—cold	**onc/o**—tumor (abnormal growth)	
cyst/o—sac of fluid	**onych/o, ungu/o**—nail (fingernail, toenail)	**tonsill/o**—tonsil (lymph tissue in the back of the oral cavity, near the back of the tongue)
diaphor/o, hidr/o—profuse sweating		
ech/o, son/o—sound	**papill/o**—nipplelike	
fibr/o—fibers, fibrous	**phleb/o, ven/o**—vein (blood vessel that carries blood from the tissues to the heart)	**tox/o**—poison
follicul/o—small glandular sac		
fung/o—fungus (yeast, mold, mushroom)		

Prefixes

Prefix—Meaning	Prefix—Meaning	Prefix—Meaning
ana-—backward	**epi-**—upon	**meta-**—beyond
apo-—off, away	**inter-**—between	**peri-**—around
de-—down, from, reversing	**intra-**—within	

Suffixes

Suffix—Meaning	Suffix—Meaning	Suffix—Meaning
-blast—immature	**-metry**—process of measuring	**-stomy**—a new permanent opening, artificial opening
-ectomy—removal, excision	**-oma**—tumor, mass	
-edema—swelling	**-phobia**—abnormal fear	**-therapy**—treatment
-ium—membrane	**-plasia, -plasm**—formation, growth	**-tome**—cutting instrument
-meter—instrument used to measure	**-stenosis**—narrowing stricture	**-tomy**—cutting into, incision

Eponyms

Eponym—Meaning

Epstein-Barr virus—the herpes virus that causes mononucleosis
Hodgkin's disease—malignant tumor of lymph tissue

Abbreviations

Abbreviation—Meaning	Abbreviation—Meaning	Abbreviation—Meaning
AIDS—acquired immune deficiency syndrome (a disease that impairs the immune system)	**crypto**—cryptococcus (an infection caused by a fungus; spreads through the lungs to the brain, skin, bones, and urinary tract)	**Ga**—gallium-67 (a radioisotope used as an IV contrast medium in diagnosis scans)
AZT—azidothymidine (a drug used to treat AIDS)		**histo**—histoplasmosis (a fungal infection from an airborne spore; attacks the immune system)
	CT, CAT—computerized tomography, also called *computerized axial tomography* (a painless method for examining structures inside the body)	
Bx, bx—biopsy (removal of a small piece of living tissue or the specimen obtained)		**HIV**—human immunodeficiency virus the virus that causes AIDS)
	DES—diethylstilbestrol (a manufactured hormone similar to estrogen)	**HSV**—herpes simplex virus (causes an infection that attacks the skin and nervous system)
C, ca—cancer		
CEA—carcinoembryonic antigen (a substance thought to be released into the bloodstream by tumors; a tumor marker)	**DNA**—deoxyribonucleic acid (carries the genetic information in a cell)	**KS**—Kaposi's sarcoma (a cancer that spreads through the lymph system)
	EBV—Epstein-Barr virus (causes mononucleosis, an infection of the immune system)	**Mets, mets**—metastases (the process by which tumor cells are spread to distant parts of the body, usually through the lymph system)
chemo—chemotherapy (treatment of a disease with chemicals or drugs)		
CMV—cytomegalovirus (a large herpes-type virus that can cause many diseases; most often seen in a person with a weak or impaired immune system)	**ER**—estrogen receptor (determines if a tumor will respond to hormone therapy)	**NED**—no evidence of disease

TABLE 1-9
Word Parts for Immune System Terminology—cont'd

Abbreviations		
Abbreviation—Meaning	Abbreviation—Meaning	Abbreviation—Meaning
NHL—non-Hodgkin's lymphoma (includes all cancers of the lymph system except Hodgkin's disease)	**RNA**—ribonucleic acid (carries genetic information from the DNA in the nucleus of a cell to the cytoplasm of the cell)	**T & A**—tonsillectomy and adenoidectomy (surgical removal of tonsils and adenoids—lymph tissue in the nasopharynx)
Pap smear—Papanicolaou smear (a cancer screening test)	**T4**—a small white blood cell of the immune system (produced by the thymus gland, it destroys or wards off foreign cells)	**TNM**—tumors, nodes, metastases
PCP—*Pneumocystis carinii* pneumonia (a lung infection from a parasite most often seen in people with a weak immune system)	**T-cell**—a lymphocyte (a small white blood cell produced by the bone marrow; it matures in the thymus and functions in immune response)	**toxo**—toxoplasmosis (a parasitic infection of the lymph nodes; it may be acquired by eating inadequately cooked meat containing the virus)
PR—partial response (tumor is one half of its original size)		**XRT**—radiation therapy (the use of radiation to treat disease; often used to treat cancer)
Prot, prot—protocol (the standard or approved method of treatment)		**ZVD**—zidovudine (a drug used to treat AIDS)
PSA—prostate specific antigen (a protein produced by the prostate gland; high levels indicate prostate disease or tumor)		

Nervous System

The **nervous system** (Figure 1-9) is made up of two distinct systems, the peripheral nervous system and the central nervous system (CNS). The CNS comprises the brain and the spinal cord. The peripheral nervous system comprises 12 pairs of cranial nerves, 31 pairs of spinal nerves, and the autonomic nervous system.

The nervous system is an electrical network organized like a computer system, and it functions in much the same way. The brain receives information from the peripheral nervous system. It stores and analyzes the information and initiates an appropriate response. The peripheral nervous system gathers and sends information to the CNS and delivers instructions from the CNS.

The brain is the primary central nervous system center for regulating and controlling body activities. The brain is divided into regions, and each region regulates and controls specific senses or body functions. The spinal cord is the "information highway" connecting the brain with the peripheral nervous system.

The cranial and spinal nerves of the peripheral nervous system are mostly voluntary nerves associated with movement and with the senses of taste, touch, sight, hearing, smell, and pain. The cranial nerves extend to the head and neck, whereas the spinal nerves extend to the rest of the body.

The autonomic nervous system regulates vital body functions by controlling involuntary muscles and involuntary responses. It is composed of sympathetic nerves that react to stress and parasympathetic nerves that balance the reactions of the sympathetic nerves to bring the body back to a normal state.

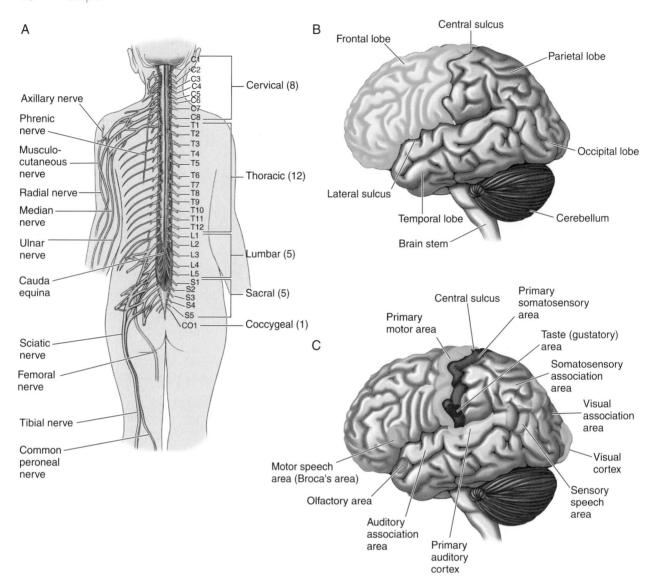

FIGURE 1-9

The nervous system. **A,** spinal nerves; **B,** lobes of the brain; **C,** functional areas of the brain. (Modified from Herlihy B and Maebius N: The Human Body in Health and Illness. Philadelphia, WB Saunders, 2000, pp. 175, 202.)

STOP & REVIEW

Answer or complete the following:

1. What part of the CNS receives, stores, and analyzes information?

_____

2. What part of the CNS serves as an information highway between the brain and the peripheral nerves?

_____

3. What part of the peripheral nervous system handles involuntary muscles and responses?

_____

4. What part of the peripheral nervous system handles voluntary nerves to the head and neck?

_____

Use Table 1-10 to define the following:

5. Hemiplegia _____

6. Radiculopathy _____

7. Neuralgia _____

8. Alzheimer's disease _____

_____

9. CVA _____

10. LP _____

TABLE 1-10
Word Parts for Nervous System Terminology

Root Words

Root—Meaning	Root—Meaning	Root—Meaning
alges/o, algesi/o—sensitivity or hypersensitivity to pain	**encephal/o**—brain	**phil/o**—love, attraction to
anxi/o—anxious, uneasy, distressed	**esthesi/o**—feeling, nervous sensation	**phren/o**—mind
arachn/o—spider	**gli/o**—glue, parts of the nervous system that support and connect	**pont/o**—pons (a region of the brain; any bridge of tissue that connects two parts of a structure or organ)
astr/o—star	**hypn/o, narc/o**—sleep	**psych/o**—mind
audi/o—sound, hearing	**iatr/o**—treatment	**pyr/o**—fire
aut/o—self	**kines/o, kinesi/o**—movement	**radicul/o**—nerve root (of spinal nerves)
caus/o—burning sensation	**lept/o**—thin, slender	**schiz/o**—split
cerebell/o—cerebellum (located beneath the posterior part of the brain)	**lex/o**—word, phrase	**somat/o**—body
cerebr/o—cerebrum (the largest part of the brain)	**mening/o, meningi/o**—meninges, membranes	**syncop/o**—to cut off or cut short
comat/o—coma, deep sleep	**ment/o**—mind	**tax/o**—order, coordination
dendr/o—dendrite, tree (the microscopic branching part of a nerve cell. It receives the nervous impulse.)	**mon/o**—one, single	**thalam/o**—thalamus (it interprets the impulses received in the brain from nerves)
dur/o—dura mater (the outermost layer of the meninges surrounding the brain and spinal column)	**my/o**—muscle	**thec/o**—sheath (refers to the meninges)
	myel/o—spinal cord (or sometimes bone marrow)	**vag/o**—vagus nerve (the tenth cranial nerve)
	neur/o—nerve	
	olig/o—few	

Prefixes

Prefix—Meaning	Prefix—Meaning	Prefix—Meaning
a-, an-—no, not	**hemi-**—half	**para-**—abnormal
cata-—down	**hypo-**—below, deficient, less than	**quadri-**—four
contra-—against	**idio-**—individual	**semi-**—half, partly
di-—twice	**inter-**—between	

Suffixes

Suffix—Meaning	Suffix—Meaning	Suffix—Meaning
-algesia—sensitivity or hypersensitivity to pain	**-leptic**—to seize hold of	**-phoria**—feeling, bearing
-algia—pain	**-mania**—obsessive preoccupation	**-phylaxis**—protection
-esthesia—feeling, nervous sensation	**-paresis**—less than total paralysis	**-plegia**—paralysis (loss of ability to move body parts)
-genic—produced by	**-pathy**—disease	**-praxia**—action
-kinesia, -kinesis—movement	**-phasia**—speech	**-sthenia**—strength
-lepsy—seizure	**-phobia**—fear (often severe and disabling)	**-thymia**—mind

Continued.

TABLE 1-10
Word Parts for Nervous System Terminology—cont'd

Eponyms
Eponym—Meaning

Alzheimer's disease—a brain disorder marked by deterioration of mental capacity (dementia). It often starts in late middle life.
Huntington's chorea—a hereditary nervous disorder due to degenerative changes in the brain. It is characterized by abrupt, bizarre, involuntary, dancelike movements and ends in insanity.
Parkinson's disease—a slowly growing disorder caused by damage to the nerves in the brain. It usually occurs late in life and leads to tremors, muscle weakness, and slower movements.
Gilles de la Tourette syndrome—a neurological disorder marked by involuntary tics and spasmodic twitching movements, involuntary vocal noises, and obscene speech.

Abbreviations
Abbreviation—Meaning

ACh—acetycholine (a substance, present in many parts of the body, that has important psychological functions)
ADHD—attention deficit hyperactivity disorder (a misfunction of the CNS without a major nervous system or mental disorder; characterized by learning or behavior disorders; seen most often in children with normal to above-average intelligence)
ALS—amyotrophic lateral sclerosis (a degenerative disease of the nerve network that regulates muscles; also called Lou Gehrig's disease)
ANS—autonomic nervous system (the part of the nervous system that regulates involuntary body functions: circulatory system, digestive system, endocrine system)
C.A.—chronological age (the age of a person stated as the amount of time that has passed since birth)
CNS—central nervous system (composed of the brain and the spinal cord, it is the part of the nervous system that regulates the peripheral nervous system and brain activity; it is the network of coordination and control of the entire body)
CSF—cerebrospinal fluid (the fluid that flows through and protects the brain and the spinal canal)
CSM—cerebrospinal meningitis (any infection or inflammation of the membranes covering the brain and spinal cord)
CT, CAT—computerized tomography or computerized axial tomography (a painless method for examining structures inside the body)

CVA—cerebrovascular accident (stroke; a blood clot or bleeding in the brain leads to a loss of oxygen to brain tissue and results in a loss of function to the body parts regulated by that area of the brain)
DT—delirium tremens (a serious and sometimes fatal reaction to the sudden withdrawal of alcohol in an alcoholic, but it may also be triggered by a head injury or by an infection)
ECT—electroconvulsive therapy (a brief convulsion is caused by passing an electric current through the brain; it is used to treat some mental disorders)
EEG—electroencephalogram (electrodes are used to measure and record brain wave activity)
ICP—intracranial pressure (the pressure in the skull)
IQ—intelligence quotient (a number that describes a person's level of intelligence as compared to average for the person's age group)
LP—lumbar puncture (inserting a needle into the lumbar portion of the spine; may be done to obtain a fluid sample, as part of a diagnostic test, or for treatment reasons)
M.A.—mental age (the age or age group in which a person's intelligence level falls in the average range)
MAO—monoamine oxidase (an enzyme that inactivates nervous system hormones; drugs that inhibit this enzyme are used to treat depression and anxiety, and people who take these drugs must avoid certain foods)
MMPI—Minnesota Multiphasic Personality Inventory (used as an objective measure of psychological disorders in adolescents and adults)

MRI—magnetic resonance imaging (a painless, but noisy, method for examining structures inside the body)
MS—multiple sclerosis (a degenerative disease that erodes the protective covering on the nerve fibers of the brain and spinal cord)
PET—positive emission tomography (a painless method for examining structures inside the body)
PNS—peripheral nervous system (the motor and sensory nerves outside of the brain and spinal cord; the autonomic nervous system is part of the peripheral nervous system)
SNS—somatic nervous system (the part of the nervous system that regulates voluntary movement—musculoskeletal system)
TAT—thematic apperception test (reveals personality structure; pictures are used as a stimulus for making up a story)
TENS—transcutaneous electrical nerve stimulation (a battery-powered device used to relieve acute and chronic pain)
TIA—transient ischemic attack (temporary interference with the blood supply to the brain due to blood vessel damage, usually either a buildup of fats or a blood clot)
WAIS—Wechsler Adult Intelligence Scale (a standardized test to measure intelligence in adults)
WISC—Wechsler Intelligence Scale for Children (a standardized test to measure intelligence in children)

Eyes and Ears

The eyes and ears are special sense organs (Figure 1-10). Eyes enable sight and ears enable hearing and balance. There are two eyes and two ears.

Light enters the pupil of the eye and passes through the lens, and an image is projected onto the retina on the back wall inside the eye in much the same way as a movie is projected onto a screen at a movie theater. The nerve structures in the retina transmit the image to the brain for interpretation. Images from both eyes are necessary for depth perception. When everything occurs in a normal manner, the result is normal vision.

Sound enters the outer ear and vibrates the eardrum. The vibrations on the eardrum start a chain reaction. The small bones of the middle ear relay the information to the inner ear. The fluid in the inner ear carries the sound to nerve endings that relay it to the brain for interpretation. The inner ear has semicircular canals and a snail-shaped structure called a cochlea that enable the nerve endings to also send the flow patterns of the fluid in the inner ear to the brain to interpret balance. Hearing from both ears is needed to interpret the direction and other fine distinctions of sound. When everything occurs in a normal manner, the result is normal hearing and good balance.

STOP & REVIEW

Answer or complete the following:

1. In the eye, an image is projected onto the _____ on the back wall inside the eye to enable vision.

2. In the ear, sound waves bounce off the _____ to start a chain reaction that results in hearing.

3. Light enters the eye through the _____.

4. The flow of fluid in the _____ ear determines balance.

Use Table 1-11 to define the following:

5. Diplopia _____

6. Otitis _____

7. Intraocular _____

8. Ménière's disease _____

9. EENT _____

10. PERRLA _____

TABLE 1-11
Word Parts for Special Senses Terminology

Root Words		
Root—Meaning	Root—Meaning	Root—Meaning
acous/o—hearing, sound	**dacry/o, lacrim/o**—tears, tear duct	**phac/o, phak/o**—lens of the eye
ambly/o—dull, dim	**dipl/o**—double	**photo**—light
aque/o—water	**glauc/o**—gray	**presby/o**—old age
audi/o, audit/o—hearing, the sense of hearing	**ir/o, irid/o**—iris (the colored portion of the eye)	**retin/o**—retina (the multi-layered nervous membrane at the back of the eye, it contains the rods and the cones that receive visual images and transmit them to the brain)
aur/o, auricul/o—the outer ear	**mastoid/o**—mastoid process (a part of the temporal bone near the ear)	
blephar/o, palpebr/o—eyelid	**mi/o**—smaller, less	
cochle/o—cochlea (the snail-shaped tube in the inner ear)	**mydr/o**—wide, enlarge	
conjunctiv/o—conjunctiva (membranes lining the eyelids and covering the white part of the eye)	**myring/o tympan/o**—tympanic membrane (eardrum; a membrane between the external ear canal and the middle ear)	**salping/o**—tube, tubes (as in the auditory or eustachian tubes that connect the middle ear to the nasopharynx or throat)
cor/o, pupill/o—pupil (the round, black "window" of the eye through which light passes)	**nyct/o**—night	**scler/o**—sclera (the white of the eye)
corne/o, kerat/o—cornea (the transparent, dome-shaped, front of the eye)	**ocul/o, ophthalm/o**—eye	**scot/o**—darkness
	opt/o, optic/o—eye, vision	**staped/o**—stapes (the small stirrup-shaped bone in the middle ear)
cycl/o—ciliary body (the part of the eye that joins the iris with the blood supply) or ciliary muscles (control the shape of the lens in the eye)	**ossicul/o**—ossicle (small bone—as in the hammer, anvil, and stirrup, the ossicle of the middle ear)	**uve/o**—uvea (the layer of the eye that includes the iris, the ciliary body, and the choroid)
	ot/o—ear	**vitre/o**—glassy
	papill/o—nipple-like, optic disk (the tiny white spot in the retina of the eye known as the blind spot)	**xer/o**—dry

Continued.

A

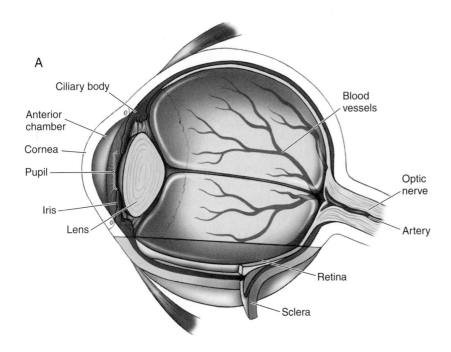

Ciliary body

Anterior chamber

Cornea

Pupil

Iris

Lens

Blood vessels

Optic nerve

Artery

Retina

Sclera

B

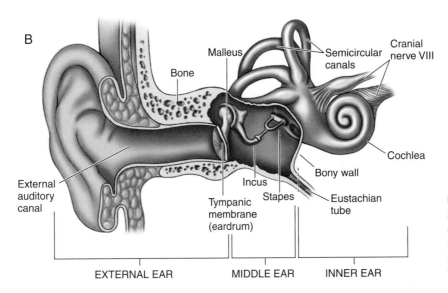

Bone

Malleus

Semicircular canals

Cranial nerve VIII

External auditory canal

Tympanic membrane (eardrum)

Incus

Stapes

Bony wall

Eustachian tube

Cochlea

EXTERNAL EAR

MIDDLE EAR

INNER EAR

FIGURE 1-10

Sensory organs. **A,** the eye; **B,** the ear. (Modified from Herlihy B and Maebius N: The Human Body in Health and Illness. Philadelphia, WB Saunders, 2000, pp. 222, 229.)

TABLE 1-11
Word Parts for Special Senses Terminology—cont'd

Prefixes

Prefix—Meaning	Prefix—Meaning	Prefix—Meaning
bi-—two **dys-**—bad, painful, difficult	**en-**—in, inside **intra-**—within	**uni-**—one

Suffixes

Suffix—Meaning	Suffix—Meaning	Suffix—Meaning
-ar—pertaining to **-cusis**—hearing	**-itis**—inflammation **-opia, -opsia**—vision	**-otia**—ear condition **-tropia**—to turn

Eponyms

Eponym—Meaning
Ménière's disease—a disorder of the labyrinth of the inner ear characterized by dizziness, nerve deafness, and buzzing or ringing of the ears.

Abbreviations

Abbreviation—Meaning	Abbreviation—Meaning	Abbreviation—Meaning
AD—auris dextra (right ear) **AS**—auris sinistra (left ear) **AU**—auris uterque (both ears) **EENT**—eyes, ears, nose, and throat **ENT**—ears, nose, and throat **IOL**—intracular lens **IOP**—intracular pressure **OD**—oculus dexter (right eye) **OS**—oculus sinister (left eye) **OU**—oculus uterque (both eye)	**PERRLA**—pupils equal, round, and react to light, accommodation (documents the condition of the eyes as being normal; includes, the size and shape of the pupils, their reaction to the light, and their ability to focus) **PE tube**—polyethylene ventilating tube (placed in the eardrum)	**VA**—visual acuity **VF**—visual field

Other Important Medical Language

SIGNS, SYMPTOMS, AND SIGNIFICANT FINDINGS

A **symptom** is something felt or noticed by the patient that helps detect a disease or disorder. Symptoms include any change or suspected change from a normal state.

A **sign** is something seen or found by an examiner that helps detect a disease or disorder. Signs often verify symptoms and may include test results.

A **significant finding** includes both significant changes from normal (signs and symptoms) and significant normal findings that help detect a disease or disorder. The absence of significant signs is just as important as the significant signs that are found by the examiner to narrow the possibilities when determining a diagnosis.

Physicians should document all significant findings from an examination, not just the abnormal findings. When a diagnosis has not yet been established, the documented signs, symptoms, and significant findings are used to determine the medical necessity for a patient visit or procedure. Word parts for signs, symptoms, and significant findings terminology are shown in Table 1-12.

CONSTITUTIONAL SIGNS AND SYMPTOMS

Constitutional signs and symptoms include **vital signs,** measurements of growth, and an assessment of the general well being of the person.

Many health professionals automatically think of temperature, pulse, respirations, and blood pressure when they hear the term *vital signs.* According to the Evaluation and Management Guidelines proposed by the American Medical Association (AMA) in June 1999, at least three of the following 10 measurements should be included when measuring vital signs:

- ❏ Sitting blood pressure
- ❏ Standing blood pressure
- ❏ Supine (lying down) blood pressure
- ❏ Heart rate and regularity
- ❏ Respiratory rate
- ❏ Temperature
- ❏ Weight
- ❏ Height
- ❏ Head circumference
- ❏ Body mass index

General appearance or general well-being includes development, nutrition, looks or physique, growth,

TABLE 1-12
Word Parts for Signs, Symptoms, and Significant Findings Terminology

Root Words

Root—Meaning	Root—Meaning	Root—Meaning
abdomin/o—abdominal	**gram/o**—to print or record	**poster/o**—posterior, back, behind
acr/o—extremities (arms and legs)	**gynec/o**—female	**proxim/o**—proximal, near
adip/o—fat	**hist/o**—tissue	**psych/o**—mind
anter/o—anterior, front	**ili/o**—ilium (upper part of the	**radi/o**—radius (a lower arm bone) or
bi/o—life, living	pelvic bone)	radiant energy (x-rays)
blephar/o—eyelid	**immun/o**—immune	**rheumat/o**—rheumatism
bol/o—to cast or throw	**infer/o**—inferior, situated below	**rhin/o**—nose
cardi/o—heart	**inguin/o**—inguinal area (groin)	**roentgen/o**—x-rays
caud/o—tail (tailbone or lower	**is/o**—same	**sacr/o**—sacrum (tailbone)
portion of body)	**kinesi/o**—movement	**sarc/o**—flesh
cephal/o—head	**laryng/o**—larynx (voice box)	**scintill/o**—spark
cervic/o—neck (upper portion of	**later/o**—side	**som/a, somat/o**—body
spine) or cervix (neck of the uterus)	**leth/o**—death	**son/o**—sound
chir/o—hand	**lumb/o**—lumbar (lower back)	**spin/o**—spine (backbone)
chondr/o—cartilage (connective	**medi/o**—medial, middle	**supr/o**—superior (uppermost, above)
tissue)	**mucos/o**—mucous membrane, mucosa	**thel/o**—nipple
chrom/o—color	**my/o**—muscle	**therapeut/o**—therapeutic, treatment
coccyg/o—coccyx (tailbone)	**neur/o**—nerve, nervous system	**thorac/o**—thorax, chest
crani/o—cranium (skull)	**onc/o**—tumor	**tox/o, toxic/o**—poison
cyan/o—blue	**ophthalm/o**—eye	**trache/o**—trachea (windpipe)
dactyl/o—digit (fingers and toes)	**opt/o, optic/o**—vision	**umbilic/o**—umbilicus, navel
dent/o, odont/o—tooth, teeth	**or/o**—mouth	**ur/o**—urine, urinary tract
derm/o, dermat/o—skin	**orth/o**—straight	**ventr/o**—ventral, belly
dist/o, tel/e—distant, far	**ot/o**—ear	**vertebr/o**—vertebrae (backbones,
dors/o—dorsal, back portion of body	**path/o**—disease	bones in spine)
electr/o—electricity	**ped/o**—child, foot	**viscer/o**—visceral (internal organs)
encephal/o—brain	**pelv/i, pelv/o**—pelvis, hip	**vitr/o**—glass
esthesi/o—feeling	**pharmaceut/o**—drug	**viv/o**—life
fluor/o—fluorescent, luminous	**physi/o**—nature	**xer/o**—dry
ger/a, ger/o, geront/o—aged	**pod/o**—foot	

Prefixes

Prefix—Meaning	Prefix—Meaning	Prefix—Meaning
an-—without	**dys-**—bad, painful, difficult	**meta-**—change
ana-—up	**echo-**—a repeated sound	**pes-**—foot
bi-—two	**en-, end-, endo-**—in, inside	**tachy-**—fast
brachy-—short, short distance	**epi-**—above	**tri-**—three
brady-—slow	**hypo-**—below	**ultra-**—beyond
cata-—down	**inter-**—between	**uni-**—one
cine-—movement	**intra-**—within	

Suffixes

Suffix—Meaning	Suffix—Meaning	Suffix—Meaning
-ac, -al, -ic—pertaining to	**-iatrics, iatry**—medicine	**-pathy**—disease
-ad—toward	**-ism**—process	**-plasm**—formation
-dynia—pain	**-itis**—inflammation	**-pnea**—breathing
-eal—pertaining to	**-logist**—one who studies	**-pod**—foot
-er, -ist—one who	**-logy**—study or science of	**-somes**—bodies
-gram—a record	**-lucent**—to shine	**-spasm**—cramp, twitching
-graph—recording instrument	**-opaque**—obscure	**-suppression**—to stop
-graphy—the process of recording	**-ose**—pertaining to, full of	**-therapy**—treatment
-ia—condition	**-osis**—condition, disease,	**-type**—picture, classification
-iac, -ior—pertaining to	or abnormal increase	

Abbreviations

Abbreviation—Meaning	Abbreviation—Meaning	Abbreviation—Meaning
Angio, angio—angiography (an x-ray procedure that uses dye to study the heart chambers and blood vessels)	**Ba**—barium (a contrast medium used for x-ray studies of the gastrointestinal tract—the tube that extends from the mouth to the anus; most of the digestive system)	**BMR**—basal metabolic rate (measures the amount of energy needed to maintain body function; an indicator of thyroid function)
AP—anteroposterior (from the front to the back of the body; direction of an x-ray beam)		

TABLE 1-12
Word Parts for Signs, Symptoms, and Significant Findings Terminology—cont'd

Abbreviations		
Abbreviation—Meaning	Abbreviation—Meaning	Abbreviation—Meaning
BSA—body surface area	**Hx**—history, history of	**RLQ**—right lower quadrant (of abdomen)
Bx, bx—biopsy	**IVP**—intravenous pyelogram (an x-ray study of the kidney using IV contrast medium)	**RUQ**—right upper quadrant (of abdomen)
C-spine—cervical spine (bones in neck)	**KUB**—kidneys, ureters, bladder (an x-ray study without contrast)	**SPECT**—single-photon emission computed tomography (radioactive substances and a computer are used to create three-dimensional images)
CXR—chest x-ray	**LAT**—lateral	
decub—decubitus (lying-down or pressure sore from lying in one position too long)	**LLQ**—left lower quadrant (of abdomen)	
DI—diagnostic imaging	**LS films**—lumbosacral films (x-rays of the lower spine)	**UGI**—upper gastrointestinal x-ray (barium contrast medium is swallowed and x-rays are taken of the esophagus, stomach, and small intestine)
DOA—dead on arrival	**LUQ**—left upper quadrant (of abdomen)	
DOB—date of birth	**OT**—occupational therapy	
Dx—diagnosis	**PA**—posteroanterior (from the back of the body to the front; direction of an x-ray beam)	**US, U/S**—ultrasound
ECG, EKG—electrocardiogram (measures heart activity)	**PE**—physical examination	**VQ**—ventilation-perfusion scan of the lungs
EEG—electroencephalogram (measures brain activity)	**PT**—physical therapy	
EMG—electromyelogram (measures nerve and muscle activity)	**Px**—physical exam	
Fx—fracture (broken bone)		
GI—gastrointestinal (the tube that extends from mouth to anus; most of the digestive system)		

skin color, deformities, any unusual physical features, attention to grooming, pattern of behavior or thought, and an assessment of the ability to communicate. Table 1-13 lists word parts for constitutional signs and symptoms terminology.

PRESCRIPTION TERMINOLOGY

A **prescription** is an order for a drug, a treatment, or a device to be dispensed. A prescription drug may only be given to the public with an order from a properly licensed professional. A prescription for a controlled drug, such as a narcotic, may only be written by a physician with a DEA (Drug Enforcement Agency) license.

A drug is any substance, usually a chemical substance, used to treat or prevent a disease. It may be swallowed, applied to the skin, or injected into a muscle, the skin, a blood vessel, or a body cavity.

A drug can have three types of names. The brand or trade name is the name given to it by the original manufacturer. It is usually an easy-to-remember, or catchy, name. No other manufacturer of the drug may use this name for its product. For example, Mexitil is a brand name.

The generic name is a descriptive name that is the legal name of the drug for scientific purposes. It is usually longer than the brand name and uses scientific word parts, instead of easy-to-remember word parts. The original manufacturer may use the generic name exclusively for 17 years, and then any

drug manufacturer may legally use it. For example, mexiletine hydrochloride is the generic name for Mexitil.

The chemical name is the chemical formula used to create the drug. This name is often long and complex, using the names of chemical substances. For example, 1-methyl-2-(2,6xylyloxy)-ethylamine hydrochloride is the chemical name of Mexitil, which has the chemical formula of $C_{11}H_{17}NO \bullet HCl$.

The route of administration is the method by which a drug is introduced into the body. *Oral administration* means the drug is taken by mouth: It is swallowed whole, or chewed and swallowed. *Sublingual administration* means the drug is dissolved under the tongue. *Rectal administration* means the drug is inserted into the rectum. *Parenteral administration* means a syringe is used to inject the drug. Drugs may be injected in the skin (intradermal), under the skin (subcutaneous), in a muscle (intramuscular), in the spinal column (intrathecal), in a blood vessel (intravenously), or in a body cavity (intracavitary), depending on the instructions given in the prescription. *Inhalation administration* means the drug is inhaled through the nose or mouth. *Topical administration* means the drug is applied directly on the skin or on a mucous membrane.

An analgesic is a drug that relieves pain. An anesthetic reduces or eliminates sensation. An "anti-" type drug acts against whatever follows the hyphen. For example, *anti*biotics act against living micro-organisms, and *anti*convulsants act against convulsions.

Drugs that name a body part in the type of drug act on that body part. For example, respiratory drugs act on the respiratory system.

Sedatives are drugs that produce calmness. Stimulants are drugs that increase alertness. Tranquilizers treat anxiety.

Prescriptions are usually written using standard medical abbreviations. Table 1-14 lists some of the most common abbreviations used in prescriptions.

UNITS OF MEASURE

Medical offices often use a combination of U.S. measurements and metric measurements. Weight and height are usually documented in the medical record in pounds/ounces and feet/inches so the patient will understand the measurements. Sometimes physicians must convert these measurements to the metric system before determining drug dosages.

TABLE 1-13
Word Parts for Constitutional Signs and Symptoms Terminology

Abbreviations		
Abbreviation—Meaning	Abbreviation—Meaning	Abbreviation—Meaning
BMI—body mass index	**ft**—foot, feet	**oz**—ounce, ounces
BP—blood pressure (measures the stress placed on walls of the veins and arteries by the pumping action of the heart)	**g, gm**—gram, grams	**T, temp**—temperature (body temperature)
	HT, ht—height	**TPR**—temperature (body temperature), pulse (heart rate), respiration (rate of breathing)
	in.—inch, inches	
C—Celsius, centigrade	**kg**—kilogram, kilograms	
circ—circumference	**lb**—pound, pounds	**WT, wt**—weight
F—Fahrenheit	**m**—meter, meters	
	mm—millimeter, millimeters	

TABLE 1-14
Word Parts for Prescription Terminology

Root Words		
Root—Meaning	Root—Meaning	Root—Meaning
aer/o—air	**esthes/o**—feeling, sensation	**pyret/o**—fever
alges/o—sensitivity to pain	**hist/o**—tissue	**thec/o**—thecal (sheath lining the brain and spinal column)
bronch/o—bronchus, bronchioles (airway tubes that lead to lungs)	**hypn/o**—sleep	
	iatr/o—treatment	
chem/o, pharmac/o—drug	**lingu/o**—tongue	**tox/o, toxic/o**—poison
cras/o—mixture	**myc/o**—mold, fungus	**vas/o**—vessel
cutane/o, derm/o—skin	**narc/o**—stupor	**ven/o**—vein
erg/o—work	**prurit/o**—itching	**vit/o**—life

Prefixes		
Prefix—Meaning	Prefix—Meaning	Prefix—Meaning
ana-—upward, excessive, again	**contra-**—against, not, opposite	**syn-**—together, with
anti-—against	**par-**—other than, apart from	

Abbreviations		
Abbreviation—Meaning	Abbreviation—Meaning	Abbreviation—Meaning
Ac, ac—before meals (ante cibum)	**OTC**—over the counter (a drug or medication that can be obtained without a prescription)	**Qns, qns**—quantity not sufficient
Ad lib, ad lib—freely, as desired (ad libitum)		**Qod, qod**—every other day
		Qpm, qpm—every evening
Aq, aq—water (aqua)	**Pc, pc**—after meals (post cibum)	**Rx**—prescription (an instruction written by a physician that directs a pharmacist to dispense a specific dose of a drug)
Bid, bid—twice a day (bis in die)	**PDR**—Physicians' Desk Reference (a guide to prescription drugs)	
c̄—with	**Prn, prn**—when requested, as needed, as desired (pro re nata)	
Caps, caps—capsule		
FDA—Food and Drug Administration	**Q, q**—every (quaque)	**s̄**—without
H, h—hour	**Qam, qam**—every morning	**Sig, sig**—let it be labeled (directions to be written on a prescription label)
hs—bedtime (hora somnolent)	**Qd, qd**—every day (quaque die)	
IM—intramuscular (into a muscle)	**Qh, qh**—every hour (quaque hora)	**Stat, stat**—immediately (statim)
IV—intravenous (into a vein)	**Qhs, qhs**—every hour of sleep, every bedtime (quaque hora somnolent)	**subcut, subq**—subcutaneous (under the skin)
Noc, noc, noct—nocturnal (night)		**Tab, tab**—tablet
NPO—nothing by mouth (nulla per os)	**Qid, qid**—four times a day (quater in die)	**Tid, tid**—three times a day (ter in die)
NSAID—nonsteroid anti-inflammatory drug		
Os, os—mouth		

This chapter does not teach mathematics, and it does not teach measurement techniques. The tables are presented to give you a general idea of the types of measurements used in a medical office. For commonly used units of measure, both U.S. and metric, please see Table 1-15. For examples of measurement conversions, please see Table 1-16. For abbreviations related to units of measure, please see Table 1-17.

TABLE 1-15
U.S.-Metric Comparison

Metric Measures	U.S. Measures
Millimeters	Fractions of an inch
Centimeters	Inches
Gram	Ounce
Kilogram	Pound
Milliliters	Fractions of teaspoon, Teaspoon, Tablespoons, Fractions of cups, Cups, Pints
Liters	Quarts
Celsius, centigrade	Fahrenheit

TABLE 1-16
Equivalent Measures

Equivalent Measures
1 centimeter = 0.39 inch
1 inch = 2.54 centimeters
1 milliliter = $\frac{1}{5}$ teaspoon
1 teaspoon = 5 milliliters
1 tablespoon = 15 milliliters
1 cup = 8 ounces = 240 milliliters
1 pint = 2 cups = 16 ounces = 480 milliliters
1 quart = 2 pints = 0.95 liter
1 gram = 0.04 ounce
1 ounce = 28.35 grams
1 kilogram = 2.20 pounds
1 pound = 0.45 kilogram

TABLE 1-17
Measurement Abbreviations

Abbreviation—Meaning	Abbreviation—Meaning	Abbreviation—Meaning
C—Celsius, centigrade	**in., ″**—inch	**pt**—pint
c—cup	**lb**—pound	**qt**—quart
cc—cubic centimeter	**kg**—kilogram	**Tbsp**—tablespoon
d—day, days	**L, l**—liter	**tsp**—teaspoon
dd—day of month expressed as two-digit number	**m**—meter	**T, temp**—temperature
F—Fahrenheit	**mg**—milligram	**WT, wt**—weight
ft, ′—foot	**min**—minute, minutes	**y**—year, years
g, gm—gram	**ml**—milliliter	**YO**—years old
gt, gtt—drop, drops	**mm**—millimeter, or month expressed as two-digit number	**yy**—year abbreviated to last two digits
h, hr—hours	**m, mo, mon**—month, months	**yyyy**—year expressed using 4 digits
HT, ht—height	**oz**—ounce	

STOP & REVIEW

Answer or complete the following:

1. A change noticed by the patient is called a _____.

2. A change noticed by an examiner is called a _____.

3. A normal finding that narrows the list of possible diagnoses is considered a _____.

4. Vital signs can include the following:
   A. Temperature, pulse, respiration, and blood pressure while lying, sitting, and/or standing
   B. Height, weight, head circumference, and body mass index
   C. All of the above
   D. None of the above

5. Constitutional signs and symptoms include at least three vital sign measurements and an assessment of general well-being.
   ____ True   ____ False

6. Prescriptions are only written for drugs.
   ____ True   ____ False

7. Only metric measurements are used in a medical office.
   ____ True   ____ False

Define the following:

8. PRN _____

9. NPO _____

10. TID _____

Chapter Review

It is important to learn about how the body functions and how to interpret medical words when you work in a medical office. The doctors and the patients must have confidence that you understand what they are saying. Word parts give clues to the meanings of medical words. The musculoskeletal system provides the framework that gives the body form, shape, and movement. It is made up of bones, joints, muscles, and connective tissue. Skin is the largest organ of the body and the first line of defense against infection. The respiratory system brings oxygen to the body by drawing air into the lungs and gets rid of carbon dioxide by exhaling air out of the lungs. The respiratory system also enables speech. The digestive system processes food to provide nutrients for the body, and it processes solid waste to be expelled by the body. The urinary system expels liquid waste from the body. The male and female reproductive systems can work together to create a human baby. The endocrine system is a system of ductless glands that produce hormones. Hormones regulate many body functions.

The circulatory system uses blood in a complex delivery system for the body. The heart pumps the blood and keeps it flowing. Blood vessels only carry blood in one direction. Arteries carry blood away from the heart, and veins carry blood back to the heart. The lymphatic system fights infection and regulates the immune responses of the body. The lymphatic system also regulates the amount of fluid in and around body cells. The nervous system is the electronic computer system for the body. It gathers, stores, and interprets information, and it initiates responses. The CNS includes the brain and the spinal cord. The peripheral nervous system includes cranial nerves, the spinal nerves, and the autonomic nervous system. The eyes and the ears are special sense organs. The eyes enable sight, and the ears enable hearing and balance.

Symptoms are changes observed by the patient. Signs are changes observed by the examiner. Significant findings include changes observed (both signs and symptoms), as well as significant normal findings that narrow the possibilities when determining a diagnosis. Constitutional signs and symptoms include measurements of vital signs and a description of general well-being. A prescription is an order for a drug, treatment, or device. Prescriptions may only be written by licensed professionals, and some require specific licenses. Measurements taken or used in a medical office may be in either the metric system or the U.S. measurement system. Conversion charts are used to translate measurements from one system to the other.

Answer or complete the following:

1. What is the largest organ and the first line of defense against infection?

2. What body system contains the voluntary and involuntary nerves as well as the body's electronic computer system?

3. What body system provides an internal defense against infection and regulates the fluid in and around the body cells?

4. What body system allows oxygen to be brought into the body and carbon dioxide to be carried out of the body?

5. What body system processes nutrients and expels solid waste?

6. What body system filters blood and expels liquid waste?

7. What body system provides the framework that gives the body form, shape, and movement?

8. Significant findings include:

9. At least three out of how many possible items should be measured when vital signs are measured?

10. Prescriptions can be written for:

Use Table 1-12 to find the terms or abbreviations from the definitions:

11. Pertaining to the lower back and sacrum

12. The process of rheumatism

13. Pertaining to between the vertebrae

14. A slow-heart condition

_____

15. The process of recording the brain's electrical
activity

_____

16. Dead on arrival

_____

17. Right lower quadrant (of the abdomen)

_____

18. Posteroanterior

_____

19. Intravenous pyelogram

_____

20. Chest x-ray

_____

2 YOU'RE PART OF A TEAM

Objectives After completing this chapter, you should be able to:

- Relate three or more responsibilities of business office personnel
- Briefly explain how each business office employee influences medical reimbursement
- Discuss legal aspects for each business office position
- Relate three or more of the responsibilities of the clinical staff
- Briefly explain clinical staff responsibilities for documentation and how it influences reimbursement
- Discuss legal aspects for each clinical staff position

Key Terms

ancillary medical providers professionals with a limited license to practice medicine and medical therapists who perform billable services.

billing manager the supervisor in charge of medical billing and collections; may or may not include medical coding.

business office personnel employees in the medical business office: office manager, billing manager, schedulers, receptionists, billers, collections employees, medical records employees, and professional medical coders.

certified coding professional someone who has met the educational and experience prerequisites and who has passed a medical coding certification test administered by a professional coding organization.

clinical staff the production employees in the medical practice: physicians, NPs, PAs, ancillary medical providers, nursing personnel, and technicians.

clinical support staff the members of the clinical staff who do not practice medicine, although some do practice nursing: RNs, LPNs, technicians, CMAs, and RMAs.

CMA certified medical assistant; an employee whose education places an emphasis on the outpatient medical office and encompasses both clinical and business office functions and who has passed a certification examination administered by the American Association of Medical Assistants (AAMA), a professional association.

collections employee an employee with responsibility for collecting payments from insurance companies and patients.

credentialing the process of verifying credentials to establish that a person has not misrepresented accomplishments, that licensure remains current, and that the person has not been excluded from participation in federal medical plans.

custodian of records the employee who is legally responsible for the care and handling of medical records for the medical practice.

DC doctor of chiropractic medicine; schooling focuses on medical health in relation to spinal alignment; fully licensed to practice chiropractic medicine.

DO doctor of osteopathy; similar to an MD, but schooling places a larger emphasis on the role of the musculoskeletal system in overall health; a graduate from an osteopathic school of medicine who is fully licensed by the state to practice medicine.

FBI Federal Bureau of Investigation; they investigate and prosecute federal offenses and criminal activity.

HIPAA Health Insurance Portability and Accountability Act of 1996; a federal law that governs many aspects of health care.

LCSW licensed clinical social worker; a limited-license mental health professional with a minimum of a bachelor's degree and who has passed a state licensure examination.

limited license the scope of medical practice has limitations; the number and the type of services are less than for a full license to practice medicine; often limited to a particular specialty and to specific services within that specialty.

LPN licensed practical nurse; a limited-license nursing professional whose education places an emphasis on the clinical aspects of nursing and who has passed a state licensure examination.

MD medical doctor; a graduate from medical school who is fully licensed by the state to practice medicine.

medical biller a medical business office employee who prepares and submits medical claim forms.

medical records employee a medical business office employee who is responsible for handling and safeguarding patient medical records.

no-show a patient who fails to arrive for a scheduled appointment and who has not called to cancel the appointment.

NP nurse practitioner; a registered nurse who has received advanced education and has passed a state certification examination to obtain a limited license to practice medicine in addition to nursing.

office manager the top-level supervisor in a medical practice whose responsibilities encompass both business office and clinical duties.

OIG/HHS Office of Inspector General, Department of Health and Human Services.

OT occupational therapist or occupational therapy; requires a minimum of a bachelor's degree and passing a state licensure examination to obtain a license in occupational therapy.

PA physician's assistant; a medical provider who has completed the required education and passed a state licensure examination to obtain a limited license to practice medicine.

patient-supplied information the billing information for the top half of the medical claim form.

physician a person who is fully licensed to practice medicine: MD or DO.

provider-supplied information the billing information for the bottom half of the medical claim form.

PT physical therapist, or physical therapy; requires a minimum of a bachelor's degree and passing a state licensure examination to obtain a license in physical therapy.

receptionist the business office employee who greets patients and obtains or verifies the patient-supplied information for the medical claim form.

RMA registered medical assistant; an employee whose education places an emphasis on the outpatient medical office and encompasses both clinical and business office functions and who has passed a certification examination administered by the American Medical Technologists (AMT), a professional association.

RN registered nurse; a fully licensed nursing professional. Must complete required education and pass a state licensure examination to obtain a license as a registered nurse.

scheduler a business office employee who schedules patient appointments.

scope of practice the legal limits of licensure or certification; the number and type of services that can be performed with a given set of credentials.

Security Standards for Health Information a law that governs the security of electronic patient records.

ST speech therapist or speech therapy. Requires a minimum of a bachelor's degree and passing a state licensure examination to obtain a license in speech therapy.

vendor a representative from another company that wishes to sell a product or a service to the medical practice.

Introduction

The rules, codes, and laws for collecting payment from medical plans and insurance companies are subject to change every year. Staying up to date and collecting payment is very time consuming. Therefore, physicians hire employees to perform these tasks.

National statistics reveal that medical offices hire an average of two full-time employees and one part-time employee per physician. That means about half the medical offices across the country have more employees per physician and about half have fewer employees per physician. Generally, one employee per physician provides clinical support and the rest work in the business office.

Every employee plays an important role in collecting and distributing information required for medical insurance billing. Clinical employees are held responsible for meeting some of the requirements and business employees are held responsible for meeting the remainder of the requirements for medical billing.

How well the team functions together to deliver and report patient services will be reflected in the payments received and will ultimately determine the overall success or failure of the practice. In a typical medical office, most of the payments are received from medical insurance companies and government medical plans, and just small portions of the payments are received from individual patients.

Business Office Personnel

Business office personnel run the business side of the medical practice, freeing physicians and clinical employees to provide patient care. In a large or very busy practice, multiple employees perform each business office function. However, in small single-physician practices, it is not unusual for a registered medical assistant **(RMA)** or a certified medical assistant **(CMA)** to be the only employee other than the physician. Therefore, it is important that every employee become proficient in medical business office duties. When you complete this course, you will have the educational background to fill any entry-level medical business office position.

Whether one person or many people are required to get the job done, each medical office position is very important and has unique responsibilities. Business office employees are responsible for collecting the **patient-supplied information** for the top half of the medical claim form, and they are responsible for processing the paperwork, submitting the claim, and collecting all payments due. One tiny piece of missing information can sometimes result in a payment of 30% or less of the amount rightfully earned by the physician, and sometimes no payment is received.

Many physicians sign insurance contracts that require specific actions from business office employees. Some insurance contracts specify who may treat the patient if the primary physician is unavailable; others specify time limits for scheduling patient visits and for filing claims, and some want specific language placed on the claim form. In addition, the physician usually agrees to accept a lower payment for each patient service. "Payment in full" usually becomes the payment amount listed in the contract, and it often includes the payment amount the contract states the physician may collect from the patient. Therefore "payment in full" for the same service may be different for each insurance plan. Collecting insurance information, filing claim forms, and tracking the results must be performed exactly as stated in the contract.

No matter how small or inconsequential it may seem, every piece of information that eventually flows onto the medical claim form is meaningful and every employee plays a critical role on the medical office team. Therefore it is essential that everyone learns about medical insurance and how to work together as a team.

OFFICE MANAGER

The **office manager** provides administrative oversight for the entire office. In larger practices, the title for this position might be the Practice or Group Administrator. The office manager is the supervisor for other employees in the medical practice, and he or she is the coordinator who ties together the clinical functions and the business functions so things flow smoothly. The organizational chart in Figure 2-1 shows the typical office manager's lines of authority, although it may vary from office to office.

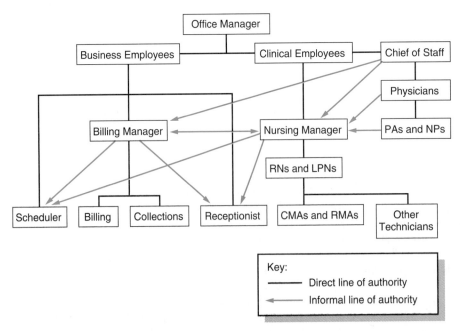

FIGURE 2-1
An organizational chart shows the official lines of authority. Medical practices differ from other businesses in that there are also informal lines of authority from physicians to employees not under their direct supervision. Physician-owners are voluntarily placed under the direct supervision of the office manager while retaining the power to hire and fire, to give directions to employees, and to make final decisions.

Office managers are responsible for employee management, business account management, insurance contract management, production management, document management, and patient account management. They do not have to personally perform each task, but they are responsible for seeing that each task is performed correctly. Only the owner(s) of a medical practice have more power, authority, and responsibility than the office manager. Let's take a closer look at each of these responsibilities.

Employee management entails recruiting, hiring, firing, orienting, training, supervising, and disciplining employees. It is the office manager's responsibility to learn the new laws, rules, and regulations that govern medical practices and to provide continuing education on these matters for the other employees.

The office manager sets an example for employees. If the office manager wears appropriate business attire, uses professional personal conduct, portrays high ethical standards, and shows that he or she values patients by treating them with the greatest respect, the other employees can be required to do the same.

The office manager is responsible for updating and enforcing the written policies and procedures of the practice. Regardless of who performs each task, the office manager is responsible for seeing that the task is performed correctly.

Business account management has four important duties:

- Payment of practice expenses (telephone, utilities, supplies, etc.)
- Payment of payroll: either by writing payroll checks and performing the payroll accounting functions or by supplying the payroll information to a designated payroll company
- Business accounting: either by performing the business accounting functions or by giving copies of the practice's income and expense records to a designated accountant
- Running productivity reports and financial reports that correlate the amount of work performed with income and expenses and that provide other important business and financial measurements. These reports are very useful when the physician sets prices or fees for services and determines which insurance contracts are profitable.

Insurance contract management includes managing existing insurance contracts and analyzing new contracts to help physicians decide which contracts to sign. Each existing contract contains information other practice employees must know. The office manager is responsible for learning the details for each contract and distributing them to employees on a need-to-know basis.

However, physicians tend to misunderstand the antitrust laws that are intended to prevent physicians from engaging in price-fixing. Under the antitrust laws, physicians are not allowed to show their insurance contracts to other physicians. As a result, many physicians lock their contracts in a file cabinet and don't share them with anyone.

Physicians are allowed to share insurance contracts with employees on a need-to-know basis. Employees must agree not to share this information with anyone else. Physicians also may share insurance contracts with accountants, consultants, and attorneys on a need-to-know basis. These professionals are obligated to keep the information confidential. They help the physician analyze contracts for profitability, for ease of meeting contract requirements, and for legal issues with insurance clauses. The office manager coordinates and distributes contracts or contract summaries as needed and meets with outside professionals who assist with contract issues.

The process of delivering medical care is considered *production*. *Productivity management* entails overseeing every practice function associated with delivering medical care. It includes many important duties:

- Scheduling patient appointments
- Coordinating procedures: making sure the necessary employees and supplies will be available
- Pulling the medical records in advance of scheduled appointments and restocking the records with any forms or blank chart notes needed
- Ordering and stocking supplies
- Greeting patients as they arrive for their appointments
- Monitoring the patient flow through the practice
- Assisting with procedures
- Reviewing any instructions with patients at checkout
- Helping patients schedule outside appointments for lab work, x-rays, specialists, etc.
- Refiling the medical records after documentation is complete

Productivity management also requires the office manager to serve as a gatekeeper for the physicians in the practice. The time each physician spends providing medical services to patients are production hours that generate revenue (income) for the practice. The time each physician spends on non–patient-care tasks does not generate revenue. Therefore the office manager oversees management of physician time by supervising the screening of telephone calls and the screening of non-patient visitors for the physicians.

Most physicians request that only telephone messages that require physician action reach them, and they often want those to be prioritized by urgency. The physician, the office manager, and the employee who takes a telephone message can all be held legally accountable to the level of their responsibility for how a telephone message is handled in a medical office. Employee responsibility for taking messages ends when the action called for by a message is completed or when responsibility for the message is turned over to the office manager. The office manager's responsibility for taking messages ends when the action called for by a message is completed or when responsibility for the message is turned over to the physician. However, many physicians appreciate follow-up reminders from the office manager until every physician-action is also completed. Documentation for some types of telephone messages should remain on file until the legal requirements for record keeping have expired. Record-keeping requirements vary from state to state, but are usually at least 7 years.

Nonpatient visitors are usually **vendors** (salesmen) for pharmaceutical companies (drug companies), software companies, medical supply companies, and office supply companies. Sometimes the office manager has the authority to make purchasing decisions. Other times the office manager filters the information so the physician can review summaries of each product and can make final decisions from a concise choice of suitable products.

Documentation management includes monitoring the quality of documentation and either appointing or personally serving as the **custodian of records** (see below). The legal requirements for medical billing are very specific, and only the level of service that is documented may be billed. Often a clinical employee is given the responsibility of monitoring the quality of documentation by checking to see if the medical record documentation for a given patient meets the legal requirements for billing each service indicated on that patient's billing documents for that visit.

The custodian of records is responsible for performing or overseeing the following duties:

❑ Maintaining the patient medical record
❑ Handling operative, procedure, lab, and x-ray reports that are delivered to the practice
❑ Handling medical records delivered to the practice from outside medical entities (hospitals, other physician offices)
❑ Determining when and how copies of medical records can be released
❑ Certifying the completeness of medical records released for legal purposes
❑ Filing loose documents after the physician is finished with them

Patient account management entails six important duties:

❑ Meeting contract requirements for patient services
❑ Obtaining authorizations when needed
❑ Preparing and filing medical insurance claims
❑ Preparing and mailing patient statements
❑ Making sure the full payment amount due has been collected from both the patient and the insurance company, as appropriate, for every patient
❑ Initiating follow-up procedures when full payment is not received

Ultimately, office managers are held accountable for how physician services are billed, regardless of who actually performs the billing task. The "Fraud and Abuse" sections in Title II of the Health Insurance Portability and Accountability Act of 1996 **(HIPAA)** state that managers and owners may be held accountable for false statements on medical claims if they *knew or should have known* that the statements were false. It is very difficult to prove that a manager or owner *should not have known* what transpired in the practice.

Depending on the seriousness of the charges, civil and/or criminal penalties may be applied. Civil penalties can include fines of up to $10,000.00 per occurrence for incorrect coding or medically unnecessary services. Criminal penalties for false statements can include imprisonment and forfeiture of property, both real estate and personal property. Fortunately, the Office of Inspector General, Department of Health and Human Services **(OIG/HHS)** representatives have publicly stated that they do not intend to target medical offices that can demonstrate an effort to comply with the laws.

There are three major professional organizations that office managers may join to enhance their skills:

Medical Group Management Association (MGMA)
Medical Office Managers Association (MOMA)
Professional Association of Health Care Office Managers (PAHCOM)

Each of these organizations can help an office manager keep up to date with current laws. Some of them offer credentials that office managers and administrators can attain. Continuing education is often required to maintain credentials and keep them current.

BILLING MANAGER

The **billing manager** provides administrative oversight for the billing department and reports directly to the office manager. The billing manager ties together the functions of billing and collections so things flow smoothly. The billing manager does not actively oversee other practice employees who collect information that is placed on the claim form, but he or she does coordinate with the other departments. The office manager mediates any disputes between the billing department and another department.

Billing managers are responsible for employee management within the billing department, and they are responsible for most aspects of patient account management. They direct both insurance and patient billing and collections. It is their responsibility to determine how to handle "problem" collections. Let's take a closer look at each of these responsibilities.

Employee management entails hiring, firing, training, supervising, and disciplining employees within the billing department. It is the billing manager's responsibility to learn the new laws, rules, and regulations that govern medical billing and collections and to provide continuing education on these matters for the other billing employees.

The billing manager is responsible for updating and enforcing the written policies and procedures for the billing department. Regardless of which billing employee performs each task, the billing manager is responsible for seeing that the task is performed correctly.

Patient account management in the billing department entails at least five important duties:

- ❑ Meeting contract requirements for billing patient services
- ❑ Preparing and filing medical insurance claims
- ❑ Preparing and mailing patient statements
- ❑ Making sure the full payment amount due has been collected from both the patient and the insurance company, as appropriate, for every patient
- ❑ Initiating follow-up procedures when full payment is not received

Obtaining required authorizations sometimes falls under the billing department and is sometimes assigned to another business office department. Converting chart information into codes for placement on the claim form is sometimes assigned to the billing office and is sometimes assigned to clinical staff members. In addition, the billing manager is usually responsible for developing a variety of routine patient letters: welcome letters, reminder letters, "no-show" letters, and collection letters.

The billing manager directs both insurance and patient billing and collections. He or she decides how to divide up the billing and collection functions between the assigned employees, and he or she determines the methods to be used for problem

collections. The billing manager enforces policies regarding when to rebill claims and when to file appeals.

The billing manager enforces policies regarding when and how often to send patient statements. Some contracts and some state laws have strict requirements regarding patient statements. When in-house collection efforts do not produce results, the billing manager determines which claims to send to a collection agency. Often physicians must give the final authorization before using a collection agency.

Ultimately, billing managers are held accountable for how physician services are billed regardless of who actually performs each billing task. The "Fraud and Abuse" sections of the HIPAA law state that managers and owners may be held accountable for false statements on medical claims if they *knew or should have known* that the statements were false. The rules and penalties are the same for all management employees.

There are six major professional organizations that billing managers may join to enhance their skills:

American Academy of Professional Coders (AAPC)
American Health Information Management Association (AHIMA)
American Medical Billing Association (AMBA)
Medical Association of Billers (MAB)
Healthcare Financial Management Association (HFMA)
American Academy of Medical Practice Analysts (AAMPA)

Each one of these organizations can help a billing manager keep up to date with current laws. Some of them offer credentials that billing managers can attain. Continuing education often is required to maintain credentials and keep them current.

SCHEDULERS

Schedulers are responsible for scheduling patient appointments. Once, this was a relatively easy task. A patient called for an appointment, and the scheduler penciled the patient's name into the first available time slot that was convenient for the patient. Payment was always a patient responsibility and the patient sought reimbursement from his or her own insurance company.

In some medical practices, especially in areas that do not have many managed care plans, appointments are still scheduled in this fashion. However, more than 80% of the patients in the United States are now covered by managed care medical insurance plans. Astonishingly, more than half these patients—and nearly as many physicians— *do not know* the medical plans are managed care

For each management position in the left column, write the letter or letters of the corresponding duties listed in the right column.

1. Office manager
   _____
   _____

2. Billing manager
   _____
   _____

A. Employee management
B. Production management
C. Patient account management
D. Insurance contract management
E. Business account management
F. Document management

Answer the following:

3. Professional organizations offer an opportunity to earn credentials, to learn about changes to laws, and to update skills.

   ____True   ____False

4. Among professional organizations, there is one clear choice for office managers and one clear choice for billing managers.

   ____True   ____False

5. Employee management includes:
   A. Hiring employees
   B. Disciplining employees
   C. Both A and B
   D. None of the above

6. Patient account management of the billing manager always includes obtaining authorizations for the services rendered.

   ____True   ____False

7. Who is the direct supervisor of the billing manager?
   A. The owner of the practice
   B. The chief of staff
   C. The office manager
   D. All of the above

8. Antitrust laws prevent:
   A. Price-fixing
   B. Sharing contracts with employees
   C. Sharing contracts with other physicians
   D. A and C, but not B

9. Productivity management includes monitoring the flow of patients through the office.

   ____True   ____False

10. Business account management includes preparing and submitting insurance claims.

    ____True   ____False

plans. All major insurance carriers, including most government carriers, now include managed care plans in the mix of medical plans offered. HMOs (health maintenance organizations) and PPOs (preferred provider organizations) are the best-known managed care plans. Chapters 8, 9, 10, and 11 cover medical insurance plans, including managed care plans, in more detail. Whether patients know they have a managed care plan or not, additional tasks must be completed at the time appointments are scheduled for these patients.

Only managed care insurance plans and government medical plans require a physician to sign a contract, and each physician is required to sign his or her own contract. Most contracts require specific actions when patients call to schedule an appointment. Therefore, schedulers today must be equipped with a list of the specific scheduling requirements for each medical plan contract and a list of each physician in the practice who is authorized to provide services under each contract. In addition, the scheduler must pay close attention to the rules for substitution coverage when the primary or authorized physician for the patient is unavailable.

The scheduler's most important responsibility is to schedule patients only with providers authorized by the patient's medical plan. The practice will not receive payment for services if an unauthorized provider sees the patient, and a provider excluded from government health plans could face fines of up to $10,000.00 per day for seeing government plan patients.

When you work as a scheduler and a patient calls for an appointment, you must first ask a number of questions to determine whether an appointment may be scheduled with the requested provider.

- ❏ You must determine whether the patient's medical plan is accepted by your practice.
- ❏ You must determine if the requested provider is authorized to provide services under the patient's medical plan.
- ❏ You must determine whether a written authorization is required, especially if you are working for a specialty practice.
- ❏ Some medical plans require you to verify patient eligibility before every appointment. Those that require continuous eligibility verification provide a system that enables you to do this quickly, while the patient is still on the phone.

Once you have determined that you can schedule an appointment for the patient with the requested physician, then you must ask the reason for the visit and determine how quickly the patient must be seen. Some medical plans have specific time requirements that must be followed, and urgent problems should always be seen as quickly as possible.

Some patients are very knowledgeable and can help determine whether a problem is urgent, but other patients are not able to help make that decision. A basic knowledge of medical terminology and a basic understanding of anatomy and physiology will make it much easier for you to become skilled at determining which problems are urgent. Some medical offices have a binder with a list of questions for each of the most common medical problems. The physician staff has approved this binder and the directions it contains. Therefore the questions you ask and the level of urgency you select is approved medical advice equivalent to passing on a message from the physician.

If you do not feel qualified to determine the urgency for a particular patient visit, ask an experienced co-worker, a member of the clinical support staff, or the office manager for help.

Most computerized schedules and most paper schedules allow space to also record the reason for the visit, a daytime telephone number, and whether the patient is new. This capability is important for numerous reasons:

❑ It enables you to determine with reasonable accuracy how much time to block off on the schedule for the visit.
❑ It enables the clinical staff to estimate the type of supplies that might be needed for the visit.
❑ If the appointment is canceled for any reason, it enables you to determine whether it is urgent to reschedule the appointment.
❑ If the patient does not show up for the scheduled appointment, it enables the clinical staff to determine whether the patient should be called.

Physicians have been found guilty of medical malpractice for failing to call patients who missed scheduled appointments *if* the seriousness of the patient's condition was such that the delay in treatment resulted in irreversible harm. Every effort you make to reschedule a canceled appointment and every effort you make to follow up if a patient does not keep a scheduled appointment *should always be documented* in the patient medical record and on the schedule if space is available. If a lawsuit were to be filed, written documentation is a better defense than memory alone.

The compliance program guidance issued by the OIG/HHS for other medical entities has stressed the importance of establishing accountability in the medical industry. In September 2000, the OIG/HHS released the final compliance guidance for solo physician offices and small group practices. All but one of the targeted items deals with accountability in the medical billing and reporting process.

Physicians must establish methods of measuring accountability for each aspect of the scheduler's job. You will be held accountable for the results of the decisions you make. Your best protection is to document thoroughly everything you do and to ask for help when necessary. Making a patient wait too long in an urgent situation can be deadly. Bringing nonurgent patients in on an urgent basis can inappropriately absorb physician time that may be needed for more urgent cases. The triage priorities (decision-making based on urgency) are:

1. Emergencies
2. Urgent problems
3. Routine visits

If you do not feel qualified to determine the urgency for a particular patient visit, ask an experienced co-worker, a member of the clinical support staff, or the office manager for help.

Public relations is another important aspect of the job for a scheduler. If your practice is to succeed, the word-of-mouth advertising must be good. Often the scheduler is the first practice employee the patient speaks with. First impressions last a long time, so telephone courtesy is extremely important. Even the most obnoxious patients must be treated with respect. Unless a patient specifically requests that you address them using a first name, always address patients formally with a title (Mr., Mrs., Miss, Ms., Dr.) and their last name. You must learn how to be firm, tactful, and polite so you don't alienate patients as you meet contract requirements and follow health care laws when scheduling appointments.

Here is an example of how to politely deal with a disgruntled patient who wants to see an unauthorized physician because his regular physician is on vacation: "Yes, Mr. Williams, I understand your frustration. I wish I could help you. Unfortunately, Dr. Anderson is on vacation for the next 2 weeks and your medical plan states that only physicians under contract with them may cover for Dr. Anderson in his absence. Dr. Wilson is not under contract with your medical plan. He is not an authorized provider. Dr. Rubin and Dr. Gomez are both authorized providers. May I schedule an appointment for you with one of them? . . . Unfortunately, your insurance will not pay for the appointment if you see Dr. Wilson; you would have to pay the entire amount yourself. . . . At least $70.00 and it could cost more if the problem is complex or if you require any tests. Would you like to do that? . . . May I give you the telephone number for your medical plan? Perhaps they can direct you to a physician you will feel more comfortable with."

Schedulers are usually given the task of calling patients with reminders the day before scheduled appointments. When a patient fails to arrive for an appointment or is very late for an appointment, there isn't time to fill the slot with another patient. Therefore, productivity and practice income go down when a patient misses a scheduled appointment. Studies have shown that "no-show" rates drop dramatically when courtesy reminder calls are given. As an added bonus, if a courtesy reminder reveals a conflict, the patient can cancel the appointment in time for the slot to be filled by another patient.

RECEPTIONISTS

The **receptionist** is the most visible employee in the practice, and patients have greater access to the receptionist than to any other member of the staff. The receptionist greets patients as they arrive and gathers or verifies the patient-supplied billing information. The receptionist evaluates this information and determines when additional forms are needed. The receptionist is the first employee in the office to visibly see the patients, and he or she must determine when a patient's condition is urgent enough to consult with the clinical staff about altering the scheduled patient-visit order. The receptionist is the first line of communication between the patients in the waiting room and the clinical staff, and he or she communicates any delays to the patients in the waiting room. The receptionist often is responsible also for answering the telephone and taking messages.

As a receptionist, you must always maintain a professional attitude and dress in a professional manner. Some patients are allergic to the scents from make-up and perfume, so keep make-up and perfume to a professional minimum. Jewelry can carry germs from the medical office to your home, so also minimize jewelry. Public relations are a very important aspect of the medical receptionist position. It is imperative to treat patients with respect, to make them feel important, and to keep them informed, even when they are unreasonable or have unrealistic expectations. As a receptionist, you usually will be the first to hear complaints. Your reaction and responsiveness to complaints will play a large role in customer satisfaction. When a patient is unhappy with the check-in experience or the experience in the waiting room, it will taint the remainder of the patient visit. On the other hand, when a patient's expectations have been met, the rest of the visit will be set up for success.

The largest portion of income in medical offices today is collected from insurance companies. When you work as a receptionist, collecting and verifying the accuracy of patient-supplied billing information is your largest contribution toward the overall success of the practice. If the patient-supplied billing information is not correct, the practice will lose money: either the practice won't receive full payment or an employee will have to be paid for the time it takes to correct the information, or both.

You must verify that the patient is the same person as is listed on the insurance card and that the patient's eligibility for the medical insurance plan has not lapsed. The best way to document this is to make a photocopy of both sides of the insurance card and to make a photocopy of a picture identification (ID) card from the patient, such as a driver's license or an official state ID. If the photocopy is not clearly legible, handwrite the information on the photocopy near the illegible item. The patient may not use a "street" name when seeking medical care. The patient must use his or her legal name because every private and every government medical plan tracks patient eligibility and health information using legal names. The name, and the spelling of the name, *as it is listed on the insurance card,* is how the patient's name should be entered into the computer system and on the medical record. The name on an insurance claim must always match both the medical record and the insurance company's records, or the claim could be denied.

As lack of insurance has become more widespread, there has been an increasing problem with patients trying to "borrow" an insurance card from a friend or relative when they need medical care. This is insurance fraud, and it gives the insured person a record of medical problems he or she doesn't really have. Therefore some medical plans have developed instant eligibility-verification programs that must be documented at the time of the visit. Some require you to swipe a card through a scanner for telephone verification just like a credit card transaction, and others have computer programs that perform this function. Most plans, however, do not yet require instant eligibility verification, and a photocopy of the insurance card and the patient ID is sufficient.

Next, you must verify that any authorizations required by the medical plan are on file, and you must verify that any patient-specific additional forms are completed.

- ❏ A *Consent to Treatment* form must be signed by each patient and must be placed in the patient's file before the doctor sees the patient.
- ❏ A *Release of Information* form and an *Assignment of Benefits* form must be signed by

the patient and placed in the patient's file if a medical plan is going to be billed. Some medical plans want only one copy of these forms on file; others want a new, dated copy for each visit.

❏ If a patient is scheduled for a service or procedure that is not covered by the patient's health plan, he or she must sign a waiver form acknowledging that:
   1. It is not a covered service and
   2. He or she will accept responsibility for payment.

❏ Some procedures also require a treatment-specific consent form.

❏ Additionally, most medical offices require patients to fill out a medical history form or to update their medical history form at check-in.

You will learn about these forms in more detail in Chapter 3. Many practices ask new patients to arrive 30 minutes before the scheduled appointment time and they ask established patients to arrive 15 minutes before the scheduled appointment time to allow adequate time to complete the check-in procedures.

Security within the physician's office should prevent a patient or a visitor from even seeing the name of another patient.

Once check-in is complete, you will notify the clinical staff that the patient has arrived. If a patient is in obvious distress, immediately ask the clinical staff to evaluate the situation—do not wait for check-in to be complete. Unlike many places of business, medical offices do not operate on a first-come, first-served basis. Scheduled appointment times are honored as much as possible, but higher levels of medical urgency sometimes take priority. Check-in procedures can be completed during checkout if medical urgency does not allow them to be completed before the appointment.

If a patient does not arrive for an appointment, you will make a notation on the schedule and inform both the clinical staff and the person assigned to follow up on **"no-shows."** It is also important to document in the patient's medical record the date and that the patient did not show up. Sometimes this becomes a very important factor when litigation (a legal action such as a lawsuit) arises at a later time.

Taking and relaying telephone messages in a medical office can literally involve life and death situations, and therefore it carries many legal responsibilities. The practice procedure manual will dictate the method to follow for your practice. Most physicians request that only the telephone messages that require physician action reach them, and they often want those to be prioritized by urgency. Most offices require all messages to be given to the office manager for assignment of action. As a receptionist,

your responsibility ends when the message is turned over to the office manager unless the office manager assigns you to carry out an action. Then it ends when both the action and any required documentation are complete.

When you take a message, you also sign or initial the message slip. Messages related to patient care and messages related to medications should not be discarded, even after the required action is complete. After action is complete, the message is filed in the patient medical record with a notation of the date and time of the call, a notation of action taken, and a signature from the person who performed the action. The physician is responsible for initialing the notation to document his or her knowledge of the action taken.

The compliance program guidance issued by the OIG/HHS for other medical entities has stressed the importance of establishing accountability in the medical industry. In September 2000, the OIG/HHS released the final compliance guidance for solo physician offices and small group practices. All but one of the items targeted deals with accountability in the medical billing and reporting process. Physicians must establish methods of measuring accountability for each aspect of the receptionist's job. You will be held accountable for the results of the decisions you make. Your best protection is to thoroughly document everything you do and to ask for help from either the clinical staff or the office manager when necessary. Always date and either sign or initial your documentation.

BILLERS, CODERS, COLLECTORS

The employees in the billing department fill out medical claim forms and submit them to medical insurance plans (Figure 2-2). The employees in the collections department receive and record payments from patients and insurance plans, and they handle any patient billing after the insurance payment has been received.

Medical coding before billing may or may not occur in the billing department. Certified coders are qualified to convert chart information into codes so physicians do not have to learn all the coding rules. Assigning responsibility for medical coding when a certified coder is not on staff is an individual practice decision. Most often physicians accept this responsibility, but sometimes the medical coding responsibility is assigned to clinical employees (e.g., medical assistants or nurses) or to billing employees.

Unless a certified professional coder has chosen the codes, you can be held accountable for the codes you place on a claim form and submit to a medical

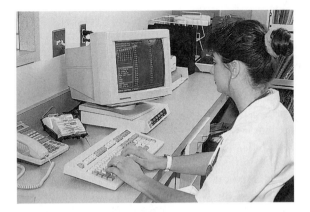

FIGURE 2-2
Before completing a claim form, the biller must verify the accuracy of insurance information entered into the computer. (From Chester G: Modern Medical Assisting. Philadelphia, WB Saunders, 1998, p. 85.)

plan. Therefore if you work in the billing department for a practice that does not employ certified coders, you will want to understand at least the basics for medical coding as presented in Chapters 5, 6, and 7 of this book.

Medicare first announced in September 1999, and has frequently reiterated since then, that "soon" they will require **certified coding professionals** to code all medical services billed to Medicare. At that time, there was a ratio of about one certified coding professional for every 100 physicians in the United States. Since then, the number of certified coders has grown tremendously, but there are still not enough certified coders available to meet the need when certification becomes a Medicare requirement, and many practices have not been able to hire certified coders. You might want to consider taking an additional medical coding course so you may take a certification exam.

The federal government holds **medical billers** responsible for double-checking the accuracy of billing information that is placed on medical claim forms. In Chapter 4, you will learn how to fill out a medical claim form. When you work as a *biller,* you must:

❑ Review the patient-supplied information to be sure it was entered correctly. The simple misspelling of a name or transposition of the numbers in an address or policy number makes the claim inaccurate and can cause the claim to be rejected.

❑ Verify that the signatures on the "Release of Information" and "Assignment of Benefits" forms are indeed on file as required.

❑ Verify that the physician-supplied information placed on the claim matches the documentation

in the patient record. It is not wise to file a claim based on the superbill alone. The medical codes placed on the claim form for diagnoses and for physician services must accurately portray the services documented in the patient medical record. *If they do not match, and you submit a claim knowing they do not match, you can be held accountable under the "Fraud and Abuse" sections of the HIPAA law.*

❑ You may not change or add to information in the patient medical record, but you may bring a discrepancy to the attention of the physician. Only the physician may amend the patient record or amend the superbill. See Chapter 14 for guidelines to follow when a physician refuses to comply with health care laws.

❑ Verify that contract requirements for billing have been met. Some contracts place time limits for submitting claims and for appealing claims. Most contracts require national standard billing rules and coding conventions and require the use of medical codes from current year codebooks. Often, contracts allow for steep penalties when these requirements are not met. See Chapter 14 for more details about insurance contracts.

As a **collections employee,** you are responsible for making a serious effort to collect the money due the physician. You will learn how to perform these tasks in Chapters 3, 13, and 14.

❑ At the time of the patient visit, you are responsible for collecting the copayment or the deductible amount due from the patient unless the patient has a secondary medical plan that covers this expense.

❑ When the practice receives payment from the insurance company, it is your responsibility to compare the payment received with the fee schedule for the contract.

❑ If full payment was not received, it is your responsibility to find out why and correct the problem. Sometimes insurance companies reduce payment by applying monetary penalties for even small errors. If further money is due from the insurance company, it is your responsibility to either re-bill or appeal using a corrected claim within the allowed time limits. Do not write off penalty amounts as uncollectable if you can correct the claim and collect an additional amount from the medical plan. Do not write off contractual discounts as uncollectable if a second medical plan may be billed for these amounts.

❑ Post each payment received.

❑ When applicable, bill the secondary insurance for the balance.

❑ After all insurance payments are received, and any remaining insurance discount is written off, you bill the patient for any remaining patient-responsibility amount. Always document your collection efforts in the patient's financial record—not the medical record.

As a collections employee, you must review the patient billing provisions of the contract with the insurance company to see whether you may balance-bill the patient. Most managed care plans and Medicare allow the physician to collect only the copayment, coinsurance, and/or deductible amount from the patient. There are a few exceptions for noncovered services, and special rules apply in those instances. All other remaining amounts represent either a penalty or an agreed-upon discount. *You may not bill patients for penalties or for agreed-upon discounts, but you may bill an additional medical plan, when available.*

❑ When payment is not received, you will use an "aging report" to identify which patients and which medical plans you will call and ask for payment. Try to collect the largest dollar amounts and the oldest claims first. See Chapter 13 for additional details about using aging reports.

❑ After a serious effort to collect payment has taken place and is documented, the physician may choose to write off a bad debt or to send the debt to a collection agency. Be careful not to send balances that represent contracted discounts or penalties to a collection agency. It is fraudulent to try to collect money not legally owed.

The federal government holds collections employees responsible for knowing collections laws and contract provisions. Both overbilling and underbilling patients can violate the law. Medicare requires patients to pay their portion of the bill. If you do not attempt to collect from the patient, Medicare can claim that they were illegally billed for 100% of the bill. You will not be found guilty if you can prove that you tried to collect from the patient but were unsuccessful.

Some medical plan contracts are misleading in their wording. The "allowed" amount in an insurance contract usually represents total payment for a service, but physicians commonly think it represents only the medical plan's share of the bill. When Medicare splits the fee for most services, the patient pays 20% of the Medicare-allowed amount and Medicare pays 80% of the Medicare-allowed amount. The allowed amount adds the medical plan's portion and the patient's portion to arrive at the total payment. You cannot legally accept a Medicare fee that is higher than the lowest fee you accept from anyone else (except Medicaid) for the same service. By law, the Medicare fee must be your lowest fee (except Medicaid). Therefore if your practice accepts a total payment for any service in an amount lower than the total amount the practice accepts from Medicare (except Medicaid) for the same service, it is a violation of federal law.

This sometimes happens when a physician who accepts Medicare also signs a contract with a medical plan whose allowed amount is 80% of the Medicare-allowed amount. The physician remembers that Medicare pays 80% of the Medicare-allowed amount, but he or she forgets about the 20% the patient pays. The physician thinks he or she is signing a contract identical to Medicare, when in fact the contract is an agreement to accept a total payment that is 20% less than Medicare's total payment. Please don't allow this to happen in your practice.

The HIPAA law states that anyone who knowingly submits a claim with inaccurate information can be personally fined up to $10,000.00 for each occurrence. Incorrect coding and billing for services that are not medically necessary fall under the civil penalties section of this law. No intent to defraud is required. False statements relating to health care matters, obstruction of investigation, and theft and embezzlement fall under the criminal offense section of the law. Criminal offenses are subject to fines, imprisonment, and forfeiture of property, both real estate and personal. Congress funded enforcement of this law, and the Federal Bureau of Investigation **(FBI)** has steadily worked in conjunction with the OIG/HHS to train field investigators. Several hundred investigators are already at work diligently investigating complaints.

Do not submit claims containing information you know to be either inaccurate or false! Do not balance-bill patients in violation of contract provisions, but be sure to collect all copayments and deductibles due from the patient!

If you obtain coding credentials, you will be required to either obtain continuing education units (CEUs) or to retest periodically to keep the credentials. The AAPC and AHIMA offer coding credentials and provide educational opportunities to maintain certifications. Sometimes local chapters also are available to help meet educational needs and to provide an opportunity to network with other medical coders.

The MAB offers a credential for certification as a medical billing specialist (CMBS). AMBA offers certification as a medical reimbursement specialist (CMRS).

MEDICAL RECORDS EMPLOYEES

It is the responsibility of **medical records employees** to safeguard the security of patient medical records and to maintain confidentiality (Figure 2-3). Unauthorized people must not be given access to private medical records. Security and confidentiality within the physician's office should prevent a patient or a visitor from even seeing the name of another patient. Even personnel within the medical office should see patient information only on a "need-to-know" basis.

As a medical records employee, you will pull patient charts before the patients arrive for their appointments and file them again after the patient visit. You will also file test results and other loose documents after the physician has seen them. You must be very careful and double-check each loose document to be sure it is placed in the correct chart.

You will be responsible for knowing medical insurance contract requirements and legal requirements pertaining to privacy and confidentiality of the medical record before supplying information to insurance companies. You must not supply any information without a written "release of records" signed by the patient. This release is usually obtained during patient registration or check-in, but a photocopy of a patient-signed release supplied by the insurance company also is acceptable. Each signed release pertains only to the medical plan listed with the release signature. When insurance information changes, new releases must be signed. You must verify that the release on file is valid for the medical plan requesting a record.

The final rule of the Privacy Act, which became mandatory in April 2003, includes a provision that states that a copy of the records for a patient visit may be released for payment purposes without a patient's consent. It was intended to apply only to insurance companies, but the wording is broad enough to include both credit card companies (when the patient uses a credit card to pay a medical bill) and banks that provide loans for medical care. It is usually better to get the patient's consent before releasing records than to be placed in the position of testing the wording of a new law.

You may or may not be appointed as the custodian of records. In many practices, the office manager accepts these responsibilities if the medical records employees are not credentialed. Therefore the duties of the custodian of records are listed with the duties of the office manager.

Accountability for security of patient information and accountability for timely physician notification of test results and faxes relating to specific patients are important aspects of a medical records position. As a medical records employee, you will be responsible for receiving and distributing faxes and test results. Faxes must be sorted by priority and distributed in a timely fashion. When a fax has more than one page, paper clip or staple the pages together so they do not become separated. Test results should be sorted by priority, keeping results for a given patient together with any abnormal results on top. They also must be distributed in a timely fashion. Faxes relating to patients and patient test results should be paper-clipped to the front of the patient record before being given to the physician for review.

The physician should "date and sign" or "date and initial" test results and faxes to indicate that they have been reviewed, and the physician will provide any further instructions relating to either the fax or the test results. Once the physician has initialed faxes and test results, he or she becomes accountable for knowing the information. A signature stamp may be used to clarify the identity for initials or a signature, but it may not be used to replace initials or a signature. Once the related instructions have been completed, the test results or fax should be filed in the patient's medical record, and the record will then be re-filed.

"Security Standards for Health Information" were included in the "Administrative Simplification" section of the HIPAA law. The final rule was released

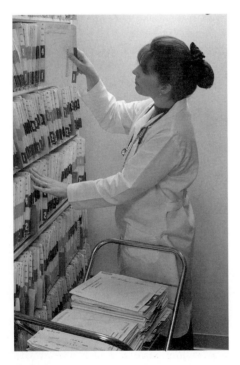

FIGURE 2-3
A medical records employee pulls charts before patients arrive for appointments.

in May 2003 with mandatory compliance in April 2005 for most health care entities (April 2006 for small health plans). The Security Standards Act governs the security of electronic records. It only applies when computers are used to store or transmit individually identifiable patient information. It clarifies boundaries for the use of patient information, including acts that constitute misuse of patient information. It details security requirements designed to protect patients from wrongful disclosure of individually identifiable health information while allowing for public access to health information in specific situations. It clarifies when individuals may have access to their own health information, and it amends the penalties when health information is mishandled or misused. Health care providers, health plans, health care employees, and clearinghouses are now subject to civil and criminal penalties (up to $25,000.00/year and 10 years in jail) for violations of the new law.

The final rule of the privacy law includes a requirement for confidentiality agreements with business associates (e.g., attorneys, accountants, consultants) who see individually identifiable health information in the course of conducting business. The final rule broadened the scope of the law as it was originally proposed to include all paper copies of medical records and spoken conversations about confidential health information. Clarifications of the final rule on privacy have been released periodically, so it is important to follow legislation and stay up to date. The websites for the Department of Health and Human Services (HHS) (www.dhhs.gov) and the Centers for Medicare and Medicaid Services (CMS) (www.cms.gov) have links that you may click on to view recent health care legislation.

AHIMA offers the credentials of registered record administrator (RRA) and accredited record technician (ART). Credentialed records employees may interpret and analyze patient data, and they may code diagnoses and review records for completeness and accuracy. To apply for these credentials, you must meet specific levels of college education in health information administration or technology, and there are continuing education requirements to maintain the credentials. AHIMA has state chapters to help their members stay up to date with new laws and regulations.

MEDICAL ASSISTANTS

CMAs and RMAs have the education required to fill every business office position. In a small office, a medical assistant might be the only employee other than the physician. Even in a large office, duties often overlap, and many times employees are cross-trained for numerous business office positions. As a new graduate, your duties might include those of a scheduler, a receptionist, a biller, a collector, or a medical records clerk. With experience, you could also become a billing manager or an office manager. You will be held accountable and must meet the responsibilities for every business office duty and every clinical duty you personally perform. When you hold a management position, you are also responsible for every duty performed by anyone under your direct supervision.

There are two major professional organizations for medical assistants:

- ❏ American Association of Medical Assistants
- ❏ American Medical Technologists

Legal Issues in the Business Office

Some insurance companies offer liability insurance to medical office employees to cover errors and omissions. If you are covered under your employer's liability plan, there is no need to purchase a private policy unless you also work in a setting that is not covered by the liability plan. If you are not covered by your employer's liability plan, consider purchasing your own policy. This insurance is designed to pay for your defense and to cover fines for unintentional errors and omissions.

Many physicians do not agree with current health care laws, and there are still a few who honestly believe they do not have to comply with the laws. However, Congress funded enforcement of HIPAA, and failure to follow it can be a serious mistake.

Errors-and-omissions insurance does not cover any action you know is improper and perform anyway, even if you are directed to do so by your employer.

You can be held accountable for every duty you perform. *Do not knowingly participate in anything improper.* Develop a plan of action to follow in case you are ever directed by an employer to do something improper, regardless of whether you believe it to be an intentional violation of a law.

If you suspect something improper is occurring, it will be important for you to document your efforts to correct the situation. Be sure to document any verbal instruction you were given and to keep a copy of any written instructions. You do not have to keep this documentation at work, but you should keep a record somewhere. Many people keep a private journal at home. Be careful not to violate the security and privacy rules. Do not include information that could identify a specific patient in a journal kept away from work.

If an official investigation reveals a problem, you will want to be able to prove what you knew, when you knew it, and what efforts you made to correct the situation. Your private documentation could be needed for your personal defense. Most

investigations cover a time span of up to 7 years, depending on state and federal laws. You can be held accountable for your actions during the time of your employment, even if you no longer work there. You will have a stronger defense if your personal records are available to support your memory of events. Keep your documentation for a minimum of 7 years after an event occurs. See Chapter 14 for additional information.

STOP & REVIEW

Match the employee positions in the right column to the duties in the left column.

1. Scheduler_____ A. Bills patients and receives all payments
2. Receptionist_____ B. Bills insurance company
3. Biller_____ C. Gives appointments to patients
4. Coder_____ D. Collects or verifies insurance plan information
5. Collector_____ E. Maintains and safeguards patient records
6. Medical records employee _____ F. Converts chart information into medical codes

Answer the following:

7. Which of the following tasks does a scheduler perform?
   A. Determines if the patient's medical plan is accepted by the practice

B. Determines if the requested physician is an authorized provider
C. Determines if any authorizations are required
D. All of the above
E. None of the above

8. Who is responsible for knowing collections laws?
   A. Schedulers
   B. Collections employees
   C. Medical records employees
   D. Receptionists

9. Who files test results and other loose documents after the physician has seen them?
   A. Schedulers
   B. Collections employees
   C. Medical records employees
   D. Receptionists

10. Who gets the "Consent to Treatment" form signed?
    A. Schedulers
    B. Collections employees
    C. Medical records employees
    D. Receptionists

Clinical Staff

The **clinical staff** in a medical office is the production team. They work together to provide and document medical care. They work directly with patients, and they carry out the primary mission of the medical business.

The production team includes:

- ❑ All fully licensed physicians and **limited-license** providers who provide medical services
- ❑ All registered and licensed nurses who provide nursing services
- ❑ All registered and certified technologists and therapists who provide ancillary medical services

- ❑ All registered or certified medical assistants who provide clinical services

The production team is responsible for:

- ❑ Diagnosing and treating medical conditions in patients
- ❑ Documenting each service rendered in the patient's medical record
- ❑ Collecting the **provider-supplied information** for the medical claim form

The provider-supplied information must accurately portray what occurred during the visit, and it must match the documentation in the medical record.

PHYSICIANS

The term **physician** usually includes all professionals who are fully licensed to practice medicine: medical doctors **(MDs),** doctors of osteopathy **(DOs),** doctors of chiropractic medicine **(DCs),** and all types of medical specialists and subspecialists who have first met the requirements as MDs, DOs, or DCs. Licensure requirements vary by state, and each physician must be licensed by the state in order to provide medical services in that state. Not all naturopaths and acupuncturists meet the requirements to become fully licensed to practice medicine, and instead they often obtain limited licenses. Every state requires physicians to meet continuing medical education (CME) requirements in order to maintain licensure.

A person who has earned an advanced college degree at the doctoral level, a PhD, is addressed with the title of "doctor." A PhD degree alone is not enough to enable a person to become fully licensed to practice medicine, and a person with a PhD in a nonmedical field cannot obtain even a limited license to practice medicine. To illustrate this difference: a psychiatrist is first fully licensed as an MD before specializing in the field of psychiatry, but a psychologist, with a PhD degree in psychology, may only obtain a limited license to practice medicine. Although both the psychiatrist and psychologist are commonly called "doctor," the **scope of practice** allowed by their licenses (the number and type of services they may legally provide), the **credentialing** requirements, and the billing requirements are different for each.

Managed care plans and government medical plans require physicians to meet specific credentialing requirements, such as proof of current state medical licensure and proof of any applicable board certifications for a specialty, before the physician is authorized to provide medical care to patients on the plan. This is a legal requirement that medical plans must meet if they want to exercise any control in determining what providers a patient may see. In addition, the physician's credentialing information must be updated periodically to enable the medical plan to verify that the physician's CME requirements have been met and that his or her state medical license remains current.

The physician's primary responsibility in the medical practice is diagnosing and treating the medical conditions of his or her patients. The physician's work can be performed in numerous locations: a private medical office, a hospital, a surgical center, an outpatient clinic, or a nursing home, just to name a few. All physician services, regardless of where they are performed, are normally billed by the physician's own billing personnel in his or her primary office.

Most medical services provided by a fully licensed physician are billable *if* the services are adequately documented in the patient medical record and *if* medical necessity requirements have been met. The documentation for each service must be detailed enough and legible enough to stand alone to meet billing requirements and to show that the service was indeed provided exactly as billed.

Documentation does not have to be in the physician's own handwriting. Notes can be dictated and typed later, someone else can write notes for the physician during the visit, or notes can be entered into a computer program. All notes, whether or not they are in the physician's own handwriting, must be dated and signed by the physician. A *secure* electronic signature is sometimes acceptable, but other types of signature stamps may not be used to replace a qualified signature. Documentation requirements for physician services are covered in more detail in Chapter 6.

Physicians are often in the unusual position of being both owners and production employees of the medical practice. As owners, they have the authority to hire and fire employees, including the office manager, and owners are ultimately held accountable for everything that occurs in the medical practice. Yet physicians seldom spend much time in an administrative capacity. Most of their time is spent as production employees, who come under the authority of the office manager. It may be tricky to balance these sometimes conflicting duties and responsibilities.

HIPAA holds the owners of a medical practice to the same standards as the managers. They must stay informed about administrative matters. In addition, physicians are held accountable for how they document services. If the superbill shows a physician is instructing billing employees to bill in a manner that is not consistent with current laws, the physician can be held personally accountable.

The first law to require specific documentation elements for specific services has been in effect only since 1995. Many physicians disagreed with the law and thought they could get it repealed through legal challenges. At the same time, Congress did not provide funding for enforcement of that law, so physicians across the nation did not personally face legal challenges about quality of documentation.

Therefore HIPAA was designed to strengthen documentation laws, and Congress provided adequate funding for enforcement. New documentation standards were released in 1996 to be effective in 1997. Physicians united and complained so loudly that the 1997 standards almost immediately began to undergo revision. Until new standards become effective, physicians are legally allowed to meet either the 1995 standards or the 1997 standards for documentation. Many physicians did not learn the 1995 standards, and they mistakenly believe they can continue to document as they did in 1995 until the next standard is released. Unfortunately, ignorance of the law is no excuse, and physicians across the nation are now personally facing legal challenges about the quality of their documentation. Some physicians already have been sentenced to prison.

If you work for a physician who does not seem to understand current billing laws, please make every effort to educate him or her gently and respectfully. Design or purchase standardized forms to make it easier for the physicians in your practice to meet current laws. Chapter 3 of this book will introduce you to forms that have been proven to be useful in helping physicians meet documentation and billing requirements. Chapter 6 explains the documentation requirements physicians must meet, and Chapter 14 discusses other methods to help noncompliant physicians become compliant. The case studies in Appendix C also use forms that have been proven effective.

In addition, physicians have always been held accountable for the outcomes of their treatments. Employees often influence the timeliness and quality of treatment. You can be held accountable for your level of involvement in each situation. The law in many states requires a physician to purchase medical malpractice insurance.

ANCILLARY PROVIDERS

Psychologists, licensed clinical social workers **(LCSWs)**, nurse practitioners **(NPs)**, midwives, and physician's assistants **(PAs)** are **ancillary medical providers.** They provide less complex medical services than physicians and are considered limited-license medical professionals. Licensure requirements vary by state, as does the scope of services each is authorized to provide. Limited-license medical professionals must meet the same documentation requirements as physicians, but the billing and credentialing requirements are not the same. All ancillary providers must meet continuing education requirements to maintain licensure.

Credentialing requirements and billing requirements vary by medical plan. Some medical plans will not pay for the services of limited-license professionals unless they are each individually credentialed with the medical plan. Others will pay for their services without credentialing as long as a fully licensed physician is on the premises and actively providing oversight. The scope of services allowed, the amount of payment received, and the method for billing services all vary depending on whether the limited-license professional is individually credentialed. Since 1999, Medicare has required individual credentialing for all PAs and NPs, but Medicare does not stipulate credentialing requirements for other limited-license medical professionals.

When the limited-license professional *is not* individually credentialed, their services are all considered to be an extension of the physician's services. Sometimes they are called physician extenders. The physician must be on the premises when care is rendered. Limited-license medical professional services are limited to providing uncomplicated follow-up care for patients first seen by the physician. They may not see new patients, and they may not treat new problems for established patients. The physician must cosign and date every entry in the medical record. An actual physician signature is required; a signature stamp alone is not enough. The services are billed in the physician's name and full payment is received as though the physician had provided the care.

When limited-license medical professionals are credentialed with the medical plan, they are allowed to see both new and established patients. The physician does not have to be on the premises when they render care. They are given much more autonomy and can provide a wider range of services. Services are billed in their own name, but payment is usually less (typically 15% to 20% less) than payment for the same services provided by the physician.

Once a limited-license professional is credentialed with a medical plan, all their services for patients in that plan must be billed as a credentialed provider. They have more autonomy and more flexibility, but all their services are reimbursed at the lower rate.

Physical therapists **(PTs)**, occupational therapists **(OTs)**, and speech therapists **(STs)** are ancillary providers also. They too are limited-license health care providers; the scope of their license is limited to one specialty, and they do not have the autonomy to order services. A therapist cannot provide services without a medical order written by someone licensed to provide medical care. Credentialed limited-license medical professionals often have this authority as well as physicians.

Billing for therapists varies depending on the ownership of the practice. When therapists own their own practices, the billing rules are similar to those for a credentialed limited-license professional. When therapists are employed by a physician's office, therapy services are considered an extension of the physician's services, so billing rules are similar to those for an uncredentialed limited-license professional. Therapy assistants are not licensed, and their services are considered to be an extension of the services provided by the therapist. Their services are billed as though the therapist provided the care.

All ancillary providers are production employees. They must meet the same documentation requirements as physicians, and they are held to the same levels of accountability for the care they render. The medical malpractice risks are less than physicians only because they provide less complex services. The HIPAA law applies to ancillary providers in much the same way as it applies to physicians, and those who hold an ownership interest in a medical practice are held accountable to the same standards as managers.

STOP & REVIEW

Answer the following:

1. Physicians are fully licensed to render medical care.

____True ____False

2. PAs and NPs are fully licensed to provide medical care.

____True ____False

3. Credentialing influences the type of care that a provider may render, but it does not affect reimbursement.

____True ____False

4. Billing for therapists is the same regardless of where they work or ownership of the practice.

____True ____False

5. Physician oversight is required for:
A. Credentialed PAs and credentialed NPs
B. Uncredentialed PAs and uncredentialed NPs
C. Credentialed PAs and uncredentialed NPs
D. Uncredentialed PAs and credentialed NPs

6. *Scope of practice* means:
A. The location of the practice
B. The number of patients
C. The number and type of services a provider may legally perform
D. All of the above

7. The physician's primary responsibility in the medical practice is diagnosing and treating the medical conditions of his or her patients.

____True ____False

8. Documentation must be in the physician's own handwriting.

____True ____False

9. A speech therapist cannot provide services without a medical order written by someone licensed to provide medical care.

____True ____False

10. Limited-license medical providers provide less complex medical services than physicians.

____True ____False

CLINICAL SUPPORT STAFF

The **clinical support staff** includes technologists, nurses, and medical assistants (MAs). Each nurse must be registered or licensed with the state, but an MA may or may not hold a certification because many states do not require them to be certified. In a medical office setting, clinical support services are considered to be an extension of the physician and are not billed separately. Licensed nurses (**RNs** and **LPNs**) and registered technicians are required to obtain continuing education units to maintain their credentials.

Technologists perform diagnostic tests within the scope of their credentials (Figure 2-4). A technologist usually is either registered or certified to perform specific tests. A registered technologist outranks a certified technologist. Medical offices most commonly employ x-ray technologists, ultrasound technologists, respiratory therapists, phlebotomists, and EKG technicians.

The nursing staff includes RNs, LPNs, CMAs, and RMAs. An RN outranks an LPN, and an LPN outranks a CMA or RMA in the line of authority within the nursing staff. However, when an RMA or CMA works in the *business office*, he or she is not part of the *clinical* staff and does not fall under RNs and LPNs in the line of authority.

Regardless of the credential held, the office manager is always at the top of the line of authority in a medical office. RNs, LPNs, CMAs, RMAs, certified coders, and billing office employees are all eligible to be appointed as office manager. See Figure 2-1 for the lines of authority.

Nursing staff employees often are required to perform technologist duties to expand the range of services available in a practice without hiring additional employees. Certification as a technician is

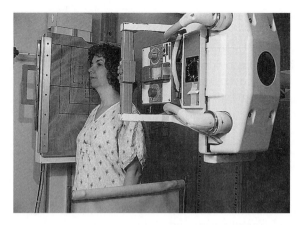

FIGURE 2-4
Technologists perform the technical component of certain procedures such as x-rays. (From Chester G: Modern Medical Assisting. Philadelphia, WB Saunders, 1998, p. 658.)

not needed when the skills required fall within the scope of your current licensure or certification, but it is wise to obtain technician credentials if the skills required would otherwise fall outside your legal scope of practice.

RNs and LPNs must be licensed by the state to provide nursing services in that state. The duties of licensed nurses in a medical office can vary widely. Sometimes they perform and document an initial physical assessment before the physician sees the patient. Often they review the plan of care with the patient at the conclusion of the office visit. Many times they draw blood for lab work, obtain cultures, administer injections, run blood pressure clinics or pacemaker clinics, and screen patient phone calls to handle as much of the workload as possible without interrupting the physician. They often call patients with lab results after the physician has seen the reports.

Registered nurses may administer controlled drugs (narcotics and medications regulated by the government), administer chemotherapy (potent drugs used to treat cancer), and administer medications directly into the bloodstream. RNs may also perform a wide variety of high-tech outpatient services, such as fetal monitoring, renal dialysis monitoring, stress test monitoring, and more. In some states, both RNs and LPNs may insert a needle into a vein and administer intravenous (IV) fluids; in other states, only an RN may perform this task. LPNs may administer some controlled drugs and may perform less complex high-tech services.

Nursing employees are often given the responsibility for triaging patients and messages (sorting them in order of urgency or importance). Although patients are seen most often by the scheduled-visit order, urgent medical conditions always take priority. Nursing employees work with schedulers to determine scheduling priority for urgent problems, and they work with receptionists to determine when a patient's condition is urgent enough to take priority over the scheduled-visit order. Nursing employees also triage messages from patients. Licensed nurses often perform a telephone assessment for urgent problems before either relaying the message to the physician or asking the patient to come in for a visit on an urgent basis.

CMAs and RMAs are very similar. Both are voluntary national credentials that are obtained by passing a certification exam. CMA is awarded by the American Association of Medical Assistants. RMA is awarded by the American Medical Technologists.

Education for either can vary from 6 months to 2 years. Most often, medical assistants have about the same number of hours of instruction as an LPN, but the focus of education differs. LPN education is strictly clinical and encompasses both inpatient and outpatient nursing care, whereas medical assistant education is geared solely toward the outpatient medical office and encompasses both clinical and administrative duties. A medical assistant may not perform any service that requires a nursing license. Most states allow CMAs and RMAs to administer some medications, and some states allow them to administer controlled drugs, but they are not usually allowed to administer intravenous fluids.

When you work as a CMA or RMA in the clinical setting, you may draw blood, give some types of injections, perform some types of tests (such as EKGs and simple x-rays, depending on state law and level of education), and assist with medical office procedures (Figure 2-5). You may record vital signs and record the patient's chief complaint, but you may not perform and document an initial physical assessment. Your notes should always be initialed or signed by you. If the physician initials your notes, your documentation of vital signs and chief complaint can be considered a part of the physician's note for documentation and billing purposes. Documentation guidelines state that in order to count an item as part of his or her notes, the physician must either rewrite the information or initial the item to prove it was considered during the encounter.

Although the entire clinical team plays a role in the collection of provider-supplied billing information, it is usually up to the clinical support employees to monitor the process and to verify that documentation does indeed match the items listed on the superbill. Clinical support employees have greater access to both the physicians and the patient's medical record than billing employees, and clinical support employees already go over chart documentation with the patient as part of their normal and routine duties at the conclusion of a patient visit. It makes sense for them to also verify that diagnoses listed on the superbill are indeed documented in the patient record, and to verify that documentation rules were met for the services listed on the superbill. Chapter 6 covers the rules for medical record documentation.

Clinical support employees also are in the best position to detect when provided services have not been included on the superbill. It is very difficult to reconstruct a patient visit at a later date in order to discover lost revenue from items or services that inadvertently were not billed or to correct documentation that was inadvertently placed on a superbill, but not entered into the patient's medical record.

As a clinical support employee, you are held accountable for every duty you perform. You are accountable under the HIPAA law for the security and confidentiality of patient information as well as for your role in the documentation of patient services and in the collection of billing information. You are also held accountable for the performance of your clinical duties according to the scope of your license or certification.

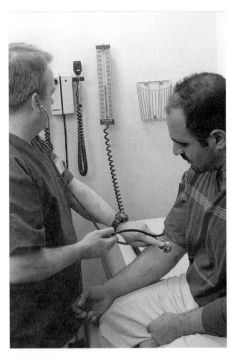

FIGURE 2-5
A medical assistant taking vital signs.

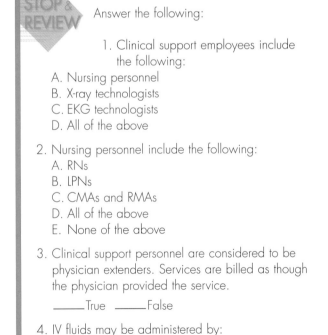

STOP & REVIEW   Answer the following:

1. Clinical support employees include the following:
   A. Nursing personnel
   B. X-ray technologists
   C. EKG technologists
   D. All of the above

2. Nursing personnel include the following:
   A. RNs
   B. LPNs
   C. CMAs and RMAs
   D. All of the above
   E. None of the above

3. Clinical support personnel are considered to be physician extenders. Services are billed as though the physician provided the service.

   _____ True _____ False

4. IV fluids may be administered by:
   A. RNs
   B. LPNs
   C. CMAs and RMAs
   D. All of the above
   E. RNs and LPNs, but not CMAs and RMAs
   F. None of the above

5. Which of the following technologists might be employed in a medical office?
   A. X-ray technologists   C. EKG technologists
   B. Ultrasound technologists   D. All of the above

6. Which clinical support employee may perform high-tech services such as monitoring renal dialysis or fetal monitoring?
   A. RMA   C. Respiratory therapist
   B. CMA   D. RN

7. Which employee(s) can be appointed as office manager?
   A. RMA   D. RN
   B. CMA   E. All of the above
   C. LPN

8. An RMA and a CMA may draw blood.

   _____ True _____ False

9. An office manager is in the middle of the line of authority.

   _____ True _____ False

10. Patients are always seen in the exact order of the scheduled visits.

    _____ True _____ False

Chapter Review

The employees of a medical office form a cohesive team. Every member performs an important function, and every member plays a role in the reimbursement process. HIPAA holds each medical office employee legally accountable for the duties he or she personally performs, and it holds managers and owners accountable for everything that occurs.

Every employee has an obligation to help keep practice expenses down and to reduce legal liability by performing his or her duties correctly and in accordance with the laws every time. When things are done correctly on a consistent basis, fewer penalties will be imposed by medical insurance plans. Full payment is more likely to be received in a timely fashion. Although providing medical care is the mission of the practice, collecting payment and achieving profitability is the ultimate goal of the practice. Legal reimbursement that was actually received is the determining factor when measuring practice success.

Answer the following:

1. What law holds medical office employees accountable for their actions?

2. Which employee position is responsible for collecting and verifying patient-supplied billing information?

3. Which employee position is responsible for matching patients with authorized providers under the patient's medical insurance plan?

4. Which employee position is responsible for safeguarding the patient's medical record?

5. Which management position has authority over both the clinical and business office employees?

6. Which employee position is responsible for submitting medical claim forms to insurance companies?

7. Which employee position is responsible for determining if the medical insurance plan paid the correct amount? _____

8. Which employees collect the provider-supplied billing information? _____

9. Who is held accountable for the medical service documentation quality in the patient medical record?

10. Which employee is responsible for coordinating billing and collection efforts?

11. The office manager is responsible for which of the following?
    A. Business account management
    B. Contract management
    C. Patient account management
    D. All of the above

12. The billing manager is responsible for which of the following?
    A. Business account management
    B. Contract management
    C. Patient account management
    D. All of the above

13. The scheduler should also record the reason for the visit.
    ____True   ____False

14. Which employee does the patient speak to first?
    A. Receptionist
    B. Billing manager
    C. Scheduler
    D. Office manager

15. Which employee does the patient see first?
    A. Office manager
    B. Receptionist
    C. Scheduler
    D. Billing manager

16. The "Release of Records" form signed during check-in allows the medical records employee to release records to the insurance company.
    ____True   ____False

17. Medical assistants may work in either the clinical side or the business office side of the medical practice.
    ____True   ____False

18. A psychologist is a fully licensed physician.
    ____True   ____False

19. All limited-license providers must be credentialed.
    ____True   ____False

20. Certification as a technologist is not needed when the skills required fall within the scope of your current licensure or certification.
    ____True   ____False

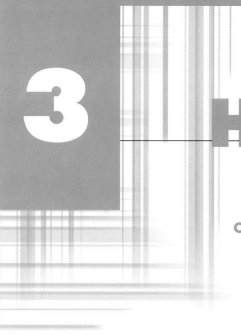

3

HOW THE MEDICAL CLAIM CYCLE WORKS

Objectives After completing this chapter, you should be able to:

- ■ Briefly explain the purpose of a medical claim
- ■ Relate what happens to claims when they reach the insurance company
- ■ Briefly explain how to complete the claim cycle after payment is received
- ■ Demonstrate how to gather the information for a medical claim
- ■ Explain how to streamline the claim cycle by using forms that collect the correct information
- ■ Demonstrate the effect on reimbursement, on practice expenses, and on profit when claims are penalized or rejected because of incorrect information

Key Terms

ABN Advance Beneficiary Notice; a Medicare waiver that notifies the patient that Medicare might not pay for a service, either because it is a noncovered service or because medical necessity, as defined by Medicare, might not be met, even though the physician believes the service is medically necessary. The patient may then choose to pay for the service if Medicare does not or may choose to decline the service. This form must be signed by the patient before the service is provided, or you cannot bill the patient if Medicare does not pay.

appeal a formal request submitted to an insurance plan to have a payment decision changed or a penalty reversed.

assignment of benefits instructs the insurance company to send payment directly to the medical practice or provider. (The patient will pay copayments and deductibles at the time of service.)

balance billing billing the patient for the balance remaining after the insurance payment has been posted.

billing address the mailing address for the patient or the mailing address for the payor.

birthday rule when a dependent child is covered by insurance plans from both parents' employers, the policy for the parent whose birthday falls earliest in the calendar year is the primary payor and is billed first.

claim audits check for duplication of services or billing that is in excess of normal.

claim edits check for completeness and accuracy of claim form.

clean claim a claim that passes payor claim edits and claim audits.

demographics statistics about a person or a population, such as name, age, gender, race, address, zip code, telephone number, and area code.

duplicate claim resubmission of an identical claim—mirror image—with no changes. Also called double billing; duplicate claims are considered fraud.

E/M evaluation and management; the process of evaluating a patient for suspected, known, or potential problems or conditions; assessing the findings; rendering an opinion; and developing and initiating a plan of action.

encounter form a fee ticket or superbill that ties reimbursement to specific encounters for line item billing.

EOB explanation of benefits; a notification of the payor's decision regarding a claim, accompanied by payment when payment is due.

EOMB explanation of Medicare benefits; a notice sent from Medicare to a beneficiary informing the beneficiary of Medicare's payment decisions and bills paid or not paid for the beneficiary.

fee ticket a record of the day's charges for a patient.

financial class a person's income or ability to pay a debt.

financial record documentation of a patient's financial transactions, i.e., billing and collections.

living will a legal document that communicates a patient's decision regarding life support measures in the event the patient is unconscious or otherwise unable to make that decision.

medical record documentation of a patient's medical visits and care rendered.

MRN Medicare remittance notice; also called remittance advice (RA); this notice is sent from Medicare to the physician (or other medical provider) giving notification of Medicare's payment decision regarding a claim, accompanied by payment when payment is due.

new patient a patient who is new to the practice or who has not been seen by a physician in the practice (or the specialty in a multi-specialty group) within the past 3 years.

patient financial responsibility the portion of the bill that the patient legally is required to pay.

payor the insurance company responsible for paying the medical claim.

penalized claim a claim that did not pass the payor's claim edits or claim audits and a penalty was applied, reducing the payment.

physical address the actual location of a building or the actual location where a person lives—not a post office box.

primary payor the insurance company that legally should be billed first when more than one insurance company can be billed.

profit the money remaining from a payment after all expenses for the service, including employee expenses, have been paid.

rebill the process of resubmitting a corrected claim.

rejected claim a claim that did not pass payor claim edits and claim audits, and no payment was sent.

release of information the patient authorizes the medical practice to send specific records, such as billing information, to a payor or to a specific person or place.

repeat claims corrected claims that have been resubmitted with information that has changed; not the same as duplicate claims.

secondary payor the insurance company that legally should be billed second for any remaining unpaid bills after the primary payor has sent payment.

superbill a tool to report chart documentation for billing purposes; part of the financial record.

unprocessable claim a claim that could not be processed by a payor because of missing key information.

write-off a discount the physician has given a patient or has authorized in a payor contract.

Introduction

The purpose of this chapter is to give you (1) an overview of how the claim cycle works, (2) an awareness of the unnecessary expense that occurs when a claim is not completed correctly the first time, and (3) the tools to gather correct information from patients and physicians for medical claims. You will need this basic understanding of the medical claim process as a foundation to build on throughout the rest of the book when you learn about claim preparation, basic billing, coding and documentation rules, types of medical insurance plans, payor-specific billing requirements, and strategies for reimbursement success, as well as what to do when things go wrong.

Medical documentation requirements have become very specific in recent years. Many physicians are struggling to meet the new, complex requirements. Insurance companies now want to know the thought processes physicians use to reach medical decisions. Therefore, much of the physician work that traditionally has been cognitive now must be documented in patient **medical records.** Well-designed forms and documents can assist physicians in meeting these complex requirements while helping you gather the correct information for billing physician services.

When the requirements are all met and the claim form is prepared correctly the first time, full payment can be received quickly. The costs for billing medical services are kept as small as possible. However, any time a reduced payment or no payment is received, the cost for billing the service rises dramatically. These extra costs reduce the **profit** for the service. Profit is the money remaining after all the expenses, including employee expenses, have been paid.

In this chapter, the lifecycle of the claim is an overview to introduce you to the claim cycle process. Each of the items is explained in more detail as the book progresses. Because the government hires private insurance companies to process government medical claims, and because the claim process is similar for both private and government medical claims, the term *insurance* in this section shall refer to both private and government medical plans. Let's take a look at the medical claim cycle from beginning to end.

Lifecycle of a Medical Claim

The potential for a medical claim begins when a person first enrolls in a medical plan (private or government). That potential increases when the person, now called a patient, calls to schedule a medical appointment. The collection of data for a medical claim begins at this time. The scheduler collects and documents insurance information in order to arrange the appointment with an authorized provider under contract with the patient's medical plan and to determine if any other requirements must be met.

The most important aspects of the medical claim cycle occur between the time the patient arrives for the appointment and the time the medical claim first arrives at the insurance company. This is such a small part of the lifecycle of a claim, as you can see from Figure 3-1, yet it determines whether correct reimbursement is received in a timely manner.

On the day of the appointment, the receptionist greets the patient and collects or verifies the patient-supplied medical billing information during patient check-in. The receptionist is held accountable for identifying all possible **payors** (insurance companies). This is done using registration forms to question the patient. The receptionist makes sure current copies of the insurance card(s) and a copy of a valid patient ID card are on file, and the receptionist obtains or verifies the signatures for the **"Release of Information"** and **"Assignment of Benefits."** The release of information allows the medical practice to send billing information to the insurance company. The assignment of benefits allows the insurance company to send payment directly to the medical practice, and the patient only pays deductible and copayment amounts at the time of the appointment. Medical claims cannot be filed

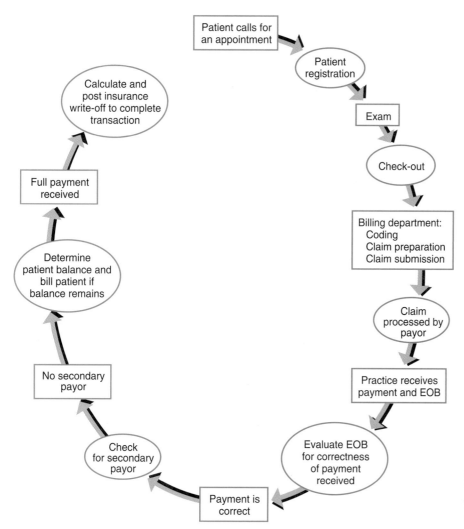

FIGURE 3-1
The lifecycle of a clean claim for a patient with one insurance plan.

without this critical information. The scheduling and patient check-in processes are described in more detail later in this chapter.

During the appointment, in addition to providing medical care, the authorized physician is responsible for (1) documenting the details of the encounter in the patient's medical record in a manner that meets legal requirements, and (2) approving the billing instructions that will be given to the billing department. Chapters 5, 6, and 7 cover the basic requirements for converting the physician's written documentation of this visit into codes that are placed first on the **superbill** (billing instructions) and then on the medical claim form. Gathering physician-supplied information is discussed in more detail later in this chapter.

At the end of the appointment, clinical support personnel (e.g., nurse or medical assistant) review the physician's instructions with the patient and they review the billing instructions. The business-office checkout personnel (often another duty of the receptionist) schedule a follow-up appointment, if needed, and verify that the patient's financial responsibility for the appointment has been met or appropriate payment arrangements have been made.

The billing department is then given the insurance billing instructions. Billing and coding personnel verify the patient-supplied and the physician-supplied billing information as they prepare the medical insurance claim. *The quality and accuracy of billing information and clinical documentation, as it flows through each department and is entered on the claim form, has the single greatest impact on the profit margin for the claim.*

The **primary payor** is the medical plan that is billed first when more than one medical plan can be billed, and the **secondary payor** is the medical plan that is billed for any remaining unpaid bills after the primary payor has sent payment.

For example: When a patient has both Medicaid and Medicare, Medicare is the primary payor because Medicaid is always the secondary payor when there are two payors. The patient's bill is sent to Medicare first. After payment is received from Medicare, the patient's bill and a copy of Medicare's payment documents are sent to Medicaid.

The biller is held accountable for determining which payor is primary. Failure to identify the correct primary payor is considered a violation of most payor contracts or agreements and is a serious breach of trust. Primary and secondary payors and payor-specific billing requirements are discussed in more detail in Chapters 8, 9, 10, and 11.

When complete, the medical claim is submitted to the payor either electronically or by mail. In Chapter 4, you will learn how to complete and submit a medical claim, and you will learn the requirements for both paper claims and electronic claims.

Payment is received a little faster with electronic submission of claims, and electronic submission eliminates the potential for data entry errors when the claim reaches the payor. However, each payor must receive electronic data in a slightly different manner to meet the requirements for payor-specific software programs. In most states, Medicare has free software you may use to send claims directly to them.

In addition, there are national claims clearinghouses that translate claim information into the format desired by the major payors for every state, and there are regional claims clearinghouses that specialize in translating claims for the majority of the payors in a particular region. You do not have to be a large practice to use a claims clearinghouse.

When an electronic medical claim is sent through a claims clearinghouse, the clearinghouse puts the claim through a series of edits before sending the claim to the payor. The edits check to see whether basic information required by the specific payor for each claim is present on the claim form. If the claim is rejected by the clearinghouse and is sent back to the medical practice, an opportunity exists to correct the claim *before* it reaches the payor. *Once the claim reaches the payor, a record of the transaction is established by the payor, and the stage is set for the remainder of the claim cycle.*

When a claim first reaches the insurance company, it is automatically subjected to a series of **claim edits** and **claim audits** established by the medical plan. Claim edits verify the completeness and accuracy of information entered on the claim form. Claim audits check for duplication of services or billing that is in "excess of normal." Excess billing could be indicated by a higher level of visit than normal for the given diagnosis, more visits than normal for the diagnosis, or a more complex procedure than normal for the diagnosis.

For example: When a patient has a simple sore throat, it normally does not take an hour for the physician to examine the patient and make the diagnosis of tonsillitis. Tonsillitis does not normally require complex diagnostic testing as does cardiac catheterization, nor does it normally require multiple follow-up visits. Claim audits detect such inconsistencies.

Chapters 5 through 14 include additional information about payor edits, payor audits, and other payor requirements. When the claim passes all of the payor edits and audits, it is called a **clean claim.** The payment amount is determined, and payment is sent to the provider, either electronically or by mail.

When the correct payment amount is received from the payor, a collections employee posts the payment by recording it in the patient ledger. If secondary insurance is responsible for an additional amount or if the patient has an outstanding balance for their portion, the account for this transaction (claim) remains open, and bills are sent out to the secondary payor, or to the patient if there is no secondary payor. When these payments are received, they are posted. As soon as no further payment is expected, the insurance **write-off** (discount), if any, is calculated and posted, and the account for this claim is closed. See Chapter 13 for detailed information on posting payments and calculating insurance write-offs.

A record of the transaction remains on file for the time specified in the payor contract or the time specified in state or federal laws, whichever is longer. The longest period is usually 7 years, so most practices choose to keep all their records for at least 7 years.

> *Note:* Some organizations are lobbying to have the laws changed so medical records are kept for the life of the patient or seven years, whichever is longer.

When the claim does *not* pass all of the edits and audits, it is not a clean claim. Then, one of two events is likely to occur: either (1) the claim is rejected and no payment is sent or (2) the claim is processed and penalties are applied, reducing the amount of payment that is sent.

An "Explanation of Benefits" **(EOB)** is sent either electronically or by mail to the physician for every claim received by the medical plan (payor). Medicare calls this form "Medicare Remittance Notice" **(MRN)** and sends the patient an explanation of Medicare benefits **(EOMB).** Payment is enclosed with the EOB or MRN when payment is authorized. The remarks on the EOB are the first indication of whether follow-up procedures are required for the claim. EOBs and payor remarks are discussed in detail in Chapter 13.

A pending claim is an outstanding claim that the payor has received, but for which the payor has not yet made a payment decision. An EOB indicates the results of a payment decision. When an EOB arrives and shows that no payment is received or when only partial payment is received, a collections employee posts the payment, but the account for the transaction remains open for further action. In most cases, the next action is to correct the claim information and either **rebill** the claim or file an **appeal.**

Rejected claims are **"unprocessable"** claims, and no payment is received. The EOB usually indicates incomplete data or incorrect data, such as "unable to identify the patient as an authorized recipient." These claims may be corrected and rebilled within time limits established by the payor contract. Most payors allow corrected claims to be submitted either electronically or on paper. However, if a claim is re-sent with no changes, it is flagged as a "mirror image" **duplicate claim** and, once again, no payment is received. Duplicate claims are, in effect, double-billing, and trying to collect twice on the same claim is considered fraud.

Penalized claims must be corrected and the payment decision must be appealed. Partial payment is usually received with these claims, though occasionally a penalized claim will receive zero payment, and the provider may even owe money due to a penalty. Appeals obtain better results when they are submitted by mail with supporting documentation. Chapter 13 covers the requirements for rebilling and filing appeals for corrected claims.

When the corrected claim is received by the payor, whether rebilled or appealed, the claim is immediately flagged for closer scrutiny. Even if the claim is now "clean" and can pass the payor's standard claim edits and claim audits, claim adjusters are seldom authorized to make payment decisions on **repeat claims;** instead, the claim is sent to the review department.

Most payor contracts have many loopholes (legal or not) that state the payor may deny or reduce payment for a wide variety of reasons. A claim review employee closely scrutinizes the claim, and every box on the claim form represents a potential reason to deny or reduce payment. Payor contract provisions often give the payor complete control and authority over claim review. The provider too often agrees in the contract to abide by the payor's decision with no requirement that the decision meet current standards of medical practice and no requirement that the decision be fair. See Chapter 14 for more information on payor contracts.

Claim review is normally performed by hand—it is not automated or computerized—and repeat claims are not subject to the payment time limits that apply to initial claims. The review process and payment decision for a repeat claim can take anywhere from 6 weeks to 6 months. Most of that time the claim just sits in a "claim review" inbox, waiting to be processed. Contested claims often must go through this process at least twice before other alternatives, such as arbitration, are available.

Once every effort has been made to collect payment from the primary medical plan, and no further payment is expected, the secondary medical plan, if any, is billed. A copy of the payment documents (EOB or MRN) received from the primary payor must accompany secondary claims. Medicare sometimes, but not always, automatically forwards the claim and the payment documents to Medigap payors that are registered in the Medicare system. See Chapter 10 for more information about Medicare billing considerations.

> In special cases the secondary medical plan may be billed without first going through the rebilling or appeal process. For example: A hearing aid might be clearly excluded from coverage with the primary plan and covered by the secondary plan only when the primary plan's denial is in writing. The primary medical plan is billed to obtain an intentional denial. The secondary insurance can then be billed immediately after receiving the written denial.

After all insurance payments are received, collections employees check to see if the patient is responsible for any of the remaining balance. More than 80% of all medical care is now subject to managed care rules and contract provisions. Most managed care contracts do not allow a provider to bill patients for anything except a deductible or copayment amount, and many specifically stipulate that penalty amounts are not a patient responsibility. Usually services that are deemed as "noncovered" services may only be billed to the patient if the patient signs a specific "NonCovered Service Payment Agreement" (Advance Beneficiary Notice [ABN] or waiver) *before* the service is rendered. ABNs and waivers are discussed later in this chapter, and examples are given at that time.

When all expected payments from all sources have been received, remaining balances are typically written off and the account for the transaction (claim) is closed. A record of the transaction remains on file for the time specified in the payor contract or the time specified in state or federal laws, whichever is longer. See Chapters 13 and 14 for more detailed information on the portion of the claim cycle that occurs after the primary payor receives the initial claim and makes a payment decision.

STOP & REVIEW

Please answer the following questions:

1. Which employee is usually the first to collect information for the claim form?

   _____

2. Which employee is responsible for identifying all possible payors? _____

   _____

3. What is a payor? _____

4. Which employee is responsible for identifying the primary payor? _____

   _____

5. Which employee is responsible for determining if full payment was received? _____

6. What is an EOB? _____

   _____

7. When are claim edits and claim audits performed?

   _____

Match the item in column A with the correct action in column B.

COLUMN A	COLUMN B
8. Clearinghouse edit	A. Checks claims for completeness and accuracy after claims reach payor
9. Claim edit	B. Checks for double claims and for services that are in "excess of normal"
10. Claim audit	C. Checks claims for completeness and accuracy before claims reach payor

---

Gathering Patient-Supplied Information

Gathering patient information for the medical claim is only a small step in the lifecycle of a claim, but it is vital, and it influences whether correct reimbursement is received in a timely manner.

Accuracy is extremely important when filing medical claims. The legal consequences for carelessness can be devastating. Therefore a system of checks and balances is built into medical office procedures. The scheduler gathers medical insurance information when the appointment is scheduled. The receptionist verifies the medical insurance information and gathers proof that the information is correct.

The physician documents medical care and approves billing instructions. The clinical support employees check to be sure the billing information includes everything, and they check the documentation to see if it matches the billing information. When clinical support employees, such as nurses or medical assistants, find an error, they bring it to the physician's attention and get it corrected immediately, before the patient leaves the office.

Then the billers and coders check the same information for accuracy one last time before completing and submitting the medical claim form. This system is designed to enable the highest level of accuracy when medical claims are filed.

The downfall of the system is that it can and often does lead to complacency. Employees don't check the data as closely as they should because they know someone else will be checking it again later. They adopt the attitude, "I really don't have time for this. If there's a mistake, the biller will find it when she verifies the information before sending out the claim." Meanwhile, the biller decides, "This information has already been checked and double-checked. I trust the other employees. They wouldn't send me information that is not accurate." Many errors slip through the system undetected, and reduced payments are mistakenly blamed on managed care rather than employee error.

Since the passage of the Health Insurance Portability and Accountability Act of 1996 (HIPAA), medical employees can no longer afford the luxury of complacency. Personal accountability for medical office employees will become mandatory when HIPAA is fully implemented. The wheels are already in motion. The final version of the "Guidance" for solo practitioners and small group practices was released in September 2000. These regulations are already in effect. You may check the status of compliance guidance for other medical entities at the website for the Office of Inspector General, Department of Health and Human Services (OIG/HHS): http://oig.hhs.gov/.

When you follow the correct procedures and check or recheck billing information for accuracy every time you should, you will establish a pattern of behavior. If the OIG/HHS receives a complaint that leads them to investigate your work, they will find you have a history of accuracy. Their stated intention is to only go after those with a history of carelessness and inaccuracy. What pattern of behavior do you want the OIG/HHS or the Federal Bureau of Investigation (FBI) to find when they arrive on your doorstep?

If your practice is computerized, each employee who enters patient information must take the time to learn what happens to the information after it is entered into the computer. Which computer screen documents information about the primary payor? Which computer screen documents information about the secondary payor? What steps are required to switch the information if the payors are accidentally entered into the computer system in the wrong order? Which computer screen documents the patient's **physical address,** and which one documents the mailing address? Which patient-address screen is used for the address that will appear on the medical claim form? What computer screen is used to document the payor's authorization number? Will the computer automatically enter this information on the claim form?

Every computer program is different, and most of them do not have help screens that tell employees "information entered here will appear in block No. 5 on the claim form." You must take the time to learn this information for yourself, and you cannot establish a record of accuracy until you do. Take a blank Centers for Medicare and Medicaid Services (CMS)-1500 claim form and identify which computer screen supplies the information for each block on the claim form. Write it down on the claim form in each block. This is your cheat sheet; don't lose it. When something is entered incorrectly on a claim form, you will know where to go in the computer system to fix the problem. Taking the time to create a claim form cheat sheet will make your job easier and greatly reduce frustration.

Sometimes it takes a few days to figure out a computer system, but once you learn how to use the management software system, a computer is very efficient. Most computer systems save patient information. You don't have to type in information that has been saved, but it is wise to review the patient address, employment, and insurance information with the patient on every visit.

SCHEDULING

The scheduler does much more than just schedule appointments. In Chapter 2 you learned that the scheduler determines whether the patient's problem is urgent or routine. The scheduler determines which physicians the patient may choose to see according to insurance plan requirements. The scheduler checks for payor-specific scheduling requirements, such as preauthorizations or time-limit requirements.

The scheduler also preregisters patients. Preregistration includes obtaining or verifying patient demographic information (address, birth date, gender, marital status, etc.) and insurance billing information (Figure 3-2). The scheduler also discusses **patient financial responsibility** (the portion of the bill due

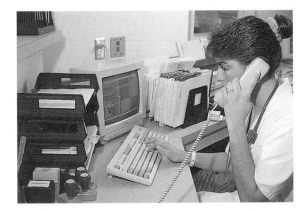

FIGURE 3-2
In booking telephone appointments, the scheduler enters insurance and demographic information into the computer system. (From Chester G: Modern Medical Assisting. Philadelphia, WB Saunders, 1998, p. 90.)

from the patient) and determines the patient's **financial class** (ability to pay).

The scheduler is the first person to gather billing information for the medical claim, and the scheduler is accountable for knowing what information to gather. When a practice is not computerized, the scheduler uses paper worksheets to schedule appointments and to record billing information. When a practice is computerized, the scheduler is accountable for knowing where each piece of information should be entered and where the computer places the information in other documents.

PATIENT CHECK-IN

The security and confidentiality of health information provisions in HIPAA mean that many medical practices must change their procedures at the registration desk. It is a breach of the Privacy Act of 2001 for a patient or visitor to see or hear any "protected health information" that could be used to identify an individual patient. Traditional check-in procedures, with sign-in sheets that also update billing information, no longer meet legal requirements. Doors and windows between employee work areas and the waiting room must remain closed to limit the potential for eavesdropping (Figure 3-3). Patient charts and computer screens must be handled in a manner that prevents patients and vendors from viewing protected health information.

Figure 3-4 is an example of a patient check-in form that meets the Privacy Act requirements and at the same time meets many of the billing requirements. The date of service is noted on the first line. The provider is identified. The patient is identified. The reason for the visit is identified. A signature is

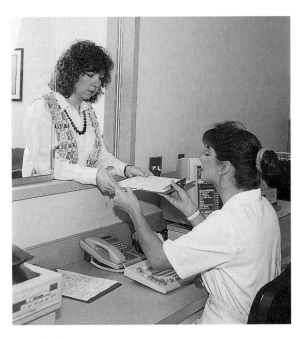

FIGURE 3-3
During check-in, the patient comes to the office window in the waiting room. The window is only open wide enough to accomplish the check-in procedure, and then it is closed again to maintain privacy. (From Chester G: Modern Medical Assisting. Philadelphia, WB Saunders, 1998, p. 67.)

obtained from either the patient or the guarantor giving written proof that the patient was indeed in the office on the specified date.

The length of time since the last visit reminds the physician that a greater level of documentation is required for payment purposes anytime it has been 3 years or more since the patient's last visit.

This form also provides a method to verify current insurance coverage, and it identifies the person responsible for charges if the insurance information is not valid. Patients are prompted give the receptionist their insurance card if their coverage has changed.

Stacks of blank forms can be left at the front desk. As patients arrive for their appointments, they sign in by completing a form and handing it to the receptionist. The receptionist attaches the check-in form to the superbill, and it becomes a part of the patient's **financial record.** The financial record is kept separate from the medical record. Insurance companies and attorneys do not usually need to see this information, but if it is included in the medical records, they will have access to it.

PATIENT REGISTRATION

New patients must also complete a full-page registration form and a patient history form. These

```
┌─────────────────────────────────────────────────────────┐
│  Patient Check-in Form        Date _____        │
│                                                           │
│  Provider:   __ Dr. Wilson   __ Dr. Anderson   __ Dr. Rubin   __ Dr. Gomez │
│              __ PA James   __ NP Lewis                     │
│                                                           │
│  Have you been seen in this office in the last three years?  __ Yes __ No │
│                                                           │
│  Patient Name: _____  │
│                                                           │
│  Reason for this visit: _____ │
│                                                           │
│  _____  │
│                                                           │
│  Insurance Plan Name: _____  │
│                                                           │
│  Is this a new insurance plan since your last visit?  __ Yes __ No │
│  If yes please provide a copy of your new insurance card.  │
│                                                           │
│  Guarantor Signature _____  │
│                                                           │
│              **Lake Eola Family Practice**                │
└─────────────────────────────────────────────────────────┘
```

FIGURE 3-4
A patient check-in form that meets Privacy Act standards while also confirming current insurance information. (Courtesy Medical Compliance Management, Inc., Orlando, Fla.)

forms establish the patient's identity and past medical history; they become a part of the patient's medical record. Copies of the registration form also are placed in the patient's financial record. Because few patients pay in full for medical care at the time of service, the registration form also serves as a credit application. By law, a credit application cannot ask for medical history. That is why medical history is on a separate sheet of paper. It should never appear on the same page as the registration form.

Many practices ask their patients to complete a new registration form once each calendar year. This is because insurance policies generally have to be renewed annually, and patients often change policies at that time. It also updates the patient's **demographics** and employment information. In the event a patient moves before meeting his or her financial responsibility, the information from the registration form enables collections employees to find the patient for billing purposes.

Patients are responsible for supplying the billing information for the top half of the claim form. The "Patient Registration Form" (Figure 3-5) is completed by the patient or the responsible party/guarantor. It serves as a written record that can be used to hold the patient or guarantor accountable for the information supplied, and it allows the practice to collect payment from the patient or the guarantor if the information is incorrect. Please refer to each section of Figure 3-5 as it is discussed in the following paragraphs.

A *new patient* is defined as one who is new to the practice (or new to the specialty in a multi-specialty group), or a patient who has not been seen by a physician in the practice (or specialty in a multi-specialty group) within the last 3 years. The documentation requirements are greater for new patients, and the fee for the visit is higher.

When a new patient has seen the physician in another location, such as the emergency room, the patient is new to the office (registration forms and history forms must be filled out), but the patient is not new to the physician for billing purposes. On the other hand, a patient who last saw the physician 3½ years ago probably would not consider himself or herself to be a new patient—the patient is not new to the office, but the patient is considered a new patient for billing purposes. Therefore the registration form in Figure 3-5 does not ask if the patient is a new patient. Instead, it asks the question in a way that allows medical office employees to determine whether the patient is "new" or "established" for billing and documentation purposes.

Living wills are legal documents that communicate a patient's decision regarding life-support measures in the event the patient is unconscious or otherwise unable to make that decision. Many patients want control of the decision about life-saving measures, so they sign documents listing their decisions while they are well. If the patient indicates that he or she has a living will, the medical office must ask for a copy to keep in the patient's medical records. Emergencies occur suddenly and unexpectedly. Families become flustered and often cannot locate important documents. Without a copy of the living will on file, the physician will not know the patient's decision in time to write orders that accurately reflect that decision.

The remaining questions in the top section of the registration form in Figure 3-5 identify the patient demographics (statistics) required for the medical claim form and/or required for patient collection procedures. Every question must be answered as completely as possible.

Lake Eola Family Practice   517860 South Pioneer Drive, Orlando, FL 32897 • 634-555-4893

Patient Registration Form

Have you been seen in this office in the past 3 years? __ **Yes**   __ **No** Do you have a living will? _____

Today's Date _____ Home Phone _____ Work Phone _____

Patient Name (Last name, First name, Middle initial) _____

Street Address _____ City _____ State _____ Zip _____

Date of Birth _____ Age _____ Gender: __Female __ Male Social Security # _____

Marital Status: __ Married __ Single __ Widowed __ Divorced __ Other   Driver's License # _____

Is the patient a student? __ Full Time __ Part Time __ No   Is the patient employed? __ Full time __ Part Time __ No

Patient's Employer Name & Address _____

School Name & Address _____

Emergency Contact Person _____ Relationship _____ Phone _____

Referring Physician Name & Phone Number _____

Insurance Plan and Responsible Party Information

Insurance Company Name _____ Address _____

City _____ State _____ Zip _____ Phone _____

Policy # _____ Group # _____ ID # _____

Policy Holder's Name _____ Address _____

City _____ State _____ Zip _____ Phone _____

Policy Holder's Date Of Birth _____ Social Security # _____ Driver License # _____

Gender: __ Male __ Female   Relationship to patient: __ Self __ Spouse __ Parent __ Guardian __ Other

Policy Holder's Employer's Name _____ Address _____

City _____ State _____ Zip _____ Phone _____

Secondary Insurance Company Name _____ Address _____

City _____ State _____ Zip _____ Phone _____

Secondary Policy # _____ Group # _____ ID # _____

Secondary Policy Holder's Name _____ Address _____

City _____ State _____ Zip _____ Phone _____

Secondary Policy Holder's Date Of Birth _____ Social Security # _____ Driver License # _____

Gender: __ Male __ Female   Relationship to patient: __ Self __ Spouse __ Parent __ Guardian __ Other

Secondary Policy Holder's Employer's Name _____ Address _____

City _____ State _____ Zip _____ Phone _____

Authorizations

It is customary to pay for all services on the date rendered unless other arrangements were made before your appointment. The patient and the guarantor are responsible for all deductibles and copays at the time of the visit and any other fees in accordance with insurance contracts. The patient and guarantor are responsible for all elective or noncovered services and any services that are not considered medically necessary.

Financially responsible person if patient is student or unemployed _____ Phone _____

I authorize the release of any medical information necessary to process this claim and I request that payment of medical benefits be made directly to Lake Eola Family Practice. I hereby acknowledge that I am fully responsible for payment as listed above.

Signed _____ Date _____ Time _____

FIGURE 3-5

Patient registration form. (Courtesy Medical Compliance Management, Inc., Orlando, Fla.)

- The patient address must be the actual physical address where the patient lives, not a P.O. box. In the event of an emergency, the practice cannot send an ambulance to a P.O. box.
- The patient may give two addresses if the **billing address** is different from the physical address, such as when the patient uses a P.O. box for mail.
- Even though many insurance ID cards do not use Social Security numbers in the patient ID section, the Social Security number is used to identify the patient to the insurance company if any of the insurance information, such as the insurance ID number or the spelling of the patient's name, is accidentally listed incorrectly. Unless the patient pays in full for each service on the day of the appointment, you must obtain the patient's Social Security number.
- Many credit card companies offer check-guarantee services to medical practices that collect money directly from patients. Check-guarantee companies (companies that guarantee payment on bounced checks) and collection agencies both require a driver's license number.

Each insurance section question must be answered as completely as possible. Medicare, Medicaid, worker's compensation, and other government medical plans are to be listed as insurance plans.

Patients who have more than one insurance plan usually list them on the registration form by premium price or by level of coverage. Patients generally do not know the laws regarding insurance billing, and it is acceptable for the patient to list them in any order on the registration form. However, there are specific laws regarding which insurance plan pays first when there is more than one plan. It is up to the medical office employees to determine which plan is the primary payor (the company that pays first) in each situation and to list the payors in the correct order in the computer system and on medical claim forms.

When a child is covered as a dependent under insurance plans from both parents, the **birthday rule** determines which plan is primary. The policy for the parent whose birthday falls earliest in the calendar year is the primary payor. For example: When the mother has a birthday on June 15, and the father has a birthday on August 10, the mother's birthday is earliest in the calendar year. In this example, the mother's insurance plan would be the primary payor for the children. Chapters 8, 9, 10, and 11 cover additional rules for primary payor/secondary payor between specific types of medical plans.

The bottom section on the registration form in Figure 3-5 covers patient payment responsibilities and provides a patient or responsible party signature for "Release of Records" and "Assignment of Benefits." At one time, it was customary for the wording in the financial responsibility section to state that the patient was responsible for all charges not paid by the insurance. The wording in the document in Figure 3-5 has been updated to reflect the wording now required by managed care contracts. If the patient gives false insurance information, all the services are "noncovered" services, and the patient or responsible party acknowledges in writing that he or she will pay for all noncovered services.

If your practice is computerized, the receptionist is accountable for knowing what information to collect, where each piece of information should be entered, and where the computer places the information in other documents.

Some medical practices want to save on paper by entering the registration information directly into the computer. There are two major concerns when direct entry is the only method for obtaining registration information.

- First, most practices do not offer enough privacy at the check-in counter. Other patients could inadvertently eavesdrop on the answers, creating a privacy violation.
- Second, the patient cannot be held accountable for the information, and an important part of the system of checks and balances is eliminated. Because there is no hardcopy to use as the authority when verifying the data entered, the practice has no method to prove whether inaccuracies are due to employee data-entry errors or to false information supplied by the patient. However, if this form is then printed out and the patient reads and signs it, it is as valid as if the entire form were handwritten.

PATIENT HISTORY AND INTERVAL HISTORY

Medical documentation laws have become complex, and physician services must meet very specific documentation requirements. Recent legal decisions have confirmed that it is acceptable for a patient to fill out a history form to meet the past history and social history documentation requirements. If a full history is already on file, it is acceptable to obtain an interval history on subsequent visits. The physician does not have to rewrite the information contained on these forms. Instead, the forms are made a permanent part of the medical record, and the physician may just note "history reviewed" or "history reviewed and updated." See Chapter 6 for detailed information about documentation requirements.

Figure 3-6 shows an example of a patient history form that is designed to meet the documentation

---

Lake Eola Family Practice   517860 South Pioneer Drive, Orlando, FL 32897 • 634-555-4893

Confidential Patient Health History

Patient Name _____ Account Number _____

Date of Birth _____ Gender: __ Male   __ Female

Please provide the following information about your general health and your health history. This will enable us to consider the best options when we manage your medical care.

Please circle P for personal history or F for family history.

P F Alcohol use/Drug use	P F Epilepsy/seizure disorder,	P F Male organ irregularity or
P F Allergies: pollen, dust, animals	convulsions	condition: prostate, impotence
P F Allergies: medications	P F Hysterectomy	P F Nervous system conditions
P F Asthma, Bronchitis	P F Female organ irregularity,	P F Mental: nervous, depression,
P F Arthritis, Gout	abnormal Pap, menstrual	anxiety
P F Eating disorder: anorexia, bulimia	P F Gallbladder	P F Migraines/Headaches
P F Bone/joint condition	P F Heart problem or condition	P F Muscle/Tendon disorders
P F Back, neck, spine, disc problem	P F Hepatitis/liver disorder	P F Prosthetic implant/ artificial limbs
or injury	P F Hernia	P F Reconstructive/Cosmetic surgery
P F Birth defects/ Deformity	P F Hypertension, blood pressure	P F Sexually transmitted diseases
P F Blood disease: anemia, leukemia	disorder	P F Skin disorders/lesions/cancer
P F Blood vessel, circulation disorder	P F Hormonal/Thyroid/Pituitary	P F Steroid use: Prednisone,
P F Breast disease	disorder	anabolic
P Breast implants (L/R)	P F HIV/AIDS	P F Stroke
P F Broken bones/ bone disease	P F Immune system disorder, Lupus	P F Tumors, cysts, polyps, growths
P F Cancer of any type	P F Stomach/ colon/ Crohn's disease	P F Ulcers, digestive disorders
P F Concussion/head injury	P F Intestinal disorders	P F Weight problems
P F Diabetes	P F Kidney/Urinary tract condition or	P F Other, explain _____
P F Ear/Nose/Throat disease or	infection	_____
infection	P F Lung condition or infection	

Details for items marked above: _____
_____
_____

Have you ever been hospitalized? If yes, please state when, where, why: _____
_____

Have you ever had surgery? If yes, please state type of surgery and when, where, why _____
_____

Have you ever been advised to have surgery, or evaluated and advised to seek treatment for something, but you declined?
If yes, please explain: _____
_____

Have you ever smoked? If yes, number of years _____ packs per day _____

If female, Date of last menstrual period _____ Are you pregnant? _____

Did another physician refer you? _____ Name of referring physician _____

Patient or guardian signature _____ Date _____

FIGURE 3-6
Confidential patient health history. (Courtesy Medical Compliance Management, Inc., Orlando, Fla.)

requirements for past history and social history. This form is intended to pick up the slack in an area in which physician documentation often falls short. The past and social histories are valid for this visit and subsequent visits, but the chief complaint changes with every visit. Therefore the chief complaint, a history item, is not listed.

A full past history includes both a personal history and a family history, and it should provide a complete review of body systems. Family past history

is important for the identification of inherited conditions. The questions are pertinent for close blood relatives: natural (biological) parents, natural grandparents, and natural children. Family social history is important for the identification of conditions related to social problems the patient has been exposed to. The questions are pertinent for family members and others who have lived with the patient.

Ideally, the patient will complete the history form during the check-in process. The physician then has

Lake Eola Family Practice   517860 South Pioneer Drive, Orlando, FL 32897 • 634-555-4893

Confidential: Patient's Check-In Form & Interim History

Today's Date _____   Have you been seen in this office in the last three years?   __ Yes   __ No

Patient Name _____   Date of Birth _____   Gender: __ Male   __ Female

Does this visit involve an auto accident? __Yes __No   If yes, please supply Auto Insurance information _____

_____

Does this visit involve a work related injury?   __Yes __No   If yes, please supply workers compensation information _____

_____

Please state the reason(s) for this visit: _____

Current Medical Plan Name: _____   Has your medical insurance plan changed recently?__Yes __No

If yes, please provide a copy of your insurance card. Have your name, address or phone number changed recently?_____

Please provide the following information about your general health and your health history since your last visit. This will enable us to consider the best options when we manage your medical care. Since your last visit to our office, have you experienced problems in any of the following areas?

__ Alcohol/Drug use	__ Hormones (hot flashes, diabetic reactions, lupus flare-up)
__ Allergic reactions (medicine, animals, plants)	__ Immune system (Hodgkin's disease, HIV)
__ Blood system (anemia, swollen glands, high or low blood counts)	__ Musculoskeletal (broken bones, sprains, strained muscles, dislocated joints)
__ Constitutional symptoms (fever, weight loss)	__ Neurological (memory, coordination, balance)
__ Ears, nose, throat, mouth (cold, virus, pain, drainage)	__ Psychiatric (orientation to time, place & person; mental; behavior)
__ Exposure to sexually transmitted diseases	
__ Eyes (vision changes, drainage, redness)	__ Respiratory (shortness of breath, wheezing)
__ Gastrointestinal (indigestion, abdominal pain, constipation, diarrhea)	__ Skin and/or breasts (rashes, sores, lumps, bumps, cuts, infections, bites)
__ Genitourinary (urinary difficulties, prostate or menstrual difficulties)	__ Cardiovascular (heart problems, palpitations, chest pain, swelling in legs or feet)

Details for items marked above: _____

_____

Have you been hospitalized since you were last seen in this office? If yes, please state when, where, why: _____

_____

Have you had surgery since you were last seen in this office? If yes, please state type of surgery and when, where, why _____

_____

Have you started or quit smoking? If yes, details _____

If female, Date of last menstrual period _____ Are you pregnant? _____

Did another physician refer you? _____ Name of referring physician _____

Is there anything else we should know about? _____

Patient or guardian signature _____ Date _____

For Office Use Only:

TPR _____ BP _____ Wt _____ Other_____

Notes _____

_____

Today's Provider: __Dr. Anderson __Dr. Wilson __Dr. Rubin __Dr. Gomez __PA James __NP Lewis   Signature _____

FIGURE 3-7

Confidential patient check-in form and interval history. (Courtesy Medical Compliance Management, Inc., Orlando, Fla.)

the opportunity to review the history, the chief complaint, and the vital signs (recorded by clinical support personnel) before he or she enters the room to examine the patient. This information is especially valuable with a new patient. The physician is able to plan the examination and use the allotted time more effectively.

Medical practices, even within the same specialty, differ in many ways. Each medical practice develops forms to fit their unique requirements. As long as legal requirements are met, many styles and variations are effective. Figure 3-7 combines the patient check-in form for established patients with the interim history form for established patients.

Although a full history is required with a new patient, the history requirements are not as stringent with established patients who have a full history readily available elsewhere in the medical record. It is not usually necessary to ask for additional family history or social history. The established-patient history need only cover history items that have changed since the last visit, usually items directly related to the patient's health. When many patients in the practice experience frequent changes in family or social history, these choices can easily be added to the interim history form.

OTHER IN-TAKE FORMS

Certain patients will also require additional forms. When it is known in advance that additional forms are required, obtaining the forms becomes part of the check-in procedure. Otherwise, obtaining the forms is the responsibility of clinical support employees.

Medicare has ruled that the financial responsibility statement on most registration forms is not specific enough to meet Medicare's requirements for billing noncovered services. Medicare requires the use of a form that includes the name of the service or procedure and specifically states that Medicare does not pay for the service(s), and the patient agrees to accept financial responsibility. Figure 3-8 is an example of an "Advance Beneficiary Notice of Non-covered Medicare Part B Services." The charge is the physician's usual fee.

Medicare has ruled that the financial responsibility statement on most registration forms is not specific enough to meet Medicare's requirements for billing services that do not meet Medicare's medical necessity requirements. If you suspect services might not meet Medicare's medical necessity requirements, the form must include the name and date of the service or procedure and state that if it does not meet Medicare's medical necessity requirements, the patient agrees to accept financial responsibility. Figure 3-9 is an example of an "Advance Beneficiary Notice of Medicare Medical Necessity." This time, however, the charge listed on the form may not exceed Medicare's allowed amount for the service.

A Medicare waiver must be signed if a physician has chosen not to participate in the Medicare program (Figure 3-10). The patient accepts personal responsibility for full payment, agrees not to send the bill to Medicare, and agrees that the provider will not bill Medicare. The physician determines the fees charged for the services, usually the standard office fee.

Lake Eola Family Practice   517860 South Pioneer Drive, Orlando, FL 32897 • 634-555-4893

Advance Beneficiary Notice of Noncovered Medicare Part B Services

I understand that _____ is always a Medicare Part B noncovered service. _____, my physician at Lake Eola Family Practice, has informed me that Medicare Part B will not pay for the service and has discussed other alternatives. I acknowledge that Medicare Part B will not pay for the service and I agree to accept personal and full financial responsibility. The cost for this service will not exceed $_____.

_____
Medicare Beneficiary Name (printed)

_____
Beneficiary Signature

_____
Representative of Lake Eola Family Practice

_____
Witnessed By

_____
Medicare ID Number (on card)

_____
Date Signed

_____
Date Signed

_____
Date Witnessed

FIGURE 3-8
Advance Beneficiary Notice of noncovered Medicare Part B services. (Courtesy Medical Compliance Management, Inc., Orlando, Fla.)

Lake Eola Family Practice   517860 South Pioneer Drive, Orlando, FL 32897 • 634-555-4893

Advance Beneficiary Notice of Medicare Medical Necessity

Medicare will pay only for services that it determines to be "reasonable and necessary" under section 1862 (a) (1) of the Medicare law. If Medicare determines that a particular service, although it would otherwise be covered, is not "reasonable and necessary" under Medicare program standards, Medicare will deny payment for the service. I believe that in your case, Medicare is likely to deny payment for the following services(s) for the reason(s) noted below:

Date	Description of service	Reason for Medicare Denial of Payment

Medicare Beneficiary Name (printed)   Health Insurance Claim Number

Provider's Signature   Date Signed

Beneficiary's acknowledgement and agreement to pay:
I have been notified by my physician that he/she believes that, in my case, Medicare is likely to deny payment for the services identified above, for the reasons stated. If Medicare denies payment, I agree accept personal and full financial responsibility. The cost for this service will not exceed $ _____ .

Medicare Beneficiary Name (printed)   Medicare ID Number (on card)

Beneficiary Signature   Date Signed

Witnessed By   Date Witnessed

FIGURE 3-9

Advance Beneficiary Notice of Medicare medical necessity. (Courtesy Medical Compliance Management, Inc., Orlando, Fla.)

You may contact Medicare directly to get more information about these forms, or you may go to one of Medicare's websites at http://medicare.gov/ or http://cms.hhs.gov/. In addition, Medicare has an educational website that includes the use of Medicare ABNs and waivers. Medicare's educational website is located at http://cms.hhs.gov/medlearn/.

By law, informed consent is required before any procedure with a significant risk of complications. The person consenting must be of legal age or must meet the legal requirements to consent on behalf of a minor: for example, parents and legal guardians. Some states make an exception to this rule for voluntary abortions.

Informed consent means the physician must provide information about risks, possible complications, and alternatives to the recommended treatment, if any. Figure 3-11 is an example of an "Informed Consent to Treatment" form. The physician's notes should accurately reflect the method by which the information was provided and give a summary of verbal information.

Some attorneys advise physicians not to list the risks and potential complications in writing on the actual consent form because of the liability that may result if an item is inadvertently omitted from the list. Instead, they advise offering the patient copies of published articles or other educational material produced by others to meet this goal and then verbally discussing the most significant risks.

Other attorneys advise developing preprinted forms for each individual treatment or procedure, listing all potential risks and potential complications. Items are not likely to be inadvertently missed if they are carefully researched and printed in advance. It is up to the individual physician (or practice) to choose or design consent forms for office treatments and procedures.

Lake Eola Family Practice   517860 South Pioneer Drive, Orlando, FL 32897 • 634-555-4893

Waiver of Medicare Part B Entitlement

I have had a thorough and deliberate discussion with my physician, Todd Wilson, M.D., at Lake Eola Family Practice regarding my medical condition. I have voluntarily decided to contract privately for his services, outside the Medicare Part B program. Neither I, nor my family, nor my heirs, nor my estate shall file any Medicare Part B claims or forms, nor do I require Todd Wilson, M.D., or his employees at Lake Eola Family Practice to do so on my behalf.

I hereby waive my entitlement to Medicare Part B benefits for all services rendered by Todd Wilson, M.D., a physician at Lake Eola Family Practice.

_____
Medicare Beneficiary Name (printed)

_____
Medicare ID Number (on card)

_____
Beneficiary Signature

_____
Date Signed

_____
Todd Wilson, M.D.

_____
Date Signed

_____
Witnessed By

_____
Date Witnessed

FIGURE 3-10
Waiver of Medicare Part B entitlement. (Courtesy Medical Compliance Management, Inc., Orlando, Fla.)

Lake Eola Family Practice   517860 South Pioneer Drive, Orlando, FL 32897 • 634-555-4893

Informed Consent to Treatment

Date of Treatment	Name and Description of Treatment	Name of Provider

I, _____, have discussed the treatment(s) listed above with my physician, _____. My physician informed me of possible risks, possible complications and alternative treatments. I understand the reason for treatment, the possible risks and possible complications. All of my questions have been answered to my satisfaction.

I consent to the listed treatment(s) on the date(s) specified, performed by the listed provider(s) and whoever he/she may designate as assistants. I consent to whatever additional treatments may be deemed necessary during the course of the procedure.

Although a satisfactory result is expected, no guarantee has been given by anyone as to the results that may be obtained. A line has been drawn diagonally through treatment lines that are blank.

_____
Patient Name (printed)

_____
Insurance ID Number (on card)

_____
Patient Signature (or Responsible Party/Relationship to Patient)

_____
Date Signed

_____
Witnessed By

_____
Date Witnessed

FIGURE 3-11
Informed consent to treatment. (Courtesy Medical Compliance Management, Inc., Orlando, Fla.)

STOP & REVIEW

Please answer the following questions:

1. When patients arrive for an appointment, they should check in by signing their name on a community sign-in sheet.

____True   ____False

2. If the scheduler entered all the registration information into the computer at the time the appointment was scheduled, a new patient does not need to fill out a patient registration form on the day of the appointment.

____True   ____False

3. Circle the correct answer. The patient history form is designed to:
   A. Report the patient's past medical history
   B. Report past medical history for blood relatives
   C. Report the patient's social history
   D. Report the social history for those who live with the patient
   E. All of the above

4. The interim history form may be used if a complete history is on file for an established patient. It reports changes since the patient's last visit.

____True   ____False

5. The patient may not list just a P.O. box address on the registration form. The physical address where the patient lives must also be listed in case an ambulance should need to be dispatched in the future.

____True   ____False

6. There is only one correct way to design a form for a medical office.

____True   ____False

Match the circumstance in column A with the form in column B:

COLUMN A	COLUMN B
7. Medicare service listed as noncovered	A. Waiver of Medicare Part B Entitlement
8. Treatment with significant risks	B. ABN of Medicare Medical Necessity
9. Provider opted out of Medicare	C. Consent to Treatment
10. Service possibly not medically necessary by Medicare's definitions	D. ABN of Noncovered Medicare Part B Services

Use the birthday rule to determine whose plan is the primary payor:

Mother's birthday is October 10; father's birthday is October 2. _____

_____

Mother's birthday is September 6; father's birthday is May 18. _____

_____

Mother's birthday is February 9; father's birthday is December 29. _____

Gathering Physician-Supplied Information

Gathering physician-supplied information for the medical claim also is only a small step in the lifecycle of a claim, but it too is vital, and it also influences whether correct reimbursement is received in a timely manner.

Just as the patient registration and check-in forms are used to document and collect patient-supplied information for the claim form, a number of forms are used to document and collect physician-supplied information for the claim form. The most common forms used are the history forms discussed above, a variety of chart documentation forms, and billing worksheets such as **fee tickets,** superbills, or **encounter forms.**

Physicians (and other providers) are responsible for supplying the information for the bottom half of the medical claim form. Physician billing information must match chart documentation as closely as possible and must reflect what actually transpired. Only the information documented in the medical record may be considered for medical billing.

CHART NOTES

Documentation in the medical record must be legible, or it may not be considered for billing purposes, and it must meet the documentation criteria for the service reported. Evaluation and management services **(E/M)** are the most common services offered in a medical office. Chapter 6 covers the documentation and billing criteria for E/M services, and Chapter 7 includes documentation and billing criteria for other types of medical services.

Clinical results (test results, lab reports, consultation reports, etc.) that are not directly referenced in the physician's notes must be dated and either initialed or signed by the physician to document that the physician is aware of the information and to document when the physician knew the information. If this does not occur, the information may not be considered for billing purposes. This also becomes a very important issue when a medical record is used in legal proceedings. Because the physician cannot know every medical record that eventually will be used in a legal proceeding, the physician should maintain all records in this manner.

The patient's medical record should be organized in a manner that allows key information to be found promptly. Dividers are usually used to separate various pieces of clinical information in each section, and the information descends in chronological order. That means the most recent information is on top and the oldest information is on the bottom under each divider. Dividers are often color coded as another tool for locating information quickly (Figure 3-12). In addition, charts are organized into either two or four sections.

For example: The left-hand side of the front section might have dividers for a Problem List, a Medication List, a Blood Pressure Flow Chart, a Growth Chart, and the Patient Registration Information. The right-hand side on the front section might have dividers for Chart Notes, Consultation Reports, Laboratory Results, Test Reports, and Operative Reports. When there are four sections, a heavy divider separates the front two sections from the back two sections. The left-hand side in the back section might be used to store carbon copies of written prescriptions and other directions given to the patient on a prescription pad. The right-hand side in the back section might be used to store original messages from the patient and correspondence related to *medical* matters about the patient, with a divider separating messages from other correspondence. Please remember, correspondence related to *financial* matters is stored in the patient's financial record, not the medical record.

The documentation requirements for medical services are very detailed and very specific. The key components for E/M services are history, examination, and medical decision-making. New-patient E/M services must meet the requirements for all three key components. Established-patient E/M services must meet the requirements for at least two of the three key components. Further details about these requirements are covered in Chapter 6.

As long as all the requirements are met, physicians may document their services as they please. Many choose to use the SOAP charting format as it naturally leads a physician to include the key components needed for billing.

"S" stands for "Subjective." Anything "stated" by the patient is documented here, including the chief complaint, or reason for the visit, and all the patient history items. This section sometimes includes statements from family members or close friends.

"O" stands for "Objective." The examiner's findings are documented here, including the *abnormal* and the *pertinent normal* findings from the examination.

"A" stands for "Assessment." The examiner's thought processes and conclusions are documented here, including a list of "significant signs, symptoms, and other significant findings"; diagnoses that were considered and ruled out during this visit; remaining

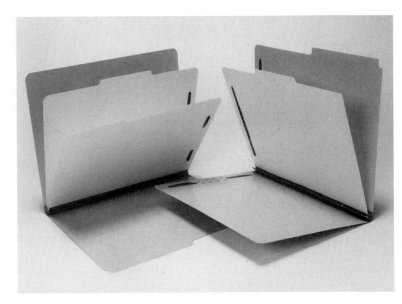

FIGURE 3-12
A new folder with four sections is ready for use as a patient medical record. Additional dividers can be added to each of the four sections. (Courtesy Bibbero Systems, Inc., Petaluma, Calif 94954; 800/242-2376; www.bibberosystems.com.)

potential diagnoses; and actual diagnoses. Only actual diagnoses and "signs, symptoms and significant findings" in the absence of an actual diagnosis may be converted into codes and placed in the diagnosis section of the medical claim form (block No. 21). However, all the physician's thought processes during assessment must now be documented in the patient's medical record because thought processes are an important component of medical decision-making and help determine the level of an E/M service. If thought processes are not documented, they cannot be considered for medical billing purposes.

Physicians (and sometimes billers and coders) often mistakenly believe that because suspected diagnoses and ruled-out diagnoses cannot be listed in the diagnosis section of the claim form, they cannot be documented in the medical record. This myth can result in failure to meet medical necessity requirements when a physician is still searching for a diagnosis. In addition, failure to document suspected and ruled-out diagnoses reduces the level of medical decision-making that can be considered for the visit and often results in payment for a lower level of service than actually occurred. Any time documentation does not match what actually occurs, the physician is at risk under HIPAA's "Fraud and Abuse" sections.

"P" stands for "Plan." The physician's plan of care is recorded here, including planned procedures, planned tests, planned treatments, ordered procedures, ordered tests, ordered treatments, ordered prescription medications, recommended over-the-counter remedies, all other directions given to the patient, and any other course of action chosen by the physician. Recommendations and orders for consultations and follow-up visits also are recorded here. This section completes the requirements for medical decision-making.

Anytime the majority of a visit is used for counseling, time becomes the determining factor for the level of service billed. The physician must document either a start time and a stop time or make an entry documenting the length of the visit in minutes or in hours and minutes. Time cannot be considered for billing unless it is documented in the medical record.

When a payor conducts an audit or otherwise investigates a claim, they only consider documentation in the medical record, and the documentation for each encounter must stand alone to meet the billing requirements. The physician must either rewrite information considered during the appointment but located elsewhere in the medical records, or the physician must state, "See complete patient history," or "See lab results" to direct an auditor to the location of other items considered during the visit.

The superbill is part of the financial record, not the medical record, and it is only a billing tool. It is *not* considered when payors look at documentation to support services billed.

Some practices want to achieve a fully electronic patient record. Physician notes are entered or scanned into the computer system. If the physician enters his or her own notes, a secure electronic signature can be attached to the notes. If someone else enters the information for the physician, the physician will have to review the information before an electronic signature can be attached.

Electronic records have many advantages:

❑ When the appropriate security measures are in place, the records can be accessed from any location. When Dr. Rubin is on-call for Lake Eola Family Practice and Miriam Gonzalez, a patient of Dr. Gomez, calls with an emergency in the middle of the night, Dr. Rubin can use his home computer to review her entire record before he calls her back. Even though Dr. Rubin has never seen her, he can make informed decisions regarding her care.
❑ Electronic records are always legible.
❑ Some computer programs organize the information in a manner that reminds physicians to include information they might otherwise miss.
❑ Specific information can be located quickly.
❑ The special forms you learned about earlier in this chapter can be designed as computer templates instead of paper forms.

There are also disadvantages to electronic records:

❑ If security measures are not in place, accessing the records from remote locations could violate health information security laws.
❑ The security requirements that apply to electronic records also apply to printed copies of electronic records.
❑ Records cannot be accessed during power failures unless the practice has an alternative source of power.
❑ If the practice does not have a current back-up and the computer crashes, the records could be lost.
❑ If an experienced computer hacker were to breach security and gain access to the records, records could be altered, and the changes might be undetectable. For this reason, paper records provide a better legal defense.

Some practices that use electronic records also print paper copies of the files at the time of service. This way they have the advantages of the electronic system and a method to detect unauthorized alterations of the files.

FORMS TO AUGMENT CHART NOTES

Many times physicians want to track specific information for a patient, and it can be very awkward and time consuming to thumb through pages and pages of notes looking for one piece of information from each past visit. Physicians need an easy reference to rapidly find and evaluate specific information compiled from many visits.

Therefore special forms are developed and designed to capture the exact information desired by the physician. These forms are usually placed in the front section of the medical record, opposite the physician notes. They allow a physician to easily find cumulative information and evaluate entries from numerous past visits. Many types of information can be tracked. Problem lists, medication lists, blood pressure records or graphs, and growth charts are common. Oncology offices (cancer specialists) often track lab results using a custom-designed form.

Figure 3-13 shows a form that captures two kinds of information in one form. It tracks current and past problems, and it tracks current and past medications. The problem list enables the physician to consider the person as a whole and to evaluate how the current problem may interact with other current or past problems. The medication list gives the physician a complete list of every medication the patient is currently taking and has taken in the past. The potential for drug interactions can be considered when the physician is evaluating the patient. Without such a tool, it would be difficult for a physician to identify and consider these important measures while evaluating a patient. A specific place for physician initials is not included, because physicians usually reference these items in their notes. Instead,

FIGURE 3-13

A combination problem list and medication list. (Courtesy Medical Compliance Management, Inc., Orlando, Fla.)

physicians are shown that the date boxes are large enough to include initials for those occasions when they do not reference the information in the body of their notes.

In Figure 3-13, the patient's name, date of birth, allergies, and allergic responses are included to reduce physician error when making decisions about medications. Although weight is also a consideration when new medications are ordered, it is a variable. It may change with every visit, and therefore would limit the usefulness of the tool if it were included on the medication form. Another form is designed to track weight when weight management is part of the treatment for the patient. Most physicians routinely document weight and other vital signs in the physician notes and do not compile the data for comparison.

Sometimes a physician must discharge a patient from his care. Usually this occurs when the patient either moves or changes insurance plans. It can also occur when the physician changes payor contracts. Occasionally the patient is noncompliant or abusive, and the physician no longer wishes to provide care.

When it is necessary to discharge a patient or withdraw from a case, the physician cannot just say goodbye and never see the patient again. Legal requirements must be met. Figure 3-14 is an example of a "Letter of Withdrawal from a Case." When the *physician* initiates the discharge, the patient must be notified in advance, and all other payor contract requirements must be met. The requirements typically include the following:

❏ The patient must be sent a formal written notice, as in Figure 3-14.
❏ The patient must be given time to find another physician, usually in the form of a deadline, such as 30 days from receipt of the letter.
❏ The letter or notice should be sent by certified mail with return receipt request, so you can prove the date the patient received the notice.
❏ A copy of the letter and the returned receipt are filed in the patient's medical record.
❏ Enforce the deadline. If the deadline is not enforced, you begin the process over again.

FEE TICKET, SUPERBILL, ENCOUNTER FORM

A fee ticket serves only to record charges so payment data regarding the day's charges may be entered into the patient accounting system. The form stays with the practice; a copy is not given to the patient.

At one time, there were different definitions for superbills and encounter forms. A superbill is a fee ticket that is modified to include enough information to serve as document for patients who have indemnity plans to bill their own insurance. Patients

---

Lake Eola Family Practice   517860 South Pioneer Drive, Orlando, FL 32897 • 634-555-4893

Letter of Withdrawal from a Case

Date_____

Dear _____:

I regret to inform you that I, together with the other physicians at Lake Eola Family Practice, must withdraw from providing services as your personal physician for the reason that the Lake Eola Family Practice physicians have withdrawn from our contracts with your medical insurance plan. Because your condition requires medical attention, I suggest you contact your medical insurance plan without delay to arrange for another primary physician. If you so desire, I will be available to provide you with medical care for a reasonable time after you receive this letter, but in no event for more than 30 days from the date on this letter.

This should give you ample time to select another competent physician from the roster at your medical plan. When you have chosen a physician, please ask for the release of records authorization form and, upon receipt of your written authorizations, I will provide your new physician with your case history and information regarding your diagnosis and the treatment you have received under my care.

Very truly yours,

_____, M.D.

FIGURE 3-14
Letter of withdrawal from a case. (Courtesy Medical Compliance Management, Inc., Orlando, Fla.)

are given a copy of the superbill. Encounter forms are superbills that also track encounters so payments can be applied to specific charges instead of just reducing the total amount owed by the patient.

In today's world, most practices are computerized, and the terms *superbill* and *encounter form* are used interchangeably. Most often, they are referred to as superbills but function as encounter forms. The simple addition of a tracking number enables this to occur.

Figure 3-15 is an example of a superbill that is set up to function like an encounter form. The tracking number is located after the superbill label at the top of the document. This example was originally prepared for a practice in which the physician did not want nursing personnel to record vital signs directly in the medical record, so a space was included at the top of the superbill for nursing personnel to record vital signs, and the physician was responsible for entering them into the medical record. A reminder was placed at the bottom of the form above the physician signature.

The information at the top of a superbill should be set up so the information is listed in the same order that the computer screens ask for the information. This will save time and increase accuracy when transcribing data.

The information in the top section of the form is detailed enough to:

❐ Identify the correct patient
❐ Identify the insurance plan to be billed as primary payor
❐ Identify elements pertinent to today's visit
❐ Remind the receptionist to ask for visit-specific details during check-in:
  ❐ Female patient's last menstrual period (pregnancy influences medication choices)
  ❐ The actual physician or provider seen today, especially when different than usual
  ❐ Payor information, especially when a *different* insurance plan is responsible for today's visit (a visit for an injury might be billed to a liability insurance plan, not a medical insurance plan)
  ❐ The referring physician, if any, including ID number

Many superbills are filled with preprinted diagnosis and procedures codes. There is nothing wrong with preprinting the codes on a superbill *if* the codes are updated annually when the codebooks change and *if* all the billing requirements are met. Unfortunately, only a few medical practices update their superbills every year.

Another problem with placing preprinted diagnosis and procedure codes on the superbill is that it can lead to a practice called pigeonholing. Pigeonholing occurs when a physician chooses the closest code match from the codes listed on the superbill rather than choosing from all available codes to find the code that most accurately reflects chart documentation. Current-year codebooks list all available codes. If a practice wants a superbill that will meet the requirements for many years, it must be designed to obtain billing information without listing information that is subject to change.

Although the definitions for E/M services change often, the codes used most often to report E/M services seldom change. Therefore Figure 3-15 lists the most common office-visit E/M codes and gives clues to the level of documentation required for each E/M code, but it does not list any other medical codes. You will learn more about documentation requirements for E/M services in Chapter 6.

Figure 3-15 is set up to allow the physician to quickly list detailed chart information for billing purposes. The physician may choose whether to code the services or describe the services so a certified coder can code the services billed. Some physicians prefer to choose their own codes. Fast-finder guides are available by specialty from codebook publishers for both diagnosis and procedure codes. In this instance, the physician writes the code choices in the appropriate blanks instead of writing a description of the service. However, be aware that the only physicians who can effectively use fast-finder guides are those who are very familiar with the codebook requirements and those who employ certified coders to make the final determination of codes placed on the claim. Most physicians should write descriptions of the services rendered.

The line items in Figure 3-15 are tailored to match the services offered by the practice, without limiting code choices. Charges for services are not preprinted, as they also change often. Line-item charges can be written in the margins by each item, and the totals can be written in at the bottom of the form.

The bottom of the superbill in Figure 3-15 is designed to give the patient reminders about future appointments and to record financial information. It includes the patient balance owed from previous visits and the amount of copayment for today's visit, so you can collect the patient's portion of the bill today.

A well-designed superbill or encounter form collects accurate billing information and does not easily become outdated. It is set up a little differently in every medical office. The superbill is a billing worksheet, a tool to report chart documentation to billing personnel. It is a part of the patient's financial record, not the patient's medical record.

Lake Eola Family Practice　　517860 South Pioneer Drive, Orlando, FL 32897 • 634-555-4893

S u p e r b i l l　#456298　　　Weight_____　BP _____　TPR _____

Account Number	Doctor		Date of Service
Patient Name		Date of Birth	LMP
Insurance	Responsible Party		Phone Number
Address	Referring Physician and ID #		
City	State	Zip	

New Patient

__ 99201　H [PF]　E [PF]　MDM [S]　10 min
__ 99202　H [EPF]　E [EPF]　MDM [S]　20 min
__ 99203　H [D]　E [D]　MDM [LC]　30 min
__ 99204　H [C]　E [C]　MDM [MC]　45 min
__ 99205　H [C]　E [C]　MDM [HC]　60 min

Established Patient

__ 99211　H [N/A]　E[N/A]　MDM [N/A]　5 min
__ 99212　H [PF]　E [PF]　MDM [S]　10 min
__ 99213　H [EPF]　E [EPF]　MDM [LC]　15 min
__ 99214　H [D]　E [D]　MDM [MC]　25 min
__ 99215　H [C]　E [C]　MDM [HC]　40 min

Reason For Visit

__ Authorization _____
　　Expiration Date _____
__ Annual exam, complex due to (history,
　　condition): _____
__ Annual exam, simple
__ Follow-up, condition _____
__ Follow-up, post procedure, no condition
　　or complication _____
　　Procedure/date _____
__ Follow-up, post procedure, with condition
　　or complication _____
　　Procedure/date _____
__ New Problem _____
__ Post-op, no condition or complication
　　Surgery/date _____
__ Post-op, with conditions or complication
　　_____
　　Surgery/date _____
__ Pre-op _____
__ Procedure _____
__ Second surgical opinion _____
__ Other (Accident, Decision for surgery)
　　_____

Procedures

⇒ Place to be done: _____
⇒ Date to be done: _____
__ Authorization _____
　　Expiration date _____
__ Biopsy,type/site_____
　　_____
__ Cautery, type/site _____
　　_____
__ Destruction of lesion(s), extensive, site:
　　_____
__ Destruction of lesion(s), simple, site:
　　_____
__ Emergency surgery, (list above), reason:
　　_____
__ Excision, type/site _____
　　_____
__ I & D abscess, type/site: _____
　　_____
__ Insertion/Removal of IUD, type _____
__ Major surgery, type/site _____
　　_____
__ Minor surgery, type/site _____
　　_____
__ Sonogram _____
__ Other _____
　　_____

Miscellaneous

__ Immunization _____
__ Injection _____
__ Supplies
__ Surgical Tray
__ Patient Teaching (Preventive medicine)
　　_____
　　_____

Other

__ Other _____
　　_____
　　_____

Outside Lab

__ Beta HCG, Serum
__ Biopsy/ Pathology
__ Biopsy, Mult./Pathology
__ CBC
__ Cholesterol
__ Culture, throat
__ Cultures (source) _____
__ Glucose, __ 1hr glucose, __ 3hr glucose
__ Estrogen
__ Herpes simplex, AB
__ Mononucleosis
__ Pap Smear
__ PT __ PTT
__ Sed rate
__ SMAC
__ Urinalysis, w/micro
__ HIV
__ Other _____
　　_____
　　_____
　　_____

Diagnosis Codes

1. _____
2. _____
3. _____
4. _____

Appointment In _____Weeks
Procedure In _____Weeks
Sent Labs to _____
Call In _____ Mos./Weeks

Previous Balance $ _____.
Co-Pay $ _____.
Paid Today Cash/Check $ _____.
Yes-No All Diagnoses, Procedures, & VS above are documented in Record

Doctor's Signature_____

New Charges $ _____.
New Balance $ _____.
Check Number _____

FIGURE 3-15

A superbill set up to function like an encounter form. (Courtesy Medical Compliance Management, Inc., Orlando, Fla.)

CAPTURING HOSPITAL INFORMATION

Hospital bills do not include fees for physician services. Physicians submit separate bills for services they render in a hospital. Yet, physician billing is required to match certain components of hospital billing. This can be a challenge for physicians. Many do not know how to communicate hospital-billing information to their billing employees.

In real life, many physicians collect napkins and scraps of paper on which they write patient names and the dates seen in the hospital. Once a month or so they fish the scraps of paper out of the pocket of their hospital lab coats, hand the jumble to the biller and say, "Here is my hospital billing for the month." They expect the biller to magically know everything else needed for billing. You may laugh now, but it will not be quite so funny when you are the biller. This really is a standard method used by many physicians, and they are very resistant to acquiring more paperwork.

Some hospitals send each admitting physician a copy of the admission slip for each patient, but this information is not automatically sent to other physicians who provide services throughout the course of the admission. Other physicians who might provide services include consultants, anesthesiologists, radiologists, pathologists, and many more.

Some office employees have coaxed physicians into at least getting a copy of the hospital face sheet for each hospitalized patient. Some physicians use pocket calendars and organizers and give copies of the notes to the billing employees. These are definite improvements over the napkin method, but they still fall short of recording the level of documentation met for each service billed.

In all likelihood, you are going to have to do some work if you want the physician to give you adequate hospital billing information. Some practice management systems have templates for hospital rounding slips. The practice just enters a list of hospitalized patients, and a customized list prints out for the physician to use when making rounds.

Figure 3-16 is an example of a hospital rounding slip. It can be used as a computerized template, or it can be preprinted. This slip is designed to accommodate three patients in the same hospital per sheet of paper. It also includes a code usage guide for the physician. You will learn how to use the guide in Chapter 6.

Complete as much information as possible for the physician in advance. When you know the names of hospitalized patients, call the hospital and get the hospital record number. Before you leave each day, prepare rounding slips for the physician to use the next day by completing the patient name, record number, and date of admission for every patient you know is hospitalized. The physician will be more cooperative when there is less required of him or her. Always include blank slips to accommodate unexpected admissions.

Ask for completed rounding slips daily. In addition, ask the physician to provide a copy of the hospital face sheet at least once per admission. The face sheet is a guide for matching your billed services to the hospital's billed services.

A surgery charge slip is another important form used to bill services performed in a hospital or an outpatient surgical center. Once again, physicians prefer the napkin and scrap-paper method of communicating surgery billing information, and you will have to work to get the proper level of billing information.

Figure 3-17 is an example of a surgery charge slip. Most surgeries are scheduled in advance. You should be able to fill out the first four lines of information in advance for scheduled surgeries. Also, give physicians blank surgery charge slips for unscheduled, emergency surgeries.

In addition to the charge slip, you will need a copy of the operative report and a copy of the hospital or facility face sheet. Insurance companies seldom pay for a physician's surgery claim until after the hospital or facility submits their claim. The payor then compares the charges before making a payment decision.

Handling Medical Claim Information

FILING MEDICAL CLAIMS

Medical claim forms are used to request payment from medical plans (payors). The top half of the medical claim form tells the payor who the patient is and what coverage applies to the claim. The bottom half of the medical claim form tells the payor what services were provided and why. It also tells the payor where to send payment.

There are two methods by which claims may be submitted to the payor. The claim may be printed out on a current version of the red CMS-1500 claim form and mailed; this is called a paper claim. Or the claim may be sent electronically, usually over the

Lake Eola Family Practice   517860 South Pioneer Drive, Orlando, FL 32897 • 634-555-4893

Hospital Rounding Slip

Initial Inpatient Care (2 of 3)

E/M	H	E	MDM	Time
99221	D or C	D or C	S or L	30
99222	C	C	M	50
99223	C	C	H	70

Subsequent Hospital Care (2 of 3)

E/M	H	E	MDM	Time
99231	PF	PF	S or L	15
99232	EPF	EPF	M	25
99233	D	D	H	35

Consultation Initial Inpatient (3 of 3)

E/M	H	E	MDM	Time
99251	PF	PF	S	20
99252	EPF	EPF	S	40
99253	D	D	L	55
99254	C	C	M	80
99255	C	C	H	110

Consultation Follow-up Inpatient (2 of 3)

E/M	H	E	MDM	Time
99261	PF	PF	S or L	10
99262	EPF	EPF	M	20
99263	D	D	H	30

Hospital Discharge Services

E/M	H	E	MDM	Time
99238	N/A	N/A	N/A	< 30
99239	N/A	N/A	N/A	> 30
99217	Observation Care Discharge			
99435	Newborn Born & Disch. Same Day			

Observation Services (3 of 3)

E/M	H	E	MDM	Time
99234	D or C	D or C	S or L	N/A
99235	C	C	M	N/A
99236	C	C	H	N/A

Notes:

Date _____ **Physician** _____ **Hospital:** _____

Patient Name	Record #
Admission Date	Discharge Date
E/M Code	Unit Time
Diagnosis	
Procedures	
Complications	
Notes	

Patient Name	Record #
Admission Date	Discharge Date
E/M Code	Unit Time
Diagnosis	
Procedures	
Complications	
Notes	

Patient Name	Record #
Admission Date	Discharge Date
E/M Code	Unit Time
Diagnosis	
Procedures	
Complications	
Notes	

FIGURE 3-16

Hospital rounding slip. (Courtesy Medical Compliance Management, Inc., Orlando, Fla.)

Lake Eola Family Practice   517860 South Pioneer Drive, Orlando, FL 32897 • 634-555-4893

Surgery Charge Slip

Patient			Hospital or Facility
Record #		Date of Admission	Inpatient Outpatient
Date of Surgery	Planned Procedure		
Pre-op Diagnosis			
Actual Procedure Done			Length (Time)
Complications and Unusual Services			
Post Operative Diagnosis			
Post Operative Condition			
Names of all Surgeons			
Name of Anesthesiologist			
Notes			

Patient			Hospital or Facility
Record #		Date of Admission	Inpatient Outpatient
Date of Surgery	Planned Procedure		
Pre-op Diagnosis			
Actual Procedure Done			Length (Time)
Complications and Unusual Services			
Post Operative Diagnosis			
Post Operative Condition			
Names of all Surgeons			
Name of Anesthesiologist			
Notes			

FIGURE 3-17
Surgery charge slip. (Courtesy Medical Compliance Management, Inc., Orlando, Fla.)

STOP & REVIEW

Answer the following questions:

1. What type of medical office service is billed most often?

   _____

2. What are the three key components for E/M services? _____

   _____

3. What is the purpose of a superbill?

   _____

4. What is the purpose of a hospital rounding slip?

   _____

5. What is the purpose of a surgery charge slip?

   _____

6. Electronic records must meet security provisions for patient privacy.

   ____True   ____False

7-10. Match the items in column A with the definitions in column B to define SOAP charting.

COLUMN A:

ELEMENT	COLUMN B: DEFINITION
7. S	A. Examiner's findings (exam requirements)
8. O	B. Plan of care (medical decision-making requirements)
9. A	C. Subjective (patient statements, history requirements)
10. P	D. Assessment (diagnoses and thought processes, medical decision-making requirements)

telephone lines; this is called an electronic claim. Chapter 4 covers the details for filling out a medical claim form. Instructions are given for both paper and electronic claims, and that chapter has an illustration of a claim form.

When paper claims arrive at the payor, most payors scan the claims into their computer system. However, if the paper claim was not prepared in a way that allows scanning, the data must be entered by hand into the computer system. Transcription errors can easily occur and cause needless rejections. Payment for scanned claims is usually received within a month of the time the claim was mailed. Claims entered by hand are processed very slowly.

Electronic claims are sent using a modem and a telephone line. Payment for electronic claims usually arrives about 2 weeks after the claim was received by the payor. Because telephone lines are a public form of communication, security measures must be used to prevent data from being seen by unauthorized people. Security programs encrypt data before it is sent, and the recipient must have a similar program to decrypt the data after it arrives. Most medical offices use a claims clearinghouse so they do not have to maintain a large number of encryption programs.

Each insurance company wants to receive claim information in a very specific manner when it is sent electronically. One reason HIPAA mandates claim transmission standards and requirements is because at the time the law was written, more than 400 different software programs were in use to transmit claims directly to payors, and there were no standards for programming language. Unless a clearinghouse is used, a practice must maintain a separate software system for each payor. Even with a clearinghouse, many claims cannot be sent electronically.

HIPAA requires every payor to accept electronic transmission of claims, and to accept every code from the authorized codebooks. In addition, only a few programming languages may be used. The last compliance deadline for payors to meet this requirement was October 16, 2003. However, other individual payor requirements still vary, so clearinghouses still provide valuable services. For example, although each payor's computer system must accept every authorized code, the medical plan is not required to provide coverage for every code. In addition, individual medical plans might have unique requirements in certain sections of the claim.

Claim clearinghouses act as translators. A practice can use one software program to send information to the clearinghouse. The clearinghouse will then translate the information into the desired format for each individual payor.

Clearinghouses also subject claims to edits similar to those used by payors. Claims that do not pass the edits are sent back to the medical office for correction before the claim reaches the payor. Fewer payor rejections occur when clearinghouses are used.

However, be aware that clearinghouse edits only check for the completeness and the accuracy of specific data on the claim form. They do not perform claim audits because they do not keep records of claim content.

Some clearinghouses are better than others. The best clearinghouses send reports when the claims arrive at the clearinghouse and again when the claims arrive at the payor. Armed with this information, you can call their bluff when a payor says the claim never arrived.

RECORDING PAYMENTS

A copy of the practice fee schedule is usually given to the scheduler, the receptionist, the biller, and the collection employees so that prices may be quoted to patients upon request and services can be billed appropriately. In most instances, every service will initially be billed using the practice fee schedule. In addition to the practice fee schedule, these employees should also be given a chart that shows specific contract provisions by payor. A managed care chart can be developed to identify contract-specific requirements.

Physicians find managed care charts to be useful when they make decisions about a patient's plan of care. Separate charts are created for each insurance contract. Sometimes every employee uses the same chart, and other times the charts separate information according to employee responsibility. The scheduler and receptionist are given information needed to schedule appointments. The billers, coders, and collection employees are given information needed to bill and collect. Job-specific charts are less complex, but if an employee fills more than one position, he or she will have to use a different set of charts for each employee function. It is up to the practice to determine the method that works best for them.

Figure 3-18 shows a template of a managed care chart. All employees use the same chart in this example. Many times a physician contract covers multiple types of insurance plans offered by one insurance carrier, so this template provides information for each type of plan included in the contract. Insurance plans can be added or taken away as needed. Employees can easily discover which services are covered by each plan, when an authorization is needed, special billing rules for specific services, and other plan-specific information.

When payments are received from insurance plans, they are accompanied by payment documents

MANAGED CARE NAME:

Office Services	Cov Serv			Auth Req			Coverage Limits			Provide Service In House			Outside Facility Coding Considerations	INSURANCE NAMES:
Annual Well Woman Exams	Y	Y	Y	Y	N	N	1YR	1YR	1YR	Y	Y	Y	Must use Preventive Med Codes, Dx V72.3 only	DDD Insurance
Office Visits/Consults	Y	Y	Y	Y	N	N	N	N	N	Y	Y	Y	Do not use Confirm Consult Codes	AAA Employee Group
Diagnostic X-Rays	Y	Y	Y	Y	N	N	N	N	N	Y	Y	Y	Dx Rad Only/All Others Outside	Rad Centers:
Labs:														XYZ Radiology
Pap Smears	Y	Y	Y	Y	N	N	N	N	N	N	N	N	SKL	(407) 888-8888
Blood Draws	Y	Y	Y	Y	N	N	N	N	N	Y	Y	Y	Use Code 99000 (No Modifier 90)	ABC Radiology
Urinalysis	Y	Y	Y	Y	N	N	N	N	N	Y	Y	Y	Urinalysis 81000 Inhouse Only/All Others Out SKL	(407) 777-7777
Lab Work	N	N	N	N	N	N	N	N	N	N	N	N	Blood Draws Inhouse Only/All Others Out SKL	
Other:														
Other:														
Other:														
Other:														
Hospital Services	All inpatient services require preauthorizations													
Hospital Admissions		Y	Y	Y	Y	Y	Y	N	N	N	N	N	N	HOSPITAL NETWORK:
Hospital Visits		Y	Y	Y	Y	Y	Y	N	N	N	N	N	N	EEE Hospital
Consultations		Y	Y	Y	Y	Y	Y	N	N	N	N	N	N	FFF Hospital
Surgical Procedures		Y	Y	Y	Y	Y	Y	N	N	N	N	N	N	PHARMACY NETWORK:
Other:														Pharmacies Are Us
Other:														(407) 222-2222

MANAGED CARE NAME:

HMO Plan
PPO Plan
Indemnity Plan

FIGURE 3-18

A managed care template is a useful tool for keeping employees informed about plan-specific insurance requirements. A separate chart is developed for each payor contract. (Copyright © 1998 MD Consultative Services.)

called an EOB (explanation of benefits) or an MRN (Medicare remittance notice). As a collections employee, you will evaluate the payment documents and determine if full payment was received by comparing the amount received to the fee schedule listed in the payor contract for that payor. Since every payor uses a different fee schedule, be sure you find the correct one when you make the comparison. Fee-schedule comparison charts can be developed for tracking this information.

The simplest method to develop a comparison chart is to draw a simple table. The CPT codes used by the practice are entered in the first column, the practice's standard fee schedule in the second column, the Medicare fee schedule in the third column, and remaining payors in subsequent columns.

You find the expected payment amount for the CPT code that is listed on the EOB by looking down the first column to find the matching code. Then follow the row across the page until you come to the column for the payor. This tells you the expected fee from the specific payor for that CPT code.

Using the fee schedule in Table 3-1, the allowed amount from Aetna for CPT code 99214 should be $131.00. If the EOB shows an allowed amount of $131.00, no deductible, and a patient copayment of $10.00, the full payment due from Aetna will be $121.00. The $121.00 from Aetna plus $10.00 from the patient should equal the "allowed" amount of $131.00.

If the Aetna payment received for CPT 99214 is $85.00, full payment has not been received even if the EOB remarks state "payment is in the amount the provider agreed to in the contract." This is a technically correct, but very misleading, statement. This remark does *not* mean that the payment is in the amount earned by the physician according to the contract fee schedule. It usually means a penalty was applied in accordance with contract provisions. By signing the payor contract, the provider agreed to a penalty anytime contract provisions are not met.

Use the patient name, the dates of service, and the service billed to find the exact transaction in the patient accounting system; payment is posted for

TABLE 3-1
Fee Schedule Comparison

CPT Code	Lake Eola	Medicare	Aetna	Blue Cross Blue Shield
99213	$93.00	$44.99	$87.00	$85.00
99214	$142.00	$68.75	$131.00	$130.00
99215	$226.00	$105.93	$205.00	$202.00

Template © 1999 Medical Compliance Management, Inc.; CPT only © American Medical Association. All Rights Reserved.

the exact transaction. If there is an amount remaining, you must determine the next step to be taken.

If the Aetna payment was $121.00 and the patient previously paid the copayment of $10.00, the full amount due from Aetna for CPT 99214 has been received. The patient cannot be billed an additional amount. Yet, the account shows a remaining balance of $11.00. This amount is the discount given to Aetna in the payor contract.

If there is a secondary payor, the $11.00 and the $10.00 paid by the patient for a total of $21.00 may be billed to the secondary payor. You must send a copy of the payment documents from Aetna (the EOB) along with the claim that is sent to the secondary payor. When the secondary payment of $21.00 is received, the patient is reimbursed the $10.00 copay and there is no write-off.

If there is no secondary payor, the remaining $11.00 is subtracted from the patient account as a write-off, and the $11.00 is added to an Aetna write-off account. A write-off is a discount the physician has given a patient or has authorized in a payor contract; a payor contract write-off is sometimes called a contractual or a contractual agreement. The patient balance for this transaction is now $0.00, and the transaction or account for this claim is closed.

However, if only $85.00 was received from Aetna, the payment is posted and the account remains open. You should research the claim to see why payment was reduced. Research begins by comparing the codes billed with the patient's medical record to see if documentation requirements were met. Next, compare the claim form to the payor contract to see if contract-specific billing rules were followed. Once the error is found and the claim is corrected, you can appeal the claim in an effort to collect the remaining $36.00 due from Aetna. Only when the maximum has been collected from Aetna is consideration given, as above, to the remaining balance.

If the patient has an indemnity plan, the physician has not signed a contract with the insurance company. The full fee from the physician's fee schedule can be collected because **balance billing** is allowed. The patient is billed for the entire balance remaining after payment from the insurance company has been posted. The standard fee for CPT 99214 is $142.00. If the Lake Eola Family Practice physician does not have a contract with a small insurance company, and the insurance pays $100.00 of the bill, the patient is billed for the remaining $42.00.

STOP & REVIEW

Answer the following questions:

1. Which employee is responsible for completing the claim form?

_____

2. What are the two methods for submitting claim forms? _____

3. Which method results in faster payment?

_____

4. Which fee schedule should be used when calculating charges billed on claims?

_____

5. Which fee schedule is used when determining if full payment is received?

_____

6. When full payment is not received, the collections employee should _____ to find out why full payment was not received.

7. When full payment is received from the primary payor and a balance remains, is the secondary payor or the patient billed next? _____

_____

8. How does the collections employee find out whether or not the patient may be balance-billed?

_____

9. When can a remaining balance be written off?

_____

10. What is a write-off? _____

_____

Chapter Review

When medical claim forms are filled out correctly, using accurate information, claims can be paid in full, and payment will be received without needless delay. If a claim is either rejected or penalized, the process for receiving payment from the payor can drag on for months, and the patient can seldom be billed for the full balance due.

Medical offices use a variety of forms to collect patient-supplied billing information. These are completed during patient registration. Sometimes additional forms are required for specific purposes. Medicare requires Advance Beneficiary Notices or waivers in a variety of circumstances.

Medical offices also use a variety of forms to collect physician-supplied billing information. The claim form must accurately portray the information documented in the chart, and both the claim form and the medical record must accurately portray what actually occurred. The False Claims Act and the fraud and abuse provisions in HIPAA establish consequences when medical claims are not accurate. Anything that is not documented in the patient's medical record cannot be billed.

The superbill is not a part of the medical record; it is a part of the financial record. It is merely a billing tool used to communicate chart information to the biller. Claims may be submitted either electronically or by mail. When payments are posted, collections employees must determine whether full payment has been received, and they must determine what to do if there is a remaining balance. Much of the information introduced in this chapter is covered in more detail later in the book.

Answer the following questions:

1. An annual physical is a noncovered service for Medicare. If a Medicare patient is scheduled for an annual physical, is an ABN or a waiver required? If yes, which one? _____

_____

2. When a new patient arrives for an office visit, which of the following forms will be completed?
   A. Check-in form
   B. Registration form
   C. History form
   D. B and C only

3. When the medical claim arrives at the insurance company, it is subjected to a series of claim edits and claim audits.

   ____True   ____False

4. When a penalty was applied and a reduced payment received, should the corrected claim be resubmitted or appealed? _____

5. Does a claims clearinghouse subject claims to edits or audits? _____

6. Payment is received the fastest when claims are submitted by mail.

   ____True   ____False

7. The superbill is part of the medical record.

   ____True   ____False

8. Which of the following employees should have a copy of a payor-contract summary chart?
   A. Scheduler
   B. Biller
   C. Collector
   D. Receptionist
   E. All of the above

9. Which of the following employees should have a copy of the practice fee schedule?
   A. Scheduler
   B. Biller
   C. Collector
   D. Receptionist
   E. All of the above

10. Which of the following employees should have a copy of the fee schedule comparison chart?
    A. Scheduler
    B. Biller
    C. Collector
    D. Receptionist
    E. All of the above

11. Who is billed first?
    A. Primary payor
    B. Secondary payor
    C. Patient

12. Who is billed second?
    A. Primary payor
    B. Secondary payor
    C. Patient

13. Who is billed last?
    A. Primary payor
    B. Secondary payor
    C. Patient

14. What happens when a balance remains after full payment is received from the primary payor?
    A. Bill the secondary payor, if applicable.
    B. Bill the patient, if no secondary payor and if allowed by contract.

C. Write off the balance, if cannot collect from secondary payor or from patient.

D. All of the above.

15. What happens when a balance remains after receiving full payment from both the primary and secondary payors?

A. Balance-bill the patient.

B. Check to see if the contract allows patient balance-billing.

C. Write off the balance without checking to see if the patient has any remaining financial responsibility.

Clinical Application Exercise

Use Table 3-1 to complete the following exercises:

1. A payment of $85.00 was received from Blue Cross Blue Shield for CPT 99213. Was full payment received? If not, how much was the penalty?

_____

2. A payment of $44.99 was received from Medicare for CPT 99214. Was full payment received? If not, how much was the penalty?

_____

3. A payment of $180.00 was received from Aetna for CPT 99215. Was full payment received? If not, how much was the penalty?

_____

4. A payment of $87.00 was received from Aetna for CPT 99213. Medicare is the secondary payor. How much will be billed to Medicare?

_____

5. A payment of $202.00 was received from Blue Cross Blue Shield for CPT 99215. Aetna is the secondary payor. How much will be billed to Aetna?

_____

4

CMS-1500 CLAIM FORM

Objectives After completing this chapter, you should be able to:

- Use the CMS-1500 claim form correctly
- Discuss the requirements for each field on the CMS-1500 claim form and correctly complete at least seven claim forms for case studies found in Appendix C and on the CD-ROM
- Explain who is responsible for supplying each piece of information and where to find it
- Demonstrate field-specific billing rules by correctly completing at least seven claim forms for case studies found in Appendix C and on the CD-ROM
- Discuss legal responsibilities related to the CMS-1500 claim form

Key Terms

ANSII format a complex format used to send electronic claims. It is very versatile; the electronic medical records may be attached to the claim.

beneficiary a person entitled to benefits under an insurance policy.

CMS-1500 claim form the claim form used by physicians and other nonfacility providers to bill payors for medical charges incurred by someone covered by the medical plan.

EDI electronic data interchange; the process used to send claims electronically.

EPSDT Medicaid's early periodic screening and diagnostic testing program; a preventive medicine program for certain children covered by Medicaid.

FEIN Federal Employer Identification Number; a tax ID number issued to a business.

insured the person entitled to benefits under an insurance policy. The insured is the policyholder, the person whose name is listed in the medical plan's files as the owner of the policy. Some medical plans call the insured a "subscriber," and Medicare calls the insured a "beneficiary."

NPI National Provider Identifier; a number that Medicare began issuing in June 2005 to replace the UPIN, PIN, and provider number systems used historically before that time. A physician will have just one number to use in every location and every state to identify who he or

she is. This number may be used in blocks 17B, 24K, and sometimes 33 on the CMS-1500 claim form for physician billing and in FL 82 and FL 83 on the UB-92 claim form for hospital and facility billing.

NSF National Standard Format; a simpler format used to send electronic claims. New versions are issued periodically. Only the data on the claim form are transmitted electronically. Supporting documentation is sent under separate cover.

OCR optical character recognition; a process by which a computer "reads" information that is scanned into the computer.

outside lab a lab that bills the physician for tests the physician purchased on behalf of a patient. The physician then bills the patient's medical plan. When an outside lab is used, the lab is identified in block No. 32 on the CMS-1500 claim form.

patient account number a number assigned by the practice for internal identification of the patient's financial record.

PIN (Medicare) a practice identification number assigned to a group practice or a solo physician who has incorporated the practice. It is used in block No. 33 on the CMS-1500 claim form.

policyholder the primary person entitled to benefits under an insurance policy, and the person whose name is listed as the owner of the policy. Some medical plans call the policyholder a "subscriber," and Medicare calls the policyholder a "beneficiary." On the CMS-1500 claim form, the policyholder is the "insured."

provider number (Medicare) a number assigned by Medicare to identify individual providers in a group and to identify solo physicians who are not incorporated. For Medicare, the NPI will replace this number. Medicare began issuing NPIs in June 2005.

SSN Social Security number; a tax ID number issued to an individual.

subscriber the primary person entitled to benefits under an insurance policy. The subscriber is the policyholder— the person whose name is listed in the medical plan's files as the owner of the policy. The subscriber is the "insured" for purposes of completing a medical claim form.

UPIN (Medicare) unique physician identifier number; used by Medicare to identify a referring physician. Medicare began replacing this number with the NPI in June 2005.

Introduction

You have learned how to speak the language of a medical office. You have learned how medical office employees function together as a team to collect billing information from patients and physicians for the medical claim form. You have learned how to design or revise office forms so you collect the correct information. Now it is time to learn how to complete and file a medical claim.

In this chapter, you will learn how to correctly complete a medical claim form for physician billing, how to find the required information, how to determine the cause of past problems, and how to avoid problems in the future. Payor-specific rules, including Medicare, are included throughout the chapter.

The compliance guidance documents issued by the Office of Inspector General (OIG) for the Department of Health and Human Services (HHS) strongly recommend that job descriptions be used to assign accountability for specific tasks in the medical office. The OIG developed the compliance guidance documents to help various types of medical entities meet the "accountability" requirements of the Health Insurance Portability and Accountability Act of 1996 (Public Law 104-191) (HIPAA). Many of the OIG's recommendations relate directly to billing and collections, including assigning responsibility for gathering the information for the billing and coding of medical claims. The Medicare website for medical office education, www.cms.hhs.gov/medlearn/cbts.asp, notes how accountability is typically assigned in a medical office, and that information provided the basis on which accountability is addressed in this chapter. However, please remember that each medical office decides exactly which employee positions are assigned individual accountability for each task, and it will vary from one office to another. In addition, in a small medical office, one multiskilled professional often fills numerous employee positions.

The **CMS-1500 claim form,** previously called the HCFA-1500 claim form, was designed for Medicare but is now used universally for physician and supplier billing. The patient is always responsible for supplying current patient demographic and medical plan information for billing, but the receptionist is usually the employee held accountable for gathering patient-supplied information and identifying all possible payors. The receptionist usually enters this information in the computer system. The computer system often generates the claim form, and it pulls information entered from the patient registration form to automatically complete the top half of the CMS-1500 claim form.

Although the patient may list payors in any order in the insurance section of the registration form, the patient is not authorized to choose which payor is listed as the primary payor on the CMS-1500 claim form. Specific rules must be followed. As you learn these rules in Chapters 8, 9, 10, and 11, you will be able to determine the primary payor from the information the patient supplies. The biller is typically held accountable for determining the primary payor, for checking to see whether additional information is required for the specific payor(s), and for meeting payor-specific preferences when evaluating and sometimes correcting the information previously entered in the computer system.

The physician (or other provider) is always responsible for supplying the diagnoses and a description of services rendered. Often this information is sent to the billing department on a superbill, but the receptionist usually enters the information from the superbill into the computer system during patient checkout procedures. The computer pulls the information entered from the superbill to automatically complete the bottom half of the claim form.

The biller is usually the employee held accountable for double-checking the accuracy of all the information placed on the CMS-1500 claim forms before the claims are sent. This may be done using the preview feature in the software, or claims may be printed on plain paper and a transparency of a blank claim can be placed on top to show the fields on the claim form. The biller uses the computer system to correct any errors that are found before the claims are sent.

As you learn the coding rules in Chapters 5, 6, and 7, you will learn how to either confirm the information supplied by the physician on the billing form (e.g., superbill, encounter form) or to convert the diagnoses and procedures listed on the billing form into the correct medical codes. You will also learn to audit the medical records by comparing the billing information listed on the superbill with the documentation in the medical records to see whether it matches. In addition, you will learn to sequence the codes correctly. Following these steps increases the likelihood that correct reimbursement will be received in a timely manner from the payor. Many practices hire certified coders to perform coding functions, and those practices typically assign accountability for the codes selected to the person who performed the coding. Other practices give the responsibility for code selection to either the biller or the physician.

When payors and government officials talk about keeping medical costs low, what they really mean is negotiating contracted payment amounts that are low (e.g., with hospitals, physicians, and other health-care providers). Government payors, private payors, and managed care payors are all very conscientious about keeping medical costs as low as possible and limiting medical fraud and abuse, and they use every means at their disposal (legal or not) to reduce payments. There have been many news reports in recent years of payor/physician contracts that contained illegal clauses, and of payors who tried to enforce the illegal clauses even when presented with legal challenges. According to contract law, illegal clauses are not legally enforceable. However, payors can try to enforce contracts that physicians have signed. It is better to find these clauses and remove the illegal clauses before the contract is signed.

When submitting a medical claim, you must address even the smallest of details, and you must be accurate. When the medical claim reaches the payor, *the computer system or the assigned claims adjuster looks first for any reason not to pay the claim.* If a reason to deny payment is not found, payment is authorized. Next, the computer system or the claims adjustor looks for any reason to pay the smallest amount possible. The payors are not being mean. They are merely fulfilling one of their financial responsibilities. They are obligated to pay valid claims, but they are not obligated to pay inaccurate claims. If a physician's office sent you a bill that was not accurate, and in fact overcharged you, would you sit right down and pay it promptly without asking any questions? If you would not do it, is it reasonable to expect a payor to do it?

The explanation of benefits (EOB) or the Medicare remittance notice (MRN) that accompanies payment or denial of payment for a medical claim is supposed to explain the payment decision, but often the explanation given is very vague. An EOB may say "insufficient data" as a reason for nonpayment but not tell you which information is missing. This is because many times when information changes in one field, the requirement for information in other fields also changes. The payor usually does not know what else might be wrong. By learning claim form requirements, you will learn how to detect missing information and check for other fields that might also require changes.

Many times a minor detail, such as not answering either "yes" or "no" to a question, can cause a delay in payment. Sometimes the diagnosis and the service billed do not seem to correlate. The payor will want more information from the physician before paying the claim. Payment might be denied if the physician's written record is not an exact match for the information submitted on the claim form. Other times, a payor might decide that the service is not covered by the medical plan or the service is not medically necessary (meaning at least one diagnosis in block No. 24E is not an adequate or an appropriate reason to perform the service on that line).

The rules for completing and submitting a claim form can vary, depending on whether you send the claim electronically or on paper. When you send a paper claim, use a barcoded "dropout red" CMS-1500 claim form. Most payors scan paper claims into their computer systems. The color of the form is called dropout red because the scanner does not read or record that color; it only reads and records the information placed in each block on the claim form. The barcode tells the payor's computer how to line up the information so the computer can correctly record the information in the corresponding computer fields and then read it correctly using optical character recognition **(OCR).** Do not use correction fluid on claims that will be scanned because correction fluid smears in the scanner. Instead, use correction tape. When there is no barcode to tell the payor's computer how to line up the information or when other OCR requirements have not been met, a claims adjustor usually must enter the claim into the payor's computer manually, and this increases the possibility of an error occurring after the claim leaves your office.

Electronic claims are sent using national electronic data interchange **(EDI)** standards. Some standards are built into the claims transmission software, and others you must meet as you prepare the claim. You have the best control over claim quality when you meet EDI standards for all electronic claims and when you meet OCR requirements for all paper claims. OCR and EDI requirements, when applicable, are noted throughout the chapter.

The CMS-1500 is the universal claim form used by physicians, other providers, and suppliers to bill payors for services rendered and for supplies. The front of the claim form (Figure 4-1) contains blocks or fields that are completed to meet specific payor requirements. The back of the claim form (Figure 4-2) provides a general guideline for all medical plans, a statement of legal responsibility, and information and directions tailored for specific government medical plans.

Patient and Insurance Information

Every medical claim is a legal document. The top half of the CMS-1500 medical claim form is used to report patient demographic and medical plan billing information. The right-side margin of the CMS-1500 claim form has a note printed sideways that says *carrier* with arrows that indicate the top margin. The carrier is the primary payor. The right-side margin on the top half of the CMS-1500 claim form also says *patient and **insured** information,* printed sideways with arrows that indicate block No. 1 through block No. 13. It is the patient's responsibility to provide the most current and accurate information for every claim that is filed on his or her behalf. Knowingly supplying false or inaccurate information is considered a federal crime (fraud), punishable by fines, imprisonment, or both.

When the scheduler faithfully gathers insurance and demographic information at the time each appointment is scheduled, every patient, even new patients, will have information on file for advance verification and for comparison to the insurance card and registration documents completed during check-in.

The receptionist is usually the employee held accountable for gathering billing information from each patient during check-in and for identifying all possible payors. It is easy to become complacent with established patients, but the receptionist must verify billing information for each encounter. Established patients can and do change insurance policies from time to time, and sometimes patients fail to pay premiums or to qualify for government programs and are dropped from coverage.

Occasionally, a patient requires treatment after a new insurance policy takes effect but before the patient receives an insurance ID card for the new plan. It is acceptable to take the insurance information verbally or in handwritten form, but you should call the insurance company to verify the ID numbers, mailing address, level of coverage, and copay amounts before the appointment or before the patient leaves the office so other payment arrangements can be made if the information is not correct. Instruct the patient to send you a copy of the front and back of the card for your files when the card does arrive.

It is the biller's responsibility to compare the patient information gathered during check-in with the existing information already on file. When a discrepancy is noted, the biller must verify which information is correct and update the patient's financial record. Sometimes you must call the patient to obtain current information when that step was missed during check-in.

The primary payor is the medical plan that is responsible for paying when there is no other coverage and the medical plan that pays first when there is coverage from more than one payor. A secondary payor pays second and tertiary payor pays third when there is more than one payor.

If you want to file clean claims and receive correct payments the first time, you must learn to look at each claim through the payor's eyes. When a claim arrives at the payor, the claim editing and claim auditing processes begin immediately. The first items the claims adjustor or the payor's computer checks are those located in the top half of the claim form. When any of the following information is incorrect, there is no obligation for payment, and the claim might be rejected. The payor wants to know:

❑ Was the claim sent to the correct address as listed on the patient's insurance card? Each payor has different billing addresses for different policies. When the claim is sent to the wrong billing address for the specific policy, the payor's computer will not recognize the patient.

❑ Is the person listed as insured for each payor on the claim form covered under that plan?

❑ Is the patient covered by each listed plan?

❑ Is the insurance policy current, meaning, have the premiums been paid?

❑ Is the correct payor identified as primary payor? If not, there is no obligation for payment until correct information is submitted. A secondary payor only pays charges remaining after the

PLEASE
DO NOT
STAPLE
IN THIS
AREA

CARRIER

PICA

HEALTH INSURANCE CLAIM FORM

PICA

1. MEDICARE (Medicare #) | MEDICAID (Medicaid #) | CHAMPUS (Sponsor's SSN) | CHAMPVA (VA File #) | GROUP HEALTH PLAN (SSN or ID) | FECA BLK LUNG (SSN) | OTHER (ID)

1a. INSURED'S I.D. NUMBER (FOR PROGRAM IN ITEM 1)

2. PATIENT'S NAME (Last Name, First Name, Middle Initital)

3. PATIENT'S BIRTH DATE MM | DD | YY — SEX M F

4. INSURED'S NAME (Last Name, First Name, Middle Initial)

5. PATIENT'S ADDRESS (No., Street)

6. PATIENT RELATIONSHIP TO INSURED — Self Spouse Child Other

7. INSURED'S ADDRESS (No., Street)

CITY — STATE

8. PATIENT STATUS — Single Married Other; Employed Full-Time Student Part-Time Student

CITY — STATE

ZIP CODE — TELEPHONE (Include Area Code) ( )

ZIP CODE — TELEPHONE (INCLUDE AREA CODE) ( )

9. OTHER INSURED'S NAME (Last Name, First Name, Middle Initial)

10. IS PATIENT'S CONDITION RELATED TO:

11. INSURED'S POLICY GROUP OR FECA NUMBER

a. OTHER INSURED'S POLICY OR GROUP NUMBER

a. EMPLOYMENT? (CURRENT OR PREVIOUS) YES NO

a. INSURED'S DATE OF BIRTH MM | DD | YY — SEX M F

b. OTHER INSURED'S DATE OF BIRTH MM | DD | YY — SEX M F

b. AUTO ACCIDENT? YES NO — PLACE (State)

b. EMPLOYER'S NAME OR SCHOOL NAME

c. EMPLOYER'S NAME OR SCHOOL NAME

c. OTHER ACCIDENT? YES NO

c. INSURANCE PLAN NAME OR PROGRAM NAME

d. INSURANCE PLAN NAME OR PROGRAM NAME

10d. RESERVED FOR LOCAL USE

d. IS THERE ANOTHER HEALTH BENEFIT PLAN? YES NO *If yes*, return to and complete item 9 a-d.

READ BACK OF FORM BEFORE COMPLETING & SIGNING THIS FORM.

12. PATIENT'S OR AUTHORIZED PERSON'S SIGNATURE I authorize the release of any medical or other information necessary to process this claim. I also request payment of government benefits either to myself or to the party who accepts assignment below.

SIGNED ________ DATE ________

13. INSURED'S OR AUTHORIZED PERSON'S SIGNATURE I authorize payment of medical benefits to the undersigned physician or supplier for services described below.

SIGNED ________

PATIENT AND INSURED INFORMATION

14. DATE OF CURRENT: MM | DD | YY — ILLNESS (First symptom) OR INJURY (Accident) OR PREGNANCY(LMP)

15. IF PATIENT HAS HAD SAME OR SIMILAR ILLNESS. GIVE FIRST DATE MM | DD | YY

16. DATES PATIENT UNABLE TO WORK IN CURRENT OCCUPATION FROM MM | DD | YY TO MM | DD | YY

17. NAME OF REFERRING PHYSICIAN OR OTHER SOURCE

17a. I.D. NUMBER OF REFERRING PHYSICIAN

18. HOSPITALIZATION DATES RELATED TO CURRENT SERVICES FROM MM | DD | YY TO MM | DD | YY

19. RESERVED FOR LOCAL USE

20. OUTSIDE LAB? YES NO — $ CHARGES

21. DIAGNOSIS OR NATURE OF ILLNESS OR INJURY. (RELATE ITEMS 1,2,3 OR 4 TO ITEM 24E BY LINE)

1. ___ . __
2. ___ . __
3. ___ . __
4. ___ . __

22. MEDICAID RESUBMISSION CODE — ORIGINAL REF. NO.

23. PRIOR AUTHORIZATION NUMBER

24. A DATE(S) OF SERVICE From MM DD YY	To MM DD YY	B Place of Service	C Type of Service	D PROCEDURES, SERVICES, OR SUPPLIES (Explain Unusual Circumstances) CPT/HCPCS | MODIFIER	E DIAGNOSIS CODE	F $ CHARGES	G DAYS OR UNITS	H EPSDT Family Plan	I EMG	J COB	K RESERVED FOR LOCAL USE
1											
2											
3											
4											
5											
6											

PHYSICIAN OR SUPPLIER INFORMATION

25. FEDERAL TAX I.D. NUMBER — SSN EIN

26. PATIENT'S ACCOUNT NO.

27. ACCEPT ASSIGNMENT? (For govt. claims, see back) YES NO

28. TOTAL CHARGE $

29. AMOUNT PAID $

30. BALANCE DUE $

31. SIGNATURE OF PHYSICIAN OR SUPPLIER INCLUDING DEGREES OR CREDENTIALS (I certify that the statements on the reverse apply to this bill and are made a part thereof.)

SIGNED DATE

32. NAME AND ADDRESS OF FACILITY WHERE SERVICES WERE RENDERED (If other than home or office)

33. PHYSICIAN'S, SUPPLIER'S BILLING NAME, ADDRESS, ZIP CODE & PHONE #

PIN# GRP#

(APPROVED BY AMA COUNCIL ON MEDICAL SERVICE 8/88) **PLEASE PRINT OR TYPE** APPROVED OMB-0938-0008 FORM CMS-1500 (12-90), FORM RRB-1500, APPROVED OMB-1215-0055 FORM OWCP-1500, APPROVED OMB-0720-0001 (CHAMPUS)

FIGURE 4-1

CMS-1500 claim form, front. The CMS-1500 is the universal claim form used by physicians, other providers, and suppliers to bill payors for services rendered and for supplies. This side of the claim form contains blocks or fields that are completed to meet specific payor requirements. *Note:* A different claim form is used by facilities such as hospitals and surgicenters to bill payors for facility fees.

BECAUSE THIS FORM IS USED BY VARIOUS GOVERNMENT AND PRIVATE HEALTH PROGRAMS, SEE SEPARATE INSTRUCTIONS ISSUED BY APPLICABLE PROGRAMS.

NOTICE: Any person who knowingly files a statement of claim containing any misrepresentation or any false, incomplete or misleading information may be guilty of a criminal act punishable under law and may be subject to civil penalties.

REFERS TO GOVERNMENT PROGRAMS ONLY

MEDICARE AND CHAMPUS PAYMENTS: A patient's signature requests that payment be made and authorizes release of any information necessary to process the claim and certifies that the information provided in Blocks 1 through 12 is true, accurate and complete. In the case of a Medicare claim, the patient's signature authorizes any entity to release to Medicare medical and nonmedical information, including employment status, and whether the person has employer group health insurance, liability, no-fault, worker's compensation or insurance which is responsible to pay for the services for which the Medicare claim is made. See 42 CFR 411.24(a). If item 9 is completed, the patient's signature authorizes release of the information to the health plan or agency shown. In Medicare assigned or CHAMPUS participation cases, the physician agrees to accept the charge determination of the Medicare carrier or CHAMPUS fiscal intermediary as the full charge, and the patient is responsible only for the deductible, coinsurance and noncovered services. Coinsurance and the deductible are based upon the charge determination of the Medicare carrier or CHAMPUS fiscal intermediary if this is less than the charge submitted. CHAMPUS is not a health insurance program but makes payment for health benefits provided through certain affiliations with the Uniformed Services. Information on the patient's sponsor should be provided in those items captioned in "Insured"; i.e., items 1a, 4, 6, 7, 9, and 11.

BLACK LUNG AND FECA CLAIMS

The provider agrees to accept the amount paid by the Government as payment in full. See Black Lung and FECA instructions regarding required procedure and diagnosis coding systems.

SIGNATURE OF PHYSICIAN OR SUPPLIER (MEDICARE, CHAMPUS, FECA AND BLACK LUNG)

I certify that the services shown on this form were medically indicated and necessary for the health of the patient and were personally furnished by me or were furnished incident to my professional service by my employee under my immediate personal supervision, except as otherwise expressly permitted by Medicare or CHAMPUS regulations.

For services to be considered as "incident" to a physician's professional service, 1) they must be rendered under the physician's immediate personal supervision by his/her employee, 2) they must be an integral, although incidental part of a covered physician's service, 3) they must be of kinds commonly furnished in physician's offices, and 4) the services of nonphysicians must be included on the physician's bills.

For CHAMPUS claims, I further certify that I (or any employee) who rendered services am not an active duty member of the Uniformed Services or a civilian employee of the United States Government or a contract employee of the United States Government, either civilian or military (refer to 5 USC 5536). For Black-Lung claims, I further certify that the services performed were for a Black Lung-related disorder.

No Part B Medicare benefits may be paid unless this form is received as required by existing law and regulations (42 CFR 424.32).

NOTICE: Any one who misrepresents or falsifies essential information to receive payment from Federal funds requested by this form may upon conviction be subject to fine and imprisonment under applicable Federal laws.

NOTICE TO PATIENT ABOUT THE COLLECTION AND USE OF MEDICARE, CHAMPUS, FECA AND BLACK LUNG INFORMATION
(PRIVACY ACT STATEMENT)

We are authorized by CMS, CHAMPUS and OWCP to ask you for information needed in the administration of the Medicare, CHAMPUS, FECA, and Black Lung programs. Authority to collect information is in section 205(a), 1862, 1872, and 1874 of the Social Security Act as amended, 42 CFR 411.24(a) and 424.5(a) (6), and 44 USC 3101;41 CFR 101 et seq and 10 USC 1079 and 1086; 5 USC 8101 et seq; and 30 USC 901 et seq; 38 USC 613; E.O. 9397.

The information we obtain to complete claims under these programs is used to identify you and to determine you eligibility. It is also used to decide if the services and supplies you received are covered by these programs and to insure that proper payment is made.

The information may also be given to other providers of services, carriers, intermediaries, medical review boards, health plans, and other organizations or Federal agencies, for the effective administration of Federal provisions that require other third parties payers to pay primary to Federal program, and as otherwise necessary to administer these programs. For example, it may be necessary to disclose information about the benefits you have used to a hospital or doctor. Additional disclosures are made through routine uses for information contained in systems of records.

FOR MEDICARE CLAIMS: See the notice modifying system No. 09-70-0501, titled, 'Carrier Medicare Claims Record,' published in the <u>Federal Register</u>, Vol. 55 No. 177, page 37549, Wed. Sept. 12, 1990, or as updated and republished.

FOR OWCP CLAIMS: Department of Labor, Privacy Act of 1974, "Republication of Notice of Systems of Records, " <u>Federal Register</u> Vol. 55 No. 40, Wed Feb. 28, 1990, See ESA-5, ESA-6, ESA-12, ESA-13, ESA-30, or as updated and republished.

FOR CHAMPUS CLAIMS: <u>PRINCIPLE PURPOSE(S)</u>: To evaluate eligibility for medical care provided by civilian sources and to issue payment upon establishment of eligibility and determination that the services/supplies received are authorized by law.

<u>ROUTINE USE(S)</u>: Information from claims and related documents may be given to the Dept. of Veterans Affairs, the Dept. of Health and Human Services and/or the Dept. of Transportation consistent with their statutory administrative responsibilities under CHAMPUS/CHAMPVA; to the Dept. of Justice for representation of the Secretary of Defense in civil actions; to the Internal Revenue Service, private collection agencies, and consumer reporting agencies in connection with recoupment claims; and to Congressional Offices in response to inquiries made at the request of the person to whom a record pertains. Appropriate disclosures may be made to other federal, state, local, foreign government agencies, private business entities, and individual providers of care, on matters relating to entitlement, claims adjudication, fraud, program abuse, utilization review, quality assurance, peer review, program integrity, third-party liability, coordination of benefits, and civil and criminal litigation related to the operation of CHAMPUS.

<u>DISCLOSURES</u>: Voluntary; however, failure to provide information will result in delay in payment or may result in denial of claim. With the one exception discussed below, there are no penalties under these programs for refusing to supply information. However, failure to furnish information regarding the medical services rendered or the amount charged would prevent payment of claims under these programs. Failure to furnish any other information, such as name or claim number, would delay payment of the claim. Failure to provide medical information under FECA could be deemed an obstruction.

It is mandatory that you tell us if you know that another party is responsible for paying for your treatment. Section 1128B of the Social Security Act and 31 USC 3801–3812 provide penalties for withholding this information.

You should be aware that P.L. 100-503, the "Computer Matching and Privacy Protection Act of 1988", permits the government to verify information by way of computer matches.

MEDICAID PAYMENTS (PROVIDER CERTIFICATION)

I hereby agree to keep such records as are necessary to disclose fully the extent of services provided to individuals under the State's Title XIX plan and to furnish information regarding any payments claimed for providing such services as the State Agency or Dept. of Health and Humans Services may request.

I further agree to accept, as payment in full, the amount paid by the Medicaid program for those claims submitted for payment under that program, with the exception of authorized deductible, coinsurance, co-payment or similar cost-sharing charge.

SIGNATURE OF PHYSICIAN (OR SUPPLIER): I certify that the services listed above were medically indicated and necessary to the health of this patient and were personally furnished by me or my employee under my personal direction.

NOTICE: This is to certify that the foregoing information is true, accurate and complete. I understand that payment and satisfaction of this claim will be from Federal and State funds, and that any false claims, statements, or documents, or concealment of a material fact, may be prosecuted under applicable Federal or State laws.

According to the Paperwork Reduction Act of 1995, no persons are required to respond to a collection of information unless it displays a valid OMB control number. The valid OMB control number for this information collection is 0938-0008. The time required to complete this information collection is estimated to average 10 minutes per response, including the time to review instructions, search existing data resources, gather the data needed, and complete and review the information collection. If you have any comments concerning the accuracy of the time estimate(s) or suggestions for improving this form, please write to: CMS, N2-14-26, 7500 Security Boulevard, Baltimore, Maryland 21244-1850.

FIGURE 4-2

CMS-1500 claim form, back. This side of the claim form provides a general guideline for all medical plans, a statement of legal responsibility, and information and directions tailored for specific government medical plans.

primary payor has paid. A tertiary payor only pays charges remaining after the secondary payor has paid.

☐ Does the demographic information for both the patient and the insured match payor records? If not, the claim will be rejected until it can be verified that the patient is covered by the plan.

Let's take a closer look at specific claim requirements for the top half of the CMS-1500.

TOP MARGIN

Figure 4-3 shows the top margin of the CMS-1500 claim form. *This is a required field.* The name and mailing address of the primary payor are printed on the right half of the top margin of the CMS-1500 claim form. The left half of the top margin is reserved for the barcode.

Windowed envelopes, such as those shown in Figure 4-4, are often used to mail paper claims. The payor's name and address show through the window as "addressee," so the information recorded here must meet postal requirements.

The patient's insurance card should list a mailing address for the payor. The mailing address is often located on the back of the card. This is why you must obtain a legible photocopy of both the front and back of each insurance card for each patient. If the information on the card is illegible in the photocopy, handwrite the information on the same page next to the illegible image. You also may call a patient if you cannot read the required information on the photocopy.

Sometimes a payor/physician contract changes the mailing address for claims to a particular payor or payor(s). Therefore you should check for contract requirements, if any.

Payor name and address are required in the top margin of the claim even when claims are transmitted electronically. When electronic claims arrive at a claims clearinghouse, only the claims that meet EDI requirements can be forwarded to payors electronically. The rest are dropped to paper (printed on a paper CMS-1500 claim form) at the clearinghouse, and a machine automatically folds them, stuffs them into windowed envelopes, and mails them.

Even when the payor mailing address is missing, electronic claims that drop to paper are automatically mailed. This is done by machine. A person does not usually check to see if postal requirements are valid for every one of the thousands of claims dropping to paper each day. The post office eventually returns claims with no mailing address to the clearinghouse as undeliverable mail. The clearinghouse must then investigate to find out where each claim originated—perhaps your office. Weeks can easily pass before you learn that the payor did not receive the claim. If the payor contract has a 60-day deadline for filing "clean" claims and 60 days have already passed, you can no longer expect to receive payment for that claim.

> When a patient has more than one payor, the claim filed to the primary payor has "P" printed in the top left margin under "Please do not staple in this area" and above the three small boxes. Secondary claims have "S," and tertiary claims have "T" instead of "P." Usually computerized billing systems automatically generate this information based on the manner in which payors are identified for each patient. However, the biller should type in this detail when claims are prepared without the aid of a computer.

Payor-specific requirements:

TRICARE/CHAMPUS: When the patient lives in the United States and travels within the United States, claims are sent to the region for the patient's home address. When the patient lives overseas, but receives medical care in the USA, the following rules apply:

☐ If the patient is not enrolled in TRICARE Prime, the claim is sent to the TRICARE claim address for the CHAMPUS region in which the care is rendered.

☐ If the patient is enrolled in TRICARE Prime, the claim is sent to the contractor that processes all overseas claims: WPS in Madison, Wisconsin.

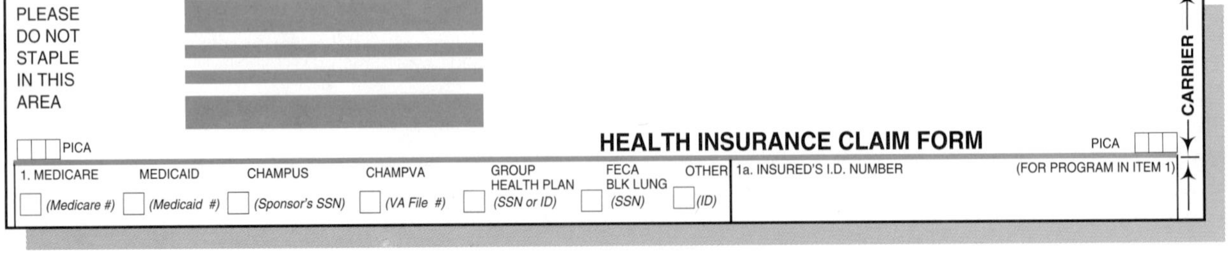

FIGURE 4-3
Top margin of the CMS-1500 and block No. 1-block No. 1a.

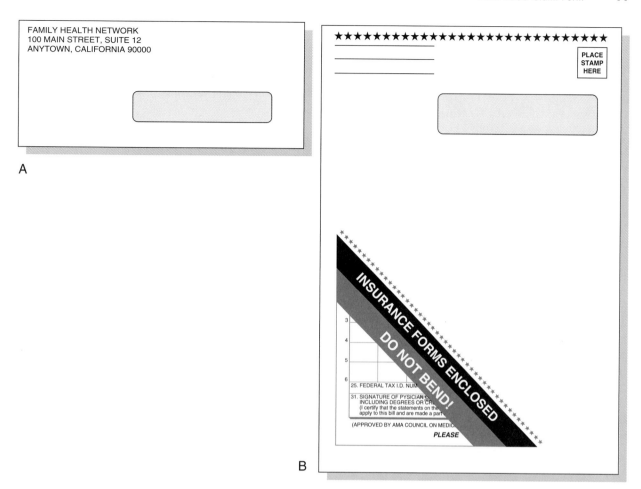

FIGURE 4-4
Windowed envelopes are often used to mail paper claims. The payor's name and address show through the window. (Courtesy Bibbero Systems, Inc., Petaluma, Calif 94954; 800/242-2376; www.bibberosystems.com.)

BLOCK NO. 1. PAYOR TYPE

Figure 4-3 shows block No. 1. *This is a required field.* The type of primary payor is indicated with an "X" placed in the box preceding the payor type. Valid selections are Medicare, Medicaid, CHAMPUS, CHAMPVA, Group Health Plan, FECA, and Other. The type of number required in block No. 1a is listed in parentheses under each payor type in this field.

Payor-specific requirements:

Medicare: Anytime Medicare is primary, even with Medicare Advantage plans (Medicare + Choice), Medicare should be marked in this field. Originally, Medicare Advantage claims were sent to Medicare, but now they are sent to the payor with whom the patient contracted for coverage. See Chapter 10 for further details about the Medicare Advantage programs.

Blue Cross Blue Shield: The traditional Blue Cross Blue Shield plans fall under "group health plan."

Managed Care: Sometimes managed care HMOs and PPOs, including Blue Cross Blue Shield HMOs and PPOs, want to be listed as a "group health plan," and sometimes they want to be listed as "other."

Workers' Compensation: For workers' compensation, mark "other."

Do not give the claims adjuster a reason to reject your claim. If you do not know the correct choice, call the payor and ask. The payor's telephone number can be found on the patient's insurance card. Often it is located on the back of the card, near the mailing address.

Document the phone call and the response in the patient's financial record so you do not have to call each time you file a claim for this patient. If you keep your own payor-specific insurance notes or notebook, also record the information there.

The Black Lung program is a federal medical program that covers qualified coal miners that suffer from anthracosis, also known as "black lung," because it is caused by coal dust in the lungs.

Block No. 1a. Insured's ID Number

Figure 4-3 shows block No. 1a. *This is a required field.* The patient-specific ID number for the primary payor goes in this field. The insured's ID number is normally found on the patient's insurance card. Sometimes it is called a member number. The payor uses this information to confirm that the patient is indeed entitled to receive benefits. Claims will not be paid without this information.

The insured is the **policyholder,** the person whose name is listed in the medical plan's files as the owner of the policy. Some medical plans call the insured the **"subscriber,"** and Medicare calls the insured the **"beneficiary."** The *employee* is the insured for an individual or a family medical plan obtained through an employer, and the *employer* is the insured for workers' compensation.

The insured's ID number is often, but not always, based on the insured's Social Security number **(SSN).** Do not make assumptions. Check the insurance card. A notation in parenthesis under the payor type in block No. 1 tells the type of number required in block No. 1a. The number listed here must be valid for the insurance plan indicated in block No. 1 and named in block No. 11c.

If the patient is covered by a family policy, sometimes this number will be the same for all covered family members. However, this is becoming rare. More often, the insured's ID number will vary for each covered person. For example, sometimes this number will be the policyholder's SSN followed by a dash and "01" to designate the policyholder, "02" to designate the spouse, "03" to designate one child, "04" to designate the next child, and so on until each person covered by the policy has been given a unique insured's ID number. The insured's ID number is not always based on a SSN. Always get the number from the insurance card.

EDI and OCR do not recognize dashes, slashes, decimal points, and other special characters. Do not enter dashes in this box, and do not leave blank spaces unless specifically directed to do so.

Payor-specific requirements:

TRICARE/CHAMPUS: Enter the military sponsor's military ID number.

Workers' Compensation: Although the "insured" is the patient's employer, enter the patient's SSN in this field.

BLOCK NO. 2. PATIENT NAME

Figure 4-5 shows block No. 2 of the CMS-1500 claim form. *This is a required field.* Enter the name as last name, first name, middle initial (when applicable). The patient's name must be spelled exactly as it appears on the insurance card. Do not enter commas between last name and first name.

The name entered here is the name of the patient—the person who received the treatment(s) or service(s) listed on the claim form. Only one patient name may be entered on each claim form. If a parent brought two children to see the physician, and the physician looked at both of them during the same visit, a separate claim form must be submitted for each child. When you are filing a batch of claims for patients who have similar names, be very careful to verify that each piece of information is completed for the correct person.

The name entered here should be the patient's legal name. However, if the patient has changed names, such as occurs when a woman marries, do not change the name in your records until the insurance card lists the new legal name. The name in the medical record must match the name on the claim form. If the claim is filed using the new name before the payor changes their records, the payor will not recognize the patient, and the claim will be denied. However, be sure to list the correct information in block No. 8 under marital status. Also, call the payor to see if coverage changed when the patient married. A dependent daughter who marries is no longer covered under a parent's policy. Knowingly supplying false or inaccurate information is considered a federal crime and is punishable by fines, imprisonment, or both.

Be very careful with your record-keeping during the interval between the time a patient's name legally changes and the time the payor recognizes the new name. Your medical office must have a record of both

2. PATIENT'S NAME (Last Name, First Name, Middle Initital)	3. PATIENT'S BIRTH DATE MM	DD	YY	SEX	4. INSURED'S NAME (Last Name, First Name, Middle Initial)
		M ☐	F ☐	

FIGURE 4-5

Block No. 2–block No. 4 of the CMS-1500 claim form.

the old name and the new name and a method to identify that both names belong to the same person. The patient will probably call the office to schedule appointments using the new name, so you must be able to find information both ways. Remember, the old name must be listed with the current marital status on both the claim and the medical record until the new name is recognized by the payor.

BLOCK NO. 3. PATIENT BIRTH DATE AND GENDER

Figure 4-5 shows block No. 3. *This is a required field.* If either the birth date or the gender is missing, the claim could be rejected. The information entered here is used to verify the identity of the patient.

Birth Date: Enter the patient's date of birth with an eight-digit date.

The patient's birth date must be earlier than any of the other dates listed on the claim, such as date of service, date of claim, date of procedure, and/or date of accident. A pregnant woman is considered to be the patient for both herself and the unborn child she is carrying.

To meet EDI and OCR requirements, use only numbers for dates, and do not enter slashes or dashes. For OCR, the date is entered as MMDDYYYY. For example, March 7, 2005, would be entered as "03072005." For EDI, the date is entered as YYYYMMDD. For example, March 7, 2001, would be entered as "20050307." If you use a claims clearinghouse, enter all dates using OCR guidelines and the clearinghouse will translate the dates to EDI requirements for the claims that are actually sent electronically.

Gender: select the appropriate gender code, "M" for male, "F" for female. Some procedures have gender-specific codes. For example, only a female would have a vaginal exam, and only a male would have a prostate exam. When the gender marked on the claim does not match the gender documented in payor records for the covered patient, or the gender marked on the claim does not match the gender specified for the procedure, the claim will be denied.

BLOCK NO. 4. INSURED'S NAME

Figure 4-5 shows block No. 4. Enter the name of the *insured* individual. When the patient is the insured, this block may be left blank or you may write "same." This block is used only when *the patient is not the policyholder.*

A family policy is issued to one specific person even though it provides coverage for the entire family. When an employer issues a family policy, the employee to whom the policy was issued is the named insured, and the name of the employee would be listed here when another covered family member is the patient.

Payor-specific requirements:

Medicare: Medicare requires this section to be blank except in certain situations when Medicare is the secondary payor. This field is completed only when the Medicare patient is not the policyholder for the other policy.

- ❑ When a Medicare patient is also covered by their spouse's medical plan, then the spouse's medical plan is the primary payor. The name of the spouse, the policyholder for the primary payor, is entered here. (Medicare is the secondary payor; the Medicare patient is not the policyholder for the primary payor.)
- ❑ When the Medicare patient is the policyholder for the other medical plan, the primary policy, this section is left blank. (Medicare is the secondary payor; the Medicare patient is the policyholder for the primary payor.)

Workers' Compensation: List the employer as the policyholder.

TRICARE/CHAMPUS: Enter the name of the military sponsor.

BLOCK NO. 5. PATIENT ADDRESS

Figure 4-6 shows block No. 5 of the CMS-1500 claim form. *This is a required field.* Enter the patient's address, including number, street, city, state, and zip code. An address is required on all claims. List the patient's telephone number with area code.

The information in this field must match the information on file with the payor, or the payor will not recognize the patient, and the claim will be denied. If the patient has moved recently, call the payor to verify the address to be listed on the claim, and remind the patient to update his or her address with the payor.

When the patient lives in a nursing home or other extended-care facility, provide the facility's address.

Some insurance companies require a telephone number. If the patient does not have one, ask the patient for the telephone number of a close friend or relative.

If the payor requires a telephone number and the patient cannot provide one, call the payor and ask

5. PATIENT'S ADDRESS (No., Street)			6. PATIENT RELATIONSHIP TO INSURED Self ☐ Spouse ☐ Child ☐ Other ☐	7. INSURED'S ADDRESS (No., Street)	
CITY		STATE	8. PATIENT STATUS Single ☐ Married ☐ Other ☐	CITY	STATE
ZIP CODE	TELEPHONE (Include Area Code) ( )		Employed ☐ Full-Time ☐ Part-Time ☐ Student Student	ZIP CODE	TELEPHONE (INCLUDE AREA CODE) ( )

FIGURE 4-6
Block No. 5-block No. 8 of the CMS-1500 claim form.

for the telephone number listed in the payor's files for the patient.

As a last resort, when the payor requires a telephone number and no other telephone number is available, list the national information number—the patient's area code plus 555-1212.

Payor-specific requirements:

TRICARE/CHAMPUS: When the patient lives overseas but is receiving medical care in the United States, the patient's overseas home address is used on the claim.

BLOCK NO. 6. PATIENT RELATIONSHIP TO INSURED

Figure 4-6 shows block No. 6. *This is a required field.* The choices are "Self," "Spouse," "Child," or "Other." The information in this block tells the payor how the patient is related to the policyholder, so the payor may verify that the patient is covered by one of their policies. Claims are not paid without this information.

If the patient is the policyholder, choose "Self." Do not expect the insurance company to assume that the patient is the insured just because the names are the same. Many parents name their children after themselves.

When you choose "Spouse," "Child," or "Other," you are telling the payor that the policy is listed in another person's name, even when the patient and the policyholder share the same name. The payor will then look to be sure block No. 4 and block No. 7 have been completed for the policyholder. If they have not, the claim will be rejected. The EOB reason code will probably say "Patient not covered" because the payor cannot verify coverage.

Even when everything else on the form is correct (including information about the insured when different from the patient), if this section is left blank, you risk a rejection. Payors receive many claim forms that have been completed incorrectly. They will not make assumptions, and they will not make a selection for you.

Payor-specific requirements:

Workers' Compensation: Select "Other."

BLOCK NO. 7. INSURED'S ADDRESS

Figure 4-6 shows block No. 7. This field is required when block No. 4 is completed *and* the insured has a different address than the patient. If the insured and the patient have the same address, place "same" in this section.

This information must match payor records or the claim will be denied.

Some insurance companies require a telephone number. If the insured does not have one (or the patient does not know the insured's telephone number), list the patient's telephone number or list the telephone number of a close friend or relative of the insured.

If the payor requires a telephone number and the patient cannot provide one, call the payor and ask for the telephone number listed in the payor's files for the insured.

As a last resort, when the payor requires a telephone number and no other telephone number is available, list the national information number—the patient's area code plus 555-1212.

Payor-specific requirements:

TRICARE/CHAMPUS: Enter the home address for the military sponsor. If the patient does not know the military sponsor's home address (as may happen after a divorce), enter the patient's address.

Workers' Compensation: List the employer's address.

BLOCK NO. 8. PATIENT STATUS

Figure 4-6 shows block No. 8. This block records the employment, student, and marital status of the patient.

- ❏ The valid selection for employment is "Employed."
- ❏ The valid selections for student status are "Full-time student" or "Part-time student."

- ❐ The valid selections for marital status are "Single," "Married," and "Other."

Marital status: For marital status choose "Single," "Married," or "Other." The payor checks to see if this matches the information in their records. If the patient's marital status has changed, the patient is required by law to notify his or her medical plan. Claims are denied when the information does not match payor records.

Employed: If the patient is employed, put "X" in this box. If the patient is not employed, leave the box blank.

Student: If the patient is a student, select "Full-time" or "Part-time."

Most insurance companies will reject a claim if both "Employed" and "Full-time student" are selected. You may select both "Employed" and "Part-time student." This information is very important if the patient is a student older than age 18 covered under a parent's policy. Generally, a child older than age 18 is only covered under a parent's policy if he or she is a student or one who meets the disability requirements.

BLOCK NO. 9. OTHER INSURED'S NAME

Figure 4-7 shows block No. 9 of the CMS-1500 claim form. Enter the name of the insured for the secondary policy. This block is used to identify the policyholder for the second plan. When the patient is the insured for both the primary and the secondary plans, this field is left blank.

When a husband and a wife both have family policies issued by their respective employers, special rules apply. When the husband is the patient, his policy is always primary. When the wife is the patient, her policy is always primary. In both instances, the spouse's plan is secondary.

When both parents' policies cover the children, special rules apply:

- ❐ In some states, a choice must be made each time the family policies are renewed, and one policy must be designated as the primary policy for the children.
- ❐ In the remaining states (and if no choice has been made in a state that allows choice), the parent whose birthday comes earliest in the year is declared to be the primary policyholder for the children. This is called the birthday rule.

Payor-specific requirements:

Medicare: Medicare requires this section to be blank unless the patient is also covered by another plan. When block No. 9 is completed, block No. 13 must be completed. When the patient is the insured for the secondary policy (as in Medigap), enter "same" in this field.

Except for Medicaid, Medigap, and specific Medicare supplemental policies, Medicare is always the secondary payor when two health plans may be billed.

Only participating Medicare physicians and suppliers may complete block No. 9 and its subdivisions for Medicare patients, and they must have an "Assignment of Benefits" from the patient for both Medicare and the other policy. For example, when a Medicare patient is also covered by a spouse's health plan, a Medicare participating physician may complete this section when "Assignment of Benefits" is on file for both Medicare and the spouse's health plan. In this instance, the spouse's plan is primary and Medicare is secondary.

Nonparticipating Medicare physicians do not complete block No. 9 and its subdivisions. Medicare prohibits this because Medicare does not file crossover claims for nonparticipating physicians. Crossover claims occur when Medicare is the primary payor, and Medicare automatically forwards the claim with Medicare payment information to the secondary payor listed in block No. 9 and its subdivisions. Nonparticipating physicians file all secondary and tertiary claims themselves and

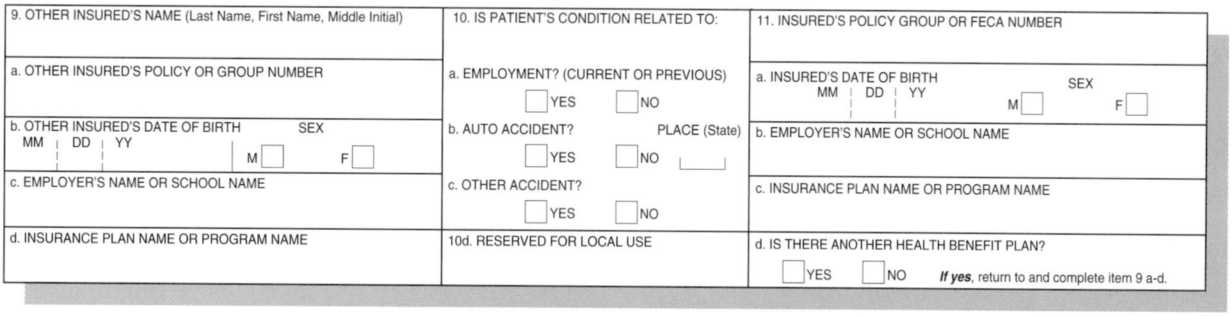
9. OTHER INSURED'S NAME (Last Name, First Name, Middle Initial)
a. OTHER INSURED'S POLICY OR GROUP NUMBER
b. OTHER INSURED'S DATE OF BIRTH MM DD YY SEX M F
c. EMPLOYER'S NAME OR SCHOOL NAME
d. INSURANCE PLAN NAME OR PROGRAM NAME
10. IS PATIENT'S CONDITION RELATED TO:
a. EMPLOYMENT? (CURRENT OR PREVIOUS) YES NO
b. AUTO ACCIDENT? PLACE (State) YES NO
c. OTHER ACCIDENT? YES NO
10d. RESERVED FOR LOCAL USE
11. INSURED'S POLICY GROUP OR FECA NUMBER
a. INSURED'S DATE OF BIRTH MM DD YY SEX M F
b. EMPLOYER'S NAME OR SCHOOL NAME
c. INSURANCE PLAN NAME OR PROGRAM NAME
d. IS THERE ANOTHER HEALTH BENEFIT PLAN? YES NO *If yes,* return to and complete item 9 a-d.

FIGURE 4-7
Block No. 9-block No. 11d of the CMS-1500 claim form.

include a copy of each MRN or EOB already received on the claim. They use the answer in block No. 11d ("Is there another health benefit plan?") combined with the letters above the PICA boxes in the top left margin of the claim form as the indicators for primary, secondary, or tertiary claim status.

Medigap: Only participating Medigap physicians and suppliers may list Medigap information in block No. 9 and its subdivisions. When block No. 9 is completed, block No. 13 must be completed.

A participating Medicare physician who is also a participating Medigap physician may complete this section when "Assignment of Benefits" is on file for both Medicare and Medigap. Anytime a patient has both Medicare and Medigap, Medicare is considered primary and Medigap is secondary.

Nonparticipating Medigap physicians do not complete block No. 9 and its subdivisions because Medicare does not file crossover claims for nonparticipating physicians. Nonparticipating Medigap physicians file all secondary claims themselves and include a copy of each MRN or EOB already received on the claim. They use the answer in block No. 11d ("Is there another health benefit plan?") combined with the letters above the PICA boxes in the top left margin of the claim form as the indicators for primary, secondary, or tertiary claim status.

Block No. 9a. Other Insured's Policy or Group Number

Figure 4-7 shows block No. 9a. This block is used to identify the secondary payor. Enter the individual or group policy number or FECA (Black Lung) number for the secondary payor. The information can be found on the insurance card for the secondary plan. If you cannot find the policy number on the insurance card, call the payor and ask them for the number. Most secondary payors require a number in this box.

To meet EDI and OCR requirements, do not enter dashes or other special characters in this box.

Payor-specific requirements:
Medicare: When Medicare is the secondary policy, enter the Medicare number here.
Medigap: The Medigap policy or group number must be preceded by the word "Medigap." For example, if the Medigap policy number is A-123-45, it should be entered as "Medigap A12345."

Block No. 9b. Other Insured's Date of Birth and Gender

Figure 4-7 shows block No. 9b. Enter the birth date and gender for the secondary policyholder or Medigap enrollee. When the patient is the insured

for both the primary and the secondary plans, this field is left blank.

Birth date: Enter the second policyholder's date of birth as an eight-digit date.

Gender: Enter the gender; "M" for male or "F" for female.

To meet EDI and OCR requirements, use only numbers for dates and do not enter slashes or dashes. For more details, see the directions for block No. 3.

Block No. 9c. Employer's Name or School Name

Figure 4-7 shows block No. 9c. If the secondary policy is from an employer, the employer's name is placed in this box. However, when the patient is a student who is old enough to be employed but who is covered by a parent's policy, the school should be listed in this box.

Payor-specific requirements:
Medicare: This field may be left blank.
Medigap: Enter the claims processing address listed on the patient's Medigap ID card. Use accepted postal abbreviations to enter an abbreviated street address, a two-letter state postal code, and a zip code.

Block No. 9d. Insurance Plan or Program Name for Second Policy

Figure 4-7 shows block No. 9d. Enter the name of the secondary insurance plan or program. This information is listed on the insurance card for the secondary payor and tells the payor the exact policy to reference for this claim.

Payor-specific requirements:
Medigap: Enter the name of the Medigap payor or the unique Medigap identifier assigned by the carrier. For Medicare crossover claims, use the Medigap identifier. This identifier is usually six letters (ABCDEF).

BLOCK NO. 10. PATIENT CONDITION

Figure 4-7 shows block No. 10. This section asks if the medical care reported on this claim form is necessary because of:

❑ A current or former work-related incident
❑ An auto accident *and* state (place) of occurrence
❑ Any other type of accident

You must check either "yes" or "no" for each one of these. This is a very important and a frequently abused section of the claim form.

The answers to these questions often determine which insurance company is responsible for covering this care. You will save much time and aggravation by filing the claim form correctly the first time. "Yes" or "no" must be selected for each choice. Do not leave this field blank.

When "yes" is selected in this section, the date of the accident or injury must be entered in block No. 14, and E-codes describing the place and cause of the accident or injury must be entered in block No. 21. Please see Chapter 5 to learn about E-codes and the diagnosis coding guidelines for injuries.

Many times a "yes" answer to one of the questions means that the primary payor should be one of the following: workers' compensation, an automobile policy, or another type of liability policy. When you list a liability payor in block No. 11 as the primary payor, the medical plan may be listed as the secondary payor.

When the claim is sent with a medical plan as primary payor and a "yes" is marked in one of these boxes, coding edits will alert the medical plan to the possibility of another payor, and the claim could be denied until payor responsibility is determined.

Payor-specific requirements:

Medicare: Medicare requires at least one E-code (explaining the accident) in block No. 21. Medicare may be billed as secondary payor for auto accidents and most types of liability insurance, and now the Medicare training website indicates that Medicare may be billed as secondary payor for workers' compensation. If payment is not received in 120 days, you may request a "conditional primary payment" from Medicare. When a Medicare conditional payment is made, special rules apply. Please see Chapter 10 for details about Medicare conditional payments.

Liability Plan: When a liability plan is billed, one of the choices in this field must be marked "yes," and payor edits will look for the date of the accident or injury in block No. 14 and an E-code describing the accident or injury in block No. 21. If any of the required information is missing or does not match payor records, the claim will be rejected.

Note: In some instances, specific medical plans want to be billed as the primary payor, with the liability plan that might be responsible listed as the secondary payor. The medical plan pays for the services initially, investigates the claim, and exercises the right of subrogation to collect from the liability plan, when applicable. TRICARE/CHAMPUS and Blue Cross Blue Shield are among the medical plans that often prefer this option.

Let's take a closer look at each of these choices.

Block No. 10a. Employment Accident

Figure 4-7 shows block No. 10a. If the medical care reported is due to a work-related incident, this box will be marked "yes." You must contact the employer involved and follow the state-specific procedures to file for workers' compensation.

When workers' compensation is denied, you are usually allowed to appeal the denial. If it continues to be denied, you may then file the claim with the patient's medical plan, attaching a copy of the denial(s). In this way, you "justify" the claim, and the medical plan is more likely to consider the claim for payment.

When an injured worker is not covered by workers' compensation, bill the applicable liability plan as primary and place "No workers' compensation" in block No. 19. The injured worker's medical plan is not billed as primary unless no other policy provides coverage.

Block No. 10b. Auto Accident

Figure 4-7 shows block No. 10b. When the medical care reported is due to an auto accident, this box is marked "yes," and you should file the claim with an automobile policy as the primary payor. Enter the two letter postal state code for the location of the accident.

If *the patient was at fault,* the patient's auto policy will be the primary payor for the claim, and the patient's medical insurance will be the secondary payor. If the *other driver was at fault,* the other driver's auto policy will be the primary payor for the claim. The patient's auto policy or the patient's medical policy, in that order, will be the secondary payor listed for the claim. Some states are considered no-fault states and different rules may apply that differ for each no-fault state. For example, in one no-fault state, the patient's insurance pays medical bills first, regardless of who was at fault. In every state, the medical plan will only provide coverage if there are still unpaid medical bills after all possible auto policies have met their obligations.

Block No. 10c. Other Accident

Figure 4-7 shows block No. 10c. If the medical care reported is due to any other accident, this box will be marked "yes."

When any other type of liability policy provides coverage, that policy should be listed as the primary payor, with the patient's medical plan as secondary payor. When no one else is liable or if liability has not yet been determined, file the claim with the patient's medical plan as the primary payor.

Any time an accident results in legal action and damages are awarded, whether by trial or by an out-of-court settlement, the payor that originally paid for the care might be entitled to reimbursement from the settlement or award for items paid through the date of the settlement or award.

Block No. 10d. Local Use

Figure 4-7 shows block No. 10d. This field is available to payors for payor-specific requirements.

> To meet EDI and OCR requirements, do not enter dashes or other special characters in this box.

Payor-specific requirements:

Medicaid: Medicaid uses this field to report the patient's Medicaid number. Because of rampant abuse in the Medicaid program, the number listed on the ID card is not always the Medicaid number used for processing claims. Call Medicaid to obtain or verify the Medicaid number used in this field.

Some states have state-specific requirements. For example, in one state, you enter the patient's 10-digit Medicaid number preceded by "MCD." For example, if the Medicaid number is 123-456-7890, enter the number as "MCD 1234567890." Call your Medicaid representative to learn the requirements for your state.

Workers' Compensation: Some states want you to enter the word "Attachments" if you have attachments to the claim.

BLOCK NO. 11. INSURED'S POLICY GROUP OR FECA NUMBER

Figure 4-7 shows block No. 11. Enter the insured's policy group or FECA number. Most insurance companies require a number in this box. The number can be found on the patient's insurance card. Payors that issue a group number require the group number to be listed in this block. When there is no group number, list the policy number.

Whereas the insured's ID number tells the payor who the patient is, the policy or group number tells the payor which type of policy the patient has. If you cannot find a group or policy number on the insurance card, please call the payor and ask for the number.

If there is no conflict with the EDI requirements for your clearinghouse or if you are filing paper claims, the field may be left blank for payors that do not issue a policy or group number.

> Many EDI systems for electronic claims require a number here as part of the tracking process. When a number is required for the EDI process, but the payor has not issued a policy or group number, use the insured's ID number from block No. 1a.

Payor-specific requirements:

Medicare: When you complete this item, it tells Medicare that you have made a good faith effort to determine whether Medicare is the secondary or primary payor.

When Medicare is the primary payor and you are filing a paper claim, enter the word "none."

If you are filing an electronic claim, verify with your EDI clearinghouse whether to enter the word "none" or to list the Medicare ID number in this section. Many medical management systems route all electronic claims through the software company. In this case, verify with the software vendor whether to enter the word "none" or whether to list the Medicare ID number in this section.

Worker's Compensation: List the policy or group number for the employer's workers' compensation plan.

Block No. 11a. Insured's Date of Birth and Gender

Figure 4-7 shows block No. 11a. This field is required when the patient is not the policyholder listed in block No. 4. Complete the insured's date of birth and gender for the policyholder identified in block No. 4. If the patient is the policyholder, leave this section blank.

Birth date: Enter the insured's date of birth as an eight-digit date.

Gender: Enter the insured's gender; "M" for male or "F" for female.

> To meet EDI and OCR requirements, use only numbers for dates and do not enter slashes or dashes. For more details, see the directions for block No. 3.

Payor-specific requirements:

Workers' Compensation: Leave this section blank.

Block No. 11b. Employer's Name or School Name

Figure 4-7 shows block No. 11b. If an employer issued the policy for the primary payor, enter the employer's name. Enter the employer's name even if the insured no longer works for this company *if* the policy is now a "continuation policy" *or* if the policy is part of a retirement package. In this case, list the company name followed by either "Former" or "Retired" and the eight-digit retirement date.

The insurance company will need this information to verify that the policy is still valid. If the patient no longer works for the company that issued the policy, and the patient either was not eligible or did not elect to purchase a continuation policy, the patient is no longer covered by the policy, and the claim will be rejected.

If the patient is a dependent student older than age 18, enter the name of the school. Generally, a child older than age 18 is only covered under a parent's policy if he or she is a student or one who meets the disability requirements.

Payor-specific requirements:
Medicare: Leave this section blank.
Workers' Compensation: Leave this section blank. (If the patient now works for another employer, the other employer's name may be entered here, but many workers' compensation payors do not require this additional information.)
Note: Some payors do not require this field.

Block No. 11c. Insurance Plan Name or Program Name

Figure 4-7 shows block No. 11c. Enter the complete name of the insurance plan or program. This information is found on the patient's insurance card. When combined with the information in block No. 1a and block No. 11a, this information pinpoints the exact insurance policy or medical plan.

Payor-specific requirements:
Workers' Compensation: List the name of the workers' compensation plan.

Block No. 11d. Are You Covered By Another Health Benefit Plan?

Figure 4-7 shows block No. 11d. Here you must enter either "yes" or "no."

Complete "yes" when a secondary payor is being billed, and complete block No. 9 and its subdivisions to record the secondary payor information.

If the answer is "no," block No. 9 and its subdivisions are left blank.

This field is often part of a payor's claim editing process. If you leave this section blank, the payor is likely to reject the claim on the grounds that they do not know whether all possible payors were identified. However, the EOB is likely to say "insufficient data," without telling you which data were missing.

Payor-specific requirements:
Medicare: You may leave this blank for Medicare when there is no secondary policy.

Workers' Compensation: Other medical plans usually exclude coverage for conditions that are covered by workers' compensation. Therefore when a claim is sent to workers' compensation, there is no secondary policy, and "no" is selected in this field.

If a claim is later submitted to another medical plan because workers' compensation denied coverage for the entire claim, the other medical plan is listed as the primary payor, and the denial from workers' compensation is attached to the claim.

BLOCK NO. 12. RELEASE OF INFORMATION

Figure 4-8 shows block No. 12 of the CMS-1500 claim form. Completion of this block indicates that the patient authorizes the physician to release medical information to the payor. Only the patient, the parent of a minor, or a legal guardian may sign a "Release of Information" statement. Some payors require an original signature for each claim; others allow a signed release to cover many claims. "Signature on file" or "SOF" may be used when the original signature on a "Release of Information" statement is on file in the patient's record.

See Figure 4-9 for an example of a label the patient may sign during check-in. Once the claim form is complete and was proofread for accuracy, the label may be applied to the claim to cover block No. 12 and block No. 13. A label such as this allows you to make sure a claim is accurate and the printer was aligned correctly before affixing the original signatures to the form.

To meet EDI requirements, "signature on file" or "SOF" is entered instead of an original signature. However, the original signature on a "Release of Information" statement must be present in the patient's record.

Some payors are beginning to require a new release form dated on each date of service. A label such as the one in Figure 4-9 could be signed during check-in and placed in the patient's record to meet this requirement for an electronic claim, or a similar statement can be added to the superbill for the patient's signature on the date of service. The payor/provider contract usually addresses issues such as this requirement.

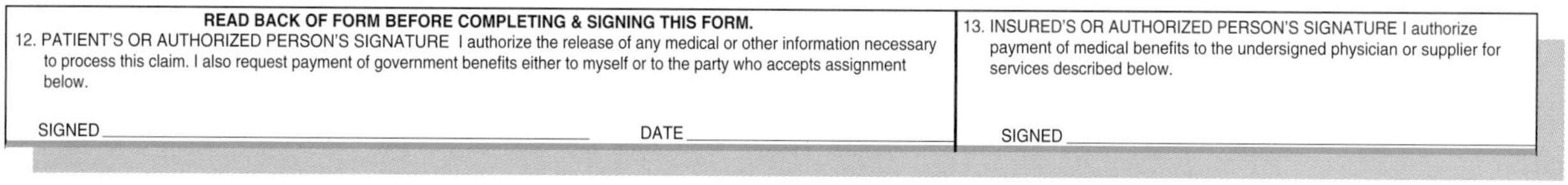

FIGURE 4-8
Block No. 12-block No. 13 of the CMS-1500 claim form.

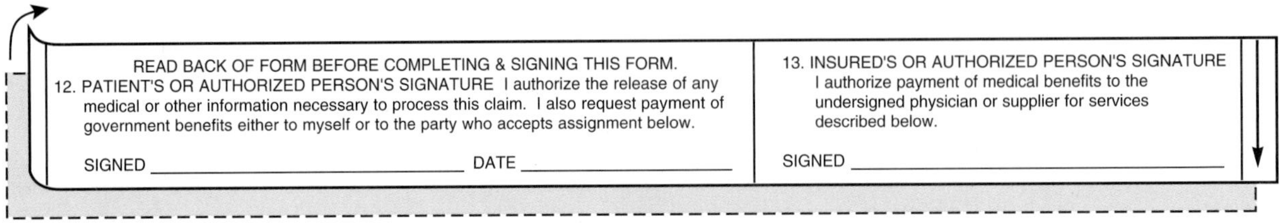

| READ BACK OF FORM BEFORE COMPLETING & SIGNING THIS FORM.
12. PATIENT'S OR AUTHORIZED PERSON'S SIGNATURE I authorize the release of any
medical or other information necessary to process this claim. I also request payment of
government benefits either to myself or to the party who accepts assignment below.

SIGNED _____ DATE _____ | 13. INSURED'S OR AUTHORIZED PERSON'S SIGNATURE
I authorize payment of medical benefits to the
undersigned physician or supplier for services
described below.

SIGNED _____ |

FIGURE 4-9

The patient may sign an insurance release label such as this during check-in. The label allows you to make sure a claim form is accurate and the printer was aligned correctly before affixing the original signatures. Carefully apply the label to cover block No. 12 and block No. 13. (Courtesy Bibbero Systems, Inc., Petaluma, Calif 94954; 800/242-2376; www.bibberosystems.com.)

> To meet EDI and OCR requirements, use only numbers for dates and do not enter slashes or dashes. For more details, see the directions for block No. 3.

BLOCK NO. 13. ASSIGNMENT OF BENEFITS

Figure 4-8 shows block No. 13. This section tells the payor where to send the check. If the patient signs an "Assignment of Benefits" statement, payment for the claim will be sent directly to the physician. If the patient does not sign this section, the payment will be sent to the patient.

Some payors require an original signature for each claim; others allow a signed release to cover many claims. "Signature on file" or "SOF" may be entered when the original signature is on file in the patient's record.

When a patient refuses to sign an "Assignment of Benefits" statement, you should collect payment-in-full at the time of service. Once the patient cashes the insurance check, it can be very difficult to collect the money due the physician.

> To meet EDI requirements, "Signature on file" is entered instead of an original signature. However, the original signature on an "Assignment of Benefits" statement must be present in the patient's record.

Payor-specific requirements:

Medicaid: In some states Medicaid requires an original "wet ink" signature.

Note: Sometimes other payors also require an original signature. An insurance release label, as pictured in Figure 4-9, is available from some vendors. The patient signs the label during check-in, and the original signatures can be attached to the paper-claim before mailing. This allows you a margin of error. You may preview the claim and correct any problems before attaching the original signatures.

STOP & REVIEW

Answer the following questions:

1. The patient has a Medicare + Choice or Medicare Advantage plan. What selection is marked in block No. 1?

2. Where do you find the insured's ID number?

3. A patient was married and changed her name since her last visit. Do you enter her new married name or her previous name on the claim form? Why?

4. Mary is covered under her husband, Paul's, insurance plan. Mary and Paul both live at 2603 State Street, Washington, IN 32853. What is entered in block No. 5?

5. Dustin is a 21-year-old college student. He attends the University of Central Florida and works for Disney World part time to earn spending money. He is not married, and he is covered under his parent's medical insurance plan. What is entered in block No. 8?

6. Using the information from question 5, what is entered in block No. 11b?

7. Madeline was treated for the flu. What is entered in block No. 10?

8. Phillip is covered by Medicare and does not have any other coverage. What is entered in block No. 9?

9. Andrew refuses to sign a "Release of Information" statement for block No. 12. Can a claim form be filed for Andrew? Why or why not?

10. The receptionist forgot to ask Xavier to sign an "Assignment of Benefits" statement. Xavier only paid his copayment amount at the time of service. What do you put in block No. 13, and where will payment be sent if you file the claim without getting an "Assignment of Benefits" statement signed?

Clinical Application Exercise

Use the patient registration form in Figure 4-10 to complete the top half of the claim form in Figure 4-11.

Physician-Supplied Information

Every medical claim is a legal document. The physician or supplier is responsible for furnishing the information recorded in the bottom half of the CMS-1500 medical claim form. The right side margin of the bottom half of the CMS-1500 claim form says "provider or supplier information," printed sideways with arrows that indicate block No. 14 through block No. 33. This half of the claim form tells the payor the "who, what, when, where, and why" for the medical service(s) reported. It tells the payor who rendered each service, what service was rendered, when it was rendered, where it was rendered, and why it was rendered. It tells the payor the credentials of the rendering provider and whether the rendering provider is an authorized contractor. It also tells the payor how much the charges are, where to send payment, and how to report the payment to the Internal Revenue Service (IRS) for income tax purposes.

Medical billers and coders often must walk a fine line between following the well-intentioned directives of their employers and following the current health care laws that regulate the billing and reporting of medical services. Most physicians use a superbill to send billing instructions to the biller. The superbill is not a part of the patient's medical record; it is a part of the patient's financial record. Legally, your billing and coding must match the documentation in the medical record, not the superbill. Therefore the medical record, not the superbill, is the source document for physician-supplied billing information reported on a medical claim form.

Lake Eola Family Practice   517860 South Pioneer Drive, Orlando, FL 32897 • 634-555-4893

Patient Registration Form

Have you been seen in this office in the past 3 years? √ **Yes**   __ **No**   Do you have a living will? _Yes_

Today's Date _Feb. 6, XX_   Home Phone _634-555-1212_   Work Phone _None_

Patient Name (Last name, First name, Middle Initial) _Parker, Wanda J._

Street Address _1679432 Joseph Ave._   City _Orlando_   State _FL_   Zip _32897_

Date of Birth _Nov. 12, 32_   Age _68_   Gender: √ Female __ Male   Social Security # _456-XX-9012_

Marital Status: √ Married __ Single __ Widowed __ Divorced __ Other   Driver's License # _None_

Is the patient a student? __ Full Time __ Part Time √ No   Is the patient employed? __ Full time __ Part Time √ No

Patient's Employer Name & Address _(Spouse Retired from AT&T) Retired 6/10/1998_

School Name & Address _None_

Emergency Contact Person _Ronald Parker_   Relationship _Husband_   Phone _634-555-1212_

Referring Physician Name & Phone Number _None_

Insurance Plan and Responsible Party Information

Insurance Company Name _Medicare_   Address _PO Box XXXX_

City _Jacksonville_   State _FL_   Zip _94187_   Phone _800-333-7586_

Policy # ____   Group # ____   ID # _456XX9012B_

Policy Holder's Name _Wanda Parker_   Address _1679432 Joseph Ave._

City _Orlando_   State _FL_   Zip _32897_   Phone _634-555-1212_

Policy Holder's Date Of Birth _Nov. 12, 32_ Social Security # _456-XX-9012_   Driver License # _None_

Gender: __ Male √ Female   Relationship to patient: √ Self __ Spouse __ Parent __ Guardian __ Other

Policy Holder's Employer's Name _None (Spouse Retired AT&T)_ Address ____

City ____   State ____   Zip ____   Phone ____

Secondary Insurance Company Name _Blue Cross/Blue Shield_   Address _PO Box YYYY_

City _Jacksonville_   State _FL_   Zip _94187_   Phone _800-555-1212_

Secondary Policy # _A6794_   Group # _B1236_   ID # _890-XX-3456-02_

Secondary Policy Holder's Name _Ronald Parker_   Phone _634-555-1212_ Address _1679432 Joseph Ave._

City _Orlando_   State _FL_   Zip _32897_   Relationship to patient: __ Self √ Spouse __ Other

Secondary Policy Holder's Date Of Birth _Feb. 6, 30_ Social Security # _890-XX-3456_   Driver License # _B650-XX-12679_

Authorizations

It is customary to pay for all services on the date rendered unless other arrangements were made before your appointment. The patient and the guarantor are responsible for all deductibles and co-pays at the time of the visit and any other fees in accordance with insurance contracts. The patient and guarantor are responsible for all elective or non-covered services and any services that are not considered medically necessary.

Financially responsible person if patient is student or unemployed _Ronald Parker_   Phone _634-555-1212_

I authorize the release of any medical information necessary to process this claim and I request that payment of medical benefits be made directly to Lake Eola Family Practice. I hereby acknowledge that I am fully responsible for payment as listed above.

Signed _Wanda Parker_   Date _Feb. 6, XX_   Time _10 AM_

FIGURE 4-10
Completed patient registration form.

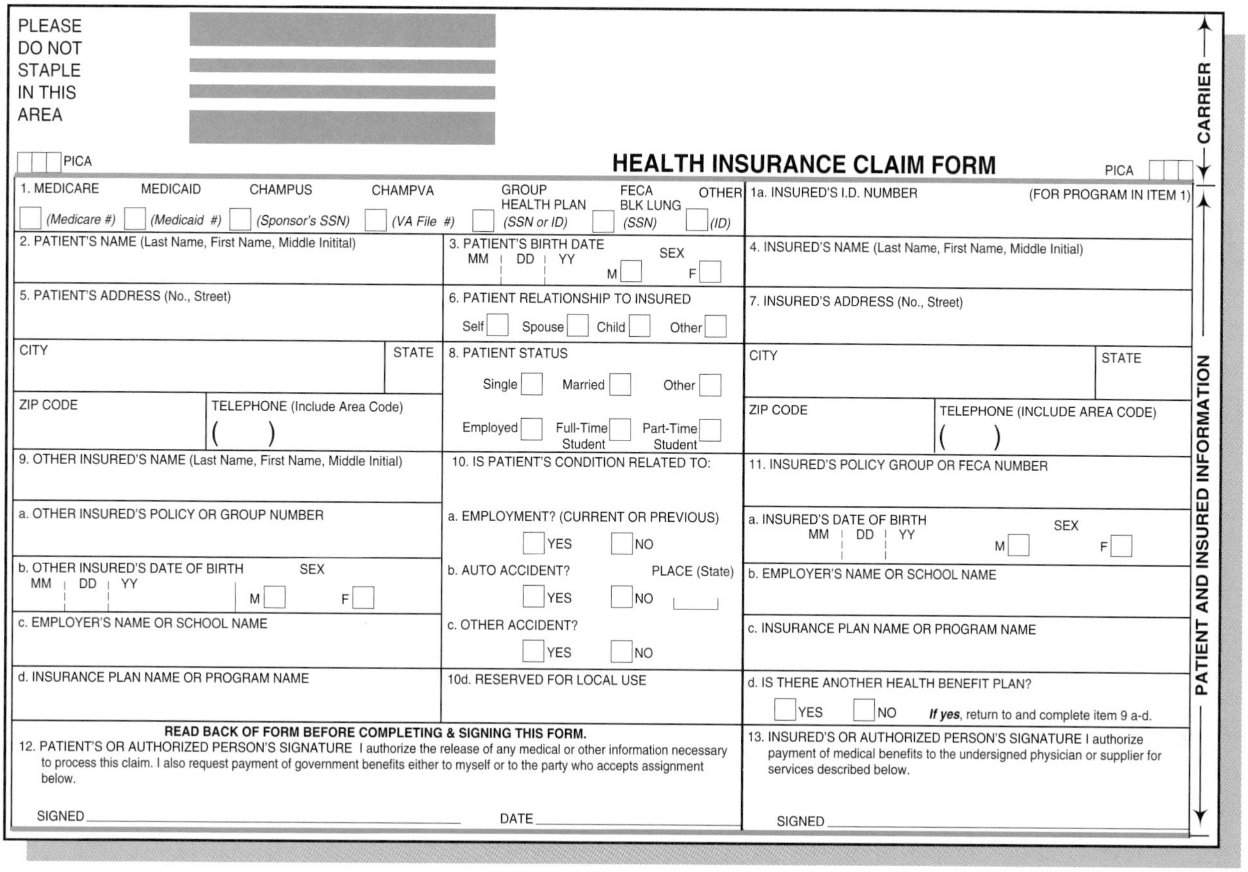
PLEASE DO NOT STAPLE IN THIS AREA

PICA HEALTH INSURANCE CLAIM FORM PICA

CARRIER

1. MEDICARE (Medicare #) MEDICAID (Medicaid #) CHAMPUS (Sponsor's SSN) CHAMPVA (VA File #) GROUP HEALTH PLAN (SSN or ID) FECA BLK LUNG (SSN) OTHER (ID)
1a. INSURED'S I.D. NUMBER (FOR PROGRAM IN ITEM 1)
2. PATIENT'S NAME (Last Name, First Name, Middle Initital)
3. PATIENT'S BIRTH DATE MM DD YY SEX M F
4. INSURED'S NAME (Last Name, First Name, Middle Initial)
5. PATIENT'S ADDRESS (No., Street)
6. PATIENT RELATIONSHIP TO INSURED Self Spouse Child Other
7. INSURED'S ADDRESS (No., Street)
CITY STATE
8. PATIENT STATUS Single Married Other Employed Full-Time Student Part-Time Student
CITY STATE
ZIP CODE TELEPHONE (Include Area Code) ( )
ZIP CODE TELEPHONE (INCLUDE AREA CODE) ( )
9. OTHER INSURED'S NAME (Last Name, First Name, Middle Initial)
10. IS PATIENT'S CONDITION RELATED TO:
11. INSURED'S POLICY GROUP OR FECA NUMBER
a. OTHER INSURED'S POLICY OR GROUP NUMBER
a. EMPLOYMENT? (CURRENT OR PREVIOUS) YES NO
a. INSURED'S DATE OF BIRTH MM DD YY SEX M F
b. OTHER INSURED'S DATE OF BIRTH MM DD YY SEX M F
b. AUTO ACCIDENT? YES NO PLACE (State)
b. EMPLOYER'S NAME OR SCHOOL NAME
c. EMPLOYER'S NAME OR SCHOOL NAME
c. OTHER ACCIDENT? YES NO
c. INSURANCE PLAN NAME OR PROGRAM NAME
d. INSURANCE PLAN NAME OR PROGRAM NAME
10d. RESERVED FOR LOCAL USE
d. IS THERE ANOTHER HEALTH BENEFIT PLAN? YES NO *If yes,* return to and complete item 9 a-d.
READ BACK OF FORM BEFORE COMPLETING & SIGNING THIS FORM.
12. PATIENT'S OR AUTHORIZED PERSON'S SIGNATURE I authorize the release of any medical or other information necessary to process this claim. I also request payment of government benefits either to myself or to the party who accepts assignment below.
SIGNED DATE
13. INSURED'S OR AUTHORIZED PERSON'S SIGNATURE I authorize payment of medical benefits to the undersigned physician or supplier for services described below.
SIGNED

PATIENT AND INSURED INFORMATION

FIGURE 4-11
Patient-supplied information section of the CMS-1500.

You may not alter physician-supplied information, but if you see an error, you may ask the physician to correct it. When you find information recorded on a superbill that is not recorded in the patient's medical record, you may not consider that information for billing and/or coding until it becomes an official part of the medical record. However, you may politely ask the physician to amend the patient record to include the missing information. Alternatively, you may send a query letter to ask the physician in writing about the missing information and to receive a written response. Only the rendering physician may amend his or her documentation in the medical record. The query letter with the written response may be included in the medical record to meet this requirement, or the physician may ask to have the record given to him or her and amend it directly.

HIPAA provides very stiff fines if you do not follow current billing rules and coding conventions when completing medical claims. These fines can be as high as $5,000 to $10,000 per line item paid incorrectly as the result of an error on a health care claim, plus three times the damages (the amount overpaid as a result of the claim). HIPAA funded government agencies with $2,500,000,000 to find and prosecute anyone who files medical claims with incorrect information. There are now more than 450 investigators trained to investigate medical claims. Currently the FBI is focusing 60% of their medical fraud and abuse efforts on government health plans and 40% of their efforts on private health plans.

In September 2000, HHS/OIG released the final version of compliance guidance for individual and small group physician practices. A copy can be found at http://oig.hhs.gov/.

You can be held liable if you submit a claim with information you know is incorrect. You must learn the claim reporting requirements, the applicable laws, and the consequences for noncompliance so that you may gently guide physicians into compliance. *Do not ever submit a claim with information you know is incorrect.*

When a physician directs you to bill a level of service not supported by documentation in the medical record, you have three choices: (1) you may wait to bill the service until the physician amends the record so it meets reporting requirements, (2) with the physician's permission, you may bill the level of service currently documented in the medical record, or (3) you may decline to complete a claim and possibly suggest the physician personally complete and send the claim for that encounter if the physician wishes to be paid for that service. If you choose the third option, you must be tactful and avoid using a disrespectful tone of voice. A regretful tone sometimes works well. "I'm really sorry, but the documentation in the medical record does not yet meet the legal requirements to submit a claim as directed. I would be happy to submit the claim once the requirements are met, but until then, my hands are tied. Of course, you always have the option of personally completing and submitting the claim."

Billing rules and medical codes change from year to year. Always use codebooks for the same year as the claim unless the claim is for workers' compensation or Medicaid. In some states, workers' compensation and Medicaid require the use of codebooks and billing rules from 1995 or 1996. Follow the state carriers' requirements for your state for Medicaid and for the state in which the work-related injury occurred for workers' compensation.

The following information is a guide to help you meet current billing rules and file clean claims. It also will help you determine the cause of past problems and help you avoid problems in the future.

If you want to file clean claims, you must learn to look at each claim through the payor's eyes. When the claim arrives at the payor, it is automatically subjected to payor edits and audits. Once the top half of the claim form passes the edits and audits, the bottom half of the claim form is targeted. When the information is not correct, there is no obligation for payment. The claim will either be penalized or rejected. Payors want to know:

❑ Were the services rendered appropriate for the age and gender of the patient?
❑ Were the services rendered appropriate for the nature of the presenting illness?
❑ Were the services rendered appropriate for each linked diagnosis?
❑ If an item is marked "yes" in block No. 10a, b, or c, does block No. 14 tell *when* the accident occurred? Does block No. 21 have an E-code or codes that tell *where* and *how* the accident occurred? If not, the payor cannot determine who the primary payor should be. The claim

will be rejected until the primary payor is determined.
❑ Does the claim show who the referring provider is, when applicable, and does it show who rendered each service?
❑ Are required modifiers present, and are they reported correctly?
❑ Are the type of service and place of service codes appropriate for the service rendered?
❑ If the type of service or place of service indicates a facility, is a facility listed in block No. 32?
❑ Are the physician's tax ID number, group or practice ID number, **provider number,** unique physician identifier number **(UPIN)** and/or National Provider Identifier **(NPI)** reported in the correct fields, and are they accurate? Each of these numbers is explained in more detail in blocks No. 17a, 24K, 25, and/or 33.
❑ Does the physician accept assignment? If not, all authorized payments will be sent to the patient.

> Most of the Medicare information that varies from state to state is located in blocks No. 19, 21, and 24D on the CMS-1500 claim form.

Let's take a closer look at specific claim requirements for the bottom half of the CMS-1500.

BLOCK NO. 14. DATE OF CURRENT ILLNESS

Figure 4-12 shows block No. 14 of the CMS-1500 claim form. This field is required for some specific visits but not for others. Use an eight-digit date.

Leave this field blank for annual exams and physicals.

It is a *required field* for accidents and injuries. With accidents and injuries, enter the date of the accident or injury. Block No. 10 must indicate the type of accident or injury, and block No. 21 must indicate where and/or how the accident or injury occurred.

It is a *required field* for pregnancy. With pregnancy, enter the patient's last menstrual period (LMP). This tells the payor when to expect the baby to be born, and the payor can determine whether the services rendered are appropriate for the stage of pregnancy.

| 14. DATE OF CURRENT:
MM   DD   YY | ◀ ILLNESS (First symptom) OR
INJURY (Accident) OR
PREGNANCY(LMP) | 15. IF PATIENT HAS HAD SAME OR SIMILAR ILLNESS.
GIVE FIRST DATE   MM   DD   YY | 16. DATES PATIENT UNABLE TO WORK IN CURRENT OCCUPATION
  MM   DD   YY   MM   DD   YY
FROM   TO |

FIGURE 4-12
Block No. 14-block No. 16 of the CMS-1500 claim form.

It is a *required field* for chiropractic claims. With chiropractic claims, enter the date of the initiation of the course of treatment and enter the x-ray date in block No. 19.

Some payors no longer require an x-ray before initiation of chiropractic services.

If your practice management computer system automatically lists today's date in block No. 14 for every claim, you must learn how to change the data entered in this field. If you cannot change it yourself, politely ask the software manufacturer to please correct the problem. Wrong information in this field can cause claim rejections and/or delays in payment.

To meet EDI and OCR requirements, use only numbers for dates and do not enter slashes or dashes. For more details, see the directions for block No. 3.

Payor-specific requirements:

Workers' Compensation: The date of the work-related injury must be listed in block No. 14.

BLOCK NO. 15. DATE OF SIMILAR ILLNESS

Figure 4-12 shows block No. 15. Most payors do not require this field. It is used to report the date of a similar illness. Use an eight-digit date.

Payors use this information, when provided, for statistical purposes. They might monitor the response to treatment this time compared to last time. They might use it to determine preexisting conditions. They might use it to track the frequency of occurrences or recurrences. They might use it to determine the severity of an illness that tends to get progressively worse over time. When you report information in this field, give the first date of the illness reported on the claim.

Note: At some point in the future, this field will probably become a requirement. However, because patients often have to change physicians every time their insurance changes, many physicians no longer have these data in their records, and patients seldom remember precise dates.

To meet EDI and OCR requirements, use only numbers for dates and do not enter slashes or dashes. For more details, see the directions for block No. 3.

Payor-specific requirements:

Medicare: Medicare does not require this information. You may leave the field blank.

BLOCK NO. 16. DATES UNABLE TO WORK

Figure 4-12 shows block No. 16. This field is used primarily by workers' compensation plans. List any dates the patient is unable to work. Include both "from" and "to" dates, when possible. The "from" date is the first day the patient is unable to work, and the "to" date is the last day the patient is unable to work. In rare instances, the patient will only miss 1 day of work. Then the "from" and "to" dates will be the same. When you do not know the date that the patient will return to work, only list the "from" date. Use eight-digit dates.

While private disability payors often request copies of office notes, the only time disability plans are ever billed directly is when the payor has requested the evaluation. Private disability payors usually require this field on claims for independent medical examinations (IMEs).

To meet EDI and OCR requirements, use only numbers for dates and do not enter slashes or dashes. For more details, see the directions for block No. 3.

Payor-specific requirements:

Medicare: When Medicare is the primary payor, leave this field blank.

BLOCK NO. 17. REFERRING PHYSICIAN NAME

Figure 4-13 shows block No. 17 of the CMS-1500 claim form. Enter the complete name of the referring physician, when applicable for the claim. The referring physician's ID number, the Medicare UPIN, or Medicare's new NPI must be included in block No. 17a.

If more than one referring physician ordered the services rendered, separate claims must be submitted

| 17. NAME OF REFERRING PHYSICIAN OR OTHER SOURCE | 17a. I.D. NUMBER OF REFERRING PHYSICIAN | 18. HOSPITALIZATION DATES RELATED TO CURRENT SERVICES |
| | | FROM MM \| DD \| YY   TO   MM \| DD \| YY |

FIGURE 4-13
Block No. 17-block No. 18 of the CMS-1500 claim form.

for the service(s) ordered by each referring physician. For example, if Dr. Smith ordered a CBC blood test for Wanda Andrews and Dr. Jones ordered a liver panel blood test for Wanda Andrews, there are two referring physicians. The lab that performs the blood tests must file two claims: one for the CBC with Dr. Smith as the referring physician and one for the liver panel with Dr. Jones as the referring physician.

Payor-specific requirements:

Managed Care: Many managed care plans (HMOs, PPOs, etc.) require this field anytime the service rendered requires an authorization. The payor edits will check block No. 23 for the authorization number, and they will check block No. 17a for the ID number to confirm that the referring physician is authorized to be a referring physician. If any of the information is missing or does not match their records, the claim will be rejected.

Block No. 17a. ID Number of the Referring Physician

Figure 4-13 shows block No. 17a. When information is listed in block No. 17, *this field is required*. List the ID number for the referring physician in block No. 17. Medicare required a Medicare UPIN until June 2005, when Medicare began to issue NPI numbers. Now the NPI for the referring provider is placed here.

It is necessary to distinguish between physicians with the same or similar names. Many payors use the physician's SSN, but some assign a physician ID number (PIN). This ID number tells the payor exactly which physician referred the patient. If you notice that a referring physician is listed, but not an ID number, do not just assume that the payor uses the physician's SSN. Call the payor and ask what type of number they want in block No. 17a before submitting the claim.

Payor-specific requirements:

Medicare: Each state Medicare carrier assigns PIN, UPIN, and PPIN numbers. The Medicare **PIN** stands for practice ID number (not physician ID number, as with other payors); it identifies the practice or group. The practice PIN could be for one incorporated physician or for a group of physicians. The Medicare PPIN stands for performing provider ID number (12345Z); it identifies the individual physician within the practice that rendered care. The Medicare UPIN stands for unique physician ID number (A12345); it identifies the individual referring physician.

In some states, Medicare UPINs are available at the state carrier's Internet site or online bulletin board.

Medicare's website (www.cms.hhs.gov) will guide you to information for each state. The Noridian website for Arizona provides UPINs for every state.

In June 2005, the Centers for Medicare and Medicaid Services (CMS) began to replace the UPIN and the PPIN numbering systems, in which each state Medicare carrier assigns their own numbers, with a single National Provider Identifier (NPI). Under the NPI numbering system, a physician who practices in more than one state will need only one number from Medicare. In addition, only one PIN will be assigned to each practice, rather than one for each work location and another for each state as was required.

The CMS also is considering developing a similar national numbering system for patients.

Medicaid: In some states Medicaid requires a referring physician Medicaid ID number in this field. Check with your state to see whether the NPI will be used for Medicaid.

Managed Care: Managed care referring physician ID numbers can be obtained from the referring physician's office. Most managed care plans do not use the physician's SSN for this field. Instead, a payor-specific ID number is issued. Often the ID number can be found in the payor/physician contract. To prevent abuse, payors often do not release these numbers to anyone except the physician to whom they were issued. If the referring physician did not make a photocopy of the contract before returning the signed contract to the payor, the physician might have to personally call the payor's physician representative and request the number or request another copy of the contract.

BLOCK NO. 18. HOSPITALIZATION DATES

Figure 4-13 shows block No. 18. Enter the dates of the hospital stay when the services in block No. 24D are *related* to a hospitalization. This includes hospital visits and routine posthospitalization check-ups that document the status (recovered, improved, unchanged, and/or deteriorated) of a condition treated during a recent hospitalization. Use eight-digit dates.

Most payors require both admission and discharge dates. "From" is the admission date, and "to" is the discharge date. When services are billed before the patient's release from the hospital, only the "from" date is included on the claim. Some specialties, such as anesthesia, do not require the discharge date.

To meet EDI and OCR requirements, use only numbers for dates and do not enter slashes or dashes. For more details, see the directions for block No. 3.

BLOCK NO. 19. LOCAL USE OR FREE FORM

Figure 4-14 shows block No. 19 of the CMS-1500 claim form. This box may be used in a variety of ways by payors.

Payor-specific requirements:
Medicare: Some of Medicare's requirements are:

❑ When a claim is submitted for routine foot care performed by a physician, enter the date the patient was last seen by their regular physician and the UPIN or NPI of the regular physician.
❑ Enter the x-ray date for chiropractic services if an x-ray was taken. By entering the x-ray date here and the initiation date of the course of treatment in block No. 14, the chiropractor is certifying that relevant documentation requirements are on file and the x-rays, when applicable, are available for review.
❑ Enter the prescription drug name and dosage when submitting a claim for not otherwise classified (NOC) drugs.
❑ When "unlisted" procedure codes are used, enter a coherent description of the procedure, if one can be given within the limits of the field. Otherwise, an attachment must be submitted on paper.
❑ Enter all applicable modifiers when modifier -99 (multiple modifiers) is used in block No. 24D. Record the line number of the procedure and the applicable modifiers. For example, if modifier -99 is entered for the procedure on line 2, the entry might be "2 = 51 52 Q6."
❑ Enter the statement "Homebound" when an independent lab renders an EKG tracing or obtains a specimen from a homebound or institutionalized patient.
❑ Enter the statement "Patient refuses to assign benefits" when the beneficiary refuses to assign benefits to a participating provider. In this case, no payment can be made on the claim.
❑ Enter the statement "Testing for hearing aid" when submitting claims to obtain an intentional denial so the hearing aid (a noncovered service) may be paid for by another payor.
❑ Enter the specific name and dosage amount for low osmolar contrast material if a current code does not convey this information.

❑ Enter the assumed and relinquishing date for a global surgery claim when providers share postoperative care.
❑ Enter the statement "Attending physician, not hospice employee" when a physician renders services to a hospice patient, but the hospice does not employ the physician.

Medicaid: In some states, Medicaid requires special codes in block No. 19 to identify the type of claim: Medipass, physician, etc. These codes are found in the Medicaid workbook for those states. In other states, Medicaid often has other specific requirements.

BLOCK NO. 20. OUTSIDE LAB

Figure 4-14 shows block No. 20. Indicate if an **outside lab** performed any lab services entered in block No. 24D.

An outside lab is one that bills the physician's office, not the payor, for tests the physician bought on behalf of the patient. The physician pays the lab, and the physician bills the payor for reimbursement.

When "yes" is marked here, the purchase price is entered on the charge line within this block, and the name of the lab is entered in block No. 32.

Any time the answer is not "yes," "no" should be marked.

Payor-specific requirements:
Medicare: If "yes," block No. 32 must be completed.

When billing for multiple purchased diagnostic tests, each test must be submitted on a separate claim form.

BLOCK NO. 21, LINES 1 TO 4. DIAGNOSIS INFORMATION

Figure 4-15 shows block No. 21 of the CMS-1500 claim form. *This is a required field.* This field conveys the diagnosis and condition information for the entire claim. Currently all providers must use current-year ICD-9-CM codes and code to the highest level of documented specificity. Enter up to four codes in priority order according to the national standard coding conventions and the official coding

19. RESERVED FOR LOCAL USE	20. OUTSIDE LAB? ☐ YES ☐ NO	$ CHARGES

FIGURE 4-14
Block No. 19-block No. 20 of the CMS-1500 claim form.

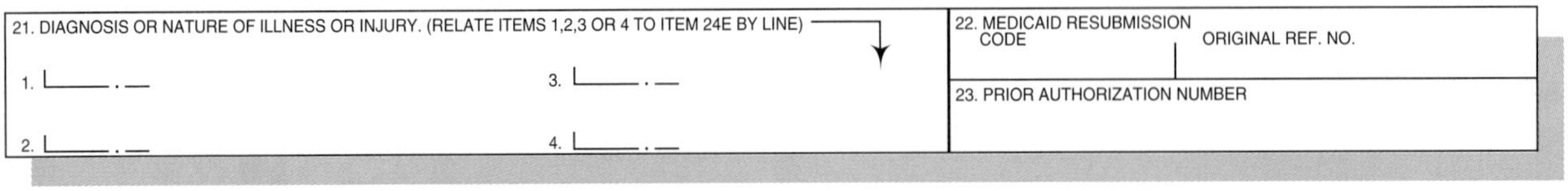
21. DIAGNOSIS OR NATURE OF ILLNESS OR INJURY. (RELATE ITEMS 1,2,3 OR 4 TO ITEM 24E BY LINE)

1. ___ . __ 3. ___ . __

2. ___ . __ 4. ___ . __

22. MEDICAID RESUBMISSION CODE | ORIGINAL REF. NO.

23. PRIOR AUTHORIZATION NUMBER

FIGURE 4-15
Block No. 21-block No. 23 of the CMS-1500 claim form.

guidelines, as found in the front of the diagnosis codebook. See Chapter 5 for the basic principles of diagnosis coding.

When rebilling or auditing, use codebooks for the same year as the date of service.

The claim form already includes the decimal point in "drop-out" red.

To meet EDI and OCR requirements, do not use decimal points (or spaces in place of decimal points) in the ICD-9-CM codes and do not enter narrative descriptions of the codes.

Many computer systems only allow five digits in this field. You may view the entire entry correctly on your computer monitor, but if you enter the decimal point (or leave a space in place of the decimal point), the code will be truncated when it prints because the computer will count the decimal point or space as one of the five digits. Your intended fifth digit will not print on the paper claim and will not be transmitted on the electronic claim.

Sometime soon, ICD-10-CM codes are expected to replace ICD-9-CM codes. These codes have more digits than the ICD-9-CM codes. If your computer system does not allow that many digits, it could truncate the codes and payment would be reduced. Upgrade to a computer system that accommodates the full code length and one that accommodates the alpha characters that are an integral part of each ICD-10-CM code before completing claims using ICD-10-CM codes.

Payor-specific requirements:

Medicare: When an item in block No. 10a, b, or c is marked "yes," an E-code is required in block No. 21, and the E-code cannot be listed first.

E-codes are used to convey the place and type of accident or injury reported on the claim. The E-code is listed last unless coding guidelines specify otherwise.

BLOCK NO. 22. MEDICAID RESUBMISSION CODE

Figure 4-15 shows block No. 22. Medicaid uses this field exclusively for the resubmission code and original reference number. When applicable, enter this information exactly as Medicaid provides it.

Payor-specific requirements:

Medicare: Medicare does not require this field. It may be left blank unless Medicaid is a secondary payor for the claim.

BLOCK NO. 23. PRIOR AUTHORIZATION NUMBER

Figure 4-15 shows block No. 23. This field is used to report prior authorization numbers, when applicable. The authorization might be required for the provider, or it might be required for the treatment or procedure. Always enter the number exactly as it is supplied by the payor receiving the claim.

Some payors load the authorizations in their systems and do not require them on the claim, so check with each payor to learn their preferences. Remember, the purpose of the claim is to meet the payor's expectations. You do not want to inadvertently trigger penalties by not following the payor's requirements.

Some payors require you to put a specific number here for rebilled claims.

Payor-specific requirements:

Medicare: Enter the professional review organization (PRO) prior authorization number for those claims requiring PRO prior approval. A mammography certification number or an investigational device exemption (IDE) number for an FDA-approved clinical trial also may be entered here. Identify IDE claims with modifier "-QA" in block No. 24D.

Medicaid: In some states, Medicaid utilizes this field. Check the Medicaid manual for your state.

Managed care: Anytime the payor requires an authorization in this field, enter the authorization number here. If the authorization number is missing or if it does not match payor records, the claim will be rejected.

Workers' Compensation: In some states, an authorization number is required for every workers' compensation service billed. Enter the claim number and authorization number.

TRICARE/CHAMPUS: Whenever a patient is admitted or whenever a procedure on the preauthorization list is performed on an outpatient basis, an authorization number is required in this field. Preauthorization is required for these services even when CHAMPUS/TRICARE is the second or third payor. If the authorization number was not obtained, a penalty is applied to the provider's payment: 50% penalty for network providers (who should know better) and 10% penalty for nonnetwork providers.

BLOCK NO. 24 (A-K), LINES 1 TO 6. PROCEDURES, SERVICES, OR SUPPLIES

This section contains billing information for services, procedures, and/or supplies. A maximum of six items may be listed per claim. Each of the six lines in this portion of the claim form consists of eleven elements. Some of the elements are required for every claim and some are not.

Let's take a closer look at each of these elements.

Block No. 24A. Date(s) of Service

Figure 4-16 shows block No. 24A of the CMS-1500 claim form. *This is a required field for every claim.* Enter both "from" and "to" dates, when applicable, using an eight-digit date. When multiple dates of service are billed on one line, they must be consecutive dates in the same calendar month. When services encompass more than one calendar month, each month's services are filed on separate claim forms.

When "from" and "to" dates are shown for a series of identical services, enter the service once in block No. 24D, and enter the number of days or units in block No. 24G.

To meet OCR requirements, only report the "from" date when the "from" and "to" dates are the same. Only use both "from" and "to" dates to report a range of dates.

To meet EDI and OCR requirements, use only numbers for dates and do not enter slashes or dashes. For more details, see the directions for block No. 3.

Payor-specific requirements:

Medicare: Claims must be filed within 1 year of the end of the fiscal year (October 1 to September 30) for the date of service reported on the claim.

For example, when a service is provided on September 30, 2000, the fiscal year is October 1, 1999 to September 30, 2000, so the claim must be filed by September 30, 2001.

However, October 1 starts a new fiscal year—October 1, 2000, to September 30, 2001. So, when the service is provided 1 day later, on October 1, 2000, the claim must be filed by September 30, 2002.

CHAMPUS/TRICARE: All claims must be filed within 1 year of the date of service for outpatient claims and within 1 year of the date of discharge for inpatient claims.

Managed Care: Many managed care contracts require clean claims to be filed within 60 days of the date of service. Read your contracts to learn the deadlines for each of your payors.

Block No. 24B. Place of Service

Figure 4-16 shows block No. 24B. *This is a required field for all claims.* This field is used to identify where the item listed on this line in block No. 24D took place. You will enter either a two-digit numeric code or a one-digit alpha or numeric code to convey this information. Code requirements vary from payor to payor.

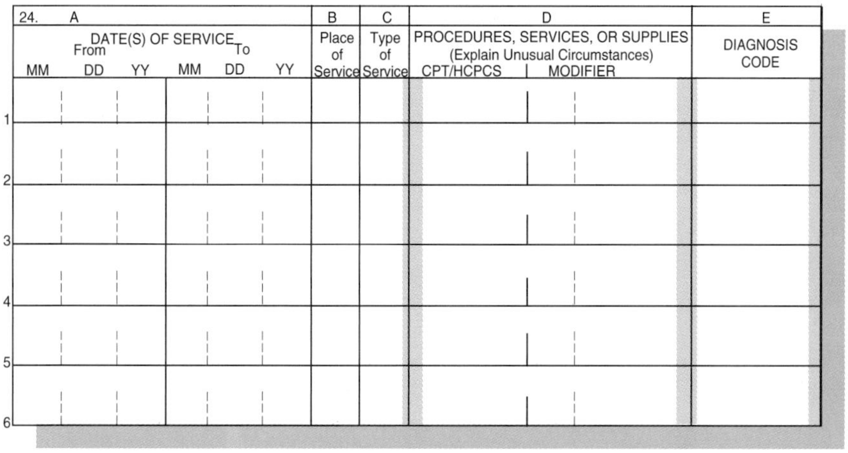

FIGURE 4-16
Block No. 24A-block No. 24E of the CMS-1500 claim form.

Claims sent on paper often require a one-digit alpha or numeric code. Check with individual payors for best results when selecting place of service codes for paper claims.

Electronic claims may be sent in either the National Standard Format **(NSF)** or the **ANSII format.** The ANSII format is more versatile, but it takes a lot of computer hard-drive space and a lot of processing power. You may attach a copy of an electronic medical record or operative report to an electronic claim when you use the ANSII format. Hospitals with large computer networks most often use the ANSII format for electronic claims.

> To meet the administrative requirements of HIPAA, eventually one format will be chosen and all claims must use the same format. It is expected that eventually all claims will use the ANSII format.

The NSF format is more restrictive because only the data completed on the actual claim form may be transmitted, but it runs well on any computer. At the writing of this book, physician offices most often use the NSF format for electronic claims, and supporting documentation, when needed, is mailed under separate cover.

Electronic claims sent in the NSF electronic format must contain the national standard two-digit numeric codes. When processing electronic claims for a payor that requires an alpha code in this field, use the two-letter national standard code to transmit the claim to your clearinghouse. The clearinghouse then converts each code into the form desired by the specific payor.

The following national standard two-digit numeric place of service codes may be used:

11-Office
12-Home
21-Hospital (inpatient)
22-Hospital (outpatient)
23-Emergency
24-ASC (ambulatory)
25-Birthing Center
26-Military Facility
31-Skilled Nursing Facility
32-Nursing Facility
33-Custodial Care
34-Hospice
41-Ambulance
42-Ambulance (land) (air/water)
50-Federal Health Clinic
51-Psych. Facility (inpatient)
52-Psych. Facility
53-Community Mental Health (partial hospitalization)
54-Intermediate Care Facility
55-Residential Facility - Substance

56-Residential Facility - Psychiatric
61-Comp. Rehabilitation - Inpatient
62-Comp. Rehabilitation - Outpatient
65-End-Stage Renal Disease
71-Public Health Clinic (state or local)
72-Health Clinic (rural)
81-Independent Laboratory
99-Other Unlisted Facility

Medicare does not recognize the following national standard codes:

5-Day Care Facility
6-Night Care Psychiatric Facility
W-Walk-In Facility

Block No. 24C. Type of Service
Figure 4-16 shows block No. 24C. Most payors require this field.

Payor-specific requirements:
   Medicare: While Medicare states they do not currently require this field, they do not reject or penalize claims that use the field. In addition, an "invalid type of service for the provider's specialty" is one of the top 10 reasons listed for denials of Medicare claims on the Noridian website for Arizona's Medicare Part B. Therefore correctly completing this field for Medicare claims might play a role in preventing denials.

The following national standard "type of service" codes are valid:

01-Medical Care
02-Surgery
03-Consultation
04-Diagnostic X-ray
05-Diagnostic Laboratory
06-Radiation Therapy
07-Anesthesia
08-Surgical Assistance
09-Other Medical
10-Blood Charges
11-Used DME
12-DME Purchase
13-ASC Facility
14-Renal Supplies in Home
15-Alternate Method
16-CDR Equipment Dialysis
17-Preadmission Testing
18-DME Rental
19-Pneumonia Vaccine
20-Second Surgical Opinion
21-Third Surgical Opinion
H*-Hospice
I*-Injections
T*-Dental

X*-Maternity
99-Other (for prescription drugs)

Block No. 24D. Procedures, Services, or Supplies

Figure 4-16 shows block No. 24D. *This is a required field for all claims.* This box is used to report procedures, services, and/or supplies using codes from current-year procedure codebooks. Procedure codes are five-digit numeric or alphanumeric codes. Always use the most specific code supported by the physician's documentation.

This element is divided into two parts: (1) CPT/HCPCS codes and (2) modifiers. The first half will contain the code number that most closely identifies the procedure, service, or supply being billed on this line, and the second half will contain the applicable modifier(s), if any. See Chapters 6 and 7 for billing guidelines and coding conventions applicable to block No. 24D.

Do not enter narrative descriptions of codes. For most payors, local codes have been replaced with Level II HCPCS codes.

Most payors allow two modifiers to be listed in the space provided. A few payors will accept three modifiers in this field when claims are sent electronically. When more modifiers are needed than the payor accepts in this field, modifier -99 is entered here and the remaining modifiers are listed in block No. 19. See Billing with Modifiers in Chapter 7 for guidelines and examples.

When rebilling or auditing, use codebooks for the same year as the date of service.

Payor-specific requirements:

Medicare: Do not send supporting documentation unless Medicare specifically requests it.

When Medicare claims are filed on paper, modifier -99 is required if more than two modifiers are used. However, when electronic claims are submitted directly to Medicare using the software provided by Medicare, up to three modifiers may be listed in block No. 24D, and modifier -99 is not required unless there are more than three modifiers. In either case, only modifier -99 appears in block No. 24D when this modifier is used on a Medicare claim. *Note:* Because Medicare now requires claims to be submitted electronically, paper claims are rarely used.

Workers' Compensation: Some states require the use of procedure codes from the 1995 or 1996 CPT codebooks. Some state carriers do not recognize some modifiers. Check with the carrier for the state in which the work-related injury occurred.

Medicaid: Some states require the use of procedure codes from the 1995 or 1996 CPT codebooks. Some states do not recognize some modifiers. Check with the Medicaid carrier for your state.

Block No. 24E. Diagnosis Code

Figure 4-16 shows block No. 24E. *This is a required field for all claims.* This field links the procedure on this line to a specific diagnosis from the choices in block No. 21. Many payors use this field to establish medical necessity for the service listed on this line.

The entire diagnosis code is not normally repeated here, just the line number. Enter the appropriate diagnosis line number (1, 2, 3, 4) from block No. 21 to identify the principal diagnosis or condition for the service reported on this line in block No. 24D. Do not include E-codes. Some payors require one linking diagnosis and others allow multiple linking diagnoses (1 3) or (13).

Payor-specific requirements:

Medicare: Medicare requires one linking diagnosis.

Medicaid: In some states, Medicaid only allows one linking diagnosis. Medicaid sometimes requires the entire diagnosis code, not the line number.

Block No. 24F. Charges

Figure 4-17 shows block No. 24F of the CMS-1500 claim form. *This is a required field for all claims, including capitation claims.* Enter the charge for the item on this line in block No. 24D.

When the physician is prepaid under the capitation system, all the charge amounts are "00." A claim is filed so both the physician and the payor may track the services rendered and analyze whether the capitation amount in the contract is appropriate for the services actually rendered each year.

To meet EDI and OCR requirements, do not include the dollar ($) sign.

F	G	H	I	J	K	
$ CHARGES	DAYS OR UNITS	EPSDT Family Plan	EMG	COB	RESERVED FOR LOCAL USE	PHYSICIAN OR SUPPLIER INFORMATION

FIGURE 4-17
Block No. 24F-block No. 24K of the CMS-1500 claim form.

Payor-specific requirements:

Medicare: You may not charge Medicare a larger fee than you accept from any other source for the same item. See the *Federal Register*, April 26, 2000, pages 24400-24419 for the final rule for "Health Care Programs, Fraud and Abuse; Revised OIG Civil Monetary Penalties Resulting From Public Law 104-191" (HIPAA).

Block No. 24G. Days or Units

Figure 4-17 shows block No. 24G. *This is a required field for all claims.* Enter the number of days or the number of units. When only one visit, service, procedure, or supply is indicated, enter the number "1."

Only whole numbers may be entered. Usually, you may round to the nearest whole number when only a fraction of a service is delivered, but do not round to zero.

Use a modifier in block No. 24D to indicate reduced services, when applicable, and adjust the fee entered on the charge line to reflect the portion of the service actually delivered.

On rare occasions, a modifier may also be used in block No. 24D to report unusual or expanded services, and the fee is increased to reflect the service actually delivered.

With medications and supplies, report each unit of medication or supply that is opened for the patient. If another patient cannot use any remaining or unused portion, the entire amount may be charged without a modifier for reduced services. For example, injectable antibiotics must be used very soon after they are mixed. Unused portions are discarded. The entire amount is charged even if only a small portion is actually used.

However, if the supply is multipatient and multiuse, only charge for the portion actually used. For example, a sterile vial of vaccine for immunizations is often multiuse in nature. Only the portion used is charged.

Oxygen gauges typically record the volume of oxygen delivered in liters. Report the volume of oxygen by using the setting on the flow gauge for the number of liters delivered.

For anesthesia, enter the number of minutes of anesthesia. Convert hours into minutes for billing purposes.

Payor-specific requirements:

Check your contracts closely for specific payor requirements. Some payors do have idiosyncrasies for this field.

For example, some payors use "010" to report "1" whole or complete service because this method allows partial services to be reported with greater specificity.

Block No. 24H. EPSDT Family Plan

Figure 4-17 shows block No. 24H. **EPSDT** stands for Medicaid's early periodic screening and diagnostic testing program.

Payor-specific requirements:

Medicaid: Medicaid uses this field to report services rendered under the EPSDT program.

Medicare: Medicare requires this field to be blank.

Block No. 24I. EMG

Figure 4-17 shows block No. 24I. This field is used by some payors when the service rendered is related to an emergency. The place of service code must also reflect the emergency nature of the care. Some payors reimburse at a higher rate for emergency services.

Payor-specific requirements:

Medicare: Medicare requires this field to be blank.

Medicaid: In some states, Medicaid requires this box for emergency room services. Check the requirements for your state.

Block No. 24J. COB

Figure 4-17 shows block No. 24J. COB stands for "coordination of benefits." Some payors require this section to identify when a second policy also provides coverage. The medical plans involved exchange information to be sure that no more than the total usual and customary charge is paid.

Payor-specific requirements:

Read your payor contracts to learn whether this field is required.

Medicare: Although Medicare currently requires this section to be blank, Medicare does use coordination of benefits to limit charges.

When Medicare is the secondary payor, Medicare pays the difference between the primary payor's "allowed" amount and the payment sent by the primary payor, up to the amount Medicare would have paid if Medicare had been the primary payor.

For example, the charge is $180.00. Plan A allowed $150.00 and paid 80%, or $120.00. Medicare's normal allowed amount for this charge is $120.00, and Medicare normally pays 50% of the allowed amount for this type of service (psychiatry). Therefore, as a secondary payor for this charge, Medicare pays up to $60.00 and the patient pays up to $60.00.

The difference between Plan A's allowed amount ($150.00) and payment ($120.00) is $30.00; $30.00 is less than $60.00, so Medicare pays the entire $30.00. The end result: Plan A pays $150.00, Medicare pays $30.00, patient pays $0.00, and the insurance write-off is $30.00.

However, if the charge remained $180.00, and Plan A allowed $150.00 but only paid 50% of the allowed amount, or $75.00, the difference between Plan A's allowed amount ($150.00) and payment ($75.00) is $75.00. As secondary payor for this charge, Medicare still pays up to $60.00, and the patient still pays up to $60.00. The end result: Plan A pays $75.00, Medicare pays $60.00, patient pays $15.00, and the insurance write-off is $30.00.

Note: When Medicare replaces the UPINs and PINs with an NPI number, it is expected that part of the NPI number will be placed in block No. 24J, and the rest of the NPI number will be placed in block No. 24K.

Medicaid: When Medicaid is the secondary payor, Medicaid often pays only the amount required for the total payment to reach Medicaid's allowed amount. For example: the charge is $180.00. Plan A allowed $150.00 and paid 80%, or $120.00. If Medicaid's allowed amount is $100.00, Medicaid will not pay an additional amount because $120.00 is more than Medicaid's allowed amount of $100.00.

However, if Medicaid's allowed amount is $130.00, Medicaid will pay $10.00 so total payment ($120.00 plus $10.00) would equal Medicaid's allowed amount ($130.00).

Block No. 24K. Reserved for Local Use

Figure 4-17 shows block No. 24k. This field is required by many payors to identify the rendering physician(s) or other provider(s) from a group practice for each item listed on the claim. Some payors require the rendering physician's SSN, and some require a payor-specific ID number.

When a payor sends payment to a practice and not to a specific physician, this element informs the payor which physician or provider actually performed each service. This is important because each physician within the medical practice signs his or her own contracts. The payor wants to verify whether the physician who performed the service is under contract with the medical plan.

Do not use the practice's Federal Employer Identification Number **(FEIN)** in this field, and do not enter the Medicare practice ID number (Medicare PIN). Only duly licensed people may render medical care; a business entity may not render medical care.

Payor-specific requirements:

Medicare: Often Medicare requires block No. 24K to be completed with a performing provider ID number (PPIN) that is unique to Medicare (12345Z). When several different physicians or suppliers within a group report services using the same group ID number, an individual performing provider ID number is issued to identify which of the physicians actually rendered each service. This provider number is entered in block No. 24K. The Medicare provider number is not the UPIN (A12345) used in block No. 17a for referring physicians, and it is not the group PIN used in block No. 33 to identify the group or practice. Beginning in June 2005, Medicare will begin issuing NPI numbers to replace both the UPIN and the PPIN.

A solo practitioner who incorporates is issued a practice ID number like a group as well as an individual provider number. The provider number is entered in block No. 24K, and the PIN is entered in block No. 33.

When a solo practitioner does not incorporate, Medicare issues a PPIN, but not a PIN. The PPIN is reported in block No. 33, but block No. 24K is left blank.

Medicaid: In some states Medicaid requires a provider number in block No. 24K. Check the Medicaid manual for your state.

BLOCK NO. 25. PROVIDER TAX ID NUMBER

Figure 4-18 shows block No. 25 of the CMS-1500 claim form. *This is a required field.* This box contains the provider's tax ID number, which may be an SSN or FEIN. The payor uses this number to tell the IRS the total amount of payments the payor sent to the physician or practice.

BLOCK NO. 26. PATIENT ACCOUNT NUMBER

Figure 4-18 shows block No. 26. *This is a required field.* The **patient account number** is a number assigned by you or by your practice management computer system for internal identification of the patient's account. Many payors use this field to link together different claims for the same patient within their computer system. The EOB also reports this

25. FEDERAL TAX I.D. NUMBER	SSN EIN	26. PATIENT'S ACCOUNT NO.	27. ACCEPT ASSIGNMENT? (For govt. claims, see back)	28. TOTAL CHARGE	29. AMOUNT PAID	30. BALANCE DUE
	☐ ☐		☐ YES ☐ NO	$	$	$

FIGURE 4-18
Block No. 25-block No. 30 of the CMS-1500 claim form.

number, enabling you to verify that payment is posted to the correct patient account.

BLOCK NO. 27. ACCEPT ASSIGNMENT?

Figure 4-18 shows block No. 27. *This is a required field.* Whereas block No. 13 indicates whether the patient is willing to assign benefits, this field indicates whether the physician is willing to accept assignment of benefits. The back of the CMS-1500 claim form contains additional directions for this field for government programs.

A "yes" in this field indicates the physician is willing to accept assignment of payments. Payor payment is mailed to the physician or practice.

A "no" in this field indicates the physician is not willing to accept assignment of benefits, and the patient must pay the physician directly. Payor payment, if any, is sent to the patient.

> Originally, this field was only used for Medicare, but now all payors use this information. You are required to complete this section, even when the claim is for a private medical plan.

Payor-specific requirements:

Medicare: "Yes" must be marked if the physician is a participating Medicare provider.

Medigap: "Yes" must be marked if the physician is a participating Medigap provider.

Managed Care: Most managed care plans require "yes" in this field.

TRICARE/CHAMPUS: The physician must file the claim when accepting assignment of benefits. By accepting assignment, the physician accepts the CHAMPUS maximum allowable charge along with the patient's deductible and cost-share as payment-in-full and may not balance bill the beneficiary for the remainder of the bill.

BLOCK NO. 28. TOTAL CHARGES

Figure 4-18 shows block No. 28. This box indicates the total charges for lines 1 through 6 in block No. 24F.

Capitation plans should enter ".00" under total charges.

> To meet EDI and OCR requirements, do not include the dollar ($) sign.

BLOCK NO. 29. AMOUNT PAID

Figure 4-18 shows block No. 29. This field is used to inform payors about payments or copayments made by patients applicable to the services reported in block No. 24D. Except in very specific instances, many payors, including Medicare, consider it fraudulent to waive the patient responsibility amount.

Patient copayments received at the time of service are entered here. If the patient has a secondary payor, this field may be left blank on the claim to the primary payor because the secondary payor usually covers these amounts.

Enter only patient payments for the covered services applicable to this claim.

Do not use this field to record payments for noncovered services.

Do not use this field to record patient payments for a balance due on other transactions.

Unless it is a capitated plan, the amount paid should not equal or exceed the amount due for the claim in block No. 28.

> To meet EDI and OCR requirements, do not include the dollar ($) sign.

Payor-specific requirements:

Medicare: Medicare will not allow you to waive the patient's portion of the charges.

Managed care: Most managed care plans require a patient copayment at the time of service. The payor contract often requires the copayment to be listed on the claim, and payor edits check this field to see if contract requirements are met. When the field is blank or records a .00 payment, a penalty may be imposed. The amount of payment could be reduced and sent with an EOB that reflects payment in "the amount agreed to in the contract."

Capitation: Capitation plans (some of the managed care HMOs and PPOs) should indicate ".00" under total charges and record the patient copayment here.

BLOCK NO. 30. BALANCE DUE

Figure 4-18 shows block No. 30. This field records the balance due for the services reported on lines 1 through 6 in block No. 24D. Except with capitation plans, the balance due is calculated by subtracting the payments received in block No. 29 from the total charges in block No. 28. For example, if the total charges were $350.00, and the patient copayments total $20.00, the balance due is $330.00.

With capitation plans, the physician is paid in advance for services rendered, so the total due is always reported as .00. Claims are filed to allow both the physician and the managed care plan to evaluate whether the amount paid to the physician each month is appropriate. That is, will it cover reasonable expenses overall for this group of patients, provide a reasonable profit for the physician, and keep medical costs down for the managed care plan?

> To meet EDI and OCR requirements, do not include the dollar ($) sign.

Payor-specific requirements:

Medicare: Medicare does not require this field. It may be left blank.

BLOCK NO. 31. PROVIDER SIGNATURE AND DATE

Figure 4-19 shows block No. 31 of the CMS-1500 claim form. *This is a required field.* This field tells the payor in writing, not numbers, who rendered the services and the date the claim was filed.

You may type the physician's name in this section only when the physician has given written permission for you to file claims in his or her name. Payor claim edits check to see if the name entered here correlates with the ID numbers listed in block No. 24K and block No. 33.

> In most of the sections that ask for a signature, you may file the claim with "signature on file" or "SOF" entered on the signature line when you have the appropriate signature(s) available in your office records. In this section, most payors will not allow the "signature on file" statement but do allow the typed name of the provider instead of an actual signature when you have written permission from the physician to file claims in his or her name.

The filing date is often different from the date services were rendered. Most payor contracts require claims to be filed within a specified number of days from the date of service. Payor claim edits check to see if contract requirements were met.

> To meet EDI and OCR requirements, use only numbers for dates and do not enter slashes or dashes. For more details, see the directions for block No. 3.

Payor-specific requirements:

Medicare: Medicare will not process claims with a typed signature unless Medicare has a copy of the physician's written permission for you to file claims in the physician's name. The information in block No. 33 must also correlate with Medicare's records.

Workers' Compensation: In some states, you do not need a signature for a workers' compensation certified physician—see the rules on the back of the CMS-1500.

Automobile: Some states require personal injury protection (PIP) to be added to every auto policy. Those states sometimes require the physician's medical license number to be entered into block No. 31 in addition to the block's normal requirements. Check the requirements for your state.

BLOCK NO. 32. NAME AND ADDRESS OF FACILITY WHERE SERVICES WERE RENDERED (IF OTHER THAN HOME OR OFFICE)

Figure 4-19 shows block No. 32. This field identifies rated facilities, such as laboratories, radiology centers, hospitals, surgical centers, emergency rooms, and more. The field is completed any time the services or procedures reported in block No. 24D were rendered in a facility, not in the patient's home and not in an office setting in which the practice is responsible for paying expenses.

If more than one facility was used, a separate claim must be submitted for the services rendered at each facility. Include the name, address, and facility ID number for each facility. This information tells the payor that a facility will be submitting a UB-92 claim form for their expenses, and the payment for the services will be split—usually 60% to the rendering physician and 40% to the facility.

The facility is only assigned a facility number when the facility processes Part B Medicare claims. The facility ID number is a two-letter code plus the nine-digit tax ID number (AL123456789). It is not the facility's Medicare provider number. Usually you may obtain the facility ID number from the facility's billing office. If they do not know the number or do not have a facility number, use the facility's tax ID number.

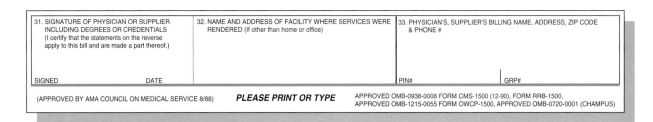

FIGURE 4-19
Block No. 31-block No. 33 on the CMS-1500 claim form.

CPT only © 2005. Current Procedural Terminology, 2006, Professional Edition, American Medical Association. All Rights Reserved.

BLOCK NO. 33. PROVIDER OR PRACTICE BILLING NAME, ADDRESS, TELEPHONE NUMBER, AND ID NUMBER

Figure 4-19 shows block No. 33. *This is a required field*. This field tells the payor the name of the physician, practice, or supplier and the address to which the claim payment will be sent. The name, address, telephone number, and ID number entered here must match the name, address, telephone number, and ID number in payor records and must correlate with payor records for the items entered in block No. 24K and block No. 31. When discrepancies are found, payment will be denied or delayed.

Payor-specific requirements:

Medicare: For a professional association, a group practice, and an incorporated practice, enter the carrier-assigned group PIN. This is not the Medicare UPIN that identifies referring physicians in block No. 17a, and it is not the Medicare PPIN that identifies each individual provider within the group or incorporated practice. The PIN identifies the group or incorporated practice.

When a solo practitioner is not incorporated, the provider number serves as the ID number for this field, and it is only reported in block No. 33. It is not reported in block No. 24K.

Answer the following questions:
1. When is block No. 14 required, and what date is entered for each item listed?

_____

2. Which payor requires the use of block No. 16?

_____

3. When is block No. 32 used?

_____

4. What is an outside lab?

_____

5. What payor requires the use of block No. 22?

_____

6. What is the purpose of block No. 24E?

_____

7. What number is placed in block No. 17a for Medicare?
   A. SSN or FEIN
   B. Medicare UPIN
   C. Medicare provider number
   D. Medicare PIN

8. What number is placed in block No. 24K for Medicare when the practice has a group ID number?
   A. SSN or FEIN
   B. Medicare UPIN
   C. Medicare provider number
   D. Medicare PIN
9. What number is placed in block No. 25 for Medicare?
   A. SSN or FEIN
   B. Medicare UPIN
   C. Medicare provider number
   D. Medicare PIN
10. What number is placed in block No. 33 for Medicare when the practice is a group?
   A. SSN or FEIN
   B. Medicare UPIN
   C. Medicare provider number
   D. Medicare PIN

Clinical Application Exercise

Use the superbill in Figure 4-20 and the physician notes in Figure 4-21 to complete the bottom half of the claim form in Figure 4-22.

SUBMISSION OF CLAIMS

Your goal is to send clean claims the first time so you do not have to research, correct, and either resubmit or appeal claims in the future. Many practice management software systems allow you to preview claims before sending them. Most allow you to print the claims on plain paper so you can use a transparency of the CMS-1500 claim form to double-check each claim for accuracy and completeness. You may want to make multiple transparencies of the claim form and highlight specific boxes that must be completed for each of your major payors so you do not overlook crucial information.

Lake Eola Family Practice
FEIN 23-XX67890   Group # 45670Y   517860 South Pioneer Drive, Orlando, FL 32897 • 634-555-4893
S u p e r b i l l   #456298   Weight _174_   BP _158/94_   TPR _98.6-92-20_

Account Number _PARW002_	Doctor _Eric Anderson MD_	Date of Service _02/06/20XX_
Patient Name _Parker, Wanda_	Date of Birth _11/12/1932_	LMP _N/A_
Insurance _BCBS/Medicare_	Responsible Party _Ronald Parker_	Phone Number _634-555-1212_
Address _PO Box YYYY_	Referring Physician and ID # _None_	
City _Jacksonville_ State _FL_	Zip _94187_	

New Patient

__ 99201 H [PF]   E [PF]   MDM [S]   10 min
__ 99202 H [EPF] E [EPF] MDM [S]   20 min
__ 99203 H [D]   E [D]   MDM [LC]   30 min
__ 99204 H [C]   E [C]   MDM [MC]   45 min
__ 99205 H [C]   E [C]   MDM [HC]   60 min

Established Patient

__ 99211 H [N/A] E[N/A]   MDM [N/A]   5 min
__ 99212 H [PF]   E [PF]   MDM [S]   10 min
__ 99213 H [EPF] E [EPF] MDM [LC]   15 min
✓ 99214 H [D]   E [D]   MDM [MC]   25 min
__ 99215 H [C]   E [C]   MDM [HC]   40 min

Reason For Visit

__ Authorization _____
      Expiration Date _____
__ Annual exam, complex due to (history,
      condition): _____
__ Annual exam, simple
✓ Follow-up, condition _Benign ↑BP_
__ Follow-up, post procedure, no condition
      or complication _____
      Procedure/date _____
__ Follow-up, post procedure, with condition
      or complication _____
      Procedure/date _____
✓ New Problem _headaches_
__ Post-op, no condition or complication
      Surgery/date _____
__ Post-op, with conditions or complication

      Surgery/date _____
__ Pre-op
__ Procedure _____
__ Second surgical opinion _____
__ Other (Accident, Decision for surgery)
      _____

Procedures

⇒ Place to be done: _____
⇒ Date to be done: _____
__ Authorization _____
      Expiration date _____
__ Biopsy,type/site_____
      _____
__ Cautery, type/site _____
      _____
__ Destruction of lesion(s), extensive, site:
      _____
__ Destruction of lesion(s), simple, site:
      _____
__ Emergency surgery, (list above), reason:
      _____
__ Excision, type/site _____
      _____
__ I & D abscess, type/site: _____
      _____
__ Insertion/Removal of IUD, type _____
__ Major surgery, type/site _____
      _____
__ Minor surgery, type/site _____
      _____
__ Sonogram _____
__ Other _____

Miscellaneous

__ Immunization _____
__ Injection _____
__ Supplies
__ Surgical Tray
__ Patient Teaching (Preventive medicine)
      _____
      _____

✓ Other _Consult Dr. Perez — please_
      conduct carotid artery studies
      _____
      _____

Outside Lab

__ Beta HCG, Serum
__ Biopsy/ Pathology
__ Biopsy, Mult./Pathology
__ CBC
__ Cholesterol
__ Culture, throat
__ Cultures (source) _____
__ Glucose, __ 1hr glucose, __ 3hr glucose
__ Estrogen
__ Herpes simplex, AB
__ Mononucleosis
__ Pap Smear
__ PT __ PTT
__ Sed rate
__ SMAC
__ Urinalysis, w/micro
__ HIV
__ Other _____
      _____
      _____
      _____

1. _401.1_
2. _784.0_
3. _437.0_
4. _____

Appointment In __1__ Weeks
Procedure In _____ Weeks
Sent Labs to _____
Call In _____ Mos./Weeks

Previous Balance $ _150.00_ .
Co-Pay $ _Secondary_ .
Paid Today Cash/Check $ _0_ .
(Yes)-No All Diagnoses, Procedures, & VS above are documented in Record

New Charges $ _120.00_ .
New Balance $ _270.00_ .
Check Number _N/A_

Doctor's Signature _Eric Anderson MD_   Provider # 78901Z

FIGURE 4-20
Completed superbill.

Name **Wanda Parker**   Date **02/06/20**XX

HPI Chief Complaint:

F/U Benign hypertension

Headaches, ↑ frequency & ↑
  severity over past month.
Does not ↑ c̄ activity.

Current Meds.:

Lasix 20 mg qd.
K Dur 10 mEq qd.
Inderal 10 mg qd.

Past/Family History

Father died from Stroke at age 54
Mother died from MI at age 58

THIS SECTION TO BE COMPLETED BY PATIENT.

Personal/Social History

Are you... ☐ single ☒ married
☐ live in partner ☐ divorced ☐ widow

Do you have children? ☒ Yes ☐ No
Ages of child(ren) **48, 44, 40**
No. of pregnancies **3** Miscarriages **0**
Occupation **Housewife**
If retired, how do you spend your time?
Active in Retirement Community

                                Yes No
a. Do you have concerns about your
  breasts? (circle): changes in size or
  shape, changes in skin color, lumps,
  tenderness, ulcerations, discharge or
  blood from nipple, inverted nipple ☐ ☒
b. Do you have menstrual bleeding? ☐ ☒
  If so, ☐ rarely ☐ monthly
      ☐ more than monthly
c. Do you take hormones (estrogen)? ☐ ☒
d. Concerns about lessions, lumps or
  swelling on your vulva or vagina? ☐ ☒
e. Do you have vaginal dryness, itching ☐ ☒
  or pain?
f. Do you have urine leakage? *not new* ☐ ☐

g. Approximate date of last pelvic exam. **6/20**XX
h. Approximate date of last pap test **6/20**XX
i. Approximate date of last mammogram **7/20**XX
                                Yes No
j. Are you sexually active now? ☒ ☐
k. Do you have other sexual concerns? ☐ ☒
l. Do you feel safe/comfortable in
  your home, with your family, and/or
  your partner relationship? ☒ ☐
m. Do you smoke or use tobacco
  products now? ☐ ☒
n. Do you use recreational drugs? ☐ ☒
o. Do you drink alcohol? ☒ ☐
  ☐ daily ☐ weekly ☒ rarely
  # of drinks **1**
  If yes, do you drink: ☐ beer, ☒ wine, ☐ liquor

Review of Systems

Are you concerned about? (circle concerns) Yes No
1. Recent changes in health status ☒ ☐
2. Eye problems: (vision,) pain, tearing ☒ ☐
3. Ears, nose, mouth, throat problems ☐ ☒
4. Heart problems: chest pain, (blood pressure) ☒ ☐

                                    Yes No
5. Lung problems: coughing, wheezing, ☐ ☒
  infections
6. Abdominal pain, stomach, bowel problems ☐ ☒
7. Kidney or bladder problems ☐ ☒
8. Muscle, bone, joint or back problems ☐ ☒
9. Skin, hair or nail problems ☐ ☒
10. Neurologic problems (headaches,) ☒ ☐
  dizziness, numbness
11. Nervousness, anxiety, depression, ☐ ☒
  suicidal thoughts
12. Excessive thirst and urine output, ☐ ☒
  recent weight changes
13. Anemia, bruising, blood clots, ☐ ☒
  swollen glands
14. Food allergies, hayfever, eczema, ☐ ☒
  asthma, decreased immunity
Do you have any other concerns? ☐ ☒

_____

_____

Wanda Parker   *Feb 6, XX*
Patient's Signature   Date

Provider Comments: Vision blurry by late in day x 1 week

HA x 1 mo, ↑ frequency, now daily, & ↑ intensity–relieved c̄ ESTylenol.
Rent ↑ causing financial stress.

☒ PFSH and ROS have been reviewed.   ☐ Unresolved problems from previous visit have been addressed.

Eric Anderson MD   *2/6/XX*
Provider's Signature   Date

Anticipatory Guidance

☐ Nutrition
☐ Calcium/Multi-vitamin
☐ Exercise/Recreation/Hobbies
☐ Dental care
☐ Sun exposure

☐ Smoking cessation
☐ Alcohol/drugs
☒ Cardiovascular risks
☐ Aspirin prophylaxis
☐ Osteoporosis risks/Estrogen
☐ Self exam. breasts, skin, oral cavity
☐ Sexual issues

☐ STD prevention
☐ Menopause
☐ Work/Retirement
☐ Family
☐ Safety/ Injury/Gun Safety
☐ Auto seat belts
☐ Smoke detectors

☐ Domestic violence
☐ Hot water <120°
☐ Fall prevention
☐ CPR for family members
☒ Stress
☒ Living Will
☒ Medical Power of Attorney

©1995 Piermed, Inc. Rev. 6/98 (800) 998-1908

500-06

Female 60+

FIGURE 4-21
Medical record entry for one visit. (Docuform courtesy Piermed, Inc., Lewisville, NC.)

Name _Wanda Parker_   DOB _11_ / _12_ / _1932_ Age _68_ Chart No. | PARW002 |

Assessment

6.a.,c. —Bruit/Thrill bilat. — carotid arteries

BP↑ $\bar{c}$ meds.

R/O CAD

R/O CVD

Chol. last month 210 — no meds.
Hx cerebal atherosclerosis

Plan

↑ Lasix to 20 mg BID
↑ Inderol to 10 mg BID
↑ K-Dur to 10 mEq BID

Consult Dr. Perez for carotid
artery Studies—
compare to studies 1 yr ago.

Eric Anderson MD _____   _1 wk_ _____
Provider's Signature   Return Visit

FOLD HERE   FOLD HERE

Physical Exam

Ht. _5' 5"_ Wt. _174_ Temp. _98^6_ Resp. _20_

B.P. sit. or stand. _158_ / _94_   Supine _150_ / _90_

Pulse rate and regularity _92 & regular_

Circle abnormal and pertinent normal findings
Describe abnormalities above.
☑ Normal   ☒ Abnormal

1. Constitutional
a.☑ gen. appear., development, body shape, nutrition, deformities, grooming

2. Eyes
a.☑ conjunctiva, lids
b.☑ pupils, irises
c.☑ fundi (optic discs, vessels, exudate, hemorr.)

3. Ears, Nose, Throat & Mouth
a.☑ appearance of ears, appearance of nose
b.☑ auditory canals, tympanic membranes
c.☑ hearing (whis. voice, finger rub, tun. fork)
d.☑ nasal mucosa, septum, turbinates
e.☑ lips, teeth, gums
f.☑ oropharynx (mucosa, saliv. glands, hard & soft palates, tongue, tonsils, post. pharynx)

4. Neck
a.☑ appearance, masses, symmetry, tracheal position, crepitus
b.☑ thyroid (enlargement, tenderness, mass)

5. Respiratory
a.☑ respiratory effort (intercostal retractions) use of accessory muscles, diaphragm move.
b.☑ percussion (dullness, flatness, hyper-reson.)
c.☑ palpation (tactile fremitus)
d.☑ auscultation (breath sounds, rhonchi, wheezes, rales, rubs)

6. Cardiovascular
a.☒ palpation (location of p.m.i., size, (thrill)
b.☑ auscultation (abnormal sounds, murmurs)
c.☒ carotid arteries (pulse amplitude, (bruits)
d.☑ abdominal aorta (size, bruits)
e.☑ femoral arteries (pulse amplitude, bruits)
f.☑ pedal pulses (pulse amplitude)
g.☑ extremities (edema, varicosities)

7. Chest (Breasts)
a.☐ inspection (size, symmetry, nipple discharge)
b.☐ palpation of breasts & axillae (masses, lumps, tenderness)

8. Gastrointestinal (Abdomen)
a.☑ examination for masses, tenderness
b.☑ examination of liver, spleen
c.☑ examination for presence or absence of hernia
d.☐ examination of (when indicated) anus, perineum, rectum: (sphincter tone, hemorrhoids, masses)
e.☐ stool for occult blood when indicated

9. Genitourinary
Pelvic Exam, (with or without specimen collection for smears or cultures), including:
a.☐ Ext. Genitalia (eg. gen. app., hair distrib., lesions) and vagina (eg. gen. app., estogen eff., lesions, pelvic support, cystocele, rectocele)
b.☐ Urethra (eg. fullness, masses, tender.)
c.☐ Bladder (eg. fullness, masses, tener.)
d.☐ Cervix (eg. gen. app., lesions, disch.)
e.☐ Uterus (eg. size, contour, position, mobility, tender., consistency, decent or support)
f.☐ Adnexia / Parametria (eg. masses, tender., organomegaly, nodularity)

10. Lymphatic
a.☑ palpation of lymph nodes in 2 or more areas: (Circle (neck (axillae) groin, other)

11. Musculoskeletal
a.☑ examination of gait and station
b.☑ inspection and/or palpation of digits & nails (clubbing, cyanosis, inflammatory conditions, petechiae, ischemia, infections, nodes)
c.☑ assessment of range of motion (pain, crepitation, contracture)
d.☑ Examination of joint, bone, & muscle of 1 or more of the following 6 areas (circle)
  • head/neck   • rt. upper extremities
  • spine, ribs, & pelvis   • lt. upper extremities
  • rt. lower extremities   • lt. lower extremities
e.☑ inspect, and/or palpation (misalign, asymmetry, crepitation, defects, tender, masses, effusion)
f.☑ assesment of stability: dislocation (luxation), subluxation or laxity
g.☑ muscle strength & tone (flaccid, cog wheel, spastic), atrophy or abnormal movement

12. Skin
a.☑ inspection of skin & sub-Q tissue (rashes, lesion, ulcers)
b.☑ palpation of skin & sub-Q tissue (induration, sub-Q nodules, tightening)

13. Neurology
a.☐ test cranial nerves: notation of deficits
b.☑ examination of DTR's with notation of pathological reflexes (eg. Babinski)
c.☑ examination of sensation (touch, pain, vibration, proprioception)

14. Psychiatric
a.☐ description of patient's judgment & insight
  Brief assessment of mental status:
b.☑ orientation to time, place, & person
c.☑ recent & remote memory
d.☑ mood & affect (depression, anxiety, agitation)
e.☐ other————————

Procedures and Immunizations

Are immunizations current? ☒ Yes ☐ No

☐ Hearing   ☐ PT   ☐ Triglyceride   ☐ Stool Guaiac
☒ Vision   ☐ TSH   ☐ CXR   ☐ Sigmoidoscopy   ☐ dT
☐ CBC   ☐ Urine   ☐ EKG   ☐ Hep B
☐ Glucose   ☐ Cholesterol ☐ PAP Test   ☐ Influenza
             ☐ HDL/LDL   ☐ Mammogram

Drug Allergies:

NKA

Female 60+   Date / Time _2/6/XX_ 11 AM   Summary 401.1 784.0 437.0   ☐ Referral

500-06

FIGURE 4-21, cont'd

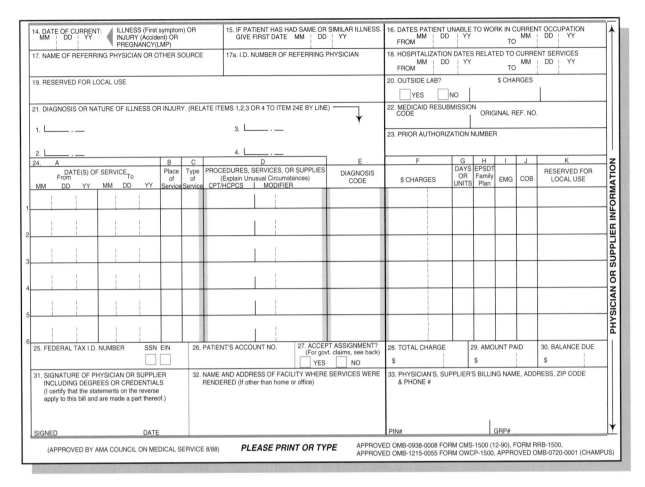

FIGURE 4-22
Physician-supplied information section of the CMS-1500.

Occasionally, you will need to correct information before submitting the claim batch. Prepare a claim form cheat-sheet showing block by block where each claim form entry is located in your practice's computer system. This way, you can easily find the practice management software's field containing the improper entry when you need to make corrections.

Electronic claims may be sent directly to each payor, or electronic claims may be sent to a clearinghouse for pre-editing before claim submission. You may expect to receive payment for clean electronic claims in approximately 14 business days.

Clearinghouse edits are similar to payor edits, and they give you the opportunity to correct a "dirty" claim before a payor record of the transaction is established. National claims clearinghouses meet payor specifications for the major payors that accept electronic claims for every state. You do not have to reside in the same state as your claims clearinghouse. If your practice is located in the United States and you have a computer with a modem, you may use any of the national claims clearinghouses to send electronic claims.

Not all clearinghouses are national, and the list of electronic payors varies for every clearinghouse. The availability of reports also varies. Some clearinghouses give you good feedback with reports to confirm claim acceptance by the payor, and some clearinghouses do not send confirmatory reports.

When you are given a choice, choose a clearinghouse that includes the majority of your payors on the electronic payor list and that confirms payor acceptance of claims. The confirmation of payor acceptance of the claim is invaluable when you are given the responsibility for following up on claims not yet paid. When you call the payor to politely request the status of the claim, you can avoid receiving the excuse, "We have no record of that transaction," by beginning your conversation with a reference to the date their computer accepted the claim.

Paper claims are printed on a barcoded "drop-out red" CMS-1500 claim form and mailed to the payor. You may expect to receive payment for clean paper claims in approximately 26 working days if the claim meets OCR requirements for scanning the claim into the payor's computer and 33 business days or longer if the claim must be hand-entered into the payor's computer system.

Regardless of whether you send the claims on paper or electronically, your computer system might not process the information in the manner you expect. Software programmers make assumptions and build them into the software systems. For example, ICD-9 codes are three, four, or five digits plus a decimal after the third digit. Often the computer system will not print or transmit more than a total of five characters and spaces, even though the system seems to accept all the information typed into the field. If you include the decimal, the computer usually will count the decimal as one of the five characters and will truncate or drop the last digit in a five-digit code when the claim is printed or transmitted.

For many years, six-digit dates were required. Some software systems allow you to enter a six-digit date, and an eight-digit date is printed on the paper claims. However, the software might continue to transmit a six-digit date. You will not know this is a problem until an EOB error report tells you. To avoid this problem, always enter an eight-digit date.

Most software systems allow a degree of customization. You may ask the software company to have their support personnel program the software to accept and transmit six digits for each line in block No. 21 so the code is not truncated if you slip up and type the decimal, but be aware that the payor's computer might still truncate the code. In addition, you may ask them to program the system to require eight-digit dates in every date field.

You may also ask for other customizations. You may ask to have the computer require a name in block No. 4 every time a choice other than "Self" is entered in block No. 6. The computer can be programmed to require a date in block No. 14 and an E-code in block No. 21 every time "Yes" is selected in 10a to 10c. The computer can be programmed to ask for an automobile insurance as primary payor anytime "Yes" is marked in block No. 10b. It can be programmed to ask for an employer's name in block No. 4 whenever "Yes" is marked in block No. 10a.

The computer can be programmed to require information in block No. 9 every time "Yes" is selected in block No. 11d. You can require a "Yes" for every claim in block No. 27. Some computers also can be programmed to warn you that certain diagnosis codes are acceptable or unacceptable with specific procedures.

Always call the software company and ask for their support personnel to make any programming changes. Some software warranties become invalid if you make unauthorized changes to the system. Do not attempt to program changes yourself unless you are directed and guided in doing so by the software company's programmer.

LEGAL ISSUES

One goal of HIPAA was to standardize and then enforce the rules for medical documentation and billing. Congress hopes medical practices will comply voluntarily when there is only one set of rules to learn. Anyone who continues to ignore health care laws risks civil and/or criminal charges should an audit occur and reveal a history of noncompliance.

Every billing error (transposed numbers, misspelled names, missing or inaccurate information) places multiple practice employees at risk—owners, managers, billers, coders, and every employee who gathers information for claims. You can be held liable if you give the biller information you know is incorrect or if you are the biller and you submit claims with information you know is incorrect. Owners and managers can also be held accountable every time they "should have known" something improper occurred.

Civil penalties may be as high as $10,000.00 per occurrence plus three times the damages (the amount paid incorrectly as a result of an error). Criminal penalties may include imprisonment and/or the confiscation of personal property purchased with proceeds (money) from improper payments. Both civil and criminal penalties may include sanctions, such as exclusion from participation in government programs for a specified period. Vendors and other payors who do business with sanctioned providers also may find themselves excluded from participation in government programs. As a result, sanctioned providers often lose all their other payor contracts and all their vendors. It is very difficult for sanctioned providers to continue to conduct business.

Although many people can and do report wrongdoing to payors or to OIG/HHS, the reported wrongdoing seldom results in an investigation *if* payor records show a provider history of clean claims (an intent to comply with the law). However, when payor records show a history of penalties and/or claim rejections, a report of wrongdoing can cause a closer look to determine whether a full-scale investigation is warranted. Claim preparation is extremely important!

Chapter Review

The CMS-1500 claim form was designed for Medicare but is now used universally for outpatient provider billing. The top half of the CMS-1500 medical claim form is used to report patient demographic and insurance billing information. When a claim arrives at the payor, the claim editing and claim auditing processes begin immediately. The first items checked are those located in the top half of the claim form.

The patient is always responsible for supplying current patient demographic and insurance information for billing, but the receptionist is usually held accountable for identifying all possible payors and gathering patient-supplied information. It is usually the biller's responsibility to compare the patient information gathered during check-in with the existing information already on file.

The physician or supplier is responsible for furnishing the information recorded in the bottom half of the CMS-1500 medical claim form. This half of the claim form tells the payor the "who, what, when, where, and why" for the medical service(s) reported. It tells the payor the credentials of the rendering provider and whether the rendering provider is an authorized contractor. It also tells the payor how much the charges are and where to send payment.

When submitting a medical claim, you must address even the smallest of details, and you must be accurate. When the medical claim reaches the payor, the computer system or the assigned claims adjuster looks first for any reason not to pay the claim. If a reason to deny payment is not found, payment is authorized. Next, the computer system or the claims adjustor looks for any reason to pay the smallest amount possible.

If you want to file clean claims, you must learn to look at each claim through the payor's eyes. Many times a minor detail, such as not answering either "yes" or "no" to a question, can cause a delay in payment. The rules for completing and submitting a claim form sometimes vary depending on whether you send the claim electronically or on paper.

You can be held liable if you submit a claim with information you know is incorrect. Legally, your billing and coding must match the documentation in the medical record, not the superbill. Therefore the medical record, not the superbill, is the source document for physician-supplied billing information. You may not alter physician-supplied information, but if you see an error, you may ask the physician to correct it. Only the rendering physician may amend his or her documentation in the medical record.

Answer the following questions:

1. Where on the claim form do you enter the date the service was rendered?

2. Where on the claim form do you enter the date the claim was filed?

3. Where on the claim form do you enter the date of a work-related injury?

4. Where on the claim form do you enter the date(s) of hospitalization?

5. When services are rendered for an unborn baby, what date of birth is entered for the patient and why?

6. Where on the claim form does the patient give permission for assignment of benefits?

7. Where on the claim form does the physician accept or decline assignment of benefits?

8. Where on the claim form is the practice tax ID entered?

9. Where on the claim form is the practice or group payor ID entered, when applicable?

10. Where on the claim form is the Medicare UPIN entered?

11. Where on the claim form is the payor-specific provider number entered?

12. When the physician receives capitation payments, what is entered in block No. 24F and block No. 30?

13. What is entered in block No. 4 for a workers' compensation claim?

14. What is entered in block No. 7 for TRICARE/CHAMPUS claims?

15. What is entered in block No. 1a for TRICARE/CHAMPUS claims?

16. Who is responsible for supplying information for the bottom half of the claim form?

    _____

17. Who is responsible for supplying information for the top half of the claim form?

    _____

18. If the patient's last name, Thirstun, is misspelled as Thurston on the insurance ID card, how should the name be spelled on the claim form?

    _____

19. Mrs. Webster cannot find the insurance card for her daughter Debbie, but she has the card for her daughter Sarah. A copy of Sarah's insurance card is in Debbie's file, and Mrs. Webster assures you that the billing information is identical; after all, they are both covered under the same family policy. May you bill the services for Debbie using information from Sarah's insurance card? Why or why not?

    _____

    _____

20. Mr. Vasquez just changed medical plans and he will not get his new insurance ID card for another month, but the effective date of the insurance was last week. Mr. Vasquez has the billing information for the medical plan, including his ID number, the group number, the plan name, the mailing address for the claim, and a toll-free telephone number for you to verify coverage. He has an urgent medical problem and should be seen today. You are the receptionist. Should you let him see the physician, or is it better to wait until he has the ID card so you can make a copy of the card? Why?

    _____

    _____

5

BASIC PRINCIPLES OF DIAGNOSIS CODING

Objectives   After completing this chapter, you should be able to:

- Demonstrate how to use the diagnosis codebook
- Relate basic rules for selecting diagnosis codes and determining code specificity
- Relate basic coding conventions for special circumstances
- Discuss the role of diagnosis coding in reimbursement
- Explain how diagnosis coding is used to establish medical necessity
- Discuss strategies for helping physicians meet diagnosis code requirements
- Discuss legal responsibilities related to diagnosis coding

Key Terms

alphabetical index an alphabetical listing of diagnoses, located in Section 1 of Volume 2 of the ICD-9-CM codebook.

alphabetical index to external causes of injury and poisoning an alphabetical listing of causes and places of injuries and poisoning, located in Section 3 of Volume 2 of the ICD-9-CM codebook, right after the table of drugs and chemicals.

category three-digit related codes within each section of a chapter in the Volume 1 tabular list of codes in the ICD-9-CM codebook.

chapter the first major division in the tabular list in Volume 1 of the ICD-9-CM codebook. Chapters represent body systems or types of conditions.

comorbidity secondary diagnoses and conditions that influence treatment; diagnoses that coexist.

downcoding a code is chosen for a less severe condition than is recorded in the patient's medical record, or for a lesser procedure than was actually performed; undercoding.

E-code an explanatory code that lists the external causes and places of occurrence for injuries and poisonings.

greatest level of specificity the code with the greatest level of detail that matches the patient's medical record with the greatest accuracy.

hypertension table a table to assist with code choices for hypertension; part of the alphabetical index in Section 1 of Volume 2 of the ICD-9-CM codebook.

ICD-9-CM *International Classification of Diseases, Ninth Revision, Clinical Modification;* the version of the diagnosis codebook used in the United States for diagnosis coding until the date ICD-10-CM is implemented.

ICD-10-CM *International Classification of Diseases, Tenth Revision, Clinical Modification;* the next version of the diagnosis codebook that will be used in the United States. It might be used for diagnosis coding as early as October 2007, but implementation could be delayed until a later year.

main term the word to look up in an alphabetical index; in ICD-9-CM, a condition, disease, or injury.

morbidity sickness or statistical incidence of disease.

mortality death or statistical incidence of death.

neoplasm table a table to assist with code selection for neoplasms; located in the alphabetical index in Section 1 of Volume 2 of the ICD-9-CM codebook.

pigeonholing the practice of using a short list of diagnosis codes and using those codes for all patients, regardless of whether the codes match actual diagnoses and conditions.

primary diagnosis the condition that prompted an outpatient visit or treatment or the underlying cause for a hospital visit.

principal diagnosis the condition that is found after study to be chiefly responsible for a hospitalization.

RBRVS resource-based relative value system; the prospective payment system used by Medicare to pay physicians. It considers the CPT code in relation to work, overhead expenses, and malpractice (risk). A geographical adjustment is then made to account for cost-of-living differences throughout the nation.

secondary diagnosis a diagnosis that contributes to a condition; for an outpatient visit, it may include the underlying cause.

section related groups of codes within a chapter in the tabular list in Volume 1 of ICD-9-CM; the major divisions within each chapter.

subcategory the fourth digit in an ICD-9-CM code; further defines the codes within a category in the Volume 1 tabular list of codes.

subclassification the fifth digit in an ICD-9-CM code; adds more specificity to distinguish between codes within a subcategory in the Volume 1 tabular list of codes.

table of drugs and chemicals a table to assist with code selections that identify drugs and other chemicals. It is located in Section 2 of Volume 2 in ICD-9-CM, right after the alphabetical index.

tabular list a numerical list of diagnosis codes presented in a format similar to a table; it is located in Volume 1 of ICD-9-CM and is arranged by body system or types of conditions.

upcoding a code is chosen for a more severe condition or for a more extensive procedure than is documented in the patient's medical record; overcoding.

V-code a supplemental code that describes reasons other than illness for which a person might encounter the health care system; many V-codes cannot be used as a principal or primary diagnosis.

Introduction

The first time diagnoses were used for statistical purposes was in England in the early to mid-1600s when John Graunt, a merchant who sold buttons, needles, and other "notions," tracked births and deaths in London. Mr. Graunt analyzed the findings with his friend, Dr. William Petty, using theories of probability that until then had only been used in games of chance (gambling). He published the findings in a book called *Natural and Political Observations Made Upon Bills of Mortality*. At least five editions of his book were published, and the *London Bills of Mortality* became an ongoing statistical study.

Graunt's book led to the development of the field of statistics and every method of risk management, including insurance. Other countries were inspired to begin their own studies. The various studies merged over the years and changed names a number of times. An organization called the World Health Organization began to track both **morbidity** (sickness) and **mortality** (death) throughout the world. In 1948, the World Health Organization gave the new study its current name, International Classification of Diseases (ICD). The study is published as a book and is revised periodically. Each revision adds a number to the name. ICD-9, the ninth revision, lists three-digit numeric diagnosis codes.

ICD-9-CM is the name of the diagnosis codebook currently used in the United States for diagnosis coding. The name means "International Classification of Diseases, Ninth Revision, Clinical Modification." The clinical modifications add fourth-digit subcategories and fifth-digit **subclassifications** used in the United States for (1) detailed billing and (2) detailed

statistical studies. With rare exceptions, ICD-9-CM is updated annually. Valid ICD-9-CM codes can have three, four, or five numeric digits.

> ICD-9-CM Volumes 1 and 2 are used for physician and provider billing.
> ICD-9-CM Volumes 1, 2, and 3 are used for hospital and facility billing.

Since 1950, diagnosis codes have been used by hospitals in the United States to:

- ❏ Track diseases
- ❏ Classify procedures
- ❏ Measure the results of medical research
- ❏ Evaluate hospital utilization

By the late 1960s to early 1970s, hospitals began to use standardized claim forms, and they began to use computers to send claims electronically. Diagnosis codes were used instead of words on electronic claims to save space because computers in those days had very limited memories.

In 1981, the first medical claim clearinghouses were formed to enable individual physicians to send claims electronically. Once again, diagnosis codes were used instead of words on electronic claims to save space on computers.

Today, hospitals and individual physicians use diagnosis codes to:

- ❏ Establish medical necessity for each treatment, procedure, and service

☐ Document the complexity of medical decision-making for each encounter

☐ Evaluate the results of specific treatments for specific conditions and diseases

☐ Evaluate all health care utilization

Medical coding becomes more complex every year, and physicians seldom know enough about current medical coding rules to *correctly* code their own services. Therefore medical coding has become a distinct specialty in the medical office.

Since 1988, physicians' offices have been required to use diagnosis codes for billing purposes. The diagnoses must be coded to the **greatest level of specificity,** and they must match chart documentation. Certified coders have passed a certification examination and are qualified to convert chart documentation into diagnosis codes so physicians do not have to learn every coding guideline and do not have to learn the semiannual updates to the codebooks.

Diagnosis coding is a complex subject that cannot be covered in detail in one chapter. The information presented in this chapter is an introduction to diagnosis coding and a broad overview of the most important diagnosis coding guidelines. It is not as comprehensive as the information presented in a medical coding course. Specialty-specific coding rules are not addressed.

The purpose of this chapter is to: (1) introduce the diagnosis codebook used for physician and provider billing, ICD-9-CM Volumes 1 and 2, (2) introduce the diagnosis codebook used for hospital and facility billing, ICD-9-CM Volumes 1, 2, and 3, and (3) lay the foundation for diagnosis coding. When you finish this course, you will be able to:

☐ Use an ICD-9-CM codebook to find diagnosis codes

☐ Match the specificity of diagnosis codes to documentation in patient medical records

☐ Apply the correct diagnosis code order for the most common situations, including common "special circumstances"

☐ Recognize when something is obviously wrong with the diagnosis codes you are given to place on a medical claim form

For example: You will know something is obviously wrong when:

☐ The code for a given diagnosis requires a second code, but you cannot find documentation in the medical record to support the second code

☐ A chronic condition is listed before an acute condition

☐ An injury is diagnosed, but there is no explanation of how or where the injury occurred

The compliance guidance documents issued by the Office of Inspector General (OIG) for the Department of Health and Human Services (HHS) strongly recommend that job descriptions be used to assign accountability for specific tasks in the medical office. The OIG developed the compliance guidance documents to help various types of medical entities meet the accountability requirements of the Health Insurance Portability and Accountability Act of 1996 (Public Law 104-191) (HIPAA). Many of the OIG's recommendations relate directly to billing and collections, including assigning responsibility for gathering the information for the billing and coding of medical claims. The Medicare website for medical office education, which is now sponsored by numerous government agencies, www.cms.hhs.gov/medlearn/cbts.asp, notes how accountability is typically assigned in a medical office, and that information provided the basis when accountability is addressed in this chapter. However, please remember that each medical office decides exactly which employee positions are assigned individual accountability for each task, and it will vary from one office to another. In addition, in a small medical office, one multiskilled professional often fills numerous employee positions.

Typically, medical billers are held accountable for the codes submitted on medical claims unless the responsibility for medical coding is clearly assigned to someone else, such as a certified professional coder (CPC, CPC-H) or a certified coding specialist (CCS, CCS-P). If the medical office you work for does not have a certified coding employee, you should consider completing a medical coding course before accepting this responsibility.

You will need a current year ICD-9-CM codebook, Volumes 1, 2, and 3, for this chapter. Open your ICD-9-CM codebook and find each item as we discuss it.

Professional edition codebooks are a little more expensive, but they contain many useful features that make coding easier.

Answer the following questions:

1. What codebook is currently used in the United States for diagnosis coding?

   _____

2. Where do you turn first when locating a diagnosis code?

   _____

3. What is the second step when locating a diagnosis code?

   _____

4. Once you have located the code in the alphabetical index in Volume 2, you are done. You can use that code.

   _____True   _____False

5. If you look up a code and find that the exact diagnosis you are coding is listed under "excludes," what is your next step?

   _____

Find the diagnosis codes for the following:

6. Obstruction of intestine due to gallstones.

   _____

7. Acute respiratory distress in an adult.

   _____

8. Third-degree AV block.

   _____

9. Osteoarthritis left hip.

   _____

10. Intractable migraine headache with an aura.

    _____

Basic ICD-9-CM Coding

GUIDELINES

Diagnosis codes are used to portray why the patient requires medical services and to indicate the severity of the condition and the amount of work required.

The official diagnosis coding guidelines are found in the ICD-9-CM codebook just before the main index in Volume 2. Please remember that the official coding guidelines can and often do change from year to year. The official guidelines may have changed since this text was written. Current-year coding guidelines always take precedence; so any time there is a discrepancy with the information in this text-book, please follow the guidelines.

A specific code order is used to convey diagnosis information in a standard format. The "general" coding guidelines tell the usual code order. The "chapter-specific" guidelines, the "inpatient" guidelines, and the "outpatient" guidelines describe special circumstances that alter the standard code order or that alter the standard rules for billing and reporting medical services.

PRINCIPAL DIAGNOSIS

The **principal diagnosis** is the condition that, after study, is found to be the main reason for a hospitalization. The principal diagnosis is listed first for inpatient coding. It is often, but not always, the same as the **primary diagnosis.**

Remember, italicized codes in the **tabular list** and codes in slanted brackets in the alphabetical index may not be listed as principal diagnoses and must be listed in the order specified.

PRIMARY DIAGNOSIS

Inpatient

The primary diagnosis is the underlying cause for a hospitalization. Sometimes the primary diagnosis is the same as the principal diagnosis. However, the principal diagnosis and the primary diagnosis *are not always* the same. Many times a chronic condition is the primary diagnosis, or underlying cause, for an acute condition that prompted the hospitalization. When they are different, the principal diagnosis is listed first and the primary diagnosis is listed second *unless* the coding guidelines or the codebook instructions direct you to a different code order.

For example:

❏ If a patient with chronic asthma is seen for an acute asthma attack, the acute asthma is the principal diagnosis and the chronic asthma is the primary diagnosis.

☐ If a patient with cerebral palsy is seen for problems related to a muscle contracture, the problem related to the muscle contracture is the principal diagnosis and the cerebral palsy is the primary diagnosis.

☐ If a patient with type 2 diabetes is admitted because home tests show sugar in the urine, glycosuria is the reason for the admission and type 2 diabetes is the underlying cause. However, the codebook specifies: code first the underlying cause, the diabetes. Remember, anytime the codebook specifies the order in which two codes are to be listed, you must list them in that order. Therefore diabetes becomes the principal diagnosis for this admission.

Outpatient

For outpatient services, the primary diagnosis is the main reason for the service(s). There is no principal diagnosis for outpatient services. When there is an underlying cause for an outpatient service, it is listed directly after the primary diagnosis *unless* the coding guidelines or the codebook instructions direct you to a different code order. For outpatients, when a definitive diagnosis has not yet been established, you code the presenting symptoms.

The official coding guidelines for outpatient services do not use the term "primary diagnosis." Instead, they simply refer to the "first-listed" diagnosis for each circumstance.

CODE LINKING

Only the physician claim form uses the concept of code linkage. In Chapter 4, you learned to use code linkage in block No. 24E of the CMS-1500 claim form to identify the main reason, or primary diagnosis, for performing a specific procedure. The field links the procedure on that line to a specific diagnosis from the choices in block No. 21. Many payors use this field to establish medical necessity for the service listed on this line.

Sometimes the diagnosis coding conventions directed you to list another diagnosis first in block No. 21, yet the primary diagnosis for each service in block No. 24 is clearly established by linking each service in block No. 24 to a line number from block No. 21 that represents the primary reason for that specific service. Each service is individually linked to the best diagnosis for that service.

The UB-92 claim form, used for reporting the hospital's charges, identifies the principal diagnosis by providing a separate field for it, FL 67. The principal diagnosis applies to the entire hospitalization and is not tied to individual services.

SECONDARY DIAGNOSES

For inpatients, secondary diagnoses contribute to the principal diagnosis or condition but are not the underlying cause. For outpatients, the first **secondary diagnosis** is the underlying cause for the primary diagnosis when it is different from the primary diagnosis.

Secondary diagnoses are also called comorbidities. They are other illnesses or conditions the patient has in addition to the main reason for the hospitalization or outpatient service. Unless codebook guidelines or specific codebook directions dictate a specific code order, secondary diagnoses are listed after the primary diagnosis in the order of impact on medical decision-making. Physicians usually list diagnoses in this order in the medical record, but the billing directions (e.g., superbill, encounter form, etc.) are usually preprinted and it is difficult to specify a particular code order.

The following is a sampling of the official coding guidelines that apply to additional diagnoses:

☐ Only code the conditions or problems that are actively managed during the visit.

☐ When both acute and chronic conditions are present and treated, both may be coded, with the acute code given first. Acute conditions are coded as long as they are present. Chronic conditions are coded only when they have an impact on medical decision-making for that visit.

☐ List applicable personal history codes or other conditions that may affect current treatment.

☐ When two codes are of equal importance, the most resource-intensive code is listed first. The most resource-intensive code is the code that took more time to evaluate or that was more expensive to evaluate if special equipment was used or if special tests were performed.

☐ Diagnoses that relate to a previous medical problem but have no bearing on the present condition are not coded or included on a medical claim.

MULTIPLE CODING

Sometimes two or more codes are needed to fully describe one diagnosis, and sometimes combination codes already list two or more diagnoses in one code. When combination codes are available, it is more correct to use the combination code than to report each item separately. However, if the combination does not fully describe both diagnoses, a second code is still needed to provide the missing details.

For example:

(1) ICD-9-CM code 482.0, pneumonia due to *Klebsiella pneumoniae,* is a combination code that fully describes both the pneumonia and the causative organism: *K. pneumoniae.* Only one code is needed.

(2) ICD-9-CM code 713.2, arthropathy associated with hematologic disorders, directs you to code first the underlying disease. Two codes are needed to fully describe the condition. Hemophilia is one of the underlying diseases that may be reported with this arthropathy code. When hemophilia is the underlying cause for your patient's arthropathy, the hemophilia diagnosis code that most closely matches your chart documentation for the visit must always be listed before arthropathy code 713.2.

(3) ICD-9-CM code 402.01, malignant hypertensive heart disease and heart failure, is a combination code. However, the directions say to use an additional code to identify the type of heart failure. In this instance, the combination code did not fully describe the type of heart failure, so a second code is needed to provide that detail.

GREATEST LEVEL OF SPECIFICITY

The diagnosis code with the greatest level of specificity is the code that most accurately portrays medical record documentation for the visit. Many times more than one code is needed, and each must show the greatest level of specificity.

Specificity in diagnosis codes is used along with the correct code order to establish or confirm:

❑ Medical necessity
❑ The complexity of medical decision-making for evaluation and management (E/M) services
❑ The amount of work performed for **RBRVS** (resource-based relative value system) payment calculations used by some payors, including Medicare

Whenever possible, read the chart documentation before looking up a diagnosis code. Do not code from a superbill alone unless frequent chart audits prove that chart documentation consistently matches the associated superbills. *Note:* Even billing agencies should perform chart audits on a routine basis to verify the accuracy of the coding received on superbills.

Always code to the greatest level of specificity. Some diagnosis codes must match the age and gender of the patient.

First, read your official coding guidelines. Then, begin with the alphabetical index, but always verify the selected code in the tabular list, reading all the associated instructions, "includes" notes and "excludes" notes.

When the codes you use fully describe each encounter, additional documentation will be required less frequently, saving time and money for both the provider's office and the payor. Penalties in the form of reduced payment are applied when coding is performed incorrectly, therefore, reimbursement is better when the diagnosis codes billed accurately portray medical record documentation.

V-CODES

V-codes are used to identify other reasons for encountering health services. They do not identify current, active diseases or injuries. You must code symptoms in the first position when they are present, even when a V-code could otherwise be used as the principal or primary diagnosis.

V-codes may only be used as the first diagnosis for the specific circumstances listed in the official coding guidelines. Examples include:

1. Preventive medicine: annual exams, vaccinations
2. Specific treatments: chemotherapy, removal of pins, casts, etc.
3. To identify that a procedure is performed due to personal or family history (cancer, heart disease, etc.): screening tests, follow-up visits

The remaining V-codes are supplemental: They provide additional information. Family history and observation codes also may be used to document specific suspected conditions.

Although "rule-out" and "probable" conditions may only be coded and billed by inpatient facilities, they should still be documented in the medical record for physician services, when applicable. They are used to meet the documentation requirements for the complexity of medical decision-making (see Chapter 6) and to document the amount of work performed for RBRVS payment calculations (see Chapters 13 and 14).

E-CODES

E-codes are used to identify the external causes and locations of poisonings, accidents, and injuries. E-codes are never used as a primary or principal diagnosis, and they are never linked to procedure codes. Except in pregnancy, E-codes always are the last code listed.

Often two or more E-codes are required to establish both the cause and the place of injury. The coding guidelines direct you to code "how" before "where." However, some payors want you to code the place of injury first because it is used in determining payor responsibility for the claim. Remember, payor contracts take legal precedence over codebook directions.

IMPORTANCE OF CODE ORDER

Code order is very important in diagnosis coding. Code order establishes medical necessity, justifies the level of medical decision-making for the evaluation and management services, and determines whether the amount of work performed was appropriate for the nature of the patient's chief complaint.

Coding guidelines and coding conventions dictate the order in which codes should be listed. Coding conventions are discussed in the next section.

Payor black box edits and patterning studies are based on diagnosis codes, code order, and the manner in which diagnosis codes are linked to procedure codes. Black box edits are considered a trade secret. They are edits programmed into the payor's computer system that direct the computer to automatically authorize or deny payment based on which diagnosis code is linked to a given procedure. Patterning studies show code usage patterns for a given physician in a given location.

Sometimes more than one claim form is required to accurately portray an encounter. Other times supporting documentation should be sent with the claim to show what occurred. Supporting documentation is sent most often for complex cases, but it is also sent for unlisted diagnoses to establish a pattern of use so specific codes can be assigned in subsequent years.

Finding Information in ICD-9-CM, Volumes 1 and 2

Most ICD-9-CM codebooks publish Volume 2, the Alphabetical Index to Diseases, at the beginning of the book, followed by Volume 1, the Tabular List of Diagnosis Codes. The proper way to use the ICD-9-CM codebook is to look up the diagnosis first in the **alphabetical index** before proceeding to the tabular list, so placing Volume 2 first makes sense.

Volume 2 of ICD-9-CM begins with **Section** 1, an alphabetical index to diseases. A **hypertension table** and a **neoplasm table** are included in Section 1, the alphabetical index. These tables allow a quick comparison of available codes, listing some of the criteria that cause similar diagnoses to have different code numbers. Hypertension is the medical term for high blood pressure. It is not just one elevated blood pressure reading; it is an actual disease process. A neoplasm is an abnormal growth or tumor. A benign neoplasm is not cancer; a malignant neoplasm is cancer.

A **table of drugs and chemicals** follows the alphabetical index and is called Section 2 of Volume 2. The last item in Volume 2 is Section 3, an **alphabetical index to external causes of injury and poisoning** (an index to E-codes).

Volume 1 of ICD-9-CM is a tabular list of diagnosis codes. The tabular list is organized numerically. **Chapters** represent body systems or types of conditions. *Sections* are related groups of topics within each chapter. *Categories* are single topics and are represented by three-digit codes within each section. Fourth-digit **subcategory** codes and fifth-digit subclassification codes add more specificity and give more information to differentiate the diagnoses included within that topic. Valid ICD-9-CM codes can have three, four, or five numeric digits.

V-codes and E-codes are valid ICD-9-CM codes that are listed in supplements to the Volume 1 tabular list. They begin with a single alpha digit (V or E) followed by two, three, or four numeric digits. They do not represent active diseases. V-codes describe other reasons for medical encounters, and E-codes describe the "how" and "where" for injuries and poisonings.

In the Volume 1 tabular list, chapters flow into one another seamlessly with new chapters sometimes starting in the middle of a page or column. The professional and expert versions of the codebook start new chapters on a separate page, and color-code the edges of the page, with each chapter a separate color. Although a number series that starts in one chapter may end in another chapter, the sections and the lower subdivisions of each section are wholly contained within a chapter.

Appendices are listed at the back of Volume 1 as follows: Appendix A–Morphology of Neoplasms (a rating scale for a scientific study of changes in neoplasms); Appendix B was deleted in 2005. Appendix B was a glossary of mental disorders that helped mental health providers convert mental health diagnoses from the criteria in the *Diagnostic and Statistical Manual of Mental Disorders, Fourth Edition* (DSM-IV) into billable ICD-9-CM codes; Appendix C–Classifications of Drugs (ICD-9-CM equivalents of American Hospital Formulary Services List Numbers); Appendix D–Classification of Industrial Accidents According to Agency; and Appendix E–List of Three-Digit Categories. Some codebook publishers provide other appendices as a unique feature for their codebook.

FINDING CODES

To find the numerical code for a diagnosis, begin by looking up the **main term** for the condition, disease, or injury in the alphabetical index or the related tables. A small sampling of valid main terms is listed in Box 5-1.

ICD-9-CM is not a user-friendly book. Many diagnoses include anatomical terms that identify the involved body parts, yet you can seldom locate a *diagnosis code* by looking up the anatomical term(s). In ICD-9-CM, anatomical terms are usually used as subterms listed under a main term that identifies the condition, disease, or injury. *Note:* Many anatomical terms are listed as a "main term" in the alphabetical index as a courtesy, but the listing usually gives directions to look up the condition rather than providing useful information.

For example:
❏ To find "knee pain," look up the condition "pain" as a main term, the anatomical subterm "joint," and the more specific anatomical subterm "knee."
❏ To find eye injury, look up the condition "injury" as a main term, and the anatomical subterm "eye."
❏ To find fractured femur, look up the condition "fracture" as a main term, the anatomical subterm "femur," and then determine whether any of the additional subterms apply.

Sometimes none of the words in the diagnosis is found in the alphabetical index. When this happens, try dividing the diagnosis into word parts. Use the word parts to determine the main term, especially word parts that identify a condition, disease, or injury.

For example: Try to look up "tibial spur." You will not find a main term "tibial" and you will not find a subterm "tibial" under the main term "spur." If you divide the word "tibial," you will find that it means *pertaining to the tibia bone.* "Bone" is a subterm under the main term "spur." A tibial spur is a bone spur located on the tibia. Then go to the tabular list to confirm the code for a bone spur on the tibia.

When dividing the diagnosis into word parts is not helpful, look up the diagnosis in a good quality medical dictionary. Use the definition to locate a main term (usually a condition, disease, or injury) and any relevant subterms.

For example: "Patella alta" cannot be found as a main term under either "patella" or "alta," and neither of these words can be divided into word parts. "Patella" means kneecap and "alta" means high. When you look up "patella alta" in a medical dictionary, you find that it is a condition in which the patellar tendon is too tight or contracted, and as a result, the kneecap is positioned higher than it should be. Look up the main term "tight" or the main term "contracted" and find the subterm "tendon." Both main terms lead you to the same code in the tabular list. Next, go to the tabular list to confirm that the definition of the code for a tight or contracted tendon is the best match for the medical dictionary's definition of patella alta.

Many times the alphabetical index does not list the fourth and fifth digit requirements for a code, and the alphabetical index never records the code definitions, notes, and the "includes" and "excludes" items that apply to each code. Codes placed on a claim form must match chart documentation closely. Therefore, each code must be confirmed in the tabular list.

After locating the main term and the subterm(s) of choice in the alphabetical index, go to the tabular list and find the code number. Read the code definition,

Box 5-1		Examples of Main Terms	
Abnormal	History	Malformation	Rupture
Anomaly	Hypertension	Malfunction	Screening
Complications	Inadequate	Malposition	Sprain
Counseling	Increased	Necrosis	State
Deficiency	Infection	Neoplasm	Status
Delivery	Inflammation	Obstruction	Swelling
Disease	Influenza	Occlusion	Symptoms
Disorder	Injury	Pain	Syndrome
Examination	Laceration	Paralysis	Test(s)
Failure, failed	Late (effect)	Perforation	Tumor
Findings	Lesion	Pregnancy	Ulcer
Fracture	Loss	Problem	Wound

the notes, and the "includes" and "excludes" items. The notes listed at the beginning of a chapter, section, **category,** or subcategory apply to all the codes in that chapter, section, category, and/or subcategory.

For example: Turn to ICD-9-CM code category 240 in the Volume 1 tabular list—the beginning of Chapter 3 in your ICD-9-CM codebook. Chapter 3, Endocrine, Nutritional and Metabolic, and Immunity Disorders (240-279), has notes and "excludes" items that apply to the entire chapter. In this instance, there are no section notes for the first section, Disorders of the Thyroid Gland (240-246), but category 242, Thyrotoxicosis with or without goiter (located in the first section) has fifth-digit subclassification requirements, notes, and "excludes" items that apply just to category 242. Each subcategory under 242 lists fourth-digit definitions. When you look up code 242.8, Thyrotoxicosis of other specified origin, there is a note that all applies just to this subcategory. Yet, the notes and the "excludes" items at the beginning of the chapter, the notes and "excludes" items at the beginning of the category, the subcategory notes, and the fifth-digit subclassification requirements, listed at the beginning of the three-digit category must all be considered. Code 242.8 is an incomplete code. A fifth digit must be applied, and all the requirements must be met, or the code cannot be used.

Be sure to read all the "includes" and "excludes" notes. "Includes" notes are a list of examples of specific diagnoses that are valid for that code. Unless a more specific code is a better match, only one diagnosis in the list needs to match your documentation to use the code. However, if even one item on the "excludes" list also matches the documentation, you may not use the code. When an item is excluded, most codebooks list a code or a range of codes to direct you to a better code choice.

Fourth and fifth digits, when available, are not optional. However, you may not add a zero (0) or

zeros to create a four- or five-digit code if none exists. There are approximately 100 valid three-digit codes and there are many valid four-digit codes. The only time a zero may be used as a filler is when a fifth digit is required on a code that does not have a fourth digit. Zero is then used for the fourth digit. However, this rarely occurs. Double-check to be sure there really is no fourth digit.

In addition, you need to review the official coding guidelines for the chapter, if any. The official guidelines are usually located just before the alphabetical index in section 1 of Volume 2. The punctuation and abbreviations in the ICD-9-CM codebook are called coding conventions and are very important (Box 5-2). Coding conventions are included at the beginning of the official coding guidelines. For the example listed above, chapter 3 did not have any chapter-specific coding guidelines, but the general coding guidelines do apply.

CODE ORDER

When two codes are required to show a cause and the resulting condition, the alphabetical index shows the required code order by listing the second code in slanted brackets ([ ]). In the tabular list, codes that are italicized are to be listed as the second code. The professional and expert editions of ICD-9-CM also have color-coded symbols to draw attention to this requirement.

When the codebook makes this distinction, usually the code for the underlying disease (the cause) is listed first and the resulting condition (the effect) is listed second. If you look up the code for the effect, the instructions will say, "code first the underlying disease" and often provide a list of possible underlying diseases with code numbers for each. The codebook draws attention in this manner because these "cause and effect" codes are an exception to

Box 5-2 ICD-9-CM Punctuation and Abbreviations	
[ ] Brackets enclose symptoms, alternate wordings, and explanatory phrases. ( ) Parentheses enclose supplementary words that may or may not be listed in the diagnosis. : Colons are used after incomplete terms to indicate that modifiers (other terms) contain additional information needed to complete the code section. { } Braces point to a series of terms, each of which is modified by the statement to the right of the brace.	NEC means "not elsewhere classified." An NEC code is used when you have the details to list a more specific condition, but a more specific code is not available. NOS means "not otherwise specified." An NOS code is a nonspecific code used primarily when you lack the details to find a more specific code.

the normal code order in which the treated condition would be listed first and the underlying cause second.

For example: Find "cardiomyopathy due to progressive muscular dystrophy" in the alphabetical index. Keep a finger in the alphabetical index and look up code number 425.8 in the tabular list: *Cardiomyopathy in other diseases classified elsewhere.* The same cause-and-effect relationship and the same code order are shown in both places.

Hospital edition codebooks sometimes also include complication and **comorbidity** exclusions (CC Excl) that are used to calculate the "typical" number of hospital days needed for a specific diagnosis.

Diagnosis codes that begin with the letter "V" are called V-codes. They are located in a supplement immediately after the tabular list in Volume 1 of the ICD-9-CM codebook.

A few V-codes can be used as the first diagnosis for patients who are not acutely ill.

Examples of V-codes that can be the first diagnosis when no other problems or symptoms are present include the following:

- ❏ Annual exam
- ❏ Immunization
- ❏ Organ donor
- ❏ Sometimes personal or family history

However, most V-codes are supplemental codes that cannot be used as the first diagnosis.

Examples of supplemental V-codes that cannot be used as the first diagnosis include the following:

- ❏ Potential health hazards related to communicable diseases
- ❏ Family history
- ❏ Conditions that influence health status (e.g., personal or family history)
- ❏ Observation for suspected conditions
- ❏ Health care related to other circumstances (economic situations, family disruptions)

The official coding guidelines contain many specific rules governing the use of V-codes.

Diagnosis codes that begin with the letter "E" are called E-codes. E-codes are used to show external causes (e.g., other events or conditions) that affect health. Some E-codes list the place of occurrence for an incident. E-codes are never used as the first diagnosis, and they are usually listed as the last diagnosis.

E-codes are used to show the cause and/or place of occurrence for:

- ❏ Injury (e.g., heavy equipment fell on arm at work causing a fractured radius)
- ❏ Poisoning (e.g., a cocaine overdose in a person found in a city park, unknown if accidental or intentional)
- ❏ Adverse reactions to medications (e.g., an allergic reaction to the correct dosage of an antibiotic taken at home)

E-codes provide additional information. Understanding how injuries occur can sometimes lead to methods of prevention. For example, many employers now require the use of back supports to prevent back injuries or the use of wrist rests to prevent carpal tunnel injuries when using a computer.

In addition, many payors require the use of the E-codes for place of occurrence to determine legal liability. Most health insurers will not pay benefits after an accident until maximum health benefits from a liability policy have been exhausted.

For example: In most states, when a patient is in an automobile accident, an automobile insurance policy is legally responsible for paying first. The medical plan only pays when unpaid bills remain after the automobile coverage has paid the policy limits.

ACCOUNTABILITY

One of the major codebook publishers advocates that coding can be done directly from their alphabetical index because they list the fourth and fifth digits in their index. However, there is no room in the alphabetical index to list all the definitions, notes, rules, inclusions, and exclusions that apply to each code, so vital information can be missed if coding is done in that manner.

Busy physicians often use cheat-sheets and fast-finder guides that list only short descriptors and omit all the details that apply to each code. *Medical business office personnel should always use the codebook and look up each code in both the alphabetical index and the tabular list.* If your job description assigns you the accountability for coding, you can legally be held more accountable for the actual codes billed than the physician. Therefore, you must develop the habit of reading every note and rule that applies to each code every time you use the code. Do not rely on your memory and do not rely on shortcuts. Occasionally, you will find that a code you use frequently excludes the exact condition you are coding today, and the codebook will direct you to a better choice.

Remember, only certified coders and certified coding specialists have passed exams proving they have the qualifications to convert chart documentation into codes. Many physicians do not have time to learn every applicable coding rule and each annual update, so they assign this task to certified coding professionals. However, anytime a physician supplies the code(s) to bill, you must discuss coding issues and get the physician's approval before changing a code to meet current coding rules. If you knowingly send an inaccurate code or if you consistently submit claims with incorrect codes, you can be held accountable for the fines, penalties, and sanctions of HIPAA.

Codebooks with color-coded symbols are very helpful in finding the most specific codes. When possible, try to purchase codebooks with extra coding clues and aids. Most medical offices purchase the required codebooks, but few medical offices are willing to purchase other books that enhance diagnosis coding. Additional resource books include medical dictionaries, books on medical abbreviations, medical terminology books, and anatomy and physiology books. You may band together with friends and coworkers to purchase additional books and share resources. If each person buys one book for everyone to share, you can all benefit from an expanded resource library.

CLINICAL APPLICATION

Clinical example: The patient, Harold, has a chief complaint of pain in the right ear and a low-grade fever. Harold has a history of chronic serous otitis media, and he is allergic to Amoxil. The limited physical exam is normal except for a fever of 100.6°F, a bulging reddened right eardrum with evidence of serous fluid in the middle ear, and a dull left eardrum with evidence of serous fluid in the middle ear. The diagnosis is listed as acute and chronic serous otitis media. The patient is given a prescription for Cephalexin (Keflex).

Code the diagnoses for this encounter: Acute conditions are coded before chronic conditions, so the primary diagnosis is acute serous otitis media. The main term "inflammation" with the subterm "ear" and the subterm "middle" directs you to see "otitis media." Therefore, use the main term "otitis."

Under the main term "otitis," you find both the subterm "acute" (no additional subterms) and the subterm "media" with more specific subterms "acute" and "serous." The first subterm "acute" directs you to the nonspecific code 382.9, unspecified otitis media. However, the subterm "media" with the more specific subterms "acute" and "serous" leads you to the more specific code of 381.01, acute serous otitis media. Confirm this code in the tabular list.

The underlying cause of the visit is chronic serous otitis media. Use the main term "otitis." Look under the subterm "chronic" and the subterm "serous" to find code 381.10. Confirm this code in the tabular list.

Lastly, look up the codes for other secondary conditions: a personal history of an allergy to Amoxil. The allergy should be coded and placed on the claim because it tells the payor why the less expensive drug, Amoxil, was not prescribed for this patient. Look up the main term "history" and the subterm "allergy." Amoxil is not specifically listed as an additional subterm, so use the code for antibiotic NEC (not elsewhere classified) to find the code V14.1. Confirm this code in the tabular list. *Note:* Although Amoxil is similar to penicillin, it is not penicillin. Therefore it should not be coded as V14.0, allergy to penicillin.

Once the codes are confirmed as the closest match to chart documentation, they will be placed on the claim as follows:

Line 1: 381.01
Line 2: 381.10
Line 3: V14.1

Clinical Application Exercise

A patient with type 1 diabetes mellitus has peripheral circulatory problems and was treated recently for early signs of gangrene in the fourth and fifth toes on the left foot. Today the patient calls to report difficulties regulating insulin, and home-tested blood sugar levels are too high. The patient is seen in the office, and the physician determines the diabetes is now uncontrolled, and the patient is in diabetic ketoacidosis. This episode was triggered by the stress placed on the body from the gangrene in the toes.

Code the diagnoses for this visit, listing them in the proper order.

1. _____ 3. _____

2. _____ 4. _____

STOP & REVIEW

Answer the following questions:

1. If both acute and chronic conditions are present and influence treatment, which should be coded first?

    _____

2. When two codes are of equal importance, which is listed first? _____

    _____

3. When are E-codes used? _____

    _____

4. What type of code is used to report family history? _____

    _____

5. What type of code lists more than one diagnosis?

    _____

    _____

Code the following diagnoses, listing the proper order (*Note:* The claim form has four diagnosis lines available, so four lines are offered for each answer; some lines will be left blank.):

6. Diabetic neuropathy, adult-onset diabetes.

    1. _____   3. _____

    2. _____   4. _____

7. Asthma with status asthmaticus and COPD.

    1. _____   3. _____

    2. _____   4. _____

8. Acute and chronic cholecystitis.

    1. _____   3. _____

    2. _____   4. _____

9. Bleeding esophageal varices with Laënnec's cirrhosis.

    1. _____   3. _____

    2. _____   4. _____

10. Pneumonia in whooping cough (*Bordetella parapertussis*).

    1. _____   3. _____

    2. _____   4. _____

Coding Special Circumstances

The rules for *diagnosis coding* (ICD-9-CM, Volumes 1 and 2) are different from the rules for *procedure coding* (ICD-9-CM, Volume 3; CPT-4; and HCPCS). Many physicians and many employees confuse the two, especially when coding special circumstances and when coding for specialties.

The basic *diagnosis* code sequencing rules for commonly encountered special circumstances are covered in this section. The basic rules for inpatient procedure coding (ICD-9-CM, Volume 3) are covered later in this chapter and the basic rules for outpatient *procedure* coding (CPT-4 and HCPCS) are covered in Chapter 7.

The information for the topics covered in this section was abstracted from the guidelines in the 2005 ICD-9-CM codebook. Please remember that the official coding guidelines can and often do change from year to year. The guidelines may have changed since this text was written. Current year coding guidelines always take precedence; so any time there is a discrepancy with the information in this textbook, please follow the official guidelines.

ANNUAL PHYSICAL/WELL-WOMAN VISITS

Examination V-codes are used for the primary diagnosis for physicals and other preventive medicine visits unless symptoms or other problems are present.

The correct sequencing of codes for annual physicals and preventive medicine is as follows:

1. Examination V-codes for the type of visit, age, and/or gender of the patient
2. Personal history V-codes for items considered during the visit, especially when screening tests are ordered primarily because of a personal history item
3. Family history V-codes for items considered during the visit, especially when screening tests are ordered primarily because of a family history item

Look up the main term "examination" followed by the subterm for the type of examination. Then look up the main term "history" followed by the subterm "personal" or the subterm "family."

When symptoms or problems are present, they are coded first, followed by the codes as listed above.

Clinical Application Exercise

A 20-year-old single woman, Veronica, is seen for her annual gynecologic examination. Her last menstrual period was 10 days ago, and it was a normal period. A Pap smear is performed as part of the examination. Because Veronica is sexually active with multiple partners and does not use any contraceptive measures, a screening test is ordered for venereal diseases. Contraception and the risks associated with the various contraceptive measures are discussed. Veronica is given a prescription for an oral contraceptive, the only method she will agree to try. Veronica has a family history of postmenopausal breast cancer. Her breast exam is normal, and a mammogram is not indicated at this time.

Code the diagnoses for this visit, listing them in the proper order.

1. _____ 3. _____

2. _____ 4. _____

OBSTETRIC CARE

Obstetric care is medical care related to a pregnancy. The *procedure* code for the management and delivery of a pregnancy, the work performed by the obstetrician, is called the global charge. It is billed after delivery and encompasses specific pregnancy-related procedures: an average number of prenatal visits, specific tests, the type of delivery, and an average number of postpartum visits. Sometimes a payor contract has a different definition for the global charge and lists a different number of items or different tests. The payor contract takes precedence over the codebook, so be sure the fee you agree to in the contract really includes each item listed there or you could lose money by giving away services.

The *diagnosis* code definitions for pregnancy are very different from the global charge definitions for pregnancy-related *procedures*. Often items that are included in the global charge for the *procedure* of a "normal delivery" are coded as "complications" for the *diagnosis*. Diagnosis code definitions apply to diagnoses and procedure code definitions apply to procedures. You must understand this distinction between the rules for diagnosis codes and the rules for procedure codes to successfully code services for a patient who is pregnant.

For example: Delivery by forceps is correctly coded as a complication of pregnancy for *diagnosis* coding even though the use of forceps is included in the global charge for "normal delivery" *procedure* coding.

The code order for the diagnosis codes can vary depending on whether the pregnancy is normal or complicated, whether this visit is normally included in the global charge for pregnancy, and whether the purpose of this visit is related to the pregnancy.

NORMAL PREGNANCY AND DELIVERY

The following code order informs the payor that this is a normal pregnancy, and the normal pregnancy global charge applies.

The correct sequencing of diagnosis codes is as follows:

1. Delivery code (antepartum care, delivered, postpartum care; vaginal or C-section)
2. V-code identifying outcome (live, stillborn; number of babies)

Look up the main term "delivery" and the subterm "completely normal." This diagnosis code is used only for vaginal deliveries that meet the exact definition of the code. The code definition instructs you to use an additional code to indicate the outcome of the delivery. Look up the main term "outcome of delivery" to find the correct V-code.

Clinical Application Exercise

Sally had a normal uneventful pregnancy with an average number of prenatal visits. She had a normal vaginal delivery of one living child with no complications.
    Code the diagnoses for the delivery.

1. _____   3. _____

2. _____   4. _____

COMPLICATED PREGNANCY AND/OR DELIVERY

The following diagnosis code order informs the payor that this visit is related to a complex pregnancy. The global pregnancy charge for a complicated pregnancy/delivery is often higher than the global charge for a completely normal pregnancy/delivery, and additional items may be billed separately. Check the definitions for the global package carefully and negotiate contract rates that truly reflect the amount of work performed.

The correct sequencing of diagnosis codes is as follows:

1. Delivery code (antepartum care, delivered, postpartum care; vaginal or C-section; primary complicating condition)

2. Other condition code(s) (other complicating conditions)
3. Any other factors that create risk or complicate the delivery in any way
4. V-code identifying outcome (live, stillborn; number of babies)

Look up the main term "delivery." Find the subterm that correctly describes the type of delivery.

To report other conditions and complications related to pregnancy, look up the main term "pregnancy" and the subterm "complicated by" and the more specific subterm for each complication. If the condition is not found there, look up the condition as a main term.

The last code listed is the V-code for the outcome of delivery. Look up the main term "outcome of delivery."

Clinical Application Exercise

Jane had a preterm delivery of a complete breech baby at 32 weeks' gestation resulting in a single live birth.
    Code the diagnoses for the delivery.

1. _____   3. _____

2. _____   4. _____

PERINATAL CODING

The actual perinatal period extends from the twenty-eighth week of gestation to 28 days after delivery. However, for coding purposes, the perinatal period for the mother is *anytime* during pregnancy to 28 days after delivery. Perinatal codes are often used during pregnancy when medical treatment *related to the pregnancy* is necessary before delivery. They are also used for complications that arise in the postpartum period after a delivery. These codes do not include normal prenatal care, and they do not include delivery. The charges are outside of the global pregnancy charge, and they are billed separately.

The correct sequencing of codes is as follows:

1. Pregnancy-related diagnoses or symptoms
2. Secondary condition(s), if applicable
3. Other conditions that impact treatment

Look up the main term "pregnancy" and the subterm "complicated by" and the subterm for each condition. Read the chapter sections in ICD-9-CM, and the coding guidelines for pregnancy closely. There are many rules relating to specificity for perinatal codes.

Clinical Application Exercise

Mary is a 25-year-old pregnant woman with a history of miscarriage. Her pregnancy is currently at 20 weeks' gestation. Today Mary is in premature labor due to an incompetent cervix. A procedure is performed to sew the cervix closed.

Code the diagnoses for this visit.

1. _____ 3. _____

2. _____ 4. _____

ANTEPARTUM CODING

This code order informs the payor that this visit is *unrelated to the pregnancy* and is not included in the global pregnancy charge.

The correct sequencing of codes is as follows:

1. Principal diagnoses, symptoms, or conditions (such as a sinus infection or a fractured arm)
2. Any additional conditions that influence treatment considerations (personal or family history)

3. Pregnancy code (V22.2 reports that the pregnancy is incidental to the visit.)

Note: For injury, follow the injury rules with the appropriate pregnancy code as the last code. Look up the main term for the injury as the principal diagnosis. Next, code any additional conditions that influence the visit. The last code identifies that the patient happens to be pregnant. Look up the main term "pregnancy." Use the code that best identifies the type of pregnancy. V22.2, pregnant state, is used when the pregnancy is incidental to the visit.

Clinical Application Exercise

Janet is a 23-year-old pregnant woman diagnosed with bronchitis.
Code the diagnoses for this visit.

1. _____ 3. _____

2. _____ 4. _____

INJURIES

Accidents are often subject to litigation. The correct sequencing of diagnosis codes establishes the correct cause and effect relationship. Fewer payor conflicts arise when codes are sequenced correctly. E-codes are used to tell the payor where and how the injury occurred. Failure to use E-codes can often cause a denial or trigger a claim review to establish the correct payor.

The correct sequencing of codes is as follows:

1. Diagnosis/symptom for each injury
2. Other diagnoses, symptoms, or conditions that affect treatment
3. E-code(s) describing the location and cause of the accident and injury
4. Other, if necessary to justify medical necessity

Look up the main term "injury" and the correct subterms for the type of injury. When multiple injuries are present, code the most severe injury first, and code the others in decreasing order of severity. Look up the main term for every additional condition that affects treatment. Then use the E-code alphabetical index (in Section 3 of Volume 2) to first look up "accident" and the subterm "occurring at" to show *where* the injury occurred, and then look up the main term for *how* the injury occurred. Box 5-3 lists a few examples of main terms for E-codes.

In cases of traumatic injury, especially when many codes are needed, include a copy of the physician notes or operative reports to further clarify what occurred. This process will ensure that you are meeting the established criteria for medical complexity and medical necessity. Sometimes more than one claim form is needed.

Box 5-3 Examples of Main Terms for E-Codes		
Accident, automobile	Hemorrhage	Reaction, abnormal
Accident, caused by	Hit by	Scalding
Accident, occurring at	Injury	Slipping
Assault	Lost at sea	Sting
Bite	Marble in nose	Stumbling
Collapse	Misadventure to patient during	Submersion
Collision	surgical or medical care	Tornado
Crushed	Object	Trapped
Explosion	Obstruction	War operations
Fall, falling	Parachuting	Wound, gunshot
Fire	Pecked by bird	
Foreign body	Poisoning	

Clinical Application Exercise

Thomas is a 14-year-old boy with a history of cerebral palsy, spastic diplegia with quadriparesis, since infancy. He normally ambulates short distances and uses a wheelchair the remainder of the time. Thomas lost his balance and fell 10 days ago while walking at home and injured his right foot. Home treatment for a sprain has proven ineffective, and he is now unable to ambulate at all. An x-ray of the foot shows a closed fracture of the fourth metatarsal and a loss of bone density in the right foot. Because of Thomas's unusual gait and the presence of osteoporosis from disuse, a decision is made to apply a cast.

Code the diagnoses for this visit.

1. _____ 3. _____

2. _____ 4. _____

BURNS

Code the type, severity, and location of each burn separately. In many burn cases, you must file multiple claim forms to provide ample coding room for box 21. The most traumatic or resource-intensive burn will be coded first, with subsequent burns listed in descending order of severity. Repeat this process in descending order of severity until all burn areas are coded. Many payors require additional documentation.

Note: The most resource-intensive burn is the one that requires either the most supplies or the most employee time for treatment.

The correct sequence of codes is as follows:

1. Site and degree of each specific burn as described using additional digits (list in descending order of severity)
2. The burn is classified according to the extent of the body surface involved (category 948)—the percentage (%) of entire burned area on the total body surface (fourth digit), and the percent of third degree burns on total body surface (fifth digit)—use the table in the codebook; some codebooks also have a diagram at the beginning of the burn chapter
3. E-codes describing where and how the burn occurred
4. Other conditions that may have an impact on treatment

First, look up the main term "burn" and the appropriate subterms. The main term "burn" with the subterm "extent" gives the percentage classifications. When medical record documentation does not list the percentage of body surface burned and the percentage with third-degree burns, you may use the rule of nines, usually depicted in a drawing in the burn section, to calculate each percentage based on the descriptions in the medical record. In the rule of nines, the body surface is divided into the following sets of 9% each: head and neck, each arm, upper front torso, lower front torso, upper back torso, lower back torso, each anterior leg, and each posterior leg. The genitalia make up the remaining 1%. The body percentages are calculated in a different manner in small children because the head makes up a larger percentage of the overall body surface.

Then use the E-code index to code where and how the injury occurred. The main term "accident" and the subterm "occurring" are used to show *where* the burn occurred. The main term "burning" and the appropriate subterm are used to show *how* the burn occurred.

Clinical example: Randy is a 30-year-old man who fell asleep while smoking in bed and his shirt caught on fire. Randy suffered third-degree burns over most of his chest and second-degree burns on most of his upper left arm.

The diagnoses are as follows:
1. 942.32 (third-degree burns on chest)
2. 943.23 (second-degree burns on upper arm)

3. 948.10 (total burns, all types, on 10% to 19% of body surface with third-degree burns on less than 10% of body surface)
4. E849.0 (accident occurring at home)

Note: When there is only room for one E-code, code the place of occurrence, because the place of occurrence is used in determining the primary payor. In the hospital setting, there is room on the U-B 92 claim form for additional E-code(s) describing how the accident occurred.

Clinical Application Exercise

Katrina, a 29-year-old pregnant woman, spilled hot coffee and scalded her right thigh. She sustained second-degree burns over an estimated 3% of her body surface.
Code the diagnoses.

1. _____   3. _____
2. _____   4. _____

LATE EFFECTS

Late effects are lingering or chronic conditions that often are the result of an accident or injury. Late effects can also occur after a disease such as polio or a medical condition such as a cerebrovascular accident (CVA). "Sequela" is a synonym for "late effect." *Late effect* and *sequela* both mean "occurring after" or "resulting from."

The symptoms usually begin at the time of the accident or illness and are called late effects when they continue for longer than the normal period of recovery. Occasionally late effects do not begin until years after an accident or injury.

Accidents are often subject to litigation and/or court proceedings. The litigation may or may not be complete at the time care is rendered for the late effect. Correct sequencing of codes establishes the correct cause-and-effect relationship. Fewer payor conflicts arise when these codes are sequenced correctly.

The correct sequencing of codes is as follows:

1. Residual effect (i.e., pain, loss of function, scarring, etc.)
2. Late effect source (late effect of a specific type of illness or injury, i.e., late effect of fractured hip)

3. For injuries only: E-code describing the cause of the original injury (late effect of a specific type of accident, i.e., late effect from fall on ice)
4. Any other condition that influences today's treatment (chronic conditions, personal history, i.e., congestive heart failure, diabetes mellitus)

First, look up the main term for the presenting problem (the residual effect) and find the correct code. Then, look up the main term "late effect," and find the correct subterm and code for the original illness or injury. (Each late effect code references a range of code numbers for the original illness or injury. Then look up the original illness or injury to confirm the correct late effect code choice.) Next, if you are coding an injury, use the E-code alphabetical index to show the cause of the original injury. Here, too, you may use the main term "late effect." (Each late effect E-code references a range of E-codes for the original injury. Look up the original injury to confirm the correct late-effect E-code choice.) Finally, go back to the main alphabetical index and look up any other conditions that influence today's treatment.

Clinical Application Exercise

A 35-year-old female patient, Debra, has an appointment today as a follow-up for long-term hip pain. Debra's hip was fractured 2 years ago in a traffic accident — she was a passenger in a moving car when another car ran a red light and struck the passenger side of her vehicle. Although the fracture appears to have healed well, the pain has never completely gone away.

Code the diagnoses for this visit.

1. _____   3. _____
2. _____   4. _____

HYPERTENSION

Hypertension (high blood pressure) can be benign, malignant, or unspecified. Benign hypertension refers to a mild elevation in blood pressure, and malignant hypertension refers to a severe elevation in blood pressure. Some types of hypertension do not have a known cause, and some are caused by other specific conditions. Some types of hypertension do not cause malfunctions elsewhere, and some types cause malfunctions in other parts of the body. An elevated blood pressure reading without a diagnosis of hypertension should be coded as a symptom.

Read the guidelines carefully as the code sequencing rules differ for each of the 11 sets of circumstances addressed in the guidelines. When hypertension is the primary reason for the visit, you must establish whether the hypertension is benign, malignant, or unspecified. Then, go to the hypertension table and find the appropriate subterms. Remember to verify the code choice in the tabular list. If the hypertension is caused by another condition, look up the main term for the causing condition and follow the hypertension guidelines for code order. Lastly, look up the main terms for other conditions that influence today's treatment. When there is room on the claim form for another diagnosis, look up the main term "history" and find the subterms for each applicable, documented personal history item.

When a physician *manages* hypertension, the unspecified codes should not be used indefinitely. At some point, the payor will expect the physician to diagnose whether the hypertension is benign or malignant, whether it is caused by another condition, and/or whether it has caused a malfunction elsewhere in the body. If the medical record documentation is nonspecific, you may show the physician the hypertension table and respectfully ask whether a more specific diagnosis has been established for this patient. If so, politely ask the physician to amend the medical record documentation so you may use the more specific code on the claim form.

When the presenting problem is not hypertension, but hypertension influences treatment, it is sequenced as a supporting diagnosis, not as a principal diagnosis. The hypertension is coded to the greatest level documented in the medical record. A consulting physician who is *not managing* the hypertension may use unspecified codes indefinitely when the exact type of hypertension is not known.

Clinical Application Exercise

Robert, a 57-year-old man, is seen for a follow-up due to elevated blood pressure. Robert currently is fighting another bout of chronic pyelonephritis with reflux neuropathy in the left ureter. The culture last week was positive for *E. coli*. Robert is diagnosed today with benign hypertension, secondary to chronic pyelonephritis.

Code the diagnoses for this visit.

1. _____   3. _____
2. _____   4. _____

MYOCARDIAL INFARCTIONS

A myocardial infarction (MI) is better known as a heart attack. It is usually caused by blockage of a heart artery that deprives an area of the heart muscle of oxygen-rich blood and results in tissue death in that area.

The correct sequencing of codes is as follows:

1. Diagnosis or presenting symptom(s) (e.g., inferior wall MI or chest pain)
2. Personal history that influences the condition or the treatment (e.g., personal history of high cholesterol or tobacco use)
3. Other, if applicable

Look up the main term "infarct, infarction" and the subterm "myocardium." When you get to the tabular list, you must select "acute" or "chronic" as a fifth-digit modifier. Select "acute" for the first 8 weeks, and select "chronic" thereafter. The fifth digit also specifies "initial" or "subsequent." Initial treatment codes may only be used once for each episode of care or once for each infarct if the infarcts do not occur during the same episode of care.

If an MI is suspected but not yet diagnosed, code the presenting symptoms instead. For substernal chest pain, look up the main term "pain," the subterm "chest," and the indented subterm "substernal."

Next, look up the main term "history" and the applicable subterm(s) for personal history items that influence the MI or the treatment. Lastly, look up the main terms for any other conditions that influence treatment.

Clinical Application Exercise

A 58-year-old man, Howard, just finished a series of radiation therapy treatments for prostate cancer. He is a two-pack-per-day smoker and has a history of hypertension and elevated cholesterol levels. Today, Howard began experiencing a crushing chest pain that radiated down the left arm. His primary physician, Dr. Rubin, sees him in the emergency room and orders an EKG and lab work. Howard's blood pressure is normal; the EKG is abnormal, and the hemoglobin and hematocrit are still low from the radiation treatments. The other lab work results, including the rest of the complete blood count (CBC), are still pending. Dr. Rubin consults with a cardiologist, who confirms the diagnosis of inferior wall MI based on the EKG tracing. Howard's medical care for the MI was turned over to the cardiologist.

Code the diagnoses for the primary physician.

1. _____   3. _____

2. _____   4. _____

CANCER/NEOPLASM

You must determine the type of neoplasm: benign (not cancer), malignant (cancer), primary malignant (the original site when cancer has metastasized, or spread to other sites), secondary malignant (not the original site when cancer has metastasized, or spread to other sites), or cancer in situ (contained in the site of origin, or has not metastasized). Occasionally, a patient will have two primary sites: the first cancer did not spread to the second site; the second site is a new, unrelated type of cancer.

If a cancer site has been eradicated or surgically excised but treatment is still directed at the site, code it using neoplasm codes. However, if it has been eradicated or excised and no further treatment is directed at the site, personal history codes are used to indicate where the site was.

The correct sequencing of codes is as follows, but please read the current-year neoplasm guidelines for the most current, precise directions and code sequencing:

1. Site and type of neoplasm treated today
2. When the first code position is a secondary site, the primary site is coded in the second position. If the first code position were a primary site, a secondary site, if applicable, would be listed in the second position. When there is more than one secondary site, list them in descending order of importance on subsequent available lines
3. Other condition(s) or history items that influence today's visit

Use the neoplasm table to find each applicable type of cancer or neoplasm. The first code position is based on which site is being treated today. When the primary site is treated, that code goes in position one with any applicable secondary sites in subsequent positions. When a secondary site is treated, that code is listed first followed by the code for the primary site. When there is more than one secondary site, list them in descending order of importance on subsequent available lines.

When the primary site is unknown, first look for the information in the patient history or from other physicians who have treated the patient. Sometimes the primary site remains unknown and nonspecific codes must be used.

After the neoplasm(s) are fully coded, look up the main term(s) for any other conditions or history items that influence today's visit.

Clinical Application Exercise

A 64-year-old male patient, Gary, is treated today for metastatic brain cancer. The primary site was determined to be a malignant lung lesion that was surgically removed from the upper lobe of his right lung 6 months ago, 3 months before the brain lesion was diagnosed. The surgical site is well healed, and tests performed several weeks ago showed no signs of lung recurrence. Gary recently completed a course of radiation therapy to the brain, and the brain lesion is much smaller. He is seen today for follow-up chemotherapy. Some chemotherapy agents cannot be considered because Gary has a history of cardiac premature ventricular contractions (PVCs), still in evidence on the most recent EKG.

Code the diagnoses for this visit.

1. _____   3. _____

2. _____   4. _____

ADVERSE REACTIONS

Adverse reaction codes are used to report adverse reactions from correct drugs, medicines, or biological substances administered correctly. Allergic reactions, nausea, and diarrhea are common types of adverse reactions.

When an adverse reaction is due to a combination of alcohol with another substance, use the poisoning codes and sequencing rules. The code sequence is different between adverse reactions and poisoning.

The correct sequencing of codes for adverse reactions is as follows:

1. Condition (rash, itching)
2. E-code describing external cause (therapeutic use; adverse reaction to correct drug administered correctly)
3. Any other condition that may influence treatment

First, look up the main term for the presenting symptoms or condition (rash; itch; irregular, action, heart; shock, anaphylactic).

Then, use the table of drugs and chemicals to find the medication and identify the "therapeutic use" E-code. For biological substances, use the E-code index to look up the main term "reaction" and the subterm for the biological substance.

Finally, look up the main term for the most significant other condition that influences today's treatment.

Clinical Application Exercise

A 4-year-old girl named Katie is seen in the morning on an urgent appointment due to complaints of ear pain. She is diagnosed with bilateral acute serous otitis media. Amoxil is prescribed. Two hours later, Katie's mother brings her back in. Within half an hour of receiving the first dose, Katie developed a raised rash, and now she is itching and scratching all over. Katie is diagnosed with an allergic reaction to Amoxil. The antibiotic is changed to cephalexin.

Code the diagnoses for the second visit.

1. _____   3. _____

2. _____   4. _____

POISONING

Poisoning codes identify the substance involved when there is a statement of poisoning, overdose, wrong substance given or taken, or intoxication. Poisoning requires a different code sequence than adverse reactions, so do not combine a "poison" code with a "therapeutic use" E-code.

Most physicians who are not mental health specialists are reluctant to list intent in poisoning cases because of the liability attached to such a diagnosis. Intent is seldom known during initial treatment.

Insurance payors vary widely in their coverage, limitations, and exclusions when poisoning is a self-inflicted injury. When care is excluded from coverage primarily because a conclusion about intent is documented, patients or their families tend to blame the physician for a "wrong" conclusion, regardless of truth. To avoid this situation, physicians tend to avoid documenting intent, even if they have obtained an answer they believe to be correct.

The poisoning codes and the associated E-codes are found using the table of drugs and chemicals in section 2 of Volume 2.

The correct code sequencing for poisoning is as follows:

1. Poison substance(s) (e.g., drug[s] and/or alcohol)
2. Symptoms/condition
3. E-code(s) describing cause (e.g., drug[s] and/or

alcohol) and intent (accident, assault, suicide, or unknown)
4. Other conditions influencing treatment

Use the table of drugs and chemicals to find the poisoning code for the substance (listed first) and to find the E-code for the cause (listed after the presenting symptoms or condition). (Do not use a "therapeutic use" E-code.) Then look up the main term for the presenting symptoms or condition (coma; confusion; agitation; alteration, mental status; nausea). Finally, look up the main term for the most significant other condition that influences today's treatment.

Clinical Application Exercise

An 18-year-old boy, Steven, is found unconscious by his parents and brought to the emergency room by ambulance. Steven's parents deny that he uses drugs, but a drug screen is positive for cocaine.

Code the diagnoses.

1. _____   3. _____

2. _____   4. _____

MENTAL DISORDERS

Mental health professionals often use the *Diagnostic and Statistical Manual of Mental Disorders, Fourth Edition* (DSM-IV), to reach a diagnosis. The definitions for DSM-IV diagnoses are often more complex than definitions for similar terms in ICD-9-CM. Most payors do not use the DSM-IV definitions; they use the ICD-9-CM definitions. Therefore DSM-IV diagnoses must be translated into ICD-9-CM codes before being placed on a claim form. Often more than one ICD-9-CM code is required to fully describe one DSM-IV diagnosis. The glossary of mental health terms once used to help mental health professionals translate or convert the codes correctly was deleted from Appendix B of ICD-9-CM in 2005.

Current-year editions of DSM-IV list applicable ICD-9-CM codes when the definitions match. *Caution:* If the DSM-IV codebook is not the most recent edition, the ICD-9-CM codes could easily be outdated.

The correct sequencing of codes is as follows:

1. Diagnosis or presenting symptoms

2. Secondary diagnosis or other conditions that influence today's treatment
3. Personal history that affects condition and treatment

Note: Many mental health codes require you to "code first the underlying condition." Sequence the codes exactly as directed by the codebook, but use block No. 24E to link the procedure to the original mental health diagnosis code indicated by the psychiatrist or psychologist to meet medical necessity.

For example: The psychiatrist you work for diagnoses a patient with "senile dementia with depressive features" and indicates that it is caused by primary parkinsonism.

Category 290 (senile and presenile organic psychotic conditions) directs you to "code first the associated neurological condition." This direction applies to the four- and five-digit codes listed in this category.

Therefore the first diagnosis code you would list is 332.0 (primary parkinsonism), and the second diagnosis code would be 290.21 (senile dementia with depressive features). To meet medical necessity, the psychiatrist's treatment code is linked to the diagnosis code on line 2.

Clinical Application Exercise

A 28-year-old male patient, Dustin, has a history of type 2 diabetes. He is in the hospital for IV antibiotic treatment for cellulitis of the left foot. On the third night of the hospital stay, Dustin suddenly jumps out of bed and starts throwing furniture around the room, endangering the other patient in the room and the hospital employees. It takes four employees to restrain him and move him into a padded room with no furniture. There Dustin is unrestrained, and he immediately begins to repeatedly bang his bandaged foot against the padded wall. His physician is called and orders a stat blood sugar. The blood sugar is dangerously low. Dustin is uncooperative and will not accept any remedy except orange juice with sugar. As his blood sugar rises, Dustin becomes more cooperative and wants to know what happened. After consulting with a psychiatrist, Dustin is diagnosed as having had acute delirium triggered by hypoglycemia. This was secondary to the cellulitis, which altered his response to his oral medication for diabetes. When stable, Dustin is returned to his original room.

Code the diagnoses for this episode.

1. _____   3. _____

2. _____   4. _____

HUMAN IMMUNODEFICIENCY VIRUS

Human immunodeficiency virus (HIV) status is superprotected health information. Therefore, the coding rules are more complex. Usually, for inpatients, suspected conditions are coded as though confirmed. This is not true for HIV. With HIV, only confirmed cases are coded for both inpatients and outpatients.

Confirmed HIV
1. 042 (HIV)
2. Any related conditions

HIV-Related Condition
1. 042 (HIV)
2. HIV-related condition

Asymptomatic HIV
1. V08 (asymptomatic HIV)

Admitted for Unrelated Condition
1. Unrelated condition

2. 042 (HIV)
3. HIV-related conditions

Inconclusive HIV Serology
1. 795.71 (Inconclusive HIV)

HIV in Pregnancy
1. 647.6x (Other specified infectious diseases in the mother classified elsewhere, but complicating pregnancy)
2. 042 (HIV) or V08 (Asymptomatic HIV)

Testing for HIV
1. V73.89 (Screening for other specified viral disease)
2. V69.8 (Other problems related to lifestyle if the patient is in a known high-risk group for HIV)

Inform of Negative Test Results
1. V65.44 (HIV counseling)

Medical Necessity

Diagnosis coding has far-reaching effects for many parties, and it is looked at more closely every year. Penalties and denials for services that would otherwise be covered are sure signs of a problem in meeting the medical necessity requirements. Payors use secret "black box" edits that tie each service and each procedure to specific diagnoses to determine the appropriateness of the service or procedure and to establish medical necessity. Some payors also use patterning studies and apply "blanket penalties" to all claims submitted by providers—and sometimes to all providers in a geographical region—who are found to regularly miscode or misreport services.

UPCODING AND DOWNCODING

Upcoding is sometimes called overcoding. A code is chosen for a more severe condition than is documented in the notes for the encounter. The patient is made to seem sicker than he or she actually is. Upcoding is often intentional to increase reimbursement, but it may be accidental if the physician and his or her medical office employees are unfamiliar with billing rules and coding conventions. Occasional upcoding is considered abuse, and consistent upcoding is considered fraud. Civil penalties and sanctions can be imposed for abuse, and criminal penalties and sanctions can be imposed for fraud.

Downcoding is sometimes called undercoding. A code is chosen for a less severe condition than is documented in the notes for the encounter. The patient is made to seem less sick than he or she actually is. Downcoding often occurs when comorbidities (secondary diagnoses) are not listed. Physician downcoding is sometimes intentional in a misguided effort to avoid charges related to upcoding. Occasional downcoding is considered abuse, and consistent downcoding is considered fraud.

Payors often downcode to pay for only the services or levels of service that meet medical necessity as established by the diagnosis codes submitted on claim forms and/or confirmed in medical record documentation. When payors downcode, the resulting reimbursement is decreased for the physician, applicable facilities such as a hospital or a surgical center, and oftentimes other providers such as medical labs, radiology centers or consulting specialists. Penalties and sanctions also may be imposed, further decreasing reimbursement. Patients sometimes end up paying a higher share of the costs.

For example: The physician performs and bills a level 4 service with a fee of $135.00. The payor determines that the diagnosis codes only meet medical necessity for a level 2 service. The payor downcodes the service to a level 2 service with an allowed amount of $60.00. Depending on the insurance plan, the patient either pays a small copay and the rest of the fee is written off as an insurance discount, or the patient pays the full remaining balance of $75.00.

When diagnosis coding does not fully describe an encounter and does not meet medical necessity:

- ❑ Physicians, facilities, and other providers become frustrated when they try to obtain fair reimbursement for services rendered.
- ❑ Patients become frustrated when they try to obtain needed care and other services that should be covered by their medical plan.
- ❑ Hospitals become frustrated when the listed diagnoses are insufficient to obtain the appropriate reimbursement for services rendered.
- ❑ Other physicians become frustrated when they provide consultative services as requested and then are not successful in obtaining reimbursement.

- ❑ Third-party payors become frustrated when patients blame the payor for not covering services that would not be needed if the patient's condition really matched the condition that was reported.
- ❑ Medical researchers become frustrated when data are not specific enough for meaningful studies.

EFFECT ON REIMBURSEMENT AND/OR EXPENSES

Because of black box edits and medical necessity requirements, diagnosis coding now has a greater influence on reimbursement than at any other time in recorded history. When the coding is performed correctly, full payments can be issued by payors and medically necessary covered services are quickly approved.

Incorrect or inaccurate diagnosis coding influences reimbursement and expenses for others as well as for the provider who initially rendered care and selected the diagnosis code(s). Let's take a closer look at how a physician's diagnosis codes influence the reimbursement and expenses of many.

Physician's Practice
Diagnosis coding determines the appropriateness (the medical necessity) for billed services and the resulting plan of care, including consultations, tests, procedures, and prescriptions for medication, equipment, and/or supplies.

Diagnosis coding supports complexity requirements for medical decision-making, and payment is only received for services considered medically necessary. At least 50% of the profit (the amount of money left after expenses are paid) for each medical claim is determined by the specificity and accuracy of the diagnosis coding.

When diagnosis coding accurately and completely portrays a medical encounter the first time:

- ❑ Employees will spend fewer hours negotiating with payors for authorizations for additional services, such as referrals, tests, supplies, and DME items.
- ❑ Claims will avoid *penalties* that could have resulted in a 60% to 100% reduction in payment, and claims will avoid *sanctions* that could have resulted in large fines and repayment in triple of any amounts wrongfully received due to incorrect coding.
- ❑ There will be fewer requests for additional supporting documentation, so employees will spend fewer hours on these tasks, leaving them free to complete other duties.

❏ Costs are decreased for labor, postage, supplies, and copying equipment (the costs associated with sending additional documentation, rebilling, and filing appeals).

Patients

Many patients purchase prepaid insurance plans, and the insurance plan is legally obligated to pay for covered services as listed in the insurance policy.

Most physician-payor contracts allow the payor to impose penalties if the physician's services are coded incorrectly, and the contracts usually state that the patient is not financially responsible for penalty amounts. The physician then receives a smaller payment than would have been due if the claim had been filed correctly. The EOB often simply says, "The physician agreed by contract to accept the enclosed rate of payment." If you then balance-bill the patient for a penalty amount, you are unlawfully asking the patient to pay a bill the patient does not owe.

Many physicians ask each patient to sign a financial responsibility statement in which the patient agrees to pay for services not covered by the insurance company. Often this form also states that the patient is responsible for payment of services that do not meet medical necessity requirements.

Financial responsibility statements obligate the patient to pay for noncovered services and to pay for optional services that the patient desires but are not medically necessary according to accepted medical standards of care. Cosmetic surgery, such as a facelift, is not usually considered medically necessary. Financial responsibility statements do not give the physician a legal right to ask a patient to pay a bill for services the insurance company would have been legally obligated to cover if the services had been billed correctly, especially if the physician agreed in writing that the patient would not be held financially responsible for payor-imposed penalties.

The patient already paid for the care when the insurance premium was paid, and the service would have been covered if the claim had been filed correctly. However, because the claim was filed incorrectly, the insurance company does not owe any additional payment. It is a contract violation, and it is fraudulent to ask a patient to pay twice for the same service. The only way to legally collect an additional amount is to correct the inaccuracies on the claim and file an appeal to the payor within the period specified in the physician-payor contract.

This situation occurs most often when diagnosis comorbidities (secondary diagnoses and conditions that influence treatment) are not listed and, as a result, the diagnosis coding does not accurately reflect the patient's medical condition.

When incorrect coding occurs in the diagnosis section:

❏ Covered services the patient is entitled to receive are often denied or inexcusably delayed.
❏ Patients seldom know the reason services are denied or delayed, and they experience frustration trying to obtain the services they have legally purchased.
❏ The increased stress can adversely affect the patient's health.

Correct medical coding greatly enhances patient satisfaction. Patients do not have to struggle to receive the services they have purchased from their health plan.

Hospitals

Hospitals are paid based on diagnosis related groups (DRGs), so hospital reimbursement is directly tied to diagnosis coding. Correct and accurate diagnosis coding enhances both the physician's revenue and the hospital's revenue for care rendered to hospital patients, but inefficient or inaccurate diagnosis coding reduces both the physician's revenue and the hospital's revenue.

Every diagnosis rendered during a hospitalization is recorded on a hospital-specific form (often the physician's discharge summary) for entry into a DRG grouper. A DRG grouper is a software program that evaluates all the diagnoses entered for a patient, compares them to the requirements for each DRG code, and assigns one DRG reimbursement code for each hospital claim. Both the DRG reimbursement code and the individual diagnoses are listed on the UB-92 claim form the hospital submits to payors for reimbursement. DRGs are discussed in more detail in Chapter 12.

Only diagnoses justified by documentation in the patient's hospital record will be considered for payment. This is true for the hospital claim and for every physician claim for services rendered to a hospital patient. When a physician submits a CMS-1500 claim for hospital services and reports a diagnosis that does not fall within the DRG code the hospital submitted on a UB-92 claim for the same dates and the same patient, both claims are flagged by the payor. Payment will be delayed until documentation is received from the hospital. Only services that are justified will be paid, and payments for miscoded services are often penalized.

Colleagues

Both diagnosis coding and documentation from the *referring* physician must confirm medical justification for each consultation and each referral given. This is true even when payors require prior authorization.

If a *referring* physician correctly completes a consult slip but fails to document in the patient's medical record the order for the consultation and the diagnosis (or the symptoms when a definitive diagnosis has not yet been reached) to justify the consultation, the payor can retroactively deny payment to the consulting specialist. Therefore, please double-check the patient's medical record documentation to be sure the order for a consultation and the diagnoses or symptoms used to obtain authorization are indeed recorded in the patient's medical record.

Consulting specialists render services in good faith that they will receive payment, and they often mistakenly blame the payors instead of their colleagues when payments are retroactively denied.

A related problem exists when the diagnoses entered into a hospital's DRG grouper for the services of a consultant are the wrong type of diagnoses for physician billing. Hospitals and facilities may submit claims using differential diagnoses ("rule-out," "possible," and "probable" diagnoses) when a definitive diagnosis has not yet been established, but physicians cannot. Physicians must submit claims with symptom codes when a definitive diagnosis has not been reached. Inpatient consultations should be ordered using symptoms if a definitive diagnosis is not yet established, and these symptoms must be reported on the form the hospital uses to enter codes into the DRG grouper.

Similarly, many radiology and laboratory procedures, both inpatient and outpatient, become unbillable for the radiologists and pathologists whenever a "rule-out" diagnosis is given to justify a test.

Please do not allow a referral, consultation, prescription for medical supplies or equipment, or an order for lab tests or radiology procedures to leave your office with a "rule-out" diagnosis attached. Encourage the physician to list symptoms when a diagnosis has not yet been established. In some instances, history V-codes may be used to establish medical necessity and justify a test or procedure.

When a payor does not require prior authorization before a visit to a specialist, the diagnosis coding of the specialist will be used alone to determine medical necessity and reimbursement for the visit.

When in doubt as to whether a payor will cover a test, you may refer to the *Radiology Cross Coder*, the *Laboratory Cross Coder*, the *Surgical Cross Coder*, the *Procedural Cross Coder*, or the *Medical Services Cross Coder*, all published by Ingenix, Inc. (St. Anthony Publishing/Medicode, Salt Lake City, Utah). These publications list diagnosis codes proven to pass medical necessity edits (black box edits) so payment

is more likely to be authorized for a given service. However, remember, different payors use different black box edits, so payment is never guaranteed.

Third-Party Payors
The quality of diagnosis coding affects payor costs in much the same way it affects practice costs. Costs are significantly higher anytime coding alone does not justify medical necessity. The payor must request and review additional documentation. Labor and supply costs rise.

To avoid this cost, many payors downcode claims and only pay for the level of service that is justified by the diagnoses submitted on the claim. In addition, payors frequently impose penalties when claims do not match medical record documentation and when claims are completed incorrectly.

Incorrect coding and inaccurate claim completion are considered abusive practices. Patterning studies identify habitual abusers, and blanket penalties may be applied to individual providers and sometimes to every provider in an entire region when abusive patterns are widespread.

Medical Researchers
Historically, insurance actuaries have always performed medical research studies as they calculate risks for the insurance company that employs them. The actuaries have access to pooled data from every insurance company that is a member of the Medical Information Bureau (MIB). Diagnosis accuracy and specificity, as well as the presence or absence of significant comorbidities, greatly influence the statistical value of medical research.

For example: A new wound management system is the subject of a study. Unfortunately, most of the medical claims submitted list only the diagnosis for the wound and only the procedure for the new treatment. Medical researchers and insurance actuaries are unable to determine how other variables, such as comorbidities (e.g., diabetes, heart disease, kidney disease) and other procedures (e.g., whirlpool treatments or wound debridement), might have influenced the study's findings.

Insurance companies use the results of medical research to determine the cost effectiveness of one treatment over another. When variables are tracked for every patient, payor coverage decisions are based on meaningful research data. However, when variables are not tracked, payor coverage decisions are based on imprecise research (faulty data that payors believe to be accurate).

Finding Information in ICD-9-CM, Volume 3

Volume 3 of ICD-9-CM lists procedures, not diagnoses. It begins with the alphabetical index and is followed by the tabular list of procedures. The index rules and standard coding conventions for Volume 3 are the same as those for Volumes 1 and 2 of ICD-9-CM.

Volume 3 of ICD-9-CM is only used to code procedures for hospital inpatients. All others code procedures from the CPT-4 and HCPCS codebooks. However, CPT/HCPCS codes have five digits, whereas ICD-9-CM Volume 3 codes have two digits followed by a decimal point and up to two additional digits.

Volume 3 codes do not report the skill of the physician. CPT codes are used for physician billing. Volume 3 codes report the overhead costs and the cost of supplies incurred by the hospital in providing the service.

Clinical Application Exercise

Find the Volume 3 codes for the following:

1. Biopsy of conjunctiva
2. Partial substernal thyroidectomy
3. Incision and drainage of cranial sinus
4. Simple mastoidectomy
5. Segmental resection of lung
6. Venous cutdown
7. Open biopsy of spleen
8. Balloon dilation of duodenum
9. Open biopsy of ureter
10. Total hip replacement

STOP & REVIEW

Answer the following questions:

1. What type of obstetric special circumstance exists when a pregnancy-related complication occurs 3 weeks after delivery?

   _____

2. Where do you look first to find the code for any type of hypertension?

   _____

3. What code is listed first in poisoning?

   _____

4. What code is listed first in adverse reactions?

   _____

5. What is a late effect?

   _____

Code the following using the proper code order:

6. Sprained left ankle, deltoid ligament, due to tripping over a rug at home.

   1. _____   3. _____
   2. _____   4. _____

7. Acute MI of the anterior wall, initial episode.

   1. _____   3. _____
   2. _____   4. _____

8. Prolonged labor (first stage) with third-degree perineal tear, delivered healthy twins.

   1. _____   3. _____
   2. _____   4. _____

9. Second-degree burns to back of right hand due to accidentally touching a hot oven at work in a restaurant.

   1. _____   3. _____
   2. _____   4. _____

10. Hodgkin's sarcoma of the intraabdominal lymph nodes.

   1. _____   3. _____
   2. _____   4. _____

Claim Form Reporting Differences for Diagnoses

The claim forms used to report physician services are quite different from the claim forms used to report hospital and facility services. A greater number of diagnoses and a wider variety of diagnoses may be listed for hospital and facility billing than physicians are allowed to list when reporting their own services. In addition, physicians must be sure that the diagnoses they submit on their own claims for services rendered in a hospital or facility are included in the codes entered into the DRG grouper by the hospital or facility.

The diagnosis sections for each type of medical claim form are as follows:

❐ CMS-1500 (physician billing):
  ❐ You may list four diagnoses per claim.
  ❐ Each CPT code must be linked to the principal diagnosis for that specific treatment, service or supply.
  ❐ When more than four diagnoses are required to adequately report services, you must either split the charges onto multiple claim forms or send supporting documentation or both.
❐ UB-92 (hospital and facility billing):
  ❐ Admitting diagnosis (1)–initial reason for admission

❐ Principal diagnosis (1)–reason determined after study to be chiefly responsible for hospitalization (inpatient only; may use selected V-codes)
❐ E-code (1)–used when there is an injury, poisoning, or adverse effect (the E-code that reports where the injury or poisoning occurred is preferred by payors in this field)
❐ Other diagnoses (8)–additional conditions that coexist at admission or develop subsequently and which affect the treatment received or the length of stay (V-codes and additional E-codes may be used; do not include diagnoses listed elsewhere.)
❐ Principal procedure (1)–the ICD-9-CM code for the principal procedure (from Volume 3, ICD-9-CM)
❐ Other procedure codes (5)–may report up to five additional ICD-9-CM procedure codes (from Volume 3, ICD-9-CM)
❐ When more additional diagnoses are required to adequately report services, the hospital or facility must either split the charges onto multiple claim forms or send supporting documentation, or both.

Legal Issues

Medical necessity is established using diagnosis codes. Therefore, diagnosis codes have the single greatest influence on medical reimbursement. *Services that are not medically justified are not paid by the payor* and in most instances cannot be billed to the patient.

Although upcoding and downcoding have long been tolerated by payors, both are considered to be abusive practices. Physicians can be prosecuted for diagnosis coding that is not consistent with the facts documented in the patient's medical record. Medical billers and coders can be prosecuted if they submit diagnoses on claims when the diagnoses do not match the documentation in the patient's medical record.

Pigeonholing occurs when a physician consistently chooses the majority of diagnoses billed from a limited selection of diagnosis codes. Pigeonholing is considered an abusive practice. Yet, many superbills encourage pigeonholing by including a list of the diagnoses the physician has chosen as his or her "most frequently used" diagnoses. Typically, a superbill that includes diagnosis codes tends to favor nonspecific codes as a way of saving space. Instead

of listing the numerous code choices for a category of codes, they only list the "unspecified" code choices. This, in turn, can lead to an inadvertent failure to justify medical necessity for nearly every service rendered. If these same codes are then used for hospital billing and are used when ordering tests, procedures, consultations, and referrals, other medical providers can also suffer financial losses.

A well-designed superbill does not lead to pigeonholing; it leads to correct coding. Instead of containing a short list of diagnoses, a superbill should guide a physician into fully describing each encounter.

The Centers for Medicare and Medicaid Services (CMS) has taken the position that *when there is evidence that "abuse" (related to the practice of medicine) occurs on a regular basis,* the "abuse" can then be reclassified as "fraud." Abuse incurs civil penalties, but fraud incurs criminal penalties.

The superbill or encounter form for physician billing and the Chargemaster for hospital or facility billing are billing worksheets; they are not part of the patient medical record. Diagnoses listed only on a billing worksheet, but not included in the patient medical record, may not be billed.

A well-designed superbill leads to correct coding. Instead of containing a short list of diagnoses, a superbill should guide a physician into fully describing each encounter.

A well-designed problem list helps physicians remember what comorbidities (secondary diagnoses and conditions that influence treatment) apply to each patient. See Chapter 3 for examples of well-designed forms.

Continuing education is very important for physicians and every employee who influences the billing process. Every diagnosis listed on the superbill for billing also must be documented in the patient's medical record. Documentation for each

encounter must stand alone to justify the medical necessity for the service rendered. Every secondary diagnosis or condition that applies to a visit should be documented in the narrative for that visit, unless the notes clearly state that the problem list was reviewed and updated. Although "rule-out," "probable," and "questionable" diagnoses may not be billed, they should be listed in the medical record to document the complexity of medical decision-making (see Chapter 6).

Review physician documentation immediately after each visit, while the physician still remembers details of the encounter. If anything is missing, politely point out what is missing and gently remind the physician that you can only bill the service as it is documented in the medical record.

STOP & REVIEW

Answer the following questions:

1. What is upcoding?

_____

2. What is downcoding?

_____

3. What is medical necessity?

_____

4. Who uses DRGs for billing?

_____

5. How does diagnosis coding influence medical research?

_____

6. Does incorrect diagnosis coding increase costs for payors? If so, why?

_____

_____

7. When a physician bills for inpatient care, his diagnosis must be included in the code billed by the hospital.

____True   ____False

8. What is pigeonholing?

_____

_____

A Preview of ICD-10-CM

The tenth revision of the *International Classification of Diseases,* ICD-10, has been in use by the World Health Organization since 1994. ICD-10 reorganizes the diagnosis categories and incorporates many of the fourth- and fifth-digit subclassifications used in the United States.

Whereas ICD-9 and ICD-9-CM primarily use numeric codes (numbers), ICD-10 uses alphanumeric codes (letters and numbers). The version of ICD-10 with clinical modifications for the United States, **ICD-10-CM,** is in the final stages of development. ICD-10-CM also adds sixth-digit and seventh-digit subclassifications.

ICD-10-CM cannot be implemented in the United States until medical software developers and manufacturers have been given sufficient time to

change the field requirements for software screens that report diagnosis codes. Medical management and claim submission software systems must be revised to accept alphanumeric codes for every diagnosis, and the field length must be expanded to accept six and seven digits. The payment systems used by Medicare and other payors must also be revised to accept the new codes.

Software and hardware updates required by the change from using a two-digit year to using a four-digit year (Y2K) pushed back the implementation date for ICD-10-CM. Publications to introduce ICD-10-CM were published in 1999, and the required minimum 2-year notification of an impending change was issued. Publications to help the medical industry get ready for the conversion process were scheduled to be published in 2000 but were not released as expected. Expect ICD-10-CM to be implemented in the United States sometime in either 2007 or 2008.

In ICD-10, the full title of the book was changed from *International Classification of Diseases* to *International Statistical Classification of Diseases and Related Health Problems*. Although it contains organizational changes and new features are added, the basic format and most of the coding conventions are unchanged.

ICD-10 Volume 1 contains the tabular list, Volume 2 contains "Rules and Guidelines for Coding," and Volume 3 contains the alphabetical index.

A final decision has not been made about including Volume 2 in ICD-10-CM, but it is possible that ICD-9-CM Volumes 1 and 2 could be replaced by ICD-10-CM Volumes 1, 2, and 3.

ICD-9-CM, Volume 3 (currently used by hospitals and facilities to report procedures), will be replaced by ICD-10-PCS. CMS is considering eliminating CPT altogether and replacing it with ICD-10-PCS. The American Medical Association (AMA) is actively developing CPT-5, and they oppose eliminating CPT. The final decision has not yet been made.

While ICD-10-CM is similar to ICD-9-CM, there are some significant differences:

❏ All ICD-10-CM codes will be alphanumeric. Every code will begin with an alpha character (A through Z, except U) followed by numeric characters. Codes will have three characters followed by a decimal and one to three additional characters, providing even greater specificity. Be careful not to confuse the letter "I" with the number "1" or the letter "O" with the number "0."

❏ In ICD-10-CM, the number of chapters increases from 17 to 21. E-codes become V-, W-, X-, and Y-codes and are placed in a chapter rather than a supplement. V-codes become Z-codes and are placed in a chapter rather than a supplement. "Eye" and "Ear" each have their own chapters.

❏ In ICD-9-CM, additional digit listings often do not include the "common" part of a code that is only printed once, with additional digit

definitions indented under it. In ICD-10-CM, additional digit listings contain the full text of the code.

❏ The rules for notes are unchanged. Expect applicable notes to be listed at the beginning of the chapter, under sections now called "blocks," under the three-character category codes, under the subcategory codes, and under the subclassification codes. Each note applies to every code in the applicable block: chapter notes apply to the entire chapter; block notes apply to the entire block; category notes apply to the entire category; subcategory notes apply to the entire subcategory; and subclassification notes apply to the entire subclassification.

❏ In ICD-9-CM, two codes are often required to list a disease and the cause (i.e., pneumonia due to streptococcus); with ICD-10-CM, one code will include both pieces of information.

❏ More combination codes will be available to include symptoms or conditions secondary to a specific disease.

❏ Expect obstetric codes to specify the trimester of the pregnancy.

❏ Expect "late effects" to be called "sequelae," the term preferred by physicians. Late effect and sequela are synonyms. They both refer to symptoms or conditions "occurring after" or "resulting from" a specific event: an injury or another condition.

❏ In ICD-10-CM, anatomic body parts may be listed as main terms, similar to CPT-4.

❏ In ICD-10-CM, many code classifications are expanded. Essential modifiers follow a comma as part of the description and must be present for the code to be valid. Nonessential modifiers are listed in parentheses and may or may not be present for the code to be valid.

❏ Categories are restructured. Some have more changes than others.

❏ Although most codes become more specific, a few of the changes decrease code specificity, so code carefully.

Table 5-1 compares the chapter differences between ICD-9-CM and ICD-10-CM.

TABLE 5-1
Chapter Comparison for ICD-9-CM—ICD-10-CM

ICD-9-CM	ICD-10-CM
1. Infectious and Parasitic Diseases (001–139)	1. Certain Infectious and Parasitic Conditions (A00–B99)
2. Neoplasms (140–239)	2. Neoplasms (C00–D48)
3. Endocrine, Nutritional, and Metabolic Disease, and Immunity Disorders (240–279)	3. Diseases of the Blood and Blood-forming Organs and Certain Disorders Involving the Immune Mechanism (D50–D89)
4. Diseases of the Blood and Blood-Forming Organs (280–289)	4. Endocrine, Nutritional, and Metabollic Diseases (E00–E90)
5. Mental Disorders (290–319)	5. Mental and Behavioral Disorders (F01–F99)
6. Diseases of the Nervous System and Sense Organs (320–389)	6. Diseases of the Nervous System (G00–G99)
7. Diseases of the Circulatory System (390–459)	7. Diseases of the Eye and Adnexa (H00–H59)
8. Diseases of the Respiratory System (460–519)	8. Diseases of the Ear and Mastold Process (H60–H99)
9. Diseases of the Digestive System (520–579)	9. Diseases of the Circulatory System (I00–I97)
10. Diseases of the Genitourinary System (580–629)	10. Diseases of the Respiratory System (J00–J99)
11. Complications of Pregnancy, Childbirth, and the Puerperium (630–677)	11. Diseases of the Digestive System (K00–K93)
12. Diseases of the Skin and Subcutaneous Tissue (680–709)	12. Diseases of the Skin and Subcutaneous Tissue (L00–L99)
13. Diseases of the Musculoskeletal System and Connective Tissue (710–739)	13. Diseases of the Musculoskeletal System and Connective Tissue (M00–M99)
14. Congenital Anomalies (740–759)	14. Diseases of the Genitourinary System (N00–N99)
15. Certain Conditions Originating in the Perinatal Period (769–779)	15. Pregnancy, Childbirth, and the Puerperium (O00–O99)
16. Symptoms, Signs, and Ill-Defined Conditions (780–799)	16. Certain Conditions Originating in the Perinatal Period (P04–P94)
17. Injury and Poisoning (800–999)	17. Congenital Malformations, Deformations and Chromosomal Abnormalities (Q00–Q94)
18. Classification of factors influencing Health Status and Contact With Health Services (V01–V82)	18. Symptoms, Signs, and Abnormal Clinical and Laboratory Findings, Not Elsewhere Classified (R00–R99)
19. Classification of External Causes of Injury and Poisoning (E800–E999)	19. Injury, Poisoning, and Certain Other Consequences of External Causes (S00–T98)
	20. External Causes of Morbidity and Mortality (V01–Y97)
	21. Factors Influencing Health Status and Contact With Health Services (Z00–Z99)

STOP & REVIEW

Answer the following questions:

1. A well-designed _____ does not contain a short list of diagnosis codes; instead, it leads the physician to describe each encounter fully.

2. A well-designed _____ helps physicians remember the secondary diagnoses and conditions that influence treatment for each patient.

3. When ICD-10-CM is implemented, are the coding conventions and billing rules expected to change significantly? _____

4. How will E-codes change when the change is made from ICD-9-CM to ICD-10-CM?

_____

_____

5. How will V-codes change when the change is made from ICD-9-CM to ICD-10-CM?

_____

_____

Chapter Review

In the United States, ICD-9-CM is the codebook currently used for diagnosis coding. ICD-9-CM stands for "International Classification of Diseases, Ninth Revision, Clinical Modification."

Volume 1 contains the tabular list and is followed by supplements for V-codes, E-codes, and five informational appendices. The information in the tabular list is divided into chapters, sections, categories, subcategories, and subclassifications. Symbols and abbreviations also are used to convey information.

Volume 2 contains the alphabetical index of diseases (the diagnosis code index), the hypertension table, the neoplasm table, a table of drugs and chemicals, and an alphabetical index to the causes of external injuries and poisoning (the E-code index).

Diagnosis coding must be performed to the highest level of specificity and must match the documentation in the medical record as closely as possible. When fourth- and fifth-digit subclassifications are available, they must be used.

The order in which diagnosis codes are reported on the claim form is used to establish medical necessity, justify the level of medical decision-making, and determine if the level of work performed was appropriate for the nature of the presenting illness. Coding conventions dictate a standard code order and a code order for commonly encountered special circumstances.

The standard code order is principal diagnosis (for inpatients), primary diagnosis (when different from the principal diagnosis; both inpatients and outpatients), and pertinent secondary diagnoses (both inpatients and outpatients).

Reimbursement today is tied to medical necessity, so diagnosis coding has a big influence on reimbursement for the physician and all subsequent care that stems from the original encounter.

Medical office employees are given the responsibility of helping physicians meet billing and coding requirements. Well-designed forms, continuing education, and timely review of documentation are the keys to helping physicians meet complex requirements.

In the near future, the codebook will change to ICD-10-CM. All codes will become alphanumeric and will be listed in chapters. Some codes will have a sixth-digit subclassification. All medical entities, including physician offices, hospitals, and other facilities, will have to upgrade computer software systems to accommodate these changes. While ICD-10-CM represents a significant change from ICD-9-CM, the coding conventions and billing rules are not expected to change dramatically.

Answer the following questions:

1. Is it possible to code accurately from the alphabetical index alone? Why or why not?

   _____

2. Which is the correct standard code order?
   A. Primary diagnosis, secondary conditions, anything else that influences treatment
   B. The order in which codes are listed in the patient's medical record
   C. Principal diagnosis, primary diagnosis, secondary diagnoses
   D. The order in which codes are listed on the superbill

3. When a patient is pregnant, what determines code order?
   A. Whether the pregnancy, through delivery, is normal or complicated
   B. Whether the care is included in the global package of pregnancy services
   C. Whether the care is related to the pregnancy
   D. All of the above

4. What is the first code when coding for cancer and neoplasm?
   A. The primary site
   B. The secondary or metastatic site
   C. The original site
   D. The site treated or evaluated today

5. What is the first code when coding for late effects?
   A. The E-code
   B. The residual effect
   C. The late effect
   D. None of the above

6. What is the code order when coding for a myocardial infarction?

   1. _____   3. _____

   2. _____   4. _____

7. What is the code order when coding for adverse reactions?

   1. _____   3. _____

   2. _____   4. _____

8. What is the code order when coding for poisoning?

   1. _____   3. _____

   2. _____   4. _____

9. What do you do if more than four diagnoses are needed to describe physician services?
   A. Use more than one CMS-1500 claim form.
   B. Send supporting documentation.
   C. List only the first diagnosis on the superbill and forget about the others.
   D. A and/or B, but not C

10. What do you do if a lab test is ordered and only a "rule-out" diagnosis is written on the order form?
    A. Nothing; this is acceptable.
    B. Ask the physician to please include the reason for the test as a diagnosis, symptom(s), or history (V-codes).
    C. Use information in the medical record to rewrite the order without bothering the physician.
    D. Use information provided by the patient to rewrite the order without bothering the physician.

11. What additional item(s) do you check when coding diagnoses for hospital services?
    A. The hospital's medical record number for the patient
    B. The DRG code billed by the hospital
    C. The patient's room number
    D. The discharge date

12. What happens to medical research when comorbid conditions and/or additional types of treatment are not listed on claim forms?
    A. The results of the research are valid for every circumstance.
    B. The results of the research are not very meaningful.
    C. Payors will be able to identify the circumstances in which one treatment obtains better results than another.
    D. Payors will not be able to identify the circumstance in which one treatment obtains better results than another.
    E. A and C only
    F. B and D only

13. Which of the following reasons do payors use to downcode services?
    A. Medical necessity not justified for the reported service or level of service
    B. Documentation not adequate for the reported service or level of service
    C. Codes reported do not match the documentation in the patient's medical record.
    D. All of the above

Code the following:

14. Pregnancy complicated by severe preeclampsia, antepartum, with preexisting benign essential hypertension.
    1. _____ 3. _____
    2. _____ 4. _____

15. Painful scarring of the hands due to old third-degree burns from a fire.
    1. _____ 3. _____
    2. _____ 4. _____

16. Malignant hypertension with congestive heart failure.
    1. _____ 3. _____
    2. _____ 4. _____

17. Metastatic carcinoma to the thoracic spine from the breast (breast surgery performed 1 year earlier with no local recurrence).
    1. _____ 3. _____
    2. _____ 4. _____

18. Bipolar affective disorder, mixed, severe with psychotic behavior.
    1. _____ 3. _____
    2. _____ 4. _____

19. A 2-year-old boy ingested several pills of an antidepressant medication (amitriptyline). He acted tired, so his grandmother put him down for a nap before discovering the open pill bottle. By the time the paramedics arrived, the child was in a coma.
    1. _____ 3. _____
    2. _____ 4. _____

20. A 45-year-old woman was prescribed ampicillin for an infected blister on her foot. She took the first dose as soon as she got home from the pharmacy. Within 20 minutes of taking the first pill, she started itching and developed raised bumps on her skin. Within 40 minutes, the itching was severe and she was having trouble breathing. She called the paramedics. In the emergency department, she was treated for upper respiratory hypersensitivity and allergic urticaria from a correct dose of medication taken correctly.
    1. _____ 3. _____
    2. _____ 4. _____

BASIC PRINCIPLES FOR EVALUATION AND MANAGEMENT (E/M) SERVICES

Objectives

After completing this chapter, you should be able to:

- Explain the purpose of documentation guidelines and discuss the role they play in E/M code selection
- Demonstrate how to use the components and requirements of the documentation guidelines when selecting physician office E/M codes
- Demonstrate how to use the components and requirements of the documentation guidelines when selecting physician hospital E/M codes
- Distinguish between a referral and a consultation
- Discuss legal responsibilities related to E/M code selection
- Discuss how E/M code selection influences reimbursement
- Discuss strategies for helping physicians meet E/M code requirements

Key Terms

amount and/or complexity of data to be reviewed documentation of the review of (1) results of diagnostic tests; (2) personal review of films or slides to confirm or augment reported results; (3) collaboration with other health professionals regarding test results or prior history; (4) review of old records or history from other sources.

associated signs and symptoms details that are included in the definition of a medical problem, or details that are used to narrow the choices when a diagnosis has not yet been established. An element of the history of present illness (HPI).

brief HPI a brief history of present illness; the medical record documentation should describe one to three elements of the present illness.

CC (1) chief complaint; a concise statement describing the reason for an outpatient visit; (2) complications and comorbidities; those additional conditions that increase the length of an inpatient stay by at least 1 day in at least 75% of patients.

complete PFSH complete past, family, and/or social history; a documented review of two or all three PFSH areas, depending on the category of E/M service. All three areas are required for comprehensive assessments.

complete ROS complete review of systems; the documented report of an inquiry about the body system(s) directly related to the problem(s) identified in the HPI plus all additional body systems (at least 10).

comprehensive exam (1) *1995 guidelines:* a general multi-system examination or a complete examination of a single organ system or body area; (2) *1997 guidelines for multi-system exam:* should include at least nine organ systems or body areas. For each system/area selected, all elements of the examination identified in a table by a bullet (•) should be performed, unless specific directions limit the content of the examination. For each area/system, documentation of at least two elements identified in a table by a bullet (•) is expected; (3) *1997 guidelines for single organ system exam:* should include performance of all elements identified in a table by a bullet (•), whether in a shaded or unshaded box. Documentation of every element in each shaded box and at least one element in each unshaded box is expected.

comprehensive history documentation must include the chief complaint, an extended HPI, a complete ROS, and complete PFSH.

consultation used when only an opinion or treatment advice is requested from the consulting physician. The consultant must send a written report to the requesting physician, or both physicians must document a telephone discussion.

context details that relate a medical problem to other factors (not timing) about other specific events (e.g., right upper quadrant abdominal pain or right shoulder pain that occurs after eating only when fatty foods are eaten). An element of HPI.

contributory elements the elements of documentation that confirm or augment the selection of codes for E/M services but that usually do not play a large enough role to make a difference in code choice. The exception is when counseling or coordination of care takes more than half the intraservice time for the encounter; then time is used to determine code selection.

detailed exam (1) *1995 guidelines:* an extended examination of the affected body areas or other symptomatic or related organ systems; (2) *1997 guidelines for multi-system exam:* should include at least six organ systems or body areas. For each system/area selected, performance and documentation of at least two elements identified in a table by a bullet (•) is expected. Alternatively, a detailed examination may include performance and documentation of at least 12 elements identified in a table by a bullet (•) in two or more organ systems or body areas; (3) *1997 guidelines for single organ system exam:* examinations other than eye or psychiatric examinations should include performance and documentation of at least 12 elements identified in a table by a bullet (•), whether in a shaded or unshaded box. Eye and psychiatric examinations should include the performance and documentation of at least nine elements identified in a table by a bullet (•), whether in a shaded or unshaded box.

detailed history documentation must include the chief complaint, an extended HPI, an extended ROS, and a pertinent PFSH.

documentation guidelines official guidelines developed by the Centers for Medicare and Medical Services (CMS) and published in the *Federal Register;* a method of evaluating physician performance by defining services and counting the items documented. All physicians are required by law to follow either the 1995 or the 1997 guidelines, or the most current guidelines once another set of guidelines is released.

duration the length of time involved for each episode or occurrence of a medical problem or symptom. An element of HPI.

established patient one who has been seen within the last 3 years by the practice or by the specialty group within a multi-specialty practice.

evaluation and management (E/M) the process of evaluating a patient for suspected, known, or potential problems or conditions; assessing the findings; rendering an opinion; and developing and initiating a plan of action.

examination the process of obtaining and recording the physician's or other health care provider's medically significant observations and findings.

expanded problem-focused exam (1) *1995 guidelines:* a limited examination of the affected body area or organ system and other symptomatic or related organ systems; (2) *1997 guidelines for multi-system exam:* performance and documentation of at least six elements identified in a table by a bullet (•) in one or more organ system(s) or body area(s); (3) *1997 guidelines for single organ system exam:* performance and documentation of at least six elements identified in a table by a bullet (•), whether in a shaded or unshaded box.

expanded problem-focused history documentation must include the chief complaint, a brief HPI, and a problem-pertinent ROS.

extended HPI the medical record documentation describes at least four elements of the present illness or describes the status of at least three chronic and/or inactive conditions.

extended ROS extended review of systems; the documented report of an inquiry about the body system(s) directly related to the problem(s) identified in the HPI and a limited number (two to nine) of additional body systems.

face-to-face time documented time spent face to face with a patient or a patient's family in an office or other outpatient setting; outpatient intraservice time.

family history a documented review of the history of medical events in the patient's family, including hereditary diseases, contagious diseases, and any other diseases or conditions that place the patient at risk.

floor/unit time documented time spent working directly on behalf of an inpatient while physically present on the patient's floor or unit; inpatient intraservice time. It includes but is not limited to face-to-face time.

high-complexity medical decision-making documentation of (1) an extensive number of diagnoses or management options; (2) an extensive amount of data or complexity of data to be reviewed; and (3) a high risk of complications and/or morbidity or mortality.

high-severity presenting problem a medical problem in which the risk of morbidity without treatment is high to extreme; there is moderate to high risk of mortality without treatment; or there is high probability of severe, prolonged functional impairment.

history of present illness (HPI) a chronological description of (1) the development of the patient's present illness or problem from the first sign or symptom or (2) the development of the patient's present illness or problem from the previous encounter to the present. It includes the following elements: location, quality, severity, duration, timing, context, associated signs and symptoms, and modifying factors.

intraservice time documented face-to-face time or floor/unit time used to calculate the level of E/M code when time is the determining factor.

key components the elements of documentation that best describe the amount of work performed and that are used to determine the code choice for E/M services.

location the anatomical location of a medical problem. An element of HPI.

low-complexity medical decision-making documentation of (1) a limited number of diagnoses or management options; (2) a limited amount of data or complexity of data to be reviewed; and (3) a low risk of complications and/or morbidity or mortality.

low-severity presenting problem a medical problem in which the risk of morbidity without treatment is low; there is little to no risk of mortality without treatment; full recovery without functional impairment is expected.

medical decision-making (MDM) documentation of the thought processes required to evaluate medical findings, documentation of the amount of work performed when evaluating medical data, and documentation of the conclusions drawn and the resulting plan of care. The amount of risk involved is also factored into the level of MDM chosen.

minimal presenting problem a medical problem that may not require the presence of a physician, but the service is provided under the physician's supervision.

moderate-complexity medical decision-making documentation of (1) multiple diagnoses or management options; (2) a moderate amount of data or complexity of data to be reviewed; and (3) a moderate risk of complications and/or morbidity or mortality.

moderate-severity presenting problem a medical problem in which the risk of morbidity without treatment is moderate; there is a moderate risk of mortality without treatment; uncertain prognosis or increased probability of prolonged functional impairment.

modifying factors details that alter the definition or scope of a medical problem (e.g., the fact that a patient smokes must be considered and it changes the scope of many medical problems). An element of HPI.

new patient a patient who is new to the practice or who has not been seen by a physician in the practice (or the specialty in a multi-specialty group) within the past 3 years.

number of diagnoses or management options documentation of (1) every diagnosis and every diagnosis option the physician thought about and considered, including new diagnoses, the status of previously established diagnoses, and rule out of possible diagnoses; and (2) every treatment and every treatment option the physician thought about and considered, including the initiation of or changes actually made in treatment and alternative treatment options discussed with the patient.

outlier payors use software programs to determine patterns of code use. They know the usual patterns for every region and every physician who submits claims. Those who fall outside the normal statistical patterns for a specialty or for a region are called outliers. Claims from outliers are scrutinized more carefully.

past history documentation of the patient's past experience with illness, operations, injuries, and/or treatments.

past, family, and/or social history (PFSH) a documented review of the patient's past history, family history, and/or age-appropriate social history and activities.

pertinent PFSH a documented review of PFSH that is directly related to the HPI. At least one item from any of the three PFSH areas must be documented.

problem-focused exam (1) *1995 guidelines:* a limited examination of the affected body area or organ system; (2) *1997 guidelines for multi-system exam:* performance and documentation of one to five elements identified in a table by a bullet (•) in one or more organ system(s) or body area(s); (3) *1997 guidelines for single organ system exam:* performance and documentation of one to five elements identified in a table by a bullet (•), whether in a shaded or unshaded box.

problem-focused history documentation must include the chief complaint and a brief HPI.

problem-pertinent ROS problem-pertinent review of systems; the documented report of an inquiry about the body system(s) directly related to the problem(s) identified in the HPI.

quality the details used to distinguish differences between similar problems (e.g., pain may be sharp, stabbing, cramping, dull, heavy, burning). An element of HPI.

referral used whenever partial or total care of the patient is transferred to another physician.

review of systems (ROS) a documented inventory of normal and abnormal subjective findings and/or symptoms reported by the patient or others.

risk of significant complications, morbidity, and/or mortality risks are based on documentation of the presenting problem(s), the procedure(s) performed, treatments ordered, and other possible management options.

self-limited or minor presenting problem a medical problem that runs a definite and prescribed course, is transient in nature, and is not likely to permanently alter heath status or has a good prognosis when treatment is given as ordered.

severity the details used to distinguish levels of seriousness for a medical problem. An element of HPI.

social history a documented, age-appropriate review of the patient's past and current activities.

straightforward medical decision-making documentation of a minimal number of diagnoses or management options, zero to minimal data or complexity of data to be reviewed, and a minimal risk of complications and/or morbidity or mortality.

timing the details that relate a medical problem to when other specific events occur, or that identify a pattern of occurrences. An element of HPI.

Introduction

Payors declare that more than 80% of all medical claims received are for **evaluation and management (E/M)** services. Therefore this chapter focuses solely on E/M services and how to code them.

Evaluation and management is the process of evaluating a patient for suspected, known, or potential problems or conditions; assessing the findings; rendering an opinion; developing a plan of action; and documenting the encounter. As appropriate, the E/M process also may include writing prescriptions for medications and ordering tests, treatments, equipment, and supplies.

E/M services only include evaluation and management activities. Procedures are governed by different rules and are coded separately. Procedure coding is covered in Chapter 7.

Medical office employees are often caught in the middle of a battle between physicians and payors about issues related to the documentation of E/M services. Legally, you are required to code and bill E/M services according to the current E/M documentation guidelines. You are personally subject to the provisions of the Health Insurance Portability and Accountability Act of 1996 (HIPAA), including the penalties of the law. Although it is becoming less of a problem, you might someday have to choose between making every effort to help your physician(s) come into compliance with the law or personally facing stiff penalties if the E/M codes you place on a medical claim form do not match chart documentation. You are more likely to succeed in inspiring a physician to change his or her documentation patterns when you understand the history and the underlying battles regarding E/M documentation.

The following excerpt is from a Medicare news release dated October 6, 2004:

> "The Healthcare Common Procedure Coding System (HCPCS) was established in 1978 to provide a standardized coding system for describing specific items and services provided in the delivery of health care. Such coding is necessary for Medicare, Medicaid, and other health insurance programs to ensure that health insurance claims are processed in an orderly and consistent manner. Initially, use of the codes was voluntary, but with the implementation of the Health Insurance Portability and Accountability Act of 1996 (HIPAA) use of the HCPCS for transactions involving healthcare information became mandatory."

In a fact sheet from the United States Department of Health and Human Services (HHS) dated October 2003, it is made clear that HIPAA required HHS to adopt national standards for health care transactions.

Later, the fact sheet states that HHS' Center for Medicare and Medicaid Services was charged with overseeing the implementation of the standards for electronic transactions and code sets.

The *Current Procedural Terminology* (CPT) codebook is the official code set for Level I of HCPCS. The HCPCS codebook is the official code set for Level II of HCPCS. E/M codes are part of the CPT codebook. When the Centers for Medicare and Medical Services (CMS) developed and released documentation guidelines for E/M services, the 1995 guidelines were mandatory for Medicare and voluntary for all others; but, under HIPAA, the 1997 guidelines became mandatory for every health care claim until the official ruling was released that suspended mandatory implementation of the 1997 Guidelines and ruled that either the 1995 or the 1997 guidelines may be used to meet the now-mandatory documentation requirements.

For many years, E/M services were purely subjective and very difficult to measure. Physicians were not under contract with insurance companies, so insurance companies had no legal basis for regulating how physicians performed and documented services.

According to George C. Halvorson in his book *Strong Medicine*, the insurance industry concluded that the *potential* for undetected fraud and abuse existed. Payors worked to develop measurable ways to uniformly define E/M services so they could better detect fraud and abuse. They began by first defining various types of E/M services. They established multiple levels for some services to provide a method to correctly identify the amount of work performed.

Initially, physicians fulfilled payor requests to better define E/M services. Since 1992, the American Medical Association (AMA) has included an E/M code section in the CPT codebook (Level I of HCPCS) to dispel payors' worries about E/M fraud and abuse. The original E/M CPT codes defined or described each service, and an appendix in the back of the CPT codebook gave examples, or scenarios, in which each code might be used if the code description matched medical record documentation. Physicians learned the new codes and began to use them to report E/M services.

Once physicians consistently used E/M codes, payors compared code usage with medical record documentation across the nation and concluded that medical coding for E/M services was not consistent. They realized that they still did not have *proof* that these services were actually performed.

In *Strong Medicine,* Halvorson, an HMO president and CEO, gives an inside look at how payors think.

Payors often suspect physicians are billing for higher levels of service than were actually performed or higher levels than were warranted by the patient's medical condition. He clearly documents why payors suspect physicians of wrongdoing, and he published numerous comments he said were made by physicians that confirmed and fueled those suspicions. His book effectively and convincingly presents payor viewpoints. Mr. Halvorson testified before Congress on health care matters. He served on the Minnesota Healthcare Commission, and he served as chairman of the Group Health Association of America.

The Health Care Financing Administration (HCFA), now called the Centers for Medicare and Medicaid Services (CMS), a federal agency that governs Medicare, Medicaid, and other federal programs, responded to payor complaints by establishing a system designed to give payors the proof they demanded. During 1994, HCFA developed documentation guidelines for E/M services, and they implemented the new requirements at the beginning of 1995. These requirements were mandatory for Medicare claims and voluntary for all others.

Documentation guidelines are a method of evaluating physician performance by defining items that must be documented for each E/M code. This allows payors to count items actually documented in the medical record to confirm the validity of an E/M code.

Although physicians accepted the use of E/M codes to better define the type and amount of work performed, physicians were deeply offended by the imposition of E/M documentation guidelines. A battle began that has yet to be resolved.

The Board of Medicine in each state closely regulates the practice of medicine. Patients and communities rely on the Board of Medicine, not the insurance industry, to set standards for care. Physicians have traditionally been respected and trusted by the community. Documentation guidelines were not developed in response to patient or community complaints. They were developed in response to insurance industry *suspicions*. By imposing E/M documentation guidelines, payors sent the message that they distrust physicians.

The legal system in the United States is based on the premise that a person is presumed innocent until proven guilty. The AMA has stated that physicians believe documentation guidelines, contrary to the rule of law, are based on the premise that physicians are presumed guilty until proven innocent. However, whether they agree with it or not, physicians are now required by law to follow current documentation guidelines.

Beginning with the 1995 edition of CPT, the AMA has included material and directions taken from the

1995 E/M documentation guidelines at the beginning of the E/M section in the CPT codebook. However, many physicians questioned the legality of the guidelines and voluntarily chose to delay using them while the AMA pursued legal channels to try to get them repealed. The use of E/M documentation guidelines was mandatory for Medicare claims beginning January 1, 1995; however, funding was not provided for enforcement. Most physicians honestly believed the law was unenforceable, and that the AMA would succeed in getting it repealed.

During 1996, the documentation requirements for E/M services were revised again by HCFA. Mandatory implementation for all medical claims, not just Medicare claims, was to occur in 1997, and because HIPAA was signed into law, ample funding was provided for enforcement.

Physicians loudly protested the 1997 version of the documentation guidelines, claiming they were too cumbersome to use. Mandatory implementation of the 1997 guidelines was suspended. Until a new version is approved, physicians may legally follow either the 1995 documentation guidelines or the 1997 documentation guidelines. The material and directions taken from 1995 guidelines continued to be published in CPT as recently as the 2005 edition of the CPT codebook. The 1997 guidelines are available from CMS but have never been included in the CPT codebooks.

For a time, claims were paid regardless of whether the guidelines were followed, but the grace period ended in 1997 when funding was made available for enforcement. Now payors are not required to pay claims unless documentation shows that the services were performed as billed.

Payors do not check documentation on every claim submitted. Instead, they periodically ask for documentation to support a particular claim, and they make broad assumptions based on claims actually reviewed. Sometimes when specific problems are found with reviewed claims, it triggers a wider audit of claims from that physician.

In addition, some payors perform "targeted reviews." Specific codes are named for review each year, and every claim with one of those codes undergoes a documentation audit.

This chapter focuses on teaching both the 1995 and the 1997 documentation guidelines as these are the versions from which billing is currently done. Please keep in mind that most physicians still dislike the imposition of documentation guidelines, and they struggle to meet even the less restrictive 1995 guidelines. Until a new version becomes official, most coding is done from the easier 1995 guidelines. Whichever guidelines your practice chooses to use, each physician must consistently use one set of guidelines. Physicians who continue to ignore all guidelines put themselves and their employees at risk of prosecution under HIPAA.

Although physicians prefer the 1995 guidelines, payors prefer the 1997 guidelines. Some payors try to penalize claims that are coded using the 1995 guidelines. You can and should challenge these penalties. The 1995 guidelines are valid and may be used until the date the next version becomes mandatory.

Medical codes are subject to annual revision, and coding becomes more complex every year. Physicians seldom know enough about current medical coding rules to *correctly* code their own services. Therefore medical coding has become a distinct specialty in the medical office.

E/M coding is a complex subject. The information presented in this chapter is an introduction to E/M coding and a broad overview of the most important documentation rules and coding conventions.

The compliance guidance documents issued by the Office of Inspector General (OIG) for the Department of Health and Human Services (HHS) strongly recommend that job descriptions be used to assign accountability for specific tasks in the medical office. The OIG developed the compliance guidance documents to help various types of medical entities meet the "accountability" requirements of HIPAA (Public Law 104-191). Many of the OIG's recommendations relate directly to billing and collections, including assigning responsibility for gathering the information for the billing and coding of medical claims. The Medicare website for medical office education, which is now sponsored by numerous government agencies, www.cms.hhs.gov/medlearn/cbts.asp, notes how accountability is typically assigned

in a medical office, and that information provided the basis on which accountability is addressed in this chapter. However, please remember that each medical office decides exactly which employee positions are assigned individual accountability for each task, and it will vary from one office to another. In addition, in a small medical office, one multiskilled professional often fills numerous employee positions.

Typically, medical billers are held accountable for the codes submitted on medical claims unless the responsibility for medical coding is clearly assigned to someone else, such as a certified professional coder (CPC, CPC-H) or a certified coding specialist (CCS, CCS-P). If the medical office you work for does not have a certified coding employee, you should consider completing a full medical coding course before accepting this responsibility.

This chapter introduces the concepts of E/M coding that every medical office employee should know in order to recognize when something is obviously wrong.

For example: You will know something is obviously wrong when:

❏ A patient who was seen by the same physician recently is assigned a **"new patient"** code.
❏ A new patient is assigned an **"established patient"** code.
❏ An outpatient is assigned an "inpatient" code.
❏ An inpatient is assigned an "office visit" code.
❏ An assigned code for a comprehensive service has only a little documentation.
❏ An assigned code for a limited service has comprehensive documentation.

1995 Documentation Guidelines for E/M Services

INTRODUCTION TO DOCUMENTATION

The information presented here is taken directly from the 1995 documentation guidelines, and much of it can be found in the section guidelines at the beginning of the E/M section within the category 1 codes (the main body of codes) in the CPT codebook. HCFA's (now CMS's) 1995 documentation guidelines begin with a definition of documentation, and the guidelines define principles of documentation.

Medical record documentation is required to record pertinent facts, findings, and observations about the patient's health history, including past and present illnesses, examinations, tests, treatments, and outcomes.

The medical record chronologically documents the care of the patient and is an important element contributing to high-quality care.

The medical record facilitates:

❏ The ability of the physician and other health care professionals to evaluate and plan the patient's immediate treatment and to monitor his/her health care over time
❏ Communication and continuity of care among physicians and other health care professionals involved in the patient's care
❏ Accurate and timely claims review and payment
❏ Appropriate utilization review and quality-of-care evaluations

❏ Collection of data that may be useful for research and education

An appropriately documented medical record can reduce many of the frustrations associated with claims processing and may serve as a legal document to authenticate the care provided, when necessary.

Because payors have a contractual obligation to enrollees, they may require documentation that services are consistent with the insurance coverage provided. They may request information to authenticate:

❏ The site of service
❏ The medical necessity and appropriateness of the diagnostic and/or therapeutic services provided
❏ That services provided have been accurately reported

PRINCIPLES OF DOCUMENTATION

Principles of documentation apply to all types of medical and surgical services in all settings. For E/M services, the nature and amount of physician work and documentation varies by type of service, place of service, and the patient's status. Therefore these principles may be modified when necessary.

1. The medical record should be complete and legible.
2. The documentation of each patient encounter should include:

   ❏ Reason for the encounter and relevant history
   ❏ Physical examination findings and prior diagnostic test results
   ❏ Assessment, clinical impression, or diagnosis
   ❏ Plan of care
   ❏ Date and legible identity of the observer

3. If not documented, the reason for ordering diagnostic or ancillary services should be easily inferred.
4. Past and present diagnoses should be available to the treating and/or consulting physician.
5. Appropriate health risk factors should be identified.
6. The patient's progress, response to treatment, changes in treatment, and revision of diagnosis should be documented.
7. The diagnosis and procedure codes reported on the health insurance claim form or billing statement should be supported by the documentation in the medical record.

RULES FOR DOCUMENTATION OF E/M SERVICES

The 1995 documentation guidelines sort documentation in the medical record into seven elements. These seven elements are then classified as either **key components** or **contributory elements.** There are three key components and four contributory elements. Key components are the items that best describe the amount of work performed and determine the code choice. Contributory elements add to or confirm the E/M code selection, but do not usually play a large enough role to make the difference between one code and another.

The seven elements are:

❏ History (key component)
❏ Examination (key component)
❏ Medical decision-making (key component)
❏ Counseling (contributory element)
❏ Coordination of care (contributory element)
❏ Nature of present problem (contributory element)
❏ Time (contributory element)

The individual E/M codes are distinguished by:

❏ New or established patients
❏ Place of service (office, hospital, surgical center, nursing home)
❏ Type of service (evaluation, treatment, consultation)
❏ Level of service within a type of service

The definition for each E/M code includes the number of the key components that must be met in order to use the code. Some E/M codes do not use any of the key components, and a few do not use any of the seven elements. Medical record documentation must meet the minimum requirements in a code definition, or you may not use the code.

Because most of the E/M codes depend on the key components, let's take a closer look at each of them.

HISTORY

History is identified as a key component when selecting an E/M service. Four types of history were established to differentiate E/M services: **problem-focused history, expanded problem-focused history, detailed history,** and **comprehensive history.**

The history section is divided into four subcomponents: (1) chief complaint; (2) history of present illness; (3) review of systems; and (4) past, family, and/or social history. Each subcomponent part is further divided to enable different levels of service.

Some types of history do not require all the subcomponents. A specific combination of subcomponents and specific levels within the requisite subcomponents portray the minimum documentation requirements to meet each type of history. Table 6-1 shows the types of history and the requirements for each.

Let's take a closer look at each history subcomponent.

Chief Complaint

The **chief complaint** (CC) is a concise statement describing the reason for the visit. Usually the chief complaint is stated as a direct quote using the patient's words. It might include the symptom(s), problem(s), condition(s), diagnoses, physician-recommended return, or any other factor that is responsible for the visit.

The chief complaint is required with every type of history. It is not subdivided into different levels.

History of Present Illness

The **history of present illness (HPI)** is a chronological description of (1) the development of the patient's present illness or problem from the first sign or symptom, *or* (2) the development of the patient's present illness or problem from the previous encounter to the present.

It includes the following elements:

☐ Location
☐ Quality
☐ Severity
☐ Duration
☐ Timing
☐ Context
☐ Associated signs and symptoms
☐ Modifying factors

Location refers to the anatomic location of the medical problem. For example, if a patient complains of chest pain, the location is the chest. Pain can stay in one location, or it can travel. Chest pain might start in the chest and travel down the left arm.

Quality indicates the details used to distinguish differences between similar medical problems. Descriptive words are often used. For example, some words used to describe the quality of pain include "dull," "aching," "sharp," "burning," "heavy," "crushing," and "throbbing."

Severity refers to the details that are used to distinguish levels of seriousness for one medical problem. Descriptive words are also used here. For example, many conditions make distinctions between mild, moderate, and severe. Pain is often rated on a scale of 1 to 10, with 1 being the mildest and 10 being the most severe.

Duration means the length of time involved for each episode or occurrence. For example, each episode of chest pain might last for 10 to 20 minutes.

Timing includes details that relate the medical problem to other specific events occurring simultaneously or that identify a pattern of occurrences. For example, chest pain could occur during exercise, after exercise, after meals, at rest, during the night, when coughing, or when lying prone. Each possibility points toward specific types of heart conditions, lung conditions, and/or gastric conditions.

Context includes details that relate the medical problem to other factors (not timing) about other specific events. For example, chest pain might occur after meals only when spicy foods are eaten or only when gas-producing foods are eaten. This information further defines the problem.

Associated signs and symptoms are factors that are included in the definition of the medical problem or that are used to narrow the choices when a diagnosis has not yet been established. For example, the chest pain might be accompanied by shortness of

TABLE 6-1
Decision Chart for History

Type of History	Chief Complaint	History of Present Illness (HPI)	Review of Systems (ROS)	Past, Family, and/or Social History (PFSH)
Problem focused	Yes	Brief (1-3 elements)	N/A	N/A
Expanded problem-focused	Yes	Brief (1-3 elements)	Problem pertinent	N/A
Detailed	Yes	Extended (4-8 elements)	Extended	Pertinent
Comprehensive	Yes	Extended (4-8 elements)	Complete	Complete

Source: U.S. Department of Health and Human Services, Centers for Medicare and Medicaid Services (CMS).

breath without exertion. The shortness of breath is characteristic of some diagnoses for chest pain but not for others.

Modifying factors include details that alter the definition or scope of a medical problem. For example, when a patient has chest pain, the fact that the patient smokes three packs of cigarettes a day expands the number of items that must be considered. Smoking is not an associated sign or symptom, but it does modify the considerations.

Brief and extended HPIs are distinguished by the amount of detail needed to accurately describe the presenting problem(s). Abnormal findings and significant normal findings for each of the elements above should be counted when determining the level of HPI.

In a **brief HPI,** the medical record should describe one to three elements of the present illness.

In an **extended HPI,** the medical record should describe at least four elements of the present illness.

Brief HPI: 8-month-old crying and tugging on ears since 8 AM. This HPI includes *location* (ears) and *duration* (since 8 AM).

Extended HPI: 8-month-old crying and tugging on ears since 8 AM. Fever of 101.6° F at 8 AM today. Given baby Tylenol. Has had a cold for 3 days. Drainage from nose for 3 days: first clear, then yellow, now green. Cough for 2 days, initially dry but now becoming croupy. Decreased appetite—baby is breast fed. Cries and pulls on ears when tries to nurse and seems to have trouble breathing when nursing.

This HPI includes *location* (ears, nose), *quality* (descriptions of cough and nasal drainage), *duration* (3 days of drainage, 2 days of cough, and crying and tugging on ears since 8 am today), *associated signs and symptoms* (fever, decreased appetite), and *context* (reactions when nursing).

Problem-focused history requires a brief HPI.

Expanded problem-focused history requires a brief HPI.

Detailed history requires an extended HPI.

Comprehensive history requires an extended HPI.

Clinical Application Exercise

Sharon is a 14-year-old girl accompanied by her mother. She reports that she has experienced intermittent abdominal pain over the past week, and the severity and duration of the pain are increasing. The pain first started 1 week ago as a dull ache in the right lower quadrant of the abdomen that lasted about 1 hour and went away. The pain occurred twice the first day, with no identified factors related to the occurrence. Gradually the severity, duration, and number of occurrences are increasing. Today each occurrence begins with a sharp, stabbing pain in the right lower quadrant of the abdomen that lasts about a minute, followed by a persistent moderate-to-severe ache (about a 7 or 8 on a scale of 1 to 10) that lasts about 2 hours. It is now occurring every 3 to 4 hours, and it woke her up during the night last night. Her last menstrual period ended 2 weeks ago. She cannot identify anything that seems to trigger the onset of the pain.

1. How many elements of the HPI were recorded?

_____

2. What level of HPI was recorded?

_____

Review of Systems

A **review of systems (ROS)** is an inventory of normal and abnormal findings *reported by the patient* regarding the functioning of body systems. The ROS is obtained through a series of verbal or written questions seeking to identify signs and/or symptoms that the patient is experiencing or has experienced. The subjective "stated" findings in the review of systems are not to be confused with the objective "hands on" findings in the examination. Items listed here may not be counted for any portion of the physician's examination.

The following systems are recognized for the ROS:

- ☐ Constitutional symptoms (e.g., fever, weight loss, high blood pressure)
- ☐ Eyes
- ☐ Ears, nose, mouth, throat
- ☐ Cardiovascular
- ☐ Respiratory
- ☐ Gastrointestinal
- ☐ Genitourinary
- ☐ Musculoskeletal
- ☐ Integumentary (skin and/or breast)
- ☐ Neurologic

❑ Psychiatric
❑ Endocrine
❑ Hematologic/lymphatic
❑ Allergic/immunologic

The patient history form and the intermittent history form, filled out by the patient during check-in, can be used to meet this requirement if the physician states "see history form" in his or her notes *and* if the history form is signed or initialed and dated by the physician. The physician must review the completed form and ask additional questions as needed. Alternatively, the patient's pertinent responses can be documented in the physician's notes for the encounter.

A **problem-pertinent ROS** inquires about the system directly related to the problem(s) identified in the HPI. The patient's positive responses and pertinent negative responses for the system related to the problem should be documented in the patient's medical record.

An **extended ROS** inquires about the system directly related to the problem(s) identified in the HPI *and* a limited number of additional systems. The patient's positive responses and pertinent negative responses for two to nine systems should be documented.

A **complete ROS** inquires about the systems(s) directly related to the problem(s) identified in the HPI *plus* all additional body systems. At least 10 organ systems must be reviewed. Those systems with positive or pertinent negative responses must be individually documented in the physician notes. For the remaining systems, a notation indicating all other systems are negative is permissible. In the absence of such a notation, at least 10 systems must be individually documented.

Problem-focused history does not require a ROS.

Expanded problem-focused history requires a problem-pertinent ROS.

Detailed history requires an extended ROS.

Comprehensive history requires a complete ROS.

Clinical Application Exercise

Sharon's mother completed the following items on Sharon's interim health history form:

___ Alcohol/Drug use

___ Allergic reactions (medicine, animals, plants)

___ Blood system (anemia, swollen glands, high or low blood counts)

X Constitutional symptoms (fever, weight loss); fever of 100.2° F

___ Ears, nose, throat, mouth (cold, virus, pain, drainage)

___ Exposure to sexually transmitted diseases

___ Eyes (vision changes, drainage, redness)

X Gastrointestinal (indigestion, abdominal pain, constipation, diarrhea)

___ Genitourinary (urinary, prostate, or menstrual difficulties)

___ Hormones (hot flashes, diabetic reactions, lupus flare-up)

___ Immune system (Hodgkin's disease, HIV)

___ Musculoskeletal (broken bones, sprains, strained muscles, dislocated joints)

___ Neurological (memory, coordination, balance)

___ Psychiatric (orientation to time, place, and person; mental; behavior)

___ Respiratory (shortness of breath, wheezing)

___ Skin and/or breasts (rashes, sores, lumps, bumps, cuts, infections, bites)

___ Cardiovascular (heart problems, palpitations, chest pain, swelling in legs or feet)

1. What level of review of systems does this interim history form meet, as it is completed, and why?

_____

_____

2. How many systems were reviewed?

_____

Past, Family, and/or Social History (PFSH)

The **past, family, and/or social history (PFSH)** consists of a review of three areas:

❑ **Past history**—the patient's past experiences with illnesses, operations, injuries, and treatments.

❑ **Family history**—a review of medical events in the patient's family, including diseases that may be hereditary or may place the patient at risk.

❑ **Social history**—an age-appropriate review of past and current activities.

A **pertinent PFSH** is a review of the PFSH area(s) directly related to the problem(s) identified in the HPI. At least one specific item from any of the three PFSH areas must be documented.

A **complete PFSH** is a review of two or all three of the PFSH areas, depending on the category of the E/M service. A review of all three history areas is required for services that, by their nature, include a comprehensive assessment or reassessment of the patient. A review of two or three history areas is sufficient for other services.

Problem-focused history does not require any elements of the PFSH.

Expanded problem-focused history does not require any elements of the PFSH.

Detailed history requires a pertinent PFSH. *Comprehensive history* requires a complete PFSH.

STOP & REVIEW

Answer the following questions:

1. How many history subcomponents are required for a problem-focused history, and which one(s)?

   _____

   _____

2. How many history subcomponents are required for a detailed history, and which one(s)?

   _____

   _____

3. How many HPI elements must be met for a brief HPI? _____

4. How many systems must be reviewed for an extended ROS? _____

   _____

5. How many PFSH elements are required for a pertinent PFSH? _____

6. Which element(s) of HPI is addressed when the patient has a dull ache?

   _____

7. Which element(s) of HPI is addressed when the patient reports running a fever? _____

   _____

8. How many organ systems must be reviewed for a complete ROS? _____

9. "An appendectomy in 1982 at Southwest Hospital" counts as what type of history item?

   _____

10. "Mother had breast cancer" counts as what type of history item? _____

EXAMINATION

Examination is identified as a key component when selecting E/M services. An examination is the process of obtaining and recording the physician's medically significant observations and findings. This is a "hands-on" examination of body systems. Do not confuse it with the verbal "stated" review of systems in the history section.

The extent of the examination performed is dependent upon clinical judgment and the nature of the presenting problem(s). Four types of examinations were established to differentiate E/M services: problem-focused exam, expanded problem-focused exam, detailed exam, and comprehensive exam.

For the purpose of examination, the following body areas are recognized:

❐ Head, including the face
❐ Neck
❐ Chest, including breasts and axilla
❐ Abdomen
❐ Genitalia, groin, buttocks
❐ Back, including the spine
❐ Each extremity

For the purpose of examination, the following organ systems are recognized:

❐ Eyes
❐ Ears, nose, mouth, and throat
❐ Cardiovascular
❐ Respiratory
❐ Gastrointestinal
❐ Genitourinary
❐ Musculoskeletal
❐ Skin
❐ Neurologic
❐ Psychiatric
❐ Hematologic/lymphatic/immunologic

Body area is used (a) if only a portion of an organ system, located entirely in one body area, is examined, such as when one extremity is examined for a greenstick fracture of a toe, or (b) if the problem is localized to one body area, but involves multiple organ systems, such as in traumatic injury of a leg that involves a skin laceration, severed nerves, blood vessels, and muscles, as well as a compound fracture of the femur (upper leg bone)—portions of four organ systems. Although multiple body areas sometimes are examined, most other examinations include entire organ systems.

Each abnormal finding and relevant normal findings of the examination of the involved body area(s) or organ system(s) must be documented. A brief statement or notation indicating "negative" or "normal" is acceptable to document normal findings in unaffected areas. However, a notation of *abnormal* without explanation is not enough. Abnormal or unexpected findings of the examination of any other body areas or organ systems must also be described.

The levels of E/M services are based on four types of examination:

- **Problem-focused exam**—a limited examination of the affected body area or organ system.
- **Expanded problem-focused exam**—a limited examination of the affected body area

or organ system and other symptomatic or related organ system(s).

- **Detailed exam**—an extended examination of the affected body area(s) and other symptomatic or related organ system(s).
- **Comprehensive exam**—a general multi-system examination or a complete examination of a single organ system. The medical record for a general multi-system examination should include information about at least eight of the organ systems.

Note: The comprehensive examination performed as part of the preventive medicine E/M service is multi-system, but its extent is based on the age and risk factors identified.

Answer the following questions:

1. Is *neck* a body area or organ system? _____

2. Is *skin* a body area or organ system? _____

3. Is *back,* including the spine, a body area or organ system? _____

4. What type of exam is a limited examination of the affected body area or organ system and other symptomatic or related organ system(s)? _____

5. Is annotation of an abnormal finding without explanation acceptable? _____

6. Is a brief statement or notation indicating "negative" or "normal" acceptable to document normal findings in unaffected areas? _____

7. What is a problem-focused exam? _____

8. The medical record for a general multi-system examination should include information about how many organ systems? _____

9. What type of exam is the following? _____

Well-nourished Hispanic female
TPR 98.6-88-16, BP 120/60
Alert, oriented ×4
HEENT: normal
Skin: warm and dry, color good
Lungs: clear
CV: heart rate reg, no gallops or murmurs, +pedal pulses
Abd: soft, nontender, +bs ×4

10. What type of exam is the following? _____

TPR 100.4-98-24, BP 118/72
Throat red with white spots on tonsils
Nose stuffy with clear drainage
Ears normal

MEDICAL DECISION-MAKING

Medical decision-making is identified as a key component when selecting E/M services. Medical decision-making includes the thought processes required to evaluate medical findings, the amount of work performed when evaluating data, the conclusions drawn, and the resulting plan of care.

Four types of medical decision-making were established to differentiate E/M services: (1) **straightforward decision-making,** (2) **low-complexity decision-making,** (3) **moderate-complexity decision-making,** and (4) **high-complexity decision-making.**

Each type of medical decision-making section is divided into three subcomponent parts: (1) number of diagnoses or management options, (2) amount and/or complexity of data to be reviewed, and (3) risk of complications and/or morbidity or mortality.

Each subcomponent part is further divided to enable different levels of service. A specific combination of subcomponent parts and specific levels within the subcomponents are required to meet each type of medical decision-making. Table 6-2 shows the types of medical decision-making and the requirements for each.

Let's take a closer look at each medical decision making subcomponent.

Number of Diagnoses or Management Options

An assessment, clinical impression, or diagnosis should be documented for each encounter. The **number of diagnoses or management options** that are documented in the patient's medical record for the visit in question determines the level for this subcomponent. Every option the physician thought about and considered during the encounter should be documented for this section.

For a presenting problem *with an established diagnosis,* the record should reflect whether the problem is:

❒ Improved, well-controlled, resolving, or resolved
❒ Inadequately controlled, worsening, or failing to change as expected

For a presenting problem *without an established diagnosis,* the assessment or clinical impression may be stated in the form of differential diagnoses:

❒ Signs, symptoms, and significant findings
❒ "Possible," "probable," and/or "rule-out" (R/O) diagnoses

Although possible, probable, and R/O diagnoses may not be listed in the diagnosis section of the claim form, they can and should be documented in the medical record to support the level of medical decision-making. Many physicians and even some professional coders do not understand this issue, and they mistakenly recommend eliminating all mention of differential diagnostic considerations.

The initiation of and changes in treatment should be documented. If referrals are made, consultations requested, or advice sought, the record should indicate the details:

❒ To whom or where the referral or consultation is made
❒ From whom the advice is requested

Straightforward decision-making requires documentation of minimal diagnoses or options.

Low-complexity decision-making requires documentation of a limited number of diagnoses or options.

Moderate-complexity decision-making requires documentation of multiple diagnoses or options.

High-complexity decision-making requires documentation of an extensive number of diagnoses or options.

Amount and/or Complexity of Data to Be Reviewed

The **amount and/or complexity of data to be reviewed** is based on (1) the types of diagnostic testing ordered or reviewed and (2) the amount of old records reviewed.

A decision to obtain history from sources other than the patient increases the amount and complexity of data to be reviewed. A discussion of contradictory or unexpected test results with the physician who performed or interpreted the tests is an indication of the complexity of data being reviewed. On occasion, the physician who ordered a test may personally review the image, tracing, or specimen to supplement information from the physician who prepared the test report or interpretation; this is another indication of the complexity of data being reviewed.

TABLE 6-2
Decision Chart for Medical Decision-Making
To qualify for each level of medical decision-making, two of the three elements in the table must be either met or exceeded.

Type of Decision-Making	Number of Diagnoses or Management Options	Amount and/or Complexity of Data to Be Reviewed	Risk of Complications and/or Morbidity or Mortality
Straightforward	Minimal	Minimal or none	Minimal
Low Complexity	Limited	Limited	Low
Moderate Complexity	Multiple	Moderate	Moderate
High Complexity	Extensive	Extensive	High

Source: U.S. Department of Health and Human Services, Centers for Medicare and Medicaid Services (CMS).

Physicians must document any diagnostic service (test or procedure) ordered, planned, scheduled, or performed at the time of the E/M encounter. They must document which lab, radiology, and/or other diagnostic tests were reviewed during the encounter. A simple notation such as "WBC elevated" or "chest x-ray unremarkable" is acceptable. Initialing and dating the report of the test results and stating "tests reviewed" in the medical record is acceptable.

Physicians must document the decision to obtain old records and/or the decision to obtain additional history from the family, caretaker, or other source. They should document any relevant findings from the review of old records and/or receipt of additional history from the family or any other source. If there is no relevant information beyond that already obtained, that fact should be documented. A notation of "old records reviewed" or "additional history obtained from family" without elaboration is not enough.

Physicians should document the results of a discussion about laboratory, radiology, or other diagnostic tests with the physician who performed or interpreted the study. They should document the direct visualization and independent interpretation of an image, tracing, or specimen previously or subsequently interpreted by another physician.

Straightforward decision-making requires documentation of no data to minimal data reviewed.

Low-complexity decision-making requires documentation of limited data reviewed.

Moderate-complexity decision-making requires documentation of moderate data reviewed.

High-complexity decision-making requires documentation of extensive data reviewed.

Risk of Significant Complications, Morbidity, and/or Mortality

The **risk of significant complications, morbidity, and/or mortality** is based on risks associated with the presenting problem(s), the diagnostic procedure(s), and the possible management options.

To meet these requirements, physicians must document comorbidities and underlying diseases that increase the risk of complications, morbidity, and/or mortality. They must document any surgical or invasive diagnostic procedure(s) ordered, planned, or scheduled at the time of an E/M encounter. They must document any surgical or invasive diagnostic procedure(s) performed at the time of the E/M encounter. In addition, they must document any referrals for or decisions to perform surgical or invasive diagnostic procedure(s) on an urgent basis.

Table 6-3 is a guide to help you determine the level of service documented for this subcomponent of medical decision-making. *The highest risk in any one category determines the overall risk.*

Straightforward decision-making documentation should meet the requirements for minimal risk.

Low-complexity decision-making documentation should meet the requirements for low risk.

Moderate-complexity decision-making documentation should meet the requirements for moderate risk.

High-complexity medical decision-making documentation should meet the requirements for high risk.

TABLE 6-3
1995-1997 Table of Risk Decision Chart
The highest level of risk in any one category determines the overall risk.

Level of Risk	Presenting Problem(s)	Diagnostic Procedure(s) Ordered	Management Options Selected
MINIMAL	• One self-limited or minor problem, e.g., cold, insect bite, tinea corporis	• Laboratory testing requiring venipuncture • Chest x-rays • EKG/EEG • Urinalysis • Ultrasound, e.g., echocardiography	• Rest • Gargles • Elastic bandages • Superficial dressings
LOW	• Two or more self-limited or minor problems • One stable chronic illness, e.g., well-controlled hypertension, non-insulin dependent diabetes, cataract, BPH • Acute uncomplicated illness or injury, e.g., cystitis, allergic rhinitis, simple sprain	• Physiologic tests not under stress, e.g., pulmonary function tests • Noncardiovascular imaging studies with contrast, e.g., barium enema • Superficial needle biopsies • Clinical laboratory tests requiring arterial puncture • Skin biopsies	• Over-the-counter drugs • Minor surgery with no identified risk factors • Physical therapy • Occupational therapy • IV fluids with additives *Continued.*

BPH, Benign prostatic hypertrophy; MI, myocardial infarction; TIA, transient ischemic attack.

TABLE 6-3
1995-1997 Table of Risk Decision Chart—cont'd
The highest level of risk in any one category determines the overall risk.

Level of Risk	Presenting Problem(s)	Diagnostic Procedure(s) Ordered	Management Options Selected
MODERATE	• One or more chronic illnesses with mild exacerbation, progression, or side effects of treatment • Two or more stable chronic illnesses • Undiagnosed new problem with uncertain prognosis, e.g., lump in breast • Acute illness with systemic symptoms, e.g., pyelonephritis, pneumonitis, colitis • Acute complicated injury, e.g., head injury with brief loss of consciousness	• Physiologic tests under stress, e.g., cardiac stress test, fetal contraction stress test • Diagnostic endoscopies with no identified risk factors • Deep needle or incisional biopsy • Cardiovascular imaging studies with contrast and no identified risk factors, e.g., arteriogram, cardiac catheterization • Obtain fluid from body cavity, e.g., lumbar puncture, thoracentesis, culdocentesis	• Minor surgery with identified risk factors • Elective minor surgery (open, percutaneous or endoscopic) with no identified risk factors • Prescription drug management • Therapeutic nuclear medicine • IV fluids with additives • Closed treatment of fracture or dislocation without manipulation
HIGH	• One or more chronic illnesses with severe exacerbation, progression, or side effects of treatment • Acute or chronic illnesses or injuries that pose a threat to life or bodily function, e.g., multiple trauma, acute MI, pulmonary embolus, severe respiratory distress, progressive severe rheumatoid arthritis, psychiatric illness with potential threat to self or others, peritonitis, acute renal failure • An abrupt change in neurological status, e.g., seizure, TIA, weakness, sensory loss	• Cardiovascular imaging studies with contrast with identified risk factors • Cardiac electrophysiological tests • Diagnostic endoscopies with identified risk factors • Discography	• Elective major surgery (open, percutaneous or endoscopic) with identified risk factors • Emergency major surgery (open, percutaneous or endoscopic) • Parenteral controlled substances • Drug therapy requiring intensive monitoring for toxicity • Decision not to resuscitate or to de-escalate care because of poor prognosis

Source: U.S. Department of Health and Human Services, Centers for Medicare and Medicaid Services (CMS).

Answer the following questions:

1. If a patient has four diagnoses but only one management option is listed, what level is met for the diagnoses or management options subcomponent?

_____

_____

2. If the physician documents that he reviewed a 2-inch-thick file of old records and talked extensively with the family but did not find anything significant to add, what level is met for the amount of data reviewed?

_____

_____

3. The physician documents that the patient had a severe exacerbation of chronic asthma. A chest x-ray is ordered, and the patient is given an injection of medication and a breathing treatment. Once the patient is stabilized, the patient is sent home with an order for a prescription medication. What level of risk is met?

_____

4. The physician documents four symptoms and the findings of three lab tests and two x-rays. The physician documents six possible diagnoses, an uncertain prognosis, and three treatment options. What type of overall medical decision-making is met?

_____

5. The physician documents that the patient has a minor scrape. The wound is cleaned and a superficial dressing is applied. What type of overall medical decision-making is met?

_____

6. The initiation of and changes in treatment are part of what decision-making subcomponent?

_____

_____

7. If a physician has a discussion of contradictory or unexpected test results with the physician who performed or interpreted the tests, may this be taken into consideration for medical decision-making, and if so, what subcomponent(s) does it fall under?

_____

_____

8. If a physician personally reviews an x-ray to supplement information from the physician who prepared the interpretation, may this be taken into consideration for medical decision-making, and if so, what subcomponent(s) does it fall under?

_____

_____

9. If a physician documents comorbidities and underlying diseases that increase the risk of complications, morbidity, and/or mortality, may this be taken into consideration for medical decision-making, and if so, what subcomponent(s) does it fall under?

_____

_____

10. Give the level for each subcomponent and the overall type of medical decision-making for the following example: The patient is seen on a follow-up visit for management of chronic back pain. The physician documents the review of an MRI report and the discussion of four possible courses of action, including elective back surgery—the excision of a herniated disk and possibly a laminectomy. The patient chooses the back surgery, and the plans for surgery are initiated. The diagnosis is chronic back pain secondary to arthritis and a herniated lumbar disk at the L4-L5 level. _____

_____

_____

CONTRIBUTORY ELEMENTS

Contributory elements play a part in code selection, but they are not required in order to use the code. Normally contributory elements are not a determining factor when selecting an E/M code, although there are some exceptions.

Time

Time is included as a contributory factor to assist physicians in selecting the appropriate level of E/M service. The time factors listed in the visit code descriptions are averages. They represent a range of times, which may be higher or lower depending on actual clinical circumstances.

Time is calculated differently for inpatient care and outpatient care. **Intraservice time** is described as **face-to-face time** for office and other outpatient visits and unit/floor time for hospital and other inpatient visits. Research has shown that there is a strong relationship between intraservice time and total length of time for E/M services.

Most of the work for *office* visits and *other outpatient* visits takes place during the time the physician is face to face with the patient or the patient's family. Research has shown the amount of work performed that does not take place during face-to-face time varies according to the amount of face-to-face time. Therefore it is already factored into the codes. Face-to-face time must be documented as spent with the patient or the patient's family, and the total amount of face-to-face time must be documented.

Medicare guidelines indicate office and outpatient face-to-face time must be spent with the patient. The patient must be present, and the patient's presence must be documented during face-to-face time, including when the only effective communication is with the family because the patient is incoherent or comatose.

Most of the work for an *inpatient* visit takes place during the time spent on the patient's floor or unit. The amount of work performed that does not take place during the **floor/unit time** usually varies according to the amount of floor/unit time. Therefore it is already factored into the codes. In a hospital or nursing facility, the amount of floor/unit time must be documented, and it includes time spent with the patient and time spent working on behalf of the patient elsewhere on the patient's floor or unit. It does not have to be performed totally at the bedside, but it may not include time spent for other patients, and it does not include work performed from other locations.

The times listed with E/M codes are averages, not hard and fast rules. Except in specific circumstances, time should not be the determining factor for E/M services. Even a low level of service occasionally involves prolonged time. The CPT codes for prolonged patient contact can be used to report time over the normal time parameters for the encounter if the other requirements to use the codes are also met. There are also CPT codes for prolonged physician services without face-to-face contact. Read the notes in the CPT codebook at the beginning of each of these subsections and follow the codebook directions when using these codes.

Time is not considered a factor for emergency department E/M services. These visits not only have varying levels of intensity, but they often involve multiple encounters with several patients over an extended period. Therefore it is very difficult for physicians in this setting to provide accurate estimates of the time spent face to face with each patient.

Time is a determining factor in E/M coding in specific circumstances, when (1) more than half the time is spent in counseling or coordination of care, or (2) there is no history or exam and all of the time is spent in counseling or coordination of care. Time must be documented for it to be billed as the determining factor. Start and stop times are advised but are not required. A simple notation of the total time involved and how much of that time was spent in counseling and/or coordination of care is acceptable.

Counseling

Counseling is a contributory element. When counseling encompasses more than half the visit, the actual intraservice time spent is used to determine the level of service.

If the physician elects to report the level of service based on counseling, the total length of intraservice time for the encounter must be documented, and the record should describe the counseling and the amount of time spent in counseling. Payors will pay for time spent in activities that are therapeutic for the patient, but they will not pay for time spent talking about unrelated matters.

> **For example**: "20 minutes of the 30-minute visit was spent in counseling on obesity and diet" is acceptable for coding based on time.

Coordination of Care

Coordination of care is a contributory element. Coordination of care includes things like arranging for home health care or arranging for various social services. When coordination of care encompasses more than half the visit, the actual intraservice time spent is used to determine the level of service.

If the physician elects to report the level of service based on the coordination of care, the total length of intraservice time for the encounter must be docu-mented, and the record should describe the activities to coordinate care. Payors will pay for time spent in activities that are therapeutic for the patient, but they will not pay for time spent talking about unrelated matters.

Nature of Presenting Problem

The presenting problem is the reason for the visit. It may be a disease, a condition, an illness, an injury, a symptom, a sign, a finding, a complaint, or any another reason for the encounter. A diagnosis may or may not be established at the time of the encounter. E/M services recognize five types of presenting problems:

1. **Minimal:** a medical problem that may not require the presence of the physician, but the service is provided under the physician's supervision
2. **Self-limited or minor:** a medical problem that runs a definite and prescribed course, is transient in nature, and is not likely to permanently alter health status *or* has a good prognosis when treatment is given as ordered
3. **Low severity:** a medical problem in which the risk of morbidity without treatment is low, there is little to no risk of mortality without treatment, and full recovery without functional impairment is expected
4. **Moderate severity:** a medical problem in which the risk of morbidity without treatment is moderate, there is a moderate risk of mortality without treatment, uncertain prognosis *or* increased probability of prolonged functional impairment
5. **High severity:** a medical problem in which the risk of morbidity without treatment is high to extreme and there is moderate to high risk of mortality without treatment, *or* high probability of severe, prolonged functional impairment

The level of E/M service chosen should be appropriate for the nature of the presenting illness. The descriptions for E/M services list the corresponding nature of presenting illness that would be typical for the code.

Some software programs make it easy to achieve a high level of documentation for every visit. Payors use the nature of presenting illness as a method to detect the type of fraud that can occur as a result of overdocumenting. If a problem is self-limited, the type of history, type of exam, and type of medical decision-making should be appropriate for a self-limited problem. A comprehensive history and a comprehensive exam are not needed to treat a simple earache in a 10-year-old child who is an established patient and who had an annual physical 7 months ago.

Answer the following questions:

1. When may a contributory element be used to determine the level of service?

_____

_____

_____

2. Documentation shows coordination of care during the office visit took 10 minutes of the total 25 minutes face-to-face time for the office visit. The coordinating activities are detailed. How is the level of service calculated?
   A. Key components
   B. Time
   C. Coordination of care
   D. Counseling

3. The documentation for the inpatient visit shows that counseling took 30 minutes of the 40 minutes total floor/unit time. The nature of the counseling is documented. How is the level of service calculated?
   A. Key components
   B. Time
   C. Coordination of care
   D. Counseling

4. Documentation shows that counseling took 20 minutes of the total 30 minutes face-to-face time for an office visit. The nature of the counseling is documented. How is the level of service calculated?
   A. Key components
   B. Time
   C. Coordination of care
   D. Counseling

5. Documentation shows coordination of care for discharge planning took 45 minutes of the 60 minutes floor/unit time for a terminally ill cancer patient. Discharge is planned later in the week. How is the level of service calculated?
   A. Key components
   B. Time
   C. Coordination of care
   D. Counseling

6. Documentation shows that extensive counseling was provided by a primary care physician, but no times are listed and the purpose of the counseling cannot be determined from the documentation. How is the level of service calculated?

   A. Key components
   B. Time
   C. Coordination of care
   D. Counseling

7. The nature of the presenting problem billed is moderate severity, but the level of service billed is appropriate for high-severity problems. If the insurance company finds the discrepancy when the edits and audits are run on the claim, what is likely to occur?
   A. The payor is likely to issue payment for the service as billed.
   B. The payor is likely to downcode and issue payment for the level of service justified by the nature of the presenting problem.
   C. The payor is likely to issue no payment and investigate the claim as potential fraud.
   D. Either B or C could occur.

8. The level of severity for the presenting problem billed is moderate severity, but the level of service billed is appropriate for low-severity problems. If the insurance company finds the discrepancy when the edits and audits are run on the claim, what is likely to occur?
   A. The payor is likely to issue payment for the service as billed.
   B. The payor is likely to downcode and issue payment for the level of service justified by the nature of the presenting problem.
   C. The payor is likely to issue no payment and investigate the claim as potential fraud.
   D. Either B or C could occur.

9. How is time measured in an office setting?
   A. Face-to-face time
   B. Floor/unit time
   C. The length of time the patient is present in the office
   D. The total length of time the physician spends during and after the visit

10. How is time measured in a hospital setting?
   A. Face-to-face time
   B. Floor/unit time
   C. The length of time the patient is present in the hospital
   D. The total length of time the physician spends during and after the visit

1997 Documentation Guidelines

The introduction to documentation, the principles of documentation, most of the history definitions, the history requirements, and the medical decision-making definitions and requirements did not change in the 1997 documentation guidelines. One history definition changed, and the examination requirements were expanded.

The following history definition changed: In an extended HPI, the medical record should describe at least four elements of the present illness *or the status of at least three chronic or inactive conditions.*

The 1997 documentation guidelines uses tables to define examination documentation requirements so physicians, coders, billers, payors, auditors, and investigators have a measurable method of determining whether examination documentation requirements were met. One table identifies documentation requirements that must be met for a general, multi-system examination, and multiple tables identify documentation requirements that must be met for examinations of each body area and each organ system. The multi-system examination table is included in this chapter, and the full set of 1997 examination tables is in Appendix A.

The 1995 history requirements still apply and the 1995 medical decision-making requirements still apply. The 1997 examination requirements changed for each single system examination and for the general multi-system examination.

GENERAL MULTI-SYSTEM EXAMINATIONS

To qualify for a general multi-system examination, the following content and documentation requirements should be met:

Problem-focused examination should include performance and documentation of one to five elements identified in a table by a bullet (•) in one or more organ system(s) or body area(s).

Expanded problem-focused examination should include performance and documentation of at least six elements identified in a table by a bullet (•) in one or more organ system(s) or body area(s).

Detailed examination should include at least six organ systems or body areas. For each system or area selected, performance and documentation of at least two elements identified in a table by a bullet (•) is

expected. Alternatively, a detailed examination may include performance and documentation of at least 12 elements identified in a table by a bullet (•) in two or more organ systems or body areas.

Comprehensive examination should include at least nine organ systems or body areas. For each system/area selected, all elements of the examination identified in a table by a bullet (•) should be performed, unless specific directions limit the content of the examination. For each area or system, documentation of at least two elements identified in a table by a bullet (•) is expected. The general multipurpose exam table is presented in Table 6-4.

SINGLE ORGAN SYSTEM EXAMINATIONS

To qualify for a given level of single organ system or body area examination, the following content and documentation requirements should be met:

Problem-focused examination should include performance and documentation of one to five elements identified in a table by a bullet (•), whether in a shaded or unshaded box.

Expanded problem-focused examination should include performance and documentation of at least six elements identified in a table by a bullet (•), whether in a shaded or unshaded box.

Detailed examination, other than eye or psychiatric examinations, should include performance and documentation of at least 12 elements identified in a table by a bullet (•), whether in a shaded or unshaded box. Eye and psychiatric examinations should include the performance and documentation of at least nine elements identified in a table by a bullet (•), whether in a shaded or unshaded box.

Comprehensive examination should include performance of all elements identified in a table by a bullet (•), whether in a shaded or unshaded box. Documentation of every element in each shaded box and at least one element in each unshaded box is expected.

The single organ system and body area examination tables for the 1997 documentation guidelines are located in Appendix A and also can be found on the Internet at www.cms.gov. The 1995-1997 comparison table for examination documentation guidelines is presented in Table 6-5.

TABLE 6-4
1997 General Multi-System Examination

Organ System/Body Area	Elements of General Multi-System Examination
Constitutional	• Measurement of any three of the following seven vital signs: 1) sitting or standing blood pressure, 2) supine blood pressure, 3) pulse rate and regularity, 4) respiration, 5) temperature, 6) height, 7) weight (may be measured and recorded by ancillary staff) • General appearance of patient (e.g., development, nutrition, body habitus, deformities, attention to grooming)
Eyes	• Inspection of conjunctiva and lids • Examination of pupils and irises (e.g., reaction to light and accommodation, size, and symmetry) • Ophthalmoscopic examination of optic discs (e.g., size, C/D ratio, appearance) and posterior segments (e.g., vessel changes, exudates, hemorrhages)
Ears, Nose, Mouth, and Throat	• External inspection of ears and nose (e.g., overall appearance, scars, lesions, masses) • Otoscopic examination of external auditory canals and tympanic membranes • Assessment of hearing (e.g., whispered voice, finger rub, tuning fork) • Inspection of nasal mucosa, septum, turbinates • Inspection of lips, teeth and gums • Examination of oropharynx: oral mucosa, salivary glands, hard and soft palates, tongue, tonsils and posterior pharynx
Neck	• Examination of neck (e.g., masses, overall appearance, symmetry, tracheal position, crepitus) • Examination of thyroid (e.g., enlargement, tenderness, mass)
Respiratory	• Assessment of respiratory effort (e.g., intercostal retractions, use of accessory muscles, diaphragmatic movement) • Percussion of chest (e.g., dullness, flatness, hyper-resonance) • Auscultation of lungs (e.g., breath sounds, adventitious sounds, rubs)

Cardiovascular	• Palpitation of heart (e.g., location, size, thrills)
	• Auscultation of heart with notation of abnormal sounds and murmurs
	• Examination of:
	  • Carotid arteries (e.g., pulse amplitude, bruits)
	  • Abdominal aorta (e.g., size, bruits)
	  • Femoral arteries (e.g., pulse amplitude, bruits)
	  • Pedal pulses (e.g., pulse amplitude)
	  • Extremities for edema and/or varicosity

Chest (Breasts)	• Inspection of breasts (e.g., symmetry, nipple discharge) • Palpation of breasts and axillae (e.g., masses, lumps, tenderness)
Gastrointestinal (Abdomen)	• Examination of abdomen with notation of presence of masses or tenderness • Examination of liver and spleen • Examination for presence or absence of hernia • Examination, when indicated, of anus, perineum and rectum, including sphincter tone, presence of hemorrhoids, rectal masses • Obtain stool sample for occult blood test when indicated

Genitourinary	MALE:
	• External examination of the scrotal contents (e.g., hydrocele, spermatocele, tenderness of cord, testicular mass)
	• Examination of the penis
	• Digital rectal examination of prostate gland (e.g., size, symmetry, nodularity, tenderness)
	FEMALE:
	• Pelvic examination (with or without specimen collection for smears and cultures), including:
	  • Examination of external genitalia (e.g., general appearance, hair distribution, lesions) and vagina (e.g., general appearance, estrogen effect, discharge, lesions, pelvic support, cystocele, rectocele)
	  • Examination of urethra (e.g., masses, tenderness, scarring)
	  • Examination of bladder (e.g., fullness, masses, tenderness)
	  • Cervix (e.g., general appearance, lesions, discharge)
	  • Uterus (e.g., size, contour, position, mobility, tenderness, consistency, descent or support)
	  • Adnexa/parametria (e.g., masses, tenderness, organomegaly, nodularity)

Lymphatic	• Palpation of lymph nodes in two or more areas:
	  • Neck
	  • Axillae
	  • Groin
	  • Other

Continued.

TABLE 6-4
1997 General Multi-System Examination—cont'd

Organ System/Body Area	Elements of General Multi-System Examination

Musculoskeletal	• Examination of gait and station
	• Inspection and/or palptation of digits and nails (e.g., clubbing, cyanosis, inflammatory conditions, petechiae, ischemia, infection, nodes)
	• Examination of joints, bones and muscles of one or more of the following six areas: 1) head and neck; 2) spine, ribs and pelvis; 3) right upper extremity; 4) left upper extremity; 5) right lower extremity; and 6) left lower extremity. The examination of a given area includes:
	  • Inspection and/or palpation with notation of presence of any misalignment, asymmetry, crepitation, defects, tenderness, masses, effusions
	  • Assessment of range of motion, with notation of any pain, crepitation or contracture
	  • Assessment of stability with notation of any dislocation (luxation), subluxation or laxity
	  • Assessment of muscle strength and tone (e.g., flaccid, cogwheel, spastic) with notation of any atrophy or abnormal movements

Skin	• Inspection of skin and subcutaneous tissue (e.g., rashes, lesions, ulcers) • Palpation of skin and subcutaneous tissue (e.g., induration, subcutaneous nodules, tightening)
Neurologic	• Test cranial nerves with notation of any deficits • Examination of deep tendon reflexes with notation of pathological reflexes (e.g., Babinski) • Examination of sensation (e.g., touch, pin, vibration, proprioception)

Psychiatric	• Description of patient's judgment and insight
	• Brief assessment of mental status, including:
	  • Orientation to time, place, and person
	  • Recent and remote memory
	  • Mood and affect (e.g., depression, anxiety, agitation)

Content and Documentation Requirements — 1997 General Multi-System Examination

Level of Exam	Perform and Document
Problem focused	One to five elements identified by a bullet
Expanded problem-focused	At least six elements identified by a bullet
Detailed	At least two elements identified by a bullet from each of six areas/systems or At least twelve elements identified by a bullet in two or more areas/systems
Comprehensive	Perform all elements identified by a bullet in at least nine organ systems or body areas and Document at least two elements identified by a bullet from each of nine areas/systems.

Source: U.S. Department of Health and Human Services, Centers for Medicare and Medicaid Services (CMS).

TABLE 6-5
1995-1997 Comparison of Documentation Guidelines Exam

Type of Exam	1995 Documentation Guidelines	1997 Documentation Guidelines
Problem-focused	A limited examination of the affected body area or organ system.	**General Multi-System** Performance and documentation of one to five elements identified in a table by a bullet (•) in one or more organ system(s) or body area(s). **Single Organ System** Performance and documentation of one to five elements identified in a table by a bullet (•), whether in a shaded or unshaded box.
Expanded problem-focused	A limited examination of the affected body area or organ system and other symptomatic or related organ systems.	**General Multi-System** Performance and documentation of at least six elements identified in a table by a bullet (•) in one or more organ system(s) or body area(s). **Single Organ System** Performance and documentation of at least six elements identified in a table by a bullet (•), whether in a shaded or unshaded box.
Detailed	An extended examination of the affected body areas or other symptomatic or related organ systems.	**General Multi-System** Should include at least six organ systems or body areas. For each system/area selected, performance and documentation of at least two elements identified in a table by a bullet (•) is expected. Alternatively, a detailed examination may include performance and documentation of at least twelve elements identified in a table by a bullet (•) in two or more organ systems or body areas.

TABLE 6-5
1995-1997 Comparison of Documentation Guidelines Exam—cont'd

Type of Exam	1995 Documentation Guidelines	1997 Documentation Guidelines
Comprehensive	A general multi-system examination or a complete examination of a single organ system.	**Single Organ System** Examinations other than eye or psychiatric examinations should include performance and documentation of at least twelve elements identified in a table by a bullet (•), whether in a shaded or unshaded box. Eye and Psychiatric examinations should include the performance and documentation of at least nine elements identified in a table by a bullet (•), whether in a shaded or unshaded box. **General Multi-System** Should include at least nine organ systems or body areas. For each system/area selected, all elements of the examination identified in a table by a bullet (•) should be performed, unless specific directions limit the content of the examination. For each area/system, documentation of at least two elements identified in a table by a bullet (•) is expected. **Single Organ System** Should include performance of all elements identified in a table by a bullet (•), whether in a shaded or unshaded box. Documentation of every element in each shaded box and at least one element in each unshaded box is expected.

Source: U.S. Department of Health and Human Services, Centers for Medicare and Medicaid Services (CMS).

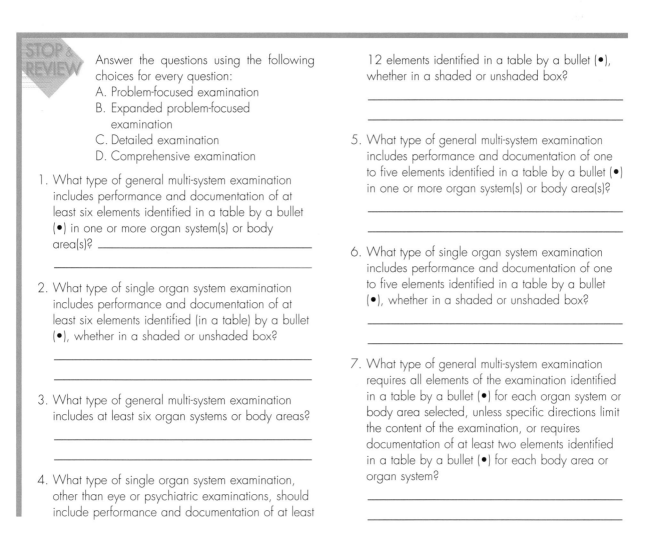

STOP & REVIEW

Answer the questions using the following choices for every question:
A. Problem-focused examination
B. Expanded problem-focused examination
C. Detailed examination
D. Comprehensive examination

1. What type of general multi-system examination includes performance and documentation of at least six elements identified in a table by a bullet (•) in one or more organ system(s) or body area(s)? _____

_____

2. What type of single organ system examination includes performance and documentation of at least six elements identified (in a table) by a bullet (•), whether in a shaded or unshaded box?

_____

_____

3. What type of general multi-system examination includes at least six organ systems or body areas?

_____

_____

4. What type of single organ system examination, other than eye or psychiatric examinations, should include performance and documentation of at least

12 elements identified in a table by a bullet (•), whether in a shaded or unshaded box?

_____

_____

5. What type of general multi-system examination includes performance and documentation of one to five elements identified in a table by a bullet (•) in one or more organ system(s) or body area(s)?

_____

_____

6. What type of single organ system examination includes performance and documentation of one to five elements identified in a table by a bullet (•), whether in a shaded or unshaded box?

_____

_____

7. What type of general multi-system examination requires all elements of the examination identified in a table by a bullet (•) for each organ system or body area selected, unless specific directions limit the content of the examination, or requires documentation of at least two elements identified in a table by a bullet (•) for each body area or organ system?

_____

_____

8. What type of single organ system examination includes performance of all elements identified in a table by a bullet (•), whether in a shaded or unshaded box, or documentation of every element in each shaded box and at least one element in each unshaded box? _____

_____

9. What type of general multi-system examination includes at least nine organ systems or body areas? _____

_____

10. What type of general multi-system examination requires performance and documentation of at least two elements identified in a table by a bullet (•) for each organ system or body area selected, or includes performance and documentation of at least 12 elements identified in a table by a bullet (•) in two or more organ systems or body areas?

_____

_____

Types of E/M Services

There are many types of E/M services. In this book, we will focus on the services most frequently billed from a physician's office, and billing considerations unique to each type of service are discussed.

OFFICE VISITS

Most office visits are distinguished by (1) whether the patient is a new patient or an established patient, and (2) what level of service is provided. Consultations and referrals can occur for both inpatient and outpatient visits, so they are discussed separately. The CPT codebook has special notes and directions at the beginning of this subsection of E/M.

New Patient

A new patient is one who has never been seen or who has not been seen within the past 3 years by the practice or by the specialty group within a multispecialty practice. Visits for new patients are more time consuming and are therefore paid at a higher rate than visits for established patients.

An established patient with a new problem is not a new patient. However, a patient who has not been seen within the past 3 years is a "new" patient for billing purposes because medical information can change so much within that time that an entirely new evaluation is needed.

There are five levels of service. The documentation must meet *all three of the three key components* in order to bill "new patient office visit" codes. In addition, the nature of the presenting problem should be appropriate for the level of service billed. Table 6-6 shows the decision chart for new office patients.

When more than 50% of the visit is spent in counseling or coordination and/or care, time becomes the determining factor for choosing the level of service. The length of the visit and the length of the counseling or coordination of care plus a summary of items discussed or performed must be included in the documentation for the visit when time is the determining factor.

Established Patient

An established patient has been seen within the last 3 years by the practice or by the specialty group within a multi-specialty practice. Services for an established patient with a new problem are billed at the established patient rates.

There are five levels of service. The documentation must meet the requirements for *two of the three key components*. In addition, the nature of the presenting problem must be appropriate for the level of service billed. Table 6-7 shows the decision chart for established office patients.

When more than 50% of the visit is spent in counseling or coordination and/or care, time becomes the determining factor for choosing the level of service. The length of the visit and the length of the counseling or coordination of care plus a summary of items discussed or performed must be included in the documentation for the visit when time is the determining factor.

INPATIENT VISITS

Hospital claims only include facility fees. Hospital claims do not include the fees for physician services, and their fees are based on diagnosis-related groups (DRGs), as discussed in Chapter 12.

Each physician office files claims for their physicians' hospital services.

Hospital E/M codes for physician services do not distinguish between new and established patients.

TABLE 6-6
Decision Chart for New Office Patients
3 of 3 key components must be met or exceeded

CPT Code	History	Exam	Decision Level	Time (min)	Presenting Problem
99201	Problem focused	Problem focused	Straightforward	10	Self-limited
99202	Expanded problem-focused	Expanded problem-focused	Straightforward	20	Low to moderate severity
99203	Detailed	Detailed	Low complexity	30	Moderate severity
99204	Comprehensive	Comprehensive	Moderate complexity	45	Moderate to high severity
99205	Comprehensive	Comprehensive	High complexity	60	Moderate to high severity

TABLE 6-7
Decision Chart for Established Office Patients
Established Patient Office or Other Outpatient Visit
2 of 3 key components must be met or exceeded

CPT Code	History	Exam	Decision Level	Time (min)	Presenting Problem
99211	N/A	N/A	N/A	5	Minimal
99212	Problem focused	Problem focused	Straightforward	10	Self-limited or minor
99213	Expanded problem-focused	Expanded problem-focused	Low complexity	15	Low to moderate severity
99214	Detailed	Detailed	Moderate complexity	25	Moderate to high severity
99215	Comprehensive	Comprehensive	High complexity	40	Moderate to high severity

Instead, they distinguish between initial and subsequent care. Initial care codes are used to report "first" inpatient encounters for the admitting physician only. Thereafter, the admitting physician uses subsequent care codes, and all others use initial inpatient consultation codes or subsequent hospital care codes, as appropriate.

Hospital Observation

Hospital observation codes have three levels of service. *All three key components* must be met in order to use these codes. The CPT codebook has special notes and directions at the beginning of this subsection of E/M.

The patient must be admitted or designated as observation status, but it is not necessary that the patient be located in a designated observation area. If a designated observation area is available in the facility, all patients placed there should be assigned the observation codes, but even then, observation patients can be located elsewhere. Observation status may not be used for postoperative recovery if the procedure performed is part of a surgical package.

When a patient is sent to an observation area from an emergency department, a physician's office, or a nursing facility, admission to observation status is treated the same as admission to the hospital. Services performed in the other locations (emergency department, physician's office, nursing facility) are rolled into the initial observation assessment and are not reported separately.

There is a designated code to use when admission and discharge occur on the same date. Therefore the observation discharge code is not reported on the same date as either hospital admission or observation admission. Medicare sets a limit on the length of observation care: a patient may be observed for 2 midnights before discharge or admission occurs.

Please note: Even though (1) the rules are similar to hospital admission rules, (2) orders may say "admit" to observation status, and (3) patients can be "discharged" from observation status, patients on "observation status" are actually hospital outpatients. They have not been formally admitted to the hospital.

Initial Hospital Care

Initial hospital care has three levels of care. *All three key components* must be met. Only the admitting physician may use these codes. All others use initial inpatient consultation codes or subsequent hospital care codes, as appropriate. The CPT codebook has special notes and directions at the beginning of this subsection of E/M. Table 6-8 shows the decision chart for initial hospital care for both new and established patients.

If the physician completes a history and physical 1 to 3 days before the actual admission (the number of days varies by payor), a comprehensive level E/M code would be reported for the office visit and the

TABLE 6-8
Decision Chart for Initial Hospital Care
Initial Hospital Care — New or Established Patients
2 of 3 key components must be met or exceeded

CPT Code	History	Exam	Decision Level	Time (min)	Presenting Problem
99221	Detailed or Comprehensive	Detailed or Comprehensive	Straightforward or Low complexity	30	Low severity
99222	Comprehensive	Comprehensive	Moderate complexity	50	Moderate severity
99223	Comprehensive	Comprehensive	High complexity	70	High severity

lowest level inpatient code would be reported on the day of admission.

When a patient is admitted to the hospital in the course of another encounter at another site of service, all the E/M services provided—regardless of where they are provided—are considered part of the initial hospital care when performed on the same date as the admission. They are all added together to select the initial care E/M code.

When there are multiple visits on the day of admission, the number of times seen, the total amount of floor time, and complexity of history, exam, and medical decision-making provided during the course of the day are all added together to select one code to bill. If multiple physicians from one practice, or one specialty in a multi-specialty group, see the patient on the day of admission, the care provided by all of them are rolled into one code and services are billed as though just one of them provided the total care.

Subsequent Hospital Care

Subsequent hospital care has three levels of care. *Two of three key components* must be met. The CPT codebook has special notes and directions at the beginning of this subsection of E/M.

When subsequent care is reported, the physician must assess the patient's response to therapy, as it is the determining factor for the level of service reported. If the level 3 code selection is inadequate for the patient's condition, consider using critical care codes when the diagnosis and extent of time fit those criteria. Table 6-9 shows the decision chart for subsequent hospital care.

These codes are only billed once per day per physician group. When there are multiple visits on the same day, the number of times seen, the total amount of floor time, and complexity of history, exam, and medical decision-making provided during the course of the day are all added together to select the one code to bill.

If multiple physicians from one practice, or one specialty in a multi-specialty group, see the patient on the same day, the care provided by all of them is rolled into one code and services are billed as though just one of them provided the total care.

Discharge management codes are time based (more or less than 30 minutes). When admission and discharge occur on the same day, use the code designated by the codebook. When a subsequent care visit and a discharge take place on the same day, even if hours apart, services are added together and only the discharge code is billed. Every service provided the day of discharge is rolled into the time factor for the discharge code.

Adult Critical Care

Critical care codes are based on time and include specific services. They are not based on key components. They have varying amounts of time, but not varying levels of service. Critical care codes are not confined to a particular site of service. They may be used anywhere and anytime the criteria are met. The CPT codebook has many special notes and directions at the beginning of this subsection of E/M.

The amount of critical care time for a specified date is added together. The total time is billed once per date. A new date begins after midnight.

Critical care is provided for an unstable patient during a life-threatening medical crisis or trauma that, if not attended to immediately, would cause some permanent damage to the functioning of the body or body parts, such as:

❑ Body system failure
❑ Central nervous system (CNS) failure
❑ Circulatory system failure
❑ Kidney failure
❑ Liver failure
❑ Respiratory system failure
❑ Shock
❑ Postoperative complications
❑ Overwhelming infection

The encounter must require constant attendance by the physician for the first hour and each subsequent 30-minute interval. The code for the first hour may be used if more than 30 minutes but less

TABLE 6-9
Decision Chart for Subsequent Hospital Care
Subsequent Hospital Care
2 of 3 Key Components must be met or exceeded

CPT Code	History	Exam	Decision Level	Time (min)	Presenting Problem
99231	Problem focused	Problem focused	Straightforward *or* Low complexity	15	Stable, recovering, *or* improving
99232	Expanded problem-focused	Expanded problem-focused	Moderate complexity	25	Inadequate response to therapy *or* minor complication
99233	Detailed	Detailed	High complexity	35	Unstable *or* significant complication *or* significant new problem

than 1 hour was spent. The additional half-hour codes may be used for each additional half-hour beyond the first hour on a given date. The last additional half-hour must account for at least 15 minutes of time. CPT states that when there is less than 30 minutes total of critical care time for a given date, you should bill the appropriate E/M code instead.

Medicare states that if the total duration of critical care time is less than 30 minutes, the higher level hospital codes should be used instead. Medicare states that only one physician may bill for a given hour of critical care, even if more than one physician is providing care to a critically ill patient.

Some payors will pay only one physician per day for critical care services. In this case, the physician whose claim reaches the payor first is the one paid. Sometimes, but not often, physicians agree to share fees paid. A few states do not allow fee sharing, so check the rules for your state.

The physician need not be constantly at the bedside but must be engaged in physician work directly related to the individual patient's care. The physician may not bill for critical care time if services were provided and billed to other patients for the same period. Patients usually have different insurance companies, but insurance companies share information through the Medical Information Bureau (MIB). Payors are well equipped to detect many types of fraud.

Medicare states there are no absolute limits on the number of critical care services that can be billed per day or per hospital stay, but documentation must support the charges billed. Payors vary on this issue. In some states, Medicaid will only cover 4 hours per 24-hour period.

Critical care services are not bundled into other E/M services for inpatients. Critical care may be provided during surgery. However, after surgery, in the postoperative period, critical care may be billed separately only for unusual complications requiring another physician and for unrelated services.

Specific procedures are included in adult critical care codes:

❑ Interpretation of cardiac output measurements
❑ Chest x-rays
❑ Blood gases
❑ Pulse oximetry
❑ Information stored in computers (e.g., EKGs, blood pressure, hematologic data)
❑ Gastric intubation
❑ Temporary transcutaneous pacing
❑ Ventilator management
❑ Vascular access procedures

Any services performed that are not listed in the codebook directions for this subsection should be reported separately. A common example is insertion of a Swan-Ganz catheter.

Other noncritical procedures performed during the physician's attendance may be reported separately, but the critical care time reporting must be suspended during the performance of these procedures (e.g., reducing or setting a fracture, suturing a laceration, lumbar puncture, bladder tap).

Start and stop times or the total time should be recorded in the physician documentation for each episode of critical care.

For example:
04/15/1999 Critical care services performed for 45 minutes or from 2130 to 2215.
04/16/1999 Critical care services performed for 1 hour and 30 minutes or from 0840 to 1010.
Note: These examples are charted using a 24-hour clock instead of a 12-hour clock. 2130 = 9:30 PM, 2215 =10:15 PM, 0840 = 8:40 AM and 1010 = 10:10 AM

If multiple physicians from one practice, or one specialty in a multi-specialty group, see the patient for critical care services on the same day, the care provided by all of them is rolled together and services are billed as though just one of them provided the total care.

Services furnished to a patient who is in the critical care unit but not critically ill at the encounter should be reported as subsequent hospital care.

Partial Hospitalization

Partial hospitalization codes are exclusive to the psychiatry subsection of the Medicine section of CPT. The CPT codebook has special notes and directions at the beginning of this subsection of the Medicine section. Some of the psychiatry codes include E/M services, but they are not located in the E/M section of the codebook; instead, they are located in the psychiatry subsection of the Medicine section. The codes are based on time, the type of therapy given, and whether or not an E/M service was also provided. Place of service indicator "52" is used on the claim form.

Partial hospitalization codes are used for:

❑ Crisis stabilization
❑ Intensive short-term daily treatment
❑ Intermediate treatment of psychiatric disorders

Do not confuse partial hospitalization with services provided by a physician in an observation area of the hospital. Medicare defines a partial hospitalization psychiatric facility as a facility for the diagnosis and treatment of mental illness that provides a planned therapeutic program for patients who do not require full-time hospitalization, but who need broader programs than are possible from outpatient visits in a hospital-based or a hospital-affiliated facility.

Emergency Department Services

Emergency department (ED) services have five levels. *All three key components* must be met. There is no distinction between new and established patients. The CPT codebook has special notes and directions at the beginning of this subsection of E/M.

Each repeat or additional evaluation during the course of the ED visit must be individually documented in the patient record. When critical care is provided in the ED, critical care codes are billed.

When two or more physicians see a patient, usually each one may bill for emergency department E/M services. However, this can vary by payor, so be sure to read your contracts or call the payor and ask.

If the attending physician admits the patient to the hospital from the ED, the attending physician will bill only the initial hospital care code.

If the patient is seen in the ED multiple times on the same day, it is essential that diagnosis codes clearly indicate the reason for each visit. Otherwise,

the payor could mistakenly consider the additional visits to represent fraudulent double billing.

A special code is used when the physician is in two-way voice communication with an ambulance. This code is for physician direction of emergency medical services (EMS) and advanced life support. The physician directs the performance of essential medical services. A partial list of included services is detailed in the CPT codebook under that subsection of E/M.

CONSULTATIONS AND REFERRALS

For billing purposes, it is very important to understand that *consultation* and *referral* are not synonyms in CPT. This is true even though the same order form is often used for both purposes, and the form is typically called a "consultation form." The requesting physician must define the intent of the visit: consultation (opinion/advice) or referral (treatment).

Most consultation and referral services have five levels of service and *all three key components* must be met. Follow-up inpatient consultations have three levels of service and *two of three key components* must be met. The CPT codebook has special notes and directions at the beginning of this subsection of E/M.

Referrals

A **referral** is used whenever partial or total care of the patient is transferred to another physician. "Evaluate and treat" indicates a referral. The accepting physician is to *manage* all or a specific portion of the patient's care. New patient office, established patient office, or subsequent-care hospital E/M codes (as appropriate) will be billed.

Consultations

A **consultation** code is used when only an opinion or treatment advice is requested from the consulting physician. The consultant must send a written report to the requesting physician, or both physicians must document a telephone discussion.

Consultations are paid at a higher rate than referrals, so consultations have stricter requirements and consultations are scrutinized more carefully for fraud and abuse. The patient's medical record should contain documentation of:

❑ The request for the consultation
❑ The consulting physician's diagnostic findings, opinion, and/or recommended treatment plan
❑ A written report or other documentation of how this information was communicated to the requesting physician

❑ Follow-up by the attending physician

If care is transferred as a result of the consultation:

❑ The opinion or advice must be communicated before the initiation of treatment.
❑ Both the referring and the receiving physician must document when the transfer of care is to be effective.
❑ The first visit is billed as a consultation, and future encounters are billed as established-patient office or subsequent care hospital visits.

The consultant may not initiate follow-up consultations. Follow-up consultations are only used when:

❑ It is necessary to complete an initial inpatient consultation.

❑ An additional request for an opinion or advice regarding the same or a new problem is received from the attending physician.

Tables 6-10, 6-11, and 6-12 show the various decision charts for consultations.

Confirmatory Consultations

Confirmatory consultations are second or even third opinions. They are sometimes paid at a lower rate than other consultations because the first consultant should have completed most of the diagnostic tests. Documentation and medical necessity are looked at closely by payors when confirmatory consultations are performed. Bill and code only the services rendered and make sure documentation backs up all the charges. Times have not been established for confirmatory consultations.

TABLE 6-10
Decision Chart for Office Consultation
Office Or Other Outpatient Consultations — New or Established Patient
3 of 3 key components must be met or exceeded

CPT Code	History	Exam	Decision Level	Time (min)	Presenting Problem
99241	Problem focused	Problem focused	Straightforward	15	Self-limited *or* minor
99242	Expanded problem-focused	Expanded problem-focused	Straightforward	30	Low severity
99243	Detailed	Detailed	Low complexity	40	Moderate severity
99244	Comprehensive	Comprehensive	Moderate complexity	60	Moderate to high severity
99245	Comprehensive	Comprehensive	High complexity	80	Moderate to high severity

TABLE 6-11
Decision Chart for Initial Inpatient Consultation
Initial Inpatient Consultations — New or Established Patient
3 of 3 key components must be met or exceeded

CPT Code	History	Exam	Decision Level	Time (min)	Presenting Problem
99251	Problem focused	Problem focused	Straightforward	20	Self-limited *or* minor
99252	Expanded problem-focused	Expanded problem-focused	Straightforward	40	Low severity
99253	Detailed	Detailed	Low complexity	55	Moderate severity
99254	Comprehensive	Comprehensive	Moderate complexity	80	Moderate to high severity
99255	Comprehensive	Comprehensive	High complexity	110	Moderate to high severity

TABLE 6-12
Decision Chart for Follow-up Inpatient Consultation
Follow-up Inpatient Consultations — Established Patient
2 of 3 key components must be met or exceeded

CPT Code	History	Exam	Decision Level	Time (min)	Presenting Problem
99261	Problem focused	Problem focused	Straightforward *or* Low complexity	10	Stable, recovering *or* improving
99262	Expanded problem-focused	Expanded problem-focused	Moderate complexity	20	Inadequate response to therapy *or* minor complication
99263	Detailed	Detailed	High complexity	30	Unstable *or* significant complication *or* significant new problem

Answer the following questions:

1. How many key components must be met or exceeded for a new office patient? _____

2. How many key components must be met or exceeded for an established office patient?

_____

3. How many key components must be met or exceeded for initial hospital care? _____

4. How many key components must be met or exceeded for subsequent hospital care? _____

_____

5. How many key components must be met or exceeded for adult critical care? _____

6. How many key components must be met or exceeded for an office consultation? _____

_____

7. How many key components must be met or exceeded for an initial inpatient consultation?

_____

8. How many key components must be met or exceeded for an inpatient follow-up consultation?

_____

9. How many key components must be met or exceeded for a confirmatory consultation?

_____

10. How many key components must be met or exceeded for emergency department services?

_____

NURSING FACILITY SERVICES

The term *nursing facility* includes:

- ❑ Skilled nursing centers
- ❑ Intermediate care centers
- ❑ Long-term care centers
- ❑ Psychiatric residential treatment centers

The CPT codebook has special notes and directions at the beginning of this subsection of E/M. Hospital discharges performed on the same date as admission to a nursing facility are reported separately.

When people use nursing facilities, they are called residents, not patients. Nursing facilities are required by law to provide a variety of periodic evaluations or assessments of each resident.

Physician services rendered in nursing facilities are governed by rules similar to inpatient settings, and there are three levels of service. Physician services are classified in two main categories: comprehensive nursing facility assessments and subsequent nursing facility care. Nursing-facility discharge codes are time based.

DOMICILIARY, REST HOME, BOARDING HOME, OR CUSTODIAL CARE FACILITIES

Domiciliary, rest home, boarding home, or custodial care facilities are not considered to be nursing facilities because they do not provide medical care. The CPT codebook has special notes and directions at the beginning of this subsection of E/M.

Physician services rendered in these settings are governed by rules similar to outpatient settings: there are three levels of service, and patients are classified as either new patients or established patients.

PREVENTIVE MEDICINE

There are distinct E/M codes exclusively for preventive medicine services, encompassing periodic examinations, preventive medicine counseling, and newborn care. Many preventive medicine codes are age based, and patients are classified as either new patients or established patients. The CPT codebook has special notes and directions at the beginning of this subsection of E/M.

Preventive medicine counseling may not be billed separately when performed the same day as a preventive medicine visit.

CPT directs that if a problem, either new or established, is evaluated in the course of a preventive medicine visit, the appropriate office or outpatient E/M code may also be billed. Not every payor honors this guidance. Medicare, for example, does not cover most preventive medicine services. With other payors, when a problem arises, is revealed, or is discovered during the course of the preventive medicine visit, a choice often must be made:

❑ If the problem is not urgent and treatment can wait until another visit, the physician performs only the preventive medicine service, and the patient returns at another time to evaluate and treat the problem.

❑ If the problem is urgent and cannot wait until another day, the physician performs the preventive medicine service and addresses the problem during the same visit. The physician bills only a regular E/M visit (not preventive care) and accepts the lower reimbursement.

❑ The physician performs the preventive medicine service and follows it with a separate visit to address the problem on the same date. The preventive medicine visit is billed on line 1 and the E/M service is billed on line 2 with modifier -25. The code requirements for history, examination, and medical decision-making must be met separately for the preventive medicine E/M service and the other E/M service. Each service must be clearly documented as a separate service.

OTHER E/M CODE SELECTION ISSUES

Covering Physician

When a "covering" physician provides E/M services, the E/M service code is chosen as though the original physician had provided the services. If the patient is an established patient for the original physician, he or she will also be an established patient for the covering physician. The physician who actually renders the service will be identified in box 24K on the claim form.

Some managed care contracts have specific requirements for covering physicians that also must be met in order to bill for the services.

Steps For Choosing E/M Codes

You have learned the requirements for each E/M key component, including subcomponents and levels of service. You have learned the requirements for the contributory elements. You have learned the most commonly used types of E/M codes. Now it is time to put it all together and learn how to select an E/M code. When selecting an E/M code, you must meet the requirements listed in the codebook for each exact code.

Step 1: Identify the type of E/M service, category, and subcategory (such as office visit, established patient; hospital care, initial; consultation, inpatient follow-up).

Step 2: Review the reporting instructions for the selected code category and subcategory.

Step 3: Review the code requirements and examples given for each code in the subcategory (such as number and extent of key components, nature of presenting problem, and time).

Step 4: Review the chart documentation. Determine the extent of history documented, the extent of examination documented, the documented complexity of medical decision-making, the nature of the presenting problem, and time, if indicated.

Step 5: Determine whether the code will be selected based on key components or based on time.

Step 6: Select the E/M code best met by chart documentation.

Example 1. A new patient office visit requires all three key components.

99201: Problem-focused history, problem-focused examination, and straightforward decision-making.

99202: Expanded problem-focused history, expanded problem-focused exam, straightforward decision-making.

99203: Detailed history, detailed exam, low-complexity decision making.

99204: Comprehensive history, comprehensive exam, moderate-complexity decision-making.

99205: Comprehensive history, comprehensive examination, and high-complexity decision-making.

If the medical record documentation meets the requirements for a detailed history, a comprehensive exam, and straightforward medical decision-making, you would bill the code 99202. The documentation does not meet all three requirements for any other code.

Example 2. An established patient office visit requires two of three key components.

99211: May not require the presence of the physician.

99212: Problem-focused history, problem-focused exam, straightforward decision-making.

99213: Expanded problem-focused history, expanded problem-focused exam, low-complexity decision-making.

99214: Detailed history, detailed exam, moderate-complexity decision-making.

99215: Comprehensive history, comprehensive exam, and high-complexity decision-making.

If medical record documentation meets the requirements for an expanded problem-focused history, a detailed exam, and straightforward decision-making, you would bill code 99213 because only two requirements must be met.

Clinical Application Exercise

Find the E/M code for the following encounter with an established office patient:

CC: 26 y.o. white ♀ w/sore throat & fever × 2 days

S: T101°-101.4°F × 2 days. Throat becoming increasingly painful. No runny nose or cough.

O: Throat red with exudative white patches on tonsils. Eyes neg. Ears neg. + ant. & post. cervical lymph nodes. Lungs clear. Heart reg. sinus rhythm. Abd. Neg.

A: Tonsillitis

P: Amoxicillin 500 mg QID × 10 days. Call if not better. Return PRN.

History: _____

Exam: _____

Medical decision-making: _____

Presenting problem: _____

Time: _____

E/M CPT code: _____

Legal Issues

The legal issues with E/M codes are similar to the legal issues with diagnosis codes. *Upcoding* takes place anytime the requirements for using a code are greater than the requirements actually met in chart documentation. The physician may actually have provided the level of service billed, but if it is not documented, it may not be billed. *Downcoding* occurs anytime the documentation in the chart justifies a higher level of service than was billed. *Payor downcoding* occurs when a payor downcodes a service to pay for only the level of service met in chart documentation.

Upcoding and downcoding are both fraudulent because they do not accurately portray chart documentation. Payors, especially private payors, do not always pursue charges of fraud when they identify upcoding and downcoding. It is much less expensive for a payor to downcode a service and

impose a penalty than to hire an attorney, and physicians often accept the penalty amount as payment-in-full, saving the payor an additional sum of money.

Payors use software programs to determine patterns of code use. They know the usual patterns for every region and every physician who submits claims. Those who fall outside the normal patterns are called **outliers.** Claims from outliers are scrutinized more carefully, and if a pattern of misuse is determined, all claims might be automatically subjected to a blanket penalty.

It is important to avoid being flagged as an outlier. The best way to do this is to consistently meet the most current documentation requirements and to code services carefully, meeting every requirement for code usage.

How to Help Physicians Meet E/M Requirements

Continuing education for physicians and medical office workers is crucial when helping physicians meet E/M documentation guidelines, and well-designed forms pave the way for correct coding.

The E/M codes listed on the superbill should also designate the required key components for each code so the physician will know what level of documentation to complete. History forms and problem lists, when they are maintained and kept current, are valuable tools to help meet the complex E/M documentation guidelines. The physician does not have to rewrite the history data and problem list data each time if the medical record documentation for the encounter tells where the information is found.

It is hard to fix documentation problems when the physicians are unaware of the problems. Regular documentation audits performed by practice personnel or performed by hired consultants provide an impartial means for physicians to become aware of documentation shortfalls. Each physician may then target individual weak points.

Figure 6-1 is an actual audit worksheet used by an independent consultant to audit physician office visits. A separate page is completed for each patient visit audited. (1) Circle the elements matched by chart documentation for each history component. (2) Select the overall level of history. (3) Circle the elements matched by chart documentation for examination. (4) Select the overall level of examination. (5) Circle the elements that match chart documentation for medical decision-making. (6) Select the overall level of medical decision-making. (7) Determine whether the patient status is new or established. (8) Circle the overall levels of history, examination, and medical decision-making for the patient status. (9) Determine the nature of presenting problem and time, if documented. (10) Select the overall level of service and the corresponding CPT code.

Figure 6-2 is also an actual audit form used by an independent consultant to summarize results from a post-payment audit of E/M services and to record other types of audit results, such as a postpayment audit of surgery coding.

Match column 1 with column 2 to show the correct steps when choosing the proper E/M code:

COLUMN 1	COLUMN 2
Step 1:	A. Review the code requirements and examples given for each code in the subcategory.
Step 2:	B. Determine whether the code will be selected based on key components or based on time.
Step 3:	C. Identify the type of E/M service, category, and subcategory.
Step 4:	D. Select the E/M code best met by chart documentation.
Step 5:	E. Review the reporting instructions for the selected code category and subcategory.
Step 6:	F. Review the chart documentation to determine the extent of history, exam, medical decision-making, presenting problem, and time.

Answer the following questions:

7. The patient is an established patient for the primary physician, but it is the first time the covering physician has seen the patient. Is the encounter billed as a new patient or an established patient? _____

8. A 25-year-old female patient is scheduled for an annual physical. Birth control options are also discussed during the appointment. May the physician bill a preventive medicine counseling E/M code in addition to the preventive medicine E/M code? _____

9. Does a physician want to be identified as an outlier when payors perform patterning studies? Why or why not? _____

_____

_____

10. Which of the following are methods to help physicians meet E/M code requirements? Choose all that apply.
   A. A superbill that lists the number and level of key components required for each E/M service listed
   B. Continuing education
   C. Documentation audits
   D. History forms
   E. Problem lists

Patient Identifier _____   Date of service _____

Documentation Guidelines for Exam

Type of Exam	1995 Documentation Guidelines	1997 Documentation Guidelines
Problem focused	A limited examination of the affected body area or organ system.	**General Multi-System** Performance and documentation of one to five elements identified in a table by a bullet (•) in one or more organ system(s) or body area(s). **Single Organ System** Performance and documentation of one to five elements identified in a table by a bullet (•), whether in a shaded or unshaded box.
Expanded problem focused	A limited examination of the affected body area or organ system and other symptomatic or related organ systems.	**General Multi-System** Performance and documentation of at least six elements identified in a table by a bullet (•) in one or more organ system(s) or body area(s). **Single Organ System** Performance and documentation of at least six elements identified in a table by a bullet (•), whether in a shaded or unshaded box.
Detailed	An extended examination of the affected body areas or other symptomatic or related organ systems.	**General Multi-System** Should include at least six organ systems or body areas. For each system/area selected, performance and documentation of at least two elements identified in a table by a bullet (•) is expected. Alternatively, a detailed examination may include performance and documentation of at least twelve elements identified in a table by a bullet (•) in two or more organ systems or body areas. **Single Organ System** Examinations other than eye or psychiatric examinations should include performance and documentation of at least twelve elements identified in a table by a bullet (•), whether in a shaded or unshaded box. Eye and psychiatric examinations should include the performance and documentation of at least nine elements identified in a table by a bullet (•), whether in a shaded or unshaded box.
Comprehensive	A general multi-system examination or a complete examination of a single organ system.	**General Multi-System** Should include at least nine organ systems or body areas. For each system/area selected, all elements of the examination identified in a table by a bullet (•) should be performed, unless specific directions limit the content of the examination. For each area/system, documentation of at least two elements identified in a table by a bullet (•) is expected. **Single Organ System** Should include performance of all elements identified in a table by a bullet (•), whether in a shaded or unshaded box. Documentation of every element in each shaded box and at least one element in each unshaded box is expected.

Decision Chart for History
Chief complaint *plus* the specified elements

Type of History	(HPI)	(ROS)	(PFSH)
Problem focused	B	N/A	N/A
Expanded problem-focused	B	Prob pert	N/A
Detailed	Ext	Ext	Pert
Comprehensive	Ext	Comp	Comp

Decision Chart for Medical Decision-Making
2 of 3 elements in the table must be either met or exceeded

Type of Decision Making	# Dx/Mgmt Options	Amt and/or Complexity of Data	Risk
Straightforward	Min	Min/none	Min
Low complexity	Lmt	Lmt	Low
Moderate complexity	Mult	Mod	Mod
High complexity	Ext	Ext	High

Decision Chart for New Office Patient
3 of 3 key components must be met or exceeded

CPT code	H	E	MDM	Time	Presenting problem
99201	PF	PF	Sfwd	10	Self limit
99202	EPF	EPF	Sfwd	20	Low/mod
99203	D	D	LC	30	Moderate
99204	C	C	MC	45	Mod/high
99205	C	C	HC	60	Mod/high

Decision Chart for Established Office Patient
2 of 3 key components must be either met or exceeded

CPT code	H	E	MDM	Time	Presenting Problem
99211	N/A	N/A	N/A	5	Min
99212	PF	PF	Sfwd	10	Self limit/minor
99213	EPF	EPF	LC	15	Low/moderate
99214	D	D	MC	25	Moderate/high
99215	C	C	HC	40	Moderate/high

FIGURE 6-1
Documentation guidelines for exam.

Audit Summary

Prepared for: _____   Provider: _____   Date: _____

	Patient Identifier:	Date of Encounter	Diagnosis Codes Billed	Diagnoses Supported by Documentation	Procedure(s) Billed	Procedure(s) Supported by Documentation	Notes	Pass Audit
1								
2								
3								
4								
5								
6								
7								
8								
9								
10								
Totals: % correct								

Other notes and observations:

Auditor: _____   Auditor Signature: _____

Date: _____

Page _____ of _____

FIGURE 6-2
Audit summary worksheet.

Chapter Review

Evaluation and management is the process of evaluating a patient for suspected, known, or potential problems or conditions; assessing the findings; rendering an opinion; and developing a plan of action. E/M services also include writing prescriptions for medications and ordering tests, treatments, equipment, and supplies.

Until a new set of documentation guidelines is implemented, coding may be performed using either the 1995 guidelines or the 1997 guidelines.

E/M documentation guidelines are intended to provide a measurable way to evaluate physician services. Key components are divided into levels to better identify the amount of work performed.

History is a key component in selection of E/M services. There are four types of history and three history subcomponents, each of which has two to three levels. A history decision chart is a tool to help select the right type of history.

Examination is a key component when selecting an E/M service. There are four types of examinations. Exams may encompass body areas or organ systems.

Medical decision-making is a key component in the selection of E/M services. There are four types of medical decision-making and three medical decision-making subcomponents, each of which has two to three levels. A medical decision-making decision chart and a table of risk decision chart are tools to help select the right type of medical decision-making.

Contributory elements should be consistent with the level of service billed, but they are not used to determine the level of service, except in specific circumstances.

The 1997 documentation guidelines had only one minor change for history and did not change medical decision-making requirements; they primarily expanded the examination requirements to make them measurable. The 1995 history requirements still apply, and the 1995 medical decision-making requirements still apply.

There are many types of E/M codes. Office visit codes can be for new or established patients. Hospital codes are for initial or subsequent care. Critical care can take place at any location. Consultations are office, initial inpatient, follow-up inpatient, or confirmatory.

Correct code selection is important. Choosing a code for a higher level of service than documented is upcoding. Choosing a code for a lower level of service than documented is downcoding.

Answer the following questions:
Identify whether each of the components listed in questions 1 to 7 is a key component or a contributory element.

1. Medical decision-making _____

2. Counseling _____

3. Coordination of care _____

4. Examination _____

5. History _____

6. Time _____

7. Nature of presenting problem _____

8. What key component(s) were not revised in the 1997 documentation guidelines?
   A. History
   B. Examination
   C. Medical decision-making
   D. A and C

9. What type of office E/M code may be billed for an established patient if the only key component met is the 1995 examination component, and no time is listed?
   A. 99211
   B. 99212
   C. 99213
   D. None of the above

10. What subcategory codes are used for inpatient physician services? Circle all that apply.
    A. New
    B. Initial
    C. Subsequent
    D. Established

11. What subcategory codes are used for consultation? Circle all that apply.
    A. New
    B. Inpatient initial
    C. Office
    D. Established
    E. Inpatient follow-up
    F. Confirmatory

12. What subcategory codes are used for office visits? Circle all that apply.
    A. New
    B. Initial
    C. Subsequent
    D. Established

13. How many history subcomponents are there?

    _____

14. How many medical decision-making subcomponents are there? _____

15. Are the 1995 exam requirements or the 1997 exam requirements more specific for a coder to use to

determine the level of exam? Why? _____

_____

_____

16. Are the 1995 exam requirements or the 1997 exam requirements easier for a physician to meet? Why?

_____

_____

_____

17. When is time a determining factor for E/M coding?

_____

_____

Use the following documentation example for the remaining questions:

Follow-up, BP 120/86

Improving. No headaches × 6 weeks. Continue BP meds. F/U 2 months.

18. What level of history is met? _____

19. What level of exam is met?

_____

20. What level of medical decision-making is met?

_____

21. Calculate the E/M code.

_____

7

BASIC PRINCIPLES OF PROCEDURE CODING

Objectives After completing this chapter, you should be able to:

- Demonstrate how to use the procedure codebooks
- Relate billing rules and coding conventions for procedure codes
- Explain the purpose of the Correct Coding Initiative (CCI)
- Demonstrate how to use modifiers
- Discuss how to link procedures to diagnoses
- Discuss how procedure coding influences reimbursement
- Discuss strategies for helping physicians meet procedure code requirements
- Discuss legal issues related to procedure coding

Key Terms

add-on codes codes used to expand the scope of a basic procedure code. Add-on codes are never used alone, and they are never listed first.

anatomic modifiers Level II HCPCS modifiers that identify specific anatomical parts of the body; they are used when the procedure code does not include that information.

comprehensive code a code that includes all the services essential to accomplishing a service or procedure; also called a bundle or a package.

Correct Coding Initiative (CCI) a Medicare editing system designed to control improper coding.

CPT *Current Procedural Terminology;* the Level I HCPCS procedure codebook updated and maintained by the American Medical Association.

fragmentation occurs when a service that is normally completed in one visit is broken apart to require two or more visits.

global period the time period during which all care related to a procedure is considered to be part of the code that reports the procedure, and it may not be billed separately.

HCPCS *HCFA Common Procedure Coding System;* the Level II HCPCS procedure codebook updated and maintained by the CMS.

indicators CCI indicators designate which codes can be pulled out of a bundle and which cannot.

modifiers used with a procedure code to report that a service or procedure has been altered by a specific circumstance.

mutually exclusive code pairs service or procedure combinations that would not or could not reasonably be performed at the same session, by the same provider, on the same patient.

place of service codes codes used to identify where a service is rendered.

single component codes codes used to bill services when only one component of a comprehensive procedure is performed.

special report a report that explains or clarifies an unusual, variable, or infrequently performed service or procedure.

starred procedures deleted in 2004, starred procedures were relatively minor surgical procedures that were not bundled and did not have a global period. All preprocedure and postprocedure work was reported separately.

type of service codes used to categorize the type of service and give a clearer picture of what occurred.

unbundling when a group of procedures covered by a single comprehensive code are each reported separately instead of using the comprehensive code.

unlisted procedure codes used when CPT does not contain an appropriate entry. They end in -9 or -99. Each section of CPT has unlisted procedure codes.

Introduction

This chapter covers the basic principles of procedure coding for services, procedures, and supplies that are not evaluation and management (E/M) services. Coding for E/M services was covered in Chapter 6.

The *HCFA Common Procedural Coding System* (**HCPCS**—pronounced "hick-picks") once was divided into three levels, but effective December 31, 2003, the third level was discontinued. The Health Care Financing Administration (HCFA—pronounced "hick-fuh") is now called the Centers for Medicare and Medicaid Services (CMS), but the "H" in HCPCS still stands for "health care."

The Level I HCPCS codes are found in the **CPT** codebook. "CPT" stands for *Current Procedural Terminology*. CPT is a registered trademark of the American Medical Association (AMA). The AMA maintains the CPT codebook and updates it annually. The fourth edition of CPT was first printed in 1977, and it has been revised every year since then. It is commonly called CPT-4. *Unless otherwise indicated, the CPT codes used throughout this textbook will refer to CPT-4 codes.*

Level I CPT is now divided into three categories of codes. The original, traditional part of CPT is called Category I, which contains the main body of procedure codes. Category I codes consist of five numeric digits, with no decimal points. In 2004, Category II was introduced. The Category II codes consist of four numeric digits followed by the letter F. They are supplemental codes that can be used for performance measurement. In 2002, Category III was introduced. The Category III codes consist of four numeric digits followed by the letter T. They are temporary codes assigned to new emerging technology.

The Level II HCPCS procedure codes are found in the HCPCS codebook. HCPCS was first developed in 1983 to provide a means to report medical supplies and medical, dental, and ancillary services not reported in CPT. HCFA developed the HCPCS codebook, and CMS updates it annually. HCPCS codes begin with a single letter (A through V), followed by four numeric digits, with no decimal points. Level I CPT codes and Level II HCPCS codes are national codes.

Level III codes were discontinued effective December 31, 2003. However, you might come across them when performing collections or audits on old claims, so you still need to know they once existed. Level III codes were local codes assigned and maintained by individual state Medicare carriers. They were found in Medicare newsletters and bulletins. Level III codes began with a single letter

(W through Z), followed by four numeric digits. They were assigned to new services and procedures on an "as needed" basis.

Medical codes are subject to annual revision, and coding becomes more complex every year. Physicians are very busy and must keep up with continuing medical education units (CMEs) to maintain their medical licenses. They seldom have time to also keep up with the changes to medical coding rules every year to *correctly* code their own services. Therefore medical coding has become a distinct specialty in the medical office, and another member of the medical office team usually performs or confirms the coding.

Procedure coding is a complex subject that cannot be fully covered in one chapter. The information presented in this chapter is an introduction to procedure coding and a broad overview of the most important coding rules. It is not as comprehensive as the information presented in a medical coding course. Specialty-specific coding rules are not addressed.

The compliance guidance documents issued by the Office of Inspector General (OIG) for the Department of Health and Human Services (HHS) strongly recommend that job descriptions be used to assign accountability for specific tasks in the medical office. The OIG developed the compliance guidance documents to help various types of medical entities meet the "accountability" requirements of the Health Insurance Portability and Accountability Act of 1996 (Public Law 104-191) (HIPAA). Many of the OIG's recommendations relate directly to billing and collections, including assigning responsibility for gathering the information for the billing and coding of medical claims. The Medicare website for medical office education, www.cms.hhs.gov/medlearn/cbts.asp, notes how accountability for given tasks is typically assigned in a medical office, and that information provided the basis of accountability as addressed in this chapter. However, please remember that each medical office decides exactly which employee positions are assigned individual accountability for each task, and it will vary from one office to another. In addition, in a small medical office, one multiskilled professional often fills numerous employee positions.

The purpose of this chapter is to introduce the procedure codebooks used for physician and provider billing and to lay the foundation for procedure coding in the physician's office. This chapter focuses on the Level I CPT and Level II HCPCS national codes for services, procedures, and supplies. When you finish this course, you will be able to:

- ❏ Use a current-year CPT codebook to look for a service, procedure, or supply code
- ❏ Use a current-year HCPCS codebook to look for a service, procedure, or supply code
- ❏ Add modifiers to procedure codes to better portray medical record documentation
- ❏ Link procedure codes with diagnosis codes
- ❏ Recognize when something is obviously wrong with procedure codes you are given to place on a medical claim form

For example: You will know something is obviously wrong if:

- ❏ A code for a procedure that can only be performed on a male is selected for a female
- ❏ A code for a procedure that can only be performed on a female is selected for a male
- ❏ A procedure that designates an age group is selected for someone not in that age group
- ❏ Routine preprocedure work, such as providing simple venous access or scrubbing the skin, is coded separately from and in addition to the procedure
- ❏ Routine postprocedure work, such as applying a dressing or monitoring vital signs, is coded separately from and in addition to the procedure
- ❏ A procedure is linked to multiple diagnosis codes

Finding Information in Procedure Codebooks

You will need a current-year CPT codebook and a current year HCPCS codebook for this chapter. Open your codebooks and find each item as we discuss it.

Each codebook publisher includes special features to entice buyers. Some codebooks provide coding tips, additional tables or appendices, expanded indexes, or enhanced cross-referencing to make the book more user friendly. Some also include color-coded symbols to alert readers to specific issues, such as "new codes," "revised codes," "services or supplies not covered by Medicare," and more.

Look at the codebooks your classmates, coworkers, friends, and colleagues use. Compare the special features and the prices when you decide which codebooks you want to purchase. Professional edition codebooks are a little more expensive, but they contain many useful features that make coding easier.

Medical procedure codes are in a constant state of change, usually based on new medical research and technologic improvements. It is vitally important to always use current-year codebooks. When codes for a particular section of the codebook are expanded, the meanings of previously assigned codes often change as well. If you are not using codes that are valid for the date of service, you could inadvertently cause penalties or denials, both of which result in a needless reduction in payment.

Do not discard your old codebooks. If you are ever audited or involved in litigation (a legal action), you will need codebooks for the years included in the audit or litigation to demonstrate the rules and code definitions that were effective on the date of service.

Note: Some commercial payors traditionally have had a 3- to 6-month lag between the effective date of new codes and the date their computer system is ready to accept them. Remember this point if an audit or litigation occurs years after the date of service. In the fall of 2004, CMS eliminated this implementation period. ICD-9-CM codes are now released twice a year with effective dates of October 1 and April 1. Level I CPT and Level II HCPCS codes are released once a year with an effective date of January 1.

Let's take a closer look at the Level I CPT and Level II HCPCS codebooks.

LEVEL I—CPT

The CPT codebook is organized into three categories. Category I, the main body of the CPT codebook, is organized into six sections. The major sections in the main body of the CPT codebook are:

- ❏ Evaluation and Management (99201-99499)
- ❏ Anesthesiology (00100-01999, 99100-99140)
- ❏ Surgery (10021-69990)
- ❏ Radiology (including Nuclear Medicine and Diagnostic Ultrasound; 70010-79999)
- ❏ Pathology and Laboratory (80048-89399)
- ❏ Medicine (except Anesthesiology; 90281-99199, 99500-99600)

In addition, there are Category II codes (0001F-6999F) and Category III codes (0001T-9999T).

CPT Category I codes consist of five numeric digits. The procedures and services are listed in numeric code order in the main body of the codebook, with one exception. The "Evaluation and Management (E/M)" section is used the most and therefore is placed at the beginning of the main body, even though the numeric order would have placed it near the end, in the middle of the Medicine section.

Each section in Category I is divided into subsections and subheadings according to body part, service, or diagnosis. Guidelines are given at the beginning of each section, and special notes and directions are given at the beginning of many subsections and subheadings to clarify how to report the information in that section, subsection, and/or subheading.

Categories II and II are still small and only have one section each. However, guidelines are given at the beginning of the sections, and special notes and directions are given at the beginning of some subsections and/or subheadings to clarify how to report the information in that section, subsection, and/or subheading.

The code narrative in the CPT codebook is not always intended to be a complete description of the service or procedure. To save space, an indented entry includes the *common portion* of a preceding entry. The *common portion* is the part of a description before the semicolon (;).

For example: "Gastrotomy;" is the common portion for the following CPT codes:

43500	Gastrotomy; with exploration or removal of foreign body
43501	with suture repair of bleeding ulcer
43502	with suture repair of pre-existing esophagogastric laceration (e.g., Mallory-Weiss)
43510	with esophageal dilation and insertion of permanent intraluminal tube (e.g., Celestin or Mousseaux-Barbin)

Add-on codes identify items that are not included in the description for a particular procedure code but that expand the scope of the service for the code. Add-on codes are never used alone, and they are not to be used with modifier -51 (multiple procedures). They are used in addition to the primary procedure code to accurately report an expanded service. The phrase in the parentheses following the add-on code tells exactly what codes the add-on code should be used with, and it may not be used with any other codes.

For example: Physical therapists and occupational therapists sometimes perform a procedure called "work hardening." If this procedure lasts more than 2 hours, an add-on code is used to report the additional time. It appears in the main body of the CPT codebook as follows:

| 97545 | Work hardening/conditioning; initial 2 hours |
| + 97546 | each additional hour (list separately in addition to code for primary procedure) (Use 97546 in conjunction with code 97545) |

Appendixes A through I and the alphabetical index follow Categories I, II, and III in the Level I CPT codebook.

Appendix A contains a complete list of Level I CPT modifiers and selected Level II modifiers (anatomic). Modifiers are used with procedure codes to report that a service or procedure has been altered by a specific circumstance. The Level I and Level II (and formerly Level III) code sets each have modifiers that may be used with code numbers in both levels. Multiple modifiers may be reported when applicable. Some modifiers have restrictions, and some apply only to specific settings. Modifiers are discussed in more detail later in this chapter.

Appendix B contains a summary of codes that have changed since the previous edition. Appendix C gives clinical examples of conditions that might warrant specific levels of E/M services when documentation requirements are also met for the code.

Appendix D is a list of valid add-on codes.

Appendix E is a list of codes exempt from modifier -51 (multiple procedures).

Appendix F is a summary of CPT codes that are exempt from modifier -63.

Appendix G is a summary of CPT codes that include conscious sedation as part of the bundle.

Appendix H is an alphabetical index of performance measures (Category II codes) by clinical condition or topic.

The alphabetical index in the CPT codebook is organized using four primary types of main terms:

- ❑ Procedure or service
- ❑ Organ or other anatomic site
- ❑ Condition
- ❑ Synonyms, eponyms, and abbreviations

Note that while anatomic locations are not included as main terms in the alphabetical index for the ICD-9-CM (diagnosis) codebook, they are one of the primary types of main terms in the alphabetical index for the Level I CPT-4 (procedure) codebook. In addition, while most publishers place the alphabetical index (Volume 2) at the beginning of the ICD-9-CM codebook, the alphabetical index in CPT-4 is located at the back of the codebook.

A main term in the alphabetic index is bolded. It can be listed alone or it can be followed by up to three levels of modifying terms, with the second and third levels of modifying terms indented to show that they only apply to the preceding modifying term.

For example: The main term "Spinal Cord" is followed by many modifying terms. The fourteenth modifying term,

"Puncture," is followed by three indented modifying terms that only pertain to "Puncture." They appear in the alphabetical index as follows:

Spinal Cord
Puncture (Tap)
    Diagnostic   62270
    Drain fluid   62272
    Lumbar   62270
Release   63200

Either a single code or a code range shows where to find the entry in the main body of the CPT codebook. When there are only two codes or the code range is nonsequential, multiple codes will be separated by a comma rather than a hyphen.

For example: The alphabetical index entry for "Radius" with the sixth subterm "excision" has both nonsequential codes, separated by a comma (,), and a sequential code range, indicated by a hyphen (-):

Radius
Excision 24130, 24136, 24145, 24152-24153

Do not code from the alphabetical index alone. Even when only one code is listed, look it up in the main body to be sure the description for the code accurately matches the service performed as it is documented in the medical record.

When the CPT description includes items not performed and a better code is not available, a modifier is required to accurately report that the entire service, as described in CPT, was not performed. Modifier -52 is appended to the CPT code to report a "reduced" service.

When additional items are performed and documented, additional codes and/or modifiers are sometimes, but not always, required to accurately report the service. Modifier -51, multiple services, is often added to additional codes, but sometimes modifier -59 is a better choice, and sometimes codes are exempt from using -51. Read modifier requirements in Appendix A carefully and codebook directions for each specific code carefully. When in doubt, call the payor and politely ask if the codes may be billed together for the same date of service. Remember to document the call: time, date, whom you spoke with, and the directions you were given.

Specific code numbers are assigned in each section of the main body for "unlisted" services or procedures related to that section. **Unlisted procedure codes** are only used when CPT does not contain an appropriate entry. Most often, they are used for new, emerging technology and for seldom-used procedures that do not get enough use to warrant a code. A **special report** is always required when an *unlisted* code is used.

A special report is a detailed description of a service or procedure and an explanation of *why* this service or procedure is the best course of action for the patient. Sometimes a special report is required to clearly identify an unusual, variable, or infrequently performed service or procedure. A special report is usually printed on letterhead stationery and signed by the physician who performed the service or procedure. Supporting documents, such as a photocopy of an article in a medical journal, may be attached to further justify medical necessity.

CPT instructs that any qualified physician may report any of the codes in the CPT codebook. The listing of a service or procedure in a particular section of the codebook does not restrict the use of the codes in that section to any particular group or specialty.

However, be aware that some payors use secret "black box" edits that monitor code selection. They consider these edits to be trade secrets. If your physician does not normally perform the reported service, the claim might be automatically flagged for closer scrutiny. This type of edit might apply when a general practice physician performs a service most often performed by a specialist, such as if an internal medicine physician reports a code for abdominal surgery. It might also apply when a specialist performs a service that is not normally in the scope of that specialty, such as when an orthopedic surgeon reports a code for bronchoscopy.

Payors know that claims that report improbable situations are most apt to occur when a biller or coder transposes two or more digits of the correct code for a service; and coding that reports an improbable situation seldom matches chart documentation. Therefore, it is wise to send supporting documentation with the claim any time you bill a service not normally performed by your provider. Secret "black box" edits are not part of the national standard billing rules and coding conventions, and specific details about them are seldom known.

LEVEL II—HCPCS

Level II HCPCS codes are national codes, and they are required when billing for government payors (Medicare and Medicaid). Each year an increasing number of commercial payors and managed care payors also provide coverage for and require the use of HCPCS codes.

Note: Since October 16, 2003, all payors are required to accept claims with HCPCS codes, but they are not required to provide coverage (payment) for them.

HCPCS codes are used to report services and supplies not included in CPT or procedure codes with more detail than included in CPT. When codes for the same service or supply are available in both CPT and HCPCS, use the HCPCS code unless the payor does not provide coverage for them.

For example:
❑ 92393 is the CPT code for the supply of an ocular prosthesis. D5916 is the HCPCS code for the supply of an ocular prosthesis. For Medicare and other payors that accept HCPCS, use D5916 to report the supply.

99070, the "supply" code in CPT, is very non-specific. The description reads, "supplies and materials (except spectacles), provided by the physician over and above those usually included in an office visit or other service rendered (list drugs, trays, supplies, or materials provided)." Most of the codes in the HCPCS codebook provide specific details about an item that would fall in this nonspecific category in the CPT codebook. For example, A4550 is for "Surgical trays" only, and the entire "J" category is for specific drugs.

HCPCS codes are organized alphabetically and numerically using alphanumeric codes. They begin with a single letter (A through V) followed by four numeric digits. In the 2004 Professional Edition HCPCS codebook published by Ingenix, the index is listed after the introduction but before the main body of codes. Seven appendices follow the main body of codes. The arrangement of information and number of appendixes may vary with other publishers and other editions of the codebook.

The codes in the HCPCS codebook are organized by alpha categories:

❑ *A-codes* report transportation services, medical and surgical supplies, and administrative, miscellaneous, and investigational services, procedures, or supplies.
❑ *B-codes* report enteral and parenteral therapy and the related equipment and supplies (feeding tubes, IV fluids, etc.).
❑ *C-codes* report codes used by Outpatient PPS, the Medicare APC classification system for outpatient hospital charges. The codes mainly represent drugs, biologicals, and devices eligible for transitional pass-through payments. When the diagnosis codes provide medical necessity, they are billed in addition to other APC services.
❑ *D-codes* report dental services and procedures, dental prosthetics, and dental supplies.
❑ *E-codes* report a wide variety of durable medical equipment and devices and related supplies and repairs.

❑ *G-codes* report temporary procedures/professional services. These codes replace many local codes for CMS and other carriers.
❑ *H-codes* report drug and alcohol abuse treatment services.
❑ *J-codes* report a limited selection of drugs and medications, primarily those reimbursed by Medicare. Each code designates routes of administration and a dosage or dosage range applicable to the specific code.
❑ *K-codes* report temporary codes assigned to Medicare's Durable Medical Equipment Regional Carriers (DMERCs) and temporary codes for wheelchairs, wheelchair accessories, spinal orthotics, immunosuppressive drugs, and miscellaneous temporary codes.
❑ *L-codes* report orthotic procedures, devices, supplies, and repairs and prosthetic procedures, devices, supplies, and repairs.
❑ *M-codes* report medical services and cardio-vascular services. These codes also are used to replace former local codes.
❑ *P-codes* report pathology and laboratory services, chemistry and toxicology tests, pathology screening tests, microbiology tests, and miscellaneous tests.
❑ *Q-codes* report temporary codes and include some medication and injection codes as well as some cast supply codes. They also replace some of the former local codes.
❑ *R-codes* report diagnostic radiology services.
❑ *S-codes* report temporary national codes. These are primarily non-Medicare medications and procedures.
❑ *T-codes* are national codes established for state Medicaid agencies. They replace many of Medicaid's local codes.
❑ *V-codes* report vision services, equipment and supplies, hearing services, and language-pathology services.

To find an item in the HCPCS codebook, you look up the item or service in the alphabetical index and confirm the code in the tabular list.

The index is listed after the codebook introduction and before the main body of codes. The alphabetical index is organized by main terms with subterms listed under the main terms. Like the CPT codebook, anatomic locations are acceptable as a main term in the index.

For example: The following is a HCPCS alphabetical index entry:

Insertion
tray, ...A4310-A4316

Please note that a physician must order the medical equipment and supplies listed in the HCPCS codebook in order for a payor to consider paying for the item. For durable medical equipment and some supplies, a certificate of medical necessity must also be completed for Medicare and some other carriers.

Appendix 1 is a complete list of Level II modifiers. HCPCS modifiers are two digits: The first is always an alpha digit, and the second may be either an alpha or a numeric digit. They are recognized by payors nationally, including payors that do not accept HCPCS codes. Some of the HCPCS modifiers are **anatomic modifiers** that identify a specific part of the body. Others clarify the credentials of the provider. Most of the others provide additional details that influence reimbursement. HCPCS modifiers are used with Level I CPT and Level II HCPCS codes.

Appendix 2 contains HCPCS abbreviations and acronyms.

Appendix 3 is a table of drugs.

Appendix 4 contains Medicare references and revisions to the CMS manual system. MCM is the Medicare Carriers' Manual. CIM is the Coverage Issues Manual. This is the largest appendix.

Appendix 5 is a list of companies that accept Level II HCPCS codes.

Appendix 6 is a list of codes for which CPT codes should be reported. Normally, when similar codes are available in both Level I CPT and Level II HCPCS, HCPCS codes override CPT codes except when the payor does not accept HCPCS codes. These codes are the exception to that rule.

Appendix 7 is a list of new, changed, or deleted codes.

STOP & REVIEW

Use a current-year CPT codebook and a current-year HCPCS codebook to answer the following:

1. What codebook is used to report a needle biopsy of a kidney? _____

2. Find the code(s) for a needle biopsy of a kidney. _____

3. What codebook is used to report a vaginal hysterectomy with removal of both fallopian tubes and both ovaries? _____

4. Find the code(s) for a vaginal hysterectomy with removal of both fallopian tubes and both ovaries. _____

5. What codebook is used to report a standard wheelchair? _____

6. Find the code(s) for a standard wheelchair. _____

7. What codebook is used to report aluminum crutches? _____

8. Find the code(s) for aluminum crutches. _____

9. What codebook is used to report a partial mastectomy? _____

10. Find the code(s) for a partial mastectomy. _____

Importance of Code Order

When more than one service or procedure code is reported for the same date of service, the order in which the codes are reported can influence the amount of reimbursement. Services listed after the first service on a particular date are usually paid at a lower rate because some of the work included in each code has already been accomplished and is not repeated. Typically, the first service or procedure code listed is reimbursed at 100%, the second code at 50%, and subsequent codes at 25% to 50%.

For example: When more than one surgical procedure is performed through the same incision during the same surgical session, the patient is admitted once, prepped for surgery once, has one incision, and goes through the recovery room once. This work is paid for in the first code and does not need to be repeated for the second surgical procedure.

Comprehensive codes are combination codes. They are available for many procedures that are commonly performed together. Some codes clearly define everything included in the bundle, and others assume that every step and sometimes every supply inherent to the procedure is included in the comprehensive code package or bundle. You must use the comprehensive code when one is available and everything included in the code has been performed and documented. When a comprehensive code is not available, the second procedure is paid at a reduced rate to accurately reflect the actual amount of work performed.

Codes for each date of service are sequenced on the claim form according to *reimbursement value*, not according to the order in which they are performed. The code with the largest reimbursement value should be listed first, followed by codes in descending order of reimbursement value.

The exact same codes are occasionally reported in a different order for different payors, depending on the payor fee schedules. For some payors, reimbursement value order only applies to surgery, but other payors use this principle for every service. The only way to know for sure is to read your contracts and watch reimbursement trends. To avoid any confusion when your contracts do vary, it is better to develop the habit of listing all codes for a specific date of service by reimbursement value.

For example: Shannon is a 12-year-old girl with a medical history of juvenile diabetes, insulin controlled, and she is recovering from a bout of pneumonia. When Shannon arrives with her mother for a follow-up office visit, a blood glucose (blood sugar) test using a reagent strip ($10.00) and a two-view chest x-ray ($25.00) are performed before the level 4 office visit ($140.00). The medical record documentation supports the level-four office visit, and the results of the blood glucose test and chest x-ray are recorded.

All work associated with each code is included in the code. Because the check-in and the check-out work are only performed once, the second and third codes are paid at a reduced rate. Shannon's insurance plan pays 100% of the first code and 50% of each subsequent code performed on the same date of service.

The level-four office visit has the highest dollar value, $140.00, so it is coded first. Look in the CPT index under "evaluation and management, office and other outpatient." Find the code range in the main body of the codebook. The level 4 office visit code for an established patient is 99214.

The chest x-ray has the second highest dollar value, $25.00, so it is coded second. Look in the CPT index under "chest, x-ray, 2-view" or under "x-ray, chest, 2-view." Confirm the code in the main body of the codebook. The code for a 2-view chest x-ray is 71020.

The blood glucose has the lowest dollar value, $10.00, so it is coded last. Look in the CPT index under "glucose, blood test." Confirm the code in the main body of the codebook. The code for blood glucose by reagent strip is 82948.

When billed correctly, the full price is billed for each code, and the reimbursement is received as follows: $140.00 (100%) + $12.50 (50%) + $5.00 (50%) for a total of $157.50.

If the codes had been billed chronologically instead of by reimbursement value, the total reimbursement received would have been $10.00 (100%) + $12.50 (50%) + $70.00 (50%) for a total of only $92.50, a needless loss of $65.00.

Clinical Application Exercise

Andrea, a 42-year-old woman, is scheduled for a laparoscopy and cholecystectomy to resolve her ongoing problem with gallstones. Presurgical tests reveal that the gallstones are all located in the gallbladder, so an exploration of the bile ducts is not anticipated.

Her surgeon first performs a diagnostic laparoscopy and discovers that Andrea also has an inflamed appendix. After the cholecystectomy is successfully completed, the surgeon also performs an appendectomy before removing the laparoscope, closing the small incisions and sending Andrea to the recovery room.

Use Table 7-1 to calculate the payment the surgeon would expect to receive if Andrea was insured by one of these payors. In each case, the first procedure is paid at 100% and the second procedure is paid at 50%. First, calculate the payment from each payor if the cholecystectomy is listed first on the claim form, and then calculate the payment from each payor if the appendectomy is listed first on the claim form. Finally, identify which procedure should be listed first for each payor.

Payor	$ Cholecystectomy first	$ Appendectomy first	First code
Medicare	$ _____	$ _____	$ _____
Aetna	$ _____	$ _____	$ _____
BCBS	$ _____	$ _____	$ _____

TABLE 7-1
Fee Schedules

Procedure CPT code	Standard Fee	Medicare	Aetna	Blue Cross Blue Shield
47562 Laparoscopic cholecystectomy	$3,500.00	$2,202.00	$2,650.00	$2,750.00
44970 Laparoscopic appendectomy	$3,000.00	$2,225.00	$2,400.00	$2,800.00

Correct Coding Initiative

In the early 1990s, the General Accounting Office (GAO) compared Medicare's software system with commercial and managed care payors' software systems that included an editing process. They concluded that software edits reduced fraud and abuse while saving money. In response, HCFA contracted with AdminaStar Federal, a Medicare carrier in Indiana, to develop software edits for Medicare. The resulting system of edits was named the **Correct Coding Initiative (CCI).** The CCI editing system went into effect on January 1, 1996.

CCI edits are based on:

❏ Coding conventions defined in the AMA's CPT-4 codebook
❏ Coding guidelines developed by national medical societies
❏ An analysis of standard medical and surgical coding practices
❏ An analysis of national and state coding policies and software edits

The resulting edits are defined in the CCI. No other payor publishes this information. Because Medicare based the CCI on the edits of other payors nationwide, a study of the CCI will provide the clearest information available about the edit process for other payors as well.

The AMA's Correct Coding Policy Committee works with the specialty societies to evaluate disputed edits and to evaluate proposed new edits. AdminaStar agreed to regularly review the suggestions it receives and make necessary corrections to the code edits.

Therefore the CCI is dynamic. The rules have changed many times over the years, with additions and deletions in each new version. It is important always to use the most current version of the CCI.

You may pay to subscribe to a quarterly update service through the National Technical Information Service (NTIS) (703-605-6060 or 800-553-6847), or you may purchase a complete copy of the CCI, with code-linking information, from NTIS and update it yourself from your carrier's Medicare updates or from the CMS website (www.cms.gov.hhs). In addition, the entire manual and the updates can be downloaded for free from the CMS website. From the main page, do a search for "CCI" and follow directions.

All the information presented here about the CCI is taken from a purchased edition of the CCI and updated from CMS resources available over the Internet.

PURPOSE

The stated purpose of the CCI is to control improper coding by *promoting* correct coding, *defining* comprehensive codes that describe multiple services commonly performed together, and *preventing* improper **"unbundling"** or **"fragmentation"** of services. The CCI defines when two codes can be billed on the same claim to completely identify a procedure, and it defines when specific code combinations cannot be billed on the same claim.

STANDARDS OF MEDICAL/SURGICAL PRACTICE

All services essential to accomplishing a service or procedure are included in that service or procedure and are part of the comprehensive code for the service or procedure. The description for the code(s) chosen must accurately describe what transpired during the patient encounter, and the code(s) must accurately portray chart documentation.

SURGICAL CODES

Surgical services typically include a specified number of days during which all care related to the procedure is considered to be part of the procedure. This is commonly referred to as the **global period.** In some cases, the global period begins as much as 3 days before the procedure (Medicare inpatients) and may extend as long as 90 days after the procedure. Most of the codes in the surgery section have either a 10-day or a 90-day follow-up period. The smaller procedures (generally those that can be performed in the office) have a 10-day follow-up period and the larger procedures (generally those that are performed in an operating room) have a 90-day follow-up period.

The CPT code 99024 is used to report postoperative follow-up visits that were included in the global charge for the surgery. Additional payment is not expected for these services. However, if a patient is seen during a global period for a visit that is not included in the global charge, modifier -24 is attached to the E/M code for the visit to notify the payor that this visit is an unrelated service, and therefore must be paid separately.

Note: Some payor contracts include different global requirements for specific codes. The payor contract then overrides the national billing guidelines and conventions for those codes for that payor.

Unless otherwise specified, services that should not be separated from a surgical comprehensive code include:

❑ Cleansing, shaving, prepping of skin
❑ Insertion of IV access for medication
❑ Draping and positioning of the patient
❑ Sedative or anesthesia administered by the physician performing the procedure (Modifier -47 is used to identify this service when it is performed.)
❑ Surgical approach, including identification of anatomic landmarks; incision; evaluation of the surgical field; lysis of simple adhesions; isolation of neurovascular, muscular, bony, or other structures limiting access to the surgical field; and muscular stimulation to identify the muscle
❑ Surgical cultures
❑ Wound irrigation
❑ Controlling intraoperative bleeding using clamps
❑ Insertion and removal of drains, suction devices, dressings, or pumps into the same site
❑ Surgical closure
❑ Application, management, and removal of postoperative dressings, including pain management devices and other devices and associated care of the sites (Trans [TENS] units may be billed separately by anesthesia.)
❑ Preoperative, intraoperative and postoperative documentation, including photographs, drawings, dictation, and transcription
❑ Surgical supplies, unless listed as an exception in an existing CMS policy

Through the end of 2003, the CPT manual used a concept called **starred procedures.** Although it is no longer a part of the CPT manual, and therefore no longer a part of the CCI, you may encounter these codes when doing collections on old claims or performing a retrospective audit on old claims. Therefore you still need to know what they were. Surgical procedures that were identified in CPT by an asterisk (*) were called starred procedures. Starred procedures were usually the smallest surgical services. The national billing conventions for starred procedures were printed in the "section guidelines" at the beginning of the surgery section of the CPT codebook.

Code definitions for starred procedures included only the procedure as listed. Preprocedure and postprocedure work varied widely and was billed separately. If complications arose, they were also billed separately.

Unless otherwise specified in a payor contract, preoperative services for starred procedures were billed as follows:

❑ When a starred procedure was performed on the same day as the initial visit for a new patient *and* the starred procedure, though small, was the largest service performed that visit, the codes for the starred procedure and CPT code 99025 were used together to report the service. An E/M code was not billed and follow-up care, if any, was billed separately. Code 99025 was deleted when the starred procedures were deleted.
❑ When a starred procedure was performed during a visit that included a significant E/M service, both services were billed, and modifier -25 was attached to the E/M service. Follow-up care, if any, was billed separately.
❑ When a starred procedure required hospitalization or occurred during a hospitalization, a hospital visit and the starred procedure were both billed. Follow-up care, if any, was billed separately.

Note: Occasionally payor contracts included global requirements for specified starred procedures. The payor contract then overrode the national billing guidelines for those codes. For example, Medicare often assigned a 10-day global period to starred procedures. Ingenix (Medicode/St. Anthony's) publishes a *Medicare Billing Guide* that lists Medicare's global requirements by procedure code. A billing guide for the same year as the claim's date of service will have the global requirements in effect on the date of service.

MEDICAL/SURGICAL PACKAGE

Most medical and surgical services have preprocedure and postprocedure work associated with them. This work is reasonably consistent among similar procedures. Once done, this work does not usually have to be repeated for additional procedures performed at the same session. Unless specifically excluded, it is considered to be included in the CPT code for the service.

❑ Most invasive procedures require vascular access (inserting an IV) and/or airway access (inserting an artificial airway). Therefore, the work associated with obtaining this access is included in the code for the procedure and should not be listed separately.

❑ When vascular access is part of the procedure, maintenance of the access also is part of the procedure and may not be reported separately. Maintaining an IV infusion includes monitoring the infusion and all IV supplies. Maintaining a heparin lock includes monitoring the site and all other supplies, including the anticoagulant.

❑ Airway access and all associated component parts are included in the codes for general anesthesia.

❑ The CPT code for intubation should be used only for emergency intubation.

❑ The CPT codes for visualization of the airway were created for coding a diagnostic or therapeutic service (nasal endoscopy, laryngoscopy, bronchoscopy) and may not be reported as part of other intubation services.

In complex situations, more invasive or more difficult access procedures are sometimes required. *When this is not typical for the procedure performed,* the more invasive or more difficult access procedure may be reported separately.

For example: When a peripheral IV site (a short IV needle/catheter inserted into a vein in an arm or a leg) cannot be established, a central venous line (a long CVP needle/catheter inserted into the largest vein in the chest cavity and advanced into the right atrium of the heart) may become necessary and may be billed separately.

SUPPLEMENTAL, ADD-ON CODES

Supplemental codes, commonly referred to as **add-on codes,** are used with another procedure code to extend the scope of the basic procedure to include

(or add on) the supplemental procedure. Add-on codes always specify the exact codes or range of codes with which they are to be used. These codes may not be used with any other codes, and they may not be used alone. A plus symbol (+) is placed before the code number to identify the code as an add-on code.

For example: 78478 is one of the add-on codes for myocardial perfusion imaging and it adds "with wall motion, qualitative or quantitative study" to the basic code definitions for the specified codes. In parentheses, the code description directs the coder to list the code separately in addition to the code for the primary procedure. Using additional parentheses, the code description further specifies that 78478 may be used with codes 78460, 78461, 78464, or 78465.

Supplemental (add-on) codes describe a separately identifiable service. Some add-on codes modify a CPT code to allow for a range of clinical situations in which the code may be used. Add-on codes are sometimes established to report advances in technology since the original code was first introduced.

Only codes designated as add-on codes may be billed as supplemental codes, and they may only be used with the codes specified in parentheses after the code. Add-on codes are not billed with modifier -51 for multiple services because that information is already built into the code.

In addition, primary procedure codes may not be submitted as "add-on" supplemental codes. When a second primary procedure is clearly a separately identifiable service, the second primary procedure is billed under the rules for multiple services by using modifier -51 with the CPT code for the second primary procedure.

UNBUNDLING

When the entire procedure is performed in one visit, the preprocedure and postprocedure work is only done once, so the comprehensive code is the correct way to convey the actual amount of work performed.

Single component codes include preprocedure and postprocedure work in each code. These codes are included in CPT and HCPCS to provide a way to bill when only one component part of a comprehensive procedure is performed.

Unbundling occurs when a group of procedures that is performed in one visit and covered by a single comprehensive code is billed separately instead of using the comprehensive code. When you bill a comprehensive procedure (performed in one visit) as separate components, you are asking to be paid for the preprocedure and postprocedure work more than once, even though the work is only performed once. Many payors, including Medicare, penalize claims by reducing payments for services they consider unbundled.

For example: When the physician orders multiple blood tests that encompass one "lab panel," the patient is registered once, and one or more vials of blood is drawn using one needlestick (the needlestick is always billed separately). The specimen is prepared once and the test is run on a machine that runs all the tests at one time. On the other hand, when each test is billed individually instead of billing for the panel, you are telling the payor that each test was run separately using separate preparation of the specimen for each test and using the equipment multiple times, once for each individual test. Payors know this is highly unlikely, so their computer system is programmed to flag these claims and automatically impose penalties to reduce payment.

EXCLUDED SERVICES

Because the CCI was originally developed solely for use with Medicare, procedures identified by Medicare as excluded or noncovered services are not addressed in the CCI. Contact your local Medicare carrier to obtain a complete list of noncovered services.

Note: Do not rely on the information in the Medicare remittance notice (MRN) or explanation of Medicare benefits (EOMB) to determine excluded or noncovered services.

An incorrectly coded claim may generate the message "not a covered service" for an item that would have been covered if coded correctly. Often this message only means that medical necessity was not clearly established by the diagnosis codes submitted on the claim.

ADVANCE BENEFICIARY NOTICE OF NONCOVERED MEDICARE SERVICES

When noncovered services are performed on Medicare patients, the patient signs an Advance Beneficiary Notice (ABN) to show that the physician discussed the issue of noncoverage with the patient. The patient acknowledges in writing that Medicare will not pay for the service, and the patient acknowledges in writing that he or she will make financial arrangements to pay for the service. You

keep the ABN in the patient's medical record in case of an audit.

When the patient wants a noncovered service but refuses to sign the ABN, the physician must document in the notes for the visit that:

- ❑ The issue on noncoverage was discussed
- ❑ The patient wants the service
- ❑ The patient refuses to sign the ABN

Medicare will then treat the service exactly as though the patient signed the ABN.

Modifiers -GY, "service not covered by Medicare," and -GA, "waiver of liability statement on file," are appended to the service on the claim form. The modifiers notify Medicare that the service was performed and the proper steps were taken. Both modifiers also are used when the patient consents to a noncovered service but refuses to sign an ABN, because Medicare treats the situation as though the patient signed the ABN.

You will not receive payment from Medicare for the noncovered service(s), but the EOMB sent to the patient will tell the patient to pay the physician's bill for the service.

Note: If a noncovered service is billed to Medicare without these modifiers, the EOMB sent to the patient will tell the patient not to pay the bill. Medicare will not pay, and the patient is not responsible for payment.

Contact your local Medicare office or visit the CMS website at www.cms.gov.hhs to obtain a current copy of ABN requirements. See Figure 3-5 in Chapter 3 for an example of an "Advance Beneficiary Notice of Noncovered Medicare Part B Services."

DESIGNATION OF GENDER

Many procedures are gender specific. Claims with the wrong patient gender for the billed procedure are automatically rejected.

For example: Most claims for OB/GYN practices are marked "female." However, many OB/GYN physicians perform circumcisions, upon request, on newborn boys. In this case, the claim should list the newborn boy as the patient, and the gender should be marked "male." A male circumcision cannot be performed on a female. If the wrong gender is marked out of habit, the claim will be rejected.

Anytime the gender section of the claim form is left blank, gender edits can cause a claim to be rejected, even if the procedure is not gender specific.

STOP & REVIEW

Answer the following questions:

1. Which physicians may perform and report services found in the "Radiology" section of the CPT codebook?
   A. Only radiologists
   B. Only pathologists
   C. Any qualified physician
   D. Only physicians who own radiology equipment

2. All services essential to accomplishing a service or procedure are included in the comprehensive code for the service or procedure.

   ____True   ____False

3. A global period defines the number of days that all care related to a procedure is part of the procedure.

   ____True   ____False

4. May cultures taken during a surgical procedure be billed separately? _____

5. Starred procedures indicate major surgeries with extra-long global periods.

   ____True   ____False

6. Is airway access included in the code for general anesthesia? _____
   _____

7. A peripheral IV is typical for a given procedure. A peripheral IV site cannot be established, and a central venous line is inserted to provide venous access for the procedure. Can the central venous line be billed separately? Why or why not?
   _____
   _____

8. Supplemental add-on codes may be used with any code or code combination.

   ____True   ____False

9. When the entire procedure is performed, reporting the component parts instead of the comprehensive code is called:
   A. Downcoding
   B. Unbundling
   C. Upcoding
   D. Bundling

10. Why is gender important on the claim form?
   _____
   _____

MOST EXTENSIVE PROCEDURE

When procedures are performed together that are basically the same, or are performed on the same site and differ only in the level of complexity, the less extensive procedure is included in the more extensive procedure.

Unless otherwise specified, the following rules apply:

- ❑ When both "simple" and "complex" CPT codes are available, the simple procedure is included in the complex procedure on the same site at the same session.

For example: 46255 is included in 46260 on the same site in the same session. They appear in CPT as follows:
46255   Hemorrhoidectomy, internal and external, simple;
46260   Hemorrhoidectomy, internal and external, complex or extensive;

- ❑ When both "limited" and "complete" CPT codes are available, the limited procedure is included in the complete procedure on the same site at the same session.

For example: 93882 is included in 93880 on the same site in the same session. They appear in CPT as follows:
93880   Duplex scan of extracranial arteries; complete bilateral study
93882   unilateral or limited study

- ❑ When both "simple" and "complicated" CPT codes are available, the simple procedure is included in the complicated procedure on the same site at the same session.

For example: 10080 is included in 10081 on the same site in the same session. They appear in CPT as follows:
10080   Incision and drainage of pilonidal cyst; simple
10081   complicated

- ❑ When "superficial" and "deep" CPT codes are both available, the superficial procedure is included in the deep procedure on the same site at the same session.

For example: 20200 is included in 20205 on the same site in the same session. They appear in CPT as follows:

20200   Muscle biopsy; superficial

20205   deep

❑ When "intermediate" and "comprehensive" CPT codes are both available, the intermediate procedure is included in the comprehensive procedure on the same site at the same session.

For example: 92002 is included in 92004 on the same site in the same session. They appear in CPT as follows:

92002   Ophthalmologic services: medical examination and evaluation with initiation of diagnostic and treatment program; intermediate, new patient

92004   comprehensive, new patient, one or more visits

❑ When "partial" and "complete" CPT codes are both available, the partial procedure is included in the complete procedure on the same site at the same session.

For example: 57106 is included in 57110 on the same site in the same session. They appear in CPT as follows:

57106   Vaginectomy, partial removal of vaginal wall

57110   Vaginectomy, complete removal of vaginal wall

❑ When "external" and "internal" CPT codes are both available, the external procedure is included in the internal procedure on the same site at the same session.

For example: 92960 is included in 92961 on the same site in the same session. They appear in CPT as follows:

92960   Cardioversion, elective, electrical conversion of arrhythmia; external

92961   internal (separate procedure)

SEQUENTIAL PROCEDURES

An initial approach to a procedure may be followed at the same encounter by a more invasive approach. The second procedure is usually performed because the initial approach was unsuccessful in accomplishing the medically necessary service.

There often are separate CPT codes describing the service for each approach. *Pay close attention to this issue.* Sometimes only the more invasive procedure is reported, and other times both procedures may be reported with a modifier. Failure to follow the rules may result in decreased reimbursement and could spark payor audits or government investigations.

Unless otherwise specified, the following rules apply:

❑ If a procedure performed through an endoscope is diagnostic and is followed by a therapeutic surgical procedure through the same endoscope at the same session, bill only the surgical procedure, not both.

For example: When both 45378 and 45380 are performed in the same session through the same scope, only the surgical procedure, the 45380, is billed.

45378   Colonoscopy, flexible, proximal to splenic flexure; diagnostic, with or without collection of specimen(s) by brushing or washing, with or without colon decompression (separate procedure)

45380   with biopsy, single or multiple

❑ If either a diagnostic or a surgical procedure performed through an endoscope is followed by an open procedure with a surgical incision, bill the open procedure as the major procedure and the endoscopic procedure as a secondary procedure with the multiple procedure modifier -51 attached.

For example: A diagnostic laparoscopy is performed to evaluate gallbladder function. A guided transhepatic cholangiography with biopsy is completed, and the surgeon determines the gallbladder must be removed. However, due to a benign abdominal wall tumor that presented a barrier to the scope, the gallbladder cannot be excised using the endoscope. An abdominal incision is required to accomplish the cholecystectomy.

Both procedures may be billed. The abdominal cholecystectomy, 47600, is listed first and the laparoscopy with guided transhepatic cholangiography with biopsy, 47561, is listed second with a -51 modifier attached to let the payor know multiple procedures were performed in the same session.

❑ Simple joint debridement and simple lysis of adhesions are generally considered incidental and are included in the code for the procedure. Therefore if an obstruction (such as an adhesion or a joint artifact) must be removed or destroyed to proceed with a procedure, it should not be billed separately. However, when the obstruction is extremely difficult or time consuming *and* a significant entry documenting the circumstances and the additional time involved is found in the operative report, the procedure may be reported separately with the multiple procedure modifier attached.

Using the gallbladder example above, if the physician documented in the operative note that the length of the procedure was extended by an hour for excision of the benign abdominal wall tumor, the excision of the abdominal wall tumor could also be billed.

The abdominal cholecystectomy procedure, 47600, is listed first. The excision of abdominal wall tumor, 22900, is listed second with a -51 modifier for multiple procedures attached. The laparoscopy with guided transhepatic cholangiography with biopsy, 47561, is listed third with a -51 modifier for multiple procedures attached.

❏ Incidental procedures are those that take so little time and so few resources that they are normally bundled into the other service(s) performed.

Before submitting a claim for an additional procedure that is sometimes considered incidental, be sure the diagnoses in the chart support medical necessity for the procedure, and verify that the medical records meet the requirements for the procedure to be billed separately. When appropriate, attach a modifier.

For example: An intramuscular (IM) injection is a very small procedure. Often the physician does not personally perform this procedure. It is not billed separately unless it is the only billable procedure performed on that date.

Note: The substance injected is billed separately.

❏ If, during an abdominal surgical procedure, an asymptomatic appendix is removed, the appendectomy is not medically necessary, and it takes so little additional time that it is considered incidental and should not be reported separately.

However, if the appendix shows significant pathology, such as inflammation, and the pathology is documented, it may be billed separately as a secondary procedure +44950. As this is an add-on code, it is modifier -51 exempt. On the other hand, when the appendix is ruptured, it is billed separately as a second procedure, 44960, with the multiple procedure modifier (-51) attached because this is not an add-on code.

❏ If a particular procedure is always done in the course of performing a major procedure or surgery, it is included in the code for the procedure and is not billed separately.

For example: If vital signs are always closely monitored using an automatic sphygmomanometer and a continuous cardiac monitor with skin electrodes during a sigmoidoscopy performed in an office setting, the monitoring procedures are bundled into the code for the sigmoidoscopy (45330 to 45345) and may not be billed separately.

Note: An instrument tray and medications are billed separately for procedures performed in an office setting, but the route of administration for medications is bundled into the procedure.

❏ If one code describes a particular procedure, and another code describes the exact same procedure with one additional component, both codes may not be used for the same site during the same session. The more comprehensive code is used alone when both components are performed.

For example: You cannot bill both 42507 and 42509. When both procedures are performed, only the more comprehensive code, 42509, is billed. They appear in CPT as follows:

42507   Parotid duct diversion, bilateral (Wilke type procedure);

42509   with excision of both submandibular glands

WITH/WITHOUT PROCEDURES

Many procedures in the CPT manuals are listed with two codes differentiated as being "with" or "without" something. The rules vary based on the circumstances.

For example:

72146   Magnetic resonance imaging, spinal canal and contents, thoracic; without contrast material

72147   with contrast material(s)

24560   Closed treatment of humeral epicondylar fracture, medial or lateral; without manipulation

24565   with manipulation

19324   Mammaplasty, augmentation; without prosthetic implant

19325   with prosthetic implant

Sometimes it is not appropriate for both the "with" and the "without" to be performed at the same session.

Other times a comprehensive code includes both the "with" and "without" procedures in one code. When available, the comprehensive code must be used when both procedures are performed and documented for the same site in the same session.

For example:

74150 Computerized axial tomography, abdomen;
        without contrast material
74160 with contrast material(s)
74170 without contrast material, followed by with
        contrast material(s) and further sections
74185 Magnetic resonance angiography, abdomen,
        with or without contrast material(s)

Unless otherwise indicated, when "with" and "without" are both performed in the same session for the same site, the "without" procedure is included in the "with" procedure. Only the "with" procedure is billed.

LABORATORY PANELS—CCI

CPT guidelines state that if chemistry tests from automated lists are performed on an individual or emergency basis, they should be coded separately, but Medicare has different requirements. Therefore the CCI states that no matter how the tests are performed, they should be bundled together and reported using the automated code. The individual tests that make up a panel may not be reported separately. It costs less to run the entire panel than to run individual tests, so Medicare wants the physician to order the entire panel, and that is all Medicare will pay for.

Software may be purchased from the National Technical Information Service (NTIS) that enables you to enter the name of a test and find every automated panel that includes that test. It also shows you which codes cannot be used together. This reduces coding errors related to incorrect application of the CCI and makes the CCI more user-friendly. Call the NTIS at 703-605-6060 or 800-553-6847 for more information.

UNLISTED SERVICES OR PROCEDURES

The CCI does not include unlisted services or procedures because of the multiple and varied procedures that can be performed using these codes. Because CCI edits cannot be created to cover procedures that have not yet been developed, Medicare evaluates each of these codes individually.

MUTUALLY EXCLUSIVE CODE PAIRS

Mutually exclusive code pairs represent services or procedures that would not or could not reasonably be performed at the same session by the same provider on the same patient. Definitions of mutually exclusive code pairs are based either upon CPT definition or standard medical practice.

For example: Dilatation of a male urethra and dilatation of a female urethra could not reasonably be performed on the same patient in the same session.

INDICATORS

Medicare has added **indicators** to the CCI to designate which codes can be pulled out of a bundle and which cannot. The indicators are found only in the CCI; they are not found in procedure codebooks.

☐ A "0" indicator means the code cannot be pulled out of a bundle in any circumstance.
☐ A "1" indicator means the code can be pulled out of a bundle with the proper modifier.
☐ A "9" indicator is used for all code pairs whose deletion date is the same as the effective date. This means the edit is no longer active, so the combination may now be billed and no modifier is required.

STOP & REVIEW

Answer the following questions:

In questions 1 through 8, how are the services billed?

1. Both limited and complete versions of a procedure are performed on the same site during the same session. _____

_____

2. Both superficial and deep versions of a procedure are performed on the same site during the same session. _____

_____

3. Both simple and complex versions of a procedure are performed on the same site during the same session. _____

_____

4. A procedure performed through an endoscope is followed by an open procedure with a surgical incision. _____

_____

5. An asymptomatic appendix is removed during another abdominal surgical procedure.

_____

_____

6. An appendix that shows significant pathology is removed during another abdominal procedure.

_____

_____

7. Both "with" and "without" versions of a procedure are performed on the same site during the same session. _____

_____

8. Tests from an automated list are performed on an individual basis during an emergency for a Medicare patient. _____

_____

9. The CCI includes unlisted services or procedures.

____True   ____False

10. CCI indicators designate which codes may be pulled out of a bundle and which cannot.

____True   ____False

Modifiers

Modifiers indicate that the service or procedure described by a code has been altered or clarified by the additional information in the description of the modifier. They are an integral part of both levels of HCPCS. Modifiers recorded in the codebooks for specific levels of HCPCS are not limited to that level. They may be used with codes from both levels.

Specific rules apply to the use of each modifier. Not every modifier may be used with every code. When multiple modifiers are used with one service or procedure code, Level I modifiers are listed first, followed by Level II modifiers.

Although this section of the chapter addresses national standard billing rules and coding conventions, please note that some payors expand the meaning of specific modifiers and restrict the use of others. Also, only the modifiers recognized by Medicare are included in the CCI.

LEVEL I MODIFIERS

Some CPT modifiers are just informational in nature and others have a specific impact on reimbursement.

CPT modifiers are used for the following purposes:

☐ To indicate that a service or procedure encompasses only the professional component (a HCPCS modifier identifies when a service or procedure encompasses only the technical component)
☐ To indicate that only part of a service or procedure was performed
☐ To indicate that an additional service was performed
☐ To indicate that a bilateral procedure was performed
☐ To indicate that a service was provided more than once
☐ To indicate that more than one physician performed the service or procedure
☐ To indicate that unusual events occurred
☐ To indicate the service or procedure was altered in some way

Some modifiers may be used only with certain sections of CPT, and some may be used only in certain places of service. Inside the front cover of a current CPT codebook, you will find a list of the current CPT modifiers with short descriptors and a list of the modifiers approved for hospital outpatient use (also used by ambulatory surgery centers). Sometimes the anatomic modifiers from Level II HCPCS also are listed inside the front cover of CPT. The full description for each modifier and the guidelines for use are found in Appendix A of the CPT codebook.

Traditionally, modifiers have not been approved for inpatient hospital billing, but that may change. Rules similar to those for hospital outpatients and ambulatory surgery centers are currently under consideration for hospital inpatients. Modifiers for hospital billing may or may not be finalized and placed in use by the time you read this textbook. When they are implemented, they are expected to be listed in the CPT codebook.

The available CPT modifiers and the guidelines for using them change from time to time. Always use current-year codebooks and read the modifier descriptions and guidelines every time you receive a new codebook.

Figure 7-1 lists utilization guidelines for Level I CPT modifiers and shows the major sections of the CPT codebook that apply to each modifier. The codes not accepted by Medicare are noted.

LEVEL II MODIFIERS

Most HCPCS modifiers are informational, but many also influence reimbursement. Some convey specific information that does not alter the service or supply, but does influence reimbursement, such as items the beneficiary has been notified about, waivers (ABNs) on file, and geographic location. Some HCPCS modifiers clarify the credentials of the provider and/or the level of involvement of the provider. Nonphysician providers are often reimbursed differently than physicians. Other HCPCS modifiers describe specific circumstances or clarify information about the service or supply, which may or may not influence reimbursement.

Anatomic modifiers are informational HCPCS modifiers. They are used to identify specific anatomic parts of the body when the procedure code does not include that information. Anatomic modifiers are very specific. They not only identify right and left, they specify each finger, each toe, and each eyelid.

When used consistently, anatomic modifiers tell the payor when the problem treated today is a new site and when the problem treated today is a previously treated site. This level of specificity influences statistical studies about the effectiveness of specific treatments as well as influencing reimbursement.

The available HCPCS modifiers and the guidelines for using them change from time to time. Please use current-year codebooks as the authoritative source for current information.

BILLING WITH MODIFIERS

When both CPT and HCPCS modifiers are used for the same service or procedure, the CPT modifier is listed first. Some payors create their own modifiers, which may be used in addition to the CPT and HCPCS modifiers. Check with the payor to learn the correct modifier order when a payor-specific modifier is included.

Modifiers are reported in the second half of block No. 24D on the CMS-1500 medical claim form. (See Figure 4-1 in Chapter 4.)

When more than two modifiers are needed to report a service, use modifier -99 in block No. 24D, and use block No. 19 to list each modifier. Block No. 19 is a multi-use field. You must identify the line number from block No. 24 for the modifiers listed here. *Note:* Some payors prefer to have two modifiers entered in block No. 24D and the remainder in block No. 19.

Presume modifiers -50, -79, -G8, and -QB all apply to line item 1 in block No. 24 of the claim form. These modifiers tell the payor that a bilateral procedure (-50) was performed during the global period from another surgery, but this procedure is unrelated to the other surgery (-79); monitored anesthesia was required due to the complex nature of the procedure (two class B findings) (-G8); and the physician provided the service in a rural HPSA (-QB). A rural HPSA is a designation from the Medicare prospective payment system. It is used to determine the geographic cost factors when calculating payment. One of the following methods is used to record the modifiers on the claim form.

- ☐ One modifier in block No. 24D and the rest in block No. 19: Modifier 99 is entered in block No. 24D, and 1 = 50 79 G8 QB is entered in block No. 19. (Hyphens are not entered on the claim form.)
- ☐ Two modifiers in block No. 24D and the rest in block No. 19: Modifiers 50 and 99 are entered in block No. 24D and 1 = 79 G8 QB is entered in block No. 19. (Hyphens are not entered on the claim form.)

When Medicare claims are filed on paper, modifier -99 is required if more than two modifiers are used. However, when electronic claims are submitted directly to Medicare using the software provided by Medicare, up to three modifiers may be listed in block No. 24D and modifier -99 is not required

Modifier Description M=Medicare does not recognize	#	EM	AN	SG	RD	LB	MD	Reimbursement Axioms and Billing Requirements When Using These Modifiers
Prolonged evaluation and management service	–21	X						Reports services greater than the highest level of E/M service. Physician determines increased revenue. Supporting documentation required. Medicare and TPP
Unusual services	–22		X	X	X	X	X	20 to 30% fee increase allowed if medical necessity is met. Medicare requires supporting documentation. Do not use to report nominal increase in time (15–20 min). May be applied to any code of a multiple procedure claim.
Unusual anesthesia	–23		X					Used to report services that normally do not require general anesthesia. TPP require supporting documentation.
Unrelated evaluation and management service by the same physician during a postoperative period	–24	X						This code should be billed with an E/M code, not a surgical code, and should link to a diagnosis unrelated to the surgery. Medicare and TPP require supporting documentation.
Significant, separately identifiable E/M service by the same physician on the same day of procedure or other service	–25	X						Do not use with minimal E/M service. Assign proper E/M code and increase fee based on level of service. Medical necessity must be met.
Professional component, M	–26			X	X	X	X	Bills the professional component only for a procedure with both a technical and a professional component.
Mandated services	–32	X	X	X	X	X	X	Bill 100% of fee schedule. Sometimes ordering agency pays and sometimes TPP pays.
Anesthesia by surgeon, M	–47		X	X				Caution, many payors will not pay for surgery and anesthesia to the same physician. Check with frequently billed payors for their instructions.
Bilateral procedure	–50			X	X			Use only when a bilateral code is not available. Bill both procedures at full price according to fee schedule and monitor reimbursement from payors. Most payors allow 50 to 100% of the second procedure when this modifier is used. Some payors list the procedure once with this modifier; others list the procedure twice with this modifier on the second code. Not used for inpatient surgery.
Multiple procedures	–51		X	X	X		X	Bill highest value procedure first, and the remainder of procedures with this modifier in descending order by value. Attach this modifier to each secondary procedure code. Do not unbundle procedures. Do not use with add-on codes.
Reduced services	–52	X		X	X	X	X	Reduce fee according to procedure reduction percentage. Do not send documentation unless requested by payor.
Discontinued procedure	–53		X	X	X	X	X	Bill from the fee schedule and monitor reimbursement. Medicare requires supporting documentation to assign final payment. Ambulatory surgical centers use modifiers –73 and –74.
Surgical care only	–54			X				Physicians negotiate percentage of global surgery fee before surgery. Surgeon bills with this modifier and includes the percentage of agreed fee.
Postoperative management only	–55			X			X	Negotiate fee with surgeon for billing. Physician bills this modifier with percentage of agreed fee.
Preoperative management only	–56			X			X	Negotiate fee with surgeon for billing. Physician bills this modifier with percentage of agreed fee.
Decision for surgery	–57	X					X	Should only be reported with E/M codes and certain ophthalmology codes. Use with major procedures. For minor (starred) procedures, use modifier –25.
Staged/related procedure by same physician during a postoperative period	–58			X	X		X	The physician must indicate the reason for the service. Modifier –58 does not alter reimbursement, and global periods still apply.
Distinct procedural service	–59		X	X	X	X	X	Bill second unrelated procedures with modifier at full fee schedule amount.
Two surgeons	–62			X	X			The fee is determined as though one surgeon provided the service. Surgeons negotiate % of fees, requires supporting documentation. All codes must be identical for both surgeons.
Procedure performed on infants	–63			X				Used for infants less than 4 kg unless the code already contains that information. Indicates an increased complexity.
Surgical team	–66			X				Same as above, all surgeons. Total charges may be increased up to 50%.
Discontinued outpatient hospital/ ambulatory surgical center procedure before administration of anesthesia	–73		X	X	X			Use for procedures discontinued before anesthesia is administered. Do not use for elective cancellations before the patient is prepped for surgery. Use modifier –53 for discontinued procedures in other locations.
Discontinued outpatient hospital/ ambulatory surgical center procedure after administration of anesthesia	–74		X	X	X			Use for procedures discontinued after anesthesia is administered. Do not use for elective cancellations before the patient is prepped for surgery. Use modifier –53 for discontinued procedures in other locations.
Repeat procedure by the same physician	–76			X	X		X	Appropriate to bill discontinued modifier on same procedure on line one, with this modifier/ procedure on line two, indicating success the second time. Requires supporting documentation. Medicare and TPP. Do not confuse with modifiers –58, –78, –79
Repeat procedure by another physician	–77			X	X		X	Medical necessity must be met. Supporting documentation advised, not required.
Return to operating room for a related procedure during postoperative period	–78			X	X		X	Medical necessity must be met. Supporting documentation advised, not required. May be performed by the initial physician or a different physician.
Unrelated procedure or service by the same physician during postoperative period	–79			X	X		X	Diagnosis codes must justify the unrelated medical necessity.
Assistant surgeon	–80			X	X			Use same codes as primary surgeon. Bill 16 to 30% of surgical Fee.
Minimum assistant surgeon	–81			X				Bill 10 to 15% of surgical fee and monitor reimbursement by payor.
Assistant surgeon — when qualified resident surgeon not available	–82			X				Bill 20 to 30% of surgical fee. Medicare requires documentation.
Reference outside laboratory, M	–90					X		For billing lab services when physicians pay the lab. Medicare does not recognize, lab must bill Medicare direct.
Repeat clinical diagnostic lab test	–91					X		Use for tests run to obtain multiple results. Do not use to rerun tests or confirm results.
Multiple modifiers	–92			X	X		X	Attach this modifier to the CPT code, and follow with multiple modifiers on subsequent lines of the claim.

EM=Evaluation/Management, AN=Anesthesia, SG=Surgery, RD=Radiology, LB=Pathology/Lab, MD=Medicine,
TPP=Third party payors

FIGURE 7-1

Modifier table. *Note:* This modifier table is not intended to replace the information in the CPT manuals. Some of the modifiers and guidelines may have changed. Please use current-year codebooks as the authoritative reference. (Modified from Holmes DL: *Practical Guide to Medical Billing,* Springfield, Va, NTIS, 1997, pp. 62-63.)

unless there are more than three modifiers. In either case, only modifier -99 appears in block No. 24D when this modifier is used on a Medicare claim.

At one time, there were a few payors who did not accept two-digit modifiers. Five-digit modifiers were available for those payors. The first three digits of a five-digit modifier were 099. Five-digit modifiers were eliminated in 2003.

For example: When a five-digit modifier was required, -51 became 09951 and -22 became 09922.

Sometimes a service is delivered in part by one medical office and completed by another. Modifiers are used to indicate who performed each part of the service.

For example: A radiologist often interprets x-rays taken in a medical office. Taking the x-ray is the technical component if the office owns the equipment, and interpreting the x-ray is the professional component. The office physician, who owns the equipment, bills the x-ray with a -TC modifier; and the radiologist bills the service with a -26 modifier. The payor splits the charge for the service accordingly.

Note: Blood work drawn in a medical office is often sent to a pathologist at a medical laboratory for interpretation, but in this case, the charge is usually different. The equipment to run the tests on the blood is located at the medical laboratory. Therefore the medical laboratory personnel perform both the technical and the professional components of the service. The medical office does not bill the blood test; they may only bill the venipuncture and, when applicable, they may bill for transporting or conveying the specimen to the laboratory. (This is not the same as using an outside lab. See Chapter 4, rules for block No. 20 on the CMS-1500 claim form.)

IMPACT ON REIMBURSEMENT

Many modifiers influence reimbursement. Figure 7-1 lists the national standard guidelines for the impact on reimbursement for Level I modifiers. Because each payor uses modifiers in a slightly different manner, the way modifiers influence reimbursement can be negotiated in payor contracts. Use Figure 7-1 as a pattern to create a table listing the modifier preferences of the major payors for your practice and include specific details from your payor contracts. You want the table to be a useful tool, so include the HCPCS modifiers used most often by your practice, and do not include modifiers that are not applicable to your practice.

Use your CPT and HCPCS codebooks to answer the following:

1. Modifier -51 is attached to:
   A. Each subsequent procedure
   B. E/M codes
   C. The first procedure
   D. The first code reported for the date of service

2. When two surgeons perform a surgery, what modifier is reported?
   A. -66
   B. -62
   C. -77
   D. -80

3. If a surgeon evaluates a patient for an unrelated matter during the global period following surgery, what modifier is used to report the service?

4. Which of the following lengths of visit would meet the requirements to use modifier -21 for a new patient office visit?

A. 22 minutes
B. 30 minutes
C. 55 minutes
D. 80 minutes

5. The same lab test, a CBC (complete blood count), is performed every 4 hours on a patient with suspected internal bleeding. What modifier is used to report the additional tests?

_____

6. Martha had a diagnostic laparotomy this morning. Her blood pressure is now dropping, and she has a weak and thready pulse. Her blood counts have also dropped, and the surgeon suspects internal bleeding. She is taken back to the operating room on an emergency basis for another laparotomy to find and correct the problem. What modifier(s) will be added to the claim for the second surgical procedure?

_____

Continued.

7. When both CPT and HCPCS modifiers are used for the same service or procedure, which are listed first? _____

_____

8. What modifier identifies a service furnished by a substitute physician under a reciprocal billing arrangement? _____

_____

9. What modifier identifies a service furnished by a locum tenens physician (a type of "covering physician" arrangement)? _____

_____

10. Timothy is an 84-year-old Medicare patient. He is scheduled for a procedure that is clearly excluded from Medicare, and he has agreed to pay for the service. Timothy signed an "Advance Beneficiary Notice of Noncovered Medicare Part B Services." When the service is reported to Medicare, what modifiers are used?

_____

_____

Procedures and E/M Services

Most of the time when procedures are performed on the same day as an E/M service, only the procedure is billed. E/M codes are generally used to bill for encounters that do not include a specific procedure. There are a few exceptions to this rule.

When a significant (Level 3 or higher), *separately identifiable* E/M service is performed on the same day as a procedure, both may be billed with modifier -25 appended to the E/M code. Modifier -25 is often used when the symptoms examined during an E/M service lead to the decision for a same-day *procedure*, and the same diagnoses may be used for both services. However, modifier -25 is not used when the visit results in a decision for *surgery*; modifier -57 is used in that instance, especially when the surgery is performed within the next 3 days. Documentation for the procedure and documentation for the E/M service must each stand alone to justify the codes billed.

Clinical Application Exercise

Office notes for Mathew Gibbons (established patient) on 12-05-2005, 10:00 AM:

S: C/O bleeding hemorrhoids, sm amt off and on × 1 year. Bleeding ↑ this AM. Denies abdominal pain. BMs—normal, 1 BM/day; stool very dark brown. Denies nausea/vomiting. Denies bloating/gas. Denies other problems. Sleeps well. Personal medical history insignificant. Denies smoking. Occasional social drinker—1-2/month. Parents alive; father Hx colon cancer.

O: TPR 98.7-84-18, BP 132/76 Well-nourished 42-year-old man, alert & oriented × 3. HEENT: WNL. Lungs: clear. HR: reg w/o murmurs or gallops. Abd: soft, flat, +BS × 4, rectal exam +: multiple small hemorrhoids & sm-mod amt fresh bleeding. Stool very dark, Hemoccult +. + pedal pulses, no pedal edema. Reflexes: WNL.

A: Multiple small internal hemorrhoids, bleeding; occult blood in stool. R/O other source of bleeding higher in GI tract.

P: Discussed options. Stat CBC. Scheduled colonoscopy this PM.

Office notes for Mathew Gibbons on 12-05-2005, 2 PM:

S: This 42-year-old male was seen this AM for internal bleeding hemorrhoids. Occult blood was found in his stool. He is here now for a colonoscopy to treat the bleeding hemorrhoids and rule out any other source of GI bleeding. Hgb 11.8, Hct 37.

O: TPR 98.6-88-20, BP 128/72. Medicated with Valium 5 mg IM. Flexible endoscope inserted through rectum. Five small hemorrhoids, each 2 cm × 3 cm noted on anterior surface of rectum, two hemorrhoids are bleeding. Cauterized using bipolar cautery.

No further bleeding noted. Endoscope advanced through descending colon—colon wall normal, no problems noted. Endoscope advanced through transverse colon—colon wall normal, no problems noted. Endoscope advanced through ascending colon—colon wall normal. No further bleeding noted.

A: Bleeding internal hemorrhoids, successfully treated with cautery. Monitored VS q15 min × 1 hr postprocedure. Stable. Tolerated the procedure well.

P: RTC 1 week. Rx Tylenol # 3, 1 tab P.O. q4h prn. Rx Proctofoam, apply in rectum qid × 7 days. Instructed to call if complications noted: bleeding, fever, unusual drainage, unusual pain.

Physician services for both visits are reported on one claim. Code the diagnoses and procedures for Mathew Gibbons on 12-05-2005.

Diagnosis codes: _____

Procedure codes with modifiers: _____

Injections

Because injections are sometimes administered without an accompanying office visit, there are three commonly accepted sets of rules for coding injections. Medicare follows these rules. Check with the individual payors for their rules on this issue.

1. When only an injection is given (as is common with antibiotic shots), bill the CPT injection code and the HCPCS J-code identifying the substance administered.
2. When an injection other than an immunization is given as part of an office visit during which an E/M service is performed, bill the CPT E/M code and the HCPCS J-code to identify the substance administered. Do not bill the injection code because that work is included in the E/M service.
3. CPT rules state that the injection is coded separately for immunizations, even when administered during an E/M visit, and CPT includes both supply and administration codes for immunizations. But remember, whenever the same supply or procedure code is listed in both CPT and HCPCS, the HCPCS code takes preference for Medicare and other payors that accept HCPCS codes.

A nurse may provide a Level 1 E/M service for an established patient if the physician is present in the office and if the E/M documentation requirements are met for a Level 1 visit. The service is billed as though the physician provided the service. These rules are found in the HCPCS codebook in Appendix 4: Medicare Carriers Manual (MCM) References under item 2049.3, the "incident to" requirements for injections and for other professional services. Rules can change from year to year. Read these rules carefully before billing "incident to" services.

Laboratory Panels–Payors Other Than Medicare

Automated or multichannel tests. All the tests in the panel must be done, and no other tests may be added to the panel. If all the tests are not done, each test should be billed separately. When chemistry tests are performed individually for immediate or emergency purposes, the chemistry codes should be used because individual tests are not automated. Medicare has different rules. Please see the CCI section of this chapter.

Organ- or disease-oriented panels. These panels were developed for coding purposes, not as clinical guidelines or clinical rules. Some panels have limited usefulness and must meet medical necessity requirements. Other tests may be performed in addition to organ- or disease-oriented panels. When adding tests to a panel, check the list of available automated tests to see if your new combination of total tests performed meets any criteria already established for another panel before reporting the added tests separately.

Chemistry tests. These codes are listed when the test is performed manually or using a different type of equipment than the automated, multichannel type of equipment.

Unlisted Services or Procedures

In each section and subsection of the CPT codebook, the last codes listed typically end in either -9 or -99 and are used to report a service that is not described anywhere else in the CPT manual. These codes are used primarily for new technology or advanced methods of performing a procedure. Frequent use of these codes is not appropriate except for research facilities. Eventually new procedures are assigned codes.

Linking Procedure Codes to Diagnosis Codes

Each procedure code must be linked to the primary diagnosis code for the service listed on that line. Payors use this information when they establish medical necessity. If even one procedure code is linked to a diagnosis that is inappropriate for the procedure, the service on that line will be denied due to "lack of medical necessity." Procedure codes are never linked to E-codes.

Block No. 24E on the CMS-1500 medical claim form is used to record this information. Most payors want you to list only the line number from block No. 21 to identify the diagnosis code, but some payors, such as Medicaid in some states, want the entire diagnosis code to be entered in block No. 24E.

Medicare stipulates that each service may be linked to only one diagnosis code. Other payors vary in their policies. Many practice management computer systems have a default that automatically links each procedure code to every listed diagnosis code or every procedure to the diagnosis listed on line 1. The primary diagnosis for an overall visit is seldom the primary diagnosis for every service reported on the claim. If your computer system has an incorrect default setting, contact the software company and ask them to fix the problem.

Medicare considers it to be an abusive practice when every procedure is linked to every diagnosis. Abuse that occurs repeatedly without correction can be reclassified as fraud. Most payors track the billing and coding history for each physician. When improper code linkage is identified as a trend, many payors automatically impose a penalty on every claim from that physician.

Clinical Application Exercise

The superbill lists the following diagnosis and procedure codes for a Medicare patient:

Diagnosis:

1) V70.0 General medical exam

2) V13.01 Personal history urinary calculi

3) V18.0 Family history of diabetes mellitus

4) V17.3 Family history of ischemic heart disease

Procedures:

1) 99214 Office visit, established patient   Links to _____

2) 93000 12 lead EKG with interpretation and report   Links to _____

3) 80053 Comprehensive metabolic panel   Links to _____

4) 80061 Lipid panel   Links to _____

5) 81001 Urinalysis with microscopy   Links to _____

Coding Surgical Procedures

Some payors require that the operative report accompany the claim form for a surgical procedure. If the contract does not address this issue, you might consider calling the payor before sending the claim to ask the payor's preferences.

An operative report includes the following information:

❑ Location of procedure performed
❑ Preoperative diagnosis
❑ Scheduled procedure(s)
❑ Date of surgery
❑ Postoperative diagnosis
❑ Procedure(s) performed

❑ Narrative description of the procedure including the approach used, a detailed description of each step taken during the procedure, normal and abnormal findings, conclusions, status of the patient at the conclusion of the procedure, and where the patient was sent after the recovery room.

You must read the operative report in order to assign the diagnosis and procedure codes for the claim. Make a photocopy of the operative report, and use a highlighter to identify the items that are important for billing.

Only the postoperative diagnoses are coded, and only the procedure(s) actually performed are coded. You must be sure the narrative description of the operative report matches the requirements for the procedure code(s) chosen. The operative report narrative often reveals a more extensive procedure than is officially listed at the top of the report. Sometimes the narrative also reveals other details that influence the code choice or modifiers and reimbursement.

Compare the codebook description of the procedure with the operative report's narrative description of the procedure. Highlight any items

included in the operative report that differ from the codebook description.

- ❏ Do any items represent a lesser service?
- ❏ Do any items represent a greater service?
- ❏ Does another code more closely match the procedure described in the operative report?
- ❏ Is an add-on code needed?
- ❏ Is an additional code needed?
- ❏ Is a modifier needed?

The codes placed on the claim form must match the actual procedure performed as closely as possible.

Clinical Application Exercise

Code the diagnoses and the surgical procedure as they would be billed by the physician's office:
Location: Lake Eola Shores Hospital
Name: Ursula Pederson
D.O.B.: 5-24-1932
Preoperative diagnosis: LUQ abdominal pain
Scheduled procedure: colonoscopy
Date: 4/15/2000
Postoperative diagnosis: colon polyp
Procedure performed: colonoscopy
Medicated with Versed 5 mg IV. The procedure began at 8:05 AM. A flexible endoscope was inserted per rectum. The sigmoid colon was observed with normal findings. The scope was advanced into the descending colon. A large polyp measuring 5 cm × 6 cm × 2 cm was visualized on

the posterior wall 20 cm into the descending colon. The polyp was successfully removed using a snare, and the specimen was sent to the lab for analysis. No bleeding noted. The scope was advanced into the transverse colon. No abnormalities were noted. The scope was advanced into the ascending colon. No abnormalities were noted. The procedure was completed, and the scope was removed at 8:27 AM. Patient tolerated the procedure well. Vital signs were monitored for an additional 30 minutes, and the patient was returned to her room in stable condition.

Diagnosis code(s): _____

Procedure code(s): _____

Role of Procedure Codes in Reimbursement

Payment for medical services is strongly influenced by the modifiers attached to the procedure codes and by code linkage to diagnosis codes. It is also strongly influenced by code sequencing and by whether the most relevant codes and modifiers are chosen. Procedure codes must accurately portray the events that occurred, and they must closely match chart documentation.

Payors word their contracts very carefully. Usually physicians agree to follow the current national standard billing rules and coding conventions. They agree to use current-year codebooks. In addition, physicians usually agree to cooperate with the payor's utilization review or quality assurance process and to accept the payor's decisions. Therefore even though it is not clearly spelled out, physicians agree in the contract to accept any payor-imposed penalties that occur as a result of the utilization

review or quality assurance process. Furthermore, physicians agree not to charge the patient for anything except the copayments and deductibles as listed in the contract. Contracted physicians are not usually allowed to balance-bill patients for payor-imposed payment reductions.

Be aware that many times a reason code on an EOB (explanation of benefits) for a reduced payment will merely state that "payment is in the amount agreed to in the contract," and it will not alert you to the fact that the payment was penalized. Very few medical practices appeal claims or contest payments when that reason code appears on an EOB. Most medical practices grumble about the low payment and feel powerless to act. In this chapter, you have learned how to choose and sequence procedure codes and modifiers. In Chapter 13 you will learn what steps you can take when payment has been reduced.

When unbundling is blatant, sometimes payors will specifically list "unbundling" on an EOB as a reason for the "allowed" amount of payment or nonpayment. Most often, reason codes on EOBs are very vague, and you must learn and follow the rules if you want to correct a problem that is influencing reimbursement.

Procedure coding has far-reaching effects for many parties.

Provider's practice. When the medical coding accurately and completely portrays the medical encounter the first time:

- ❏ There will be fewer requests for additional supporting documentation.
- ❏ Employees will spend fewer hours on these tasks, leaving them free to complete other duties.
- ❏ Claims will avoid most penalties and sanctions.
- ❏ Practice expenses associated with repeat billing and sending additional documentation are decreased (labor, postage, supplies, photocopies).
- ❏ Fewer hours are spent by employees negotiating with payors for authorization of additional services (referrals, tests, supplies, medical equipment, etc.).

Patients:

- ❏ Many patients have already prepaid their insurance plan for the services rendered. If the physician receives less revenue than expected from the payor because of incorrect coding or inaccurate claim preparation and then balance-bills the patient, the physician is asking the patient to pay twice for the same services.
- ❏ When services are not coded correctly, covered services the patient is entitled to receive are often denied or inexcusably delayed. Patients seldom know the reason services are denied or delayed, and they experience frustration trying to obtain the coverage they have purchased from their insurance plan. The increased stress can sometimes adversely affect the patient's health.
- ❏ Correct and accurate medical coding greatly enhances patient satisfaction. Patients do not have to struggle to receive the services they have purchased from their medical plan.

Third-party payors:

- ❏ Many payors will "downcode" a claim and only pay for the level of service that is justified by the medical diagnoses submitted on the claim, without requesting additional documentation.

- ❏ Payor contracts often include a section that requires coding to be done correctly and allows payors to impose penalties when this is not done correctly. The penalties are seldom clearly spelled out. Payors benefit financially from this method of conducting business.

PLACE OF SERVICE

Although both billers and coders should know all the rules, typically certified medical coders select diagnosis codes and procedure codes, whereas insurance billers select the **place of service codes** and **type of service codes** for each procedure.

Reimbursement sometimes varies, depending on where the service was performed. For example, supply trays often can be billed when a procedure is performed in a private office, but not when the same procedure is performed in a hospital or an outpatient facility that bills facility charges using a UB-92 claim form. This is because facility charges represent overhead costs incurred by the facility, and supply trays are part of those overhead costs.

Place of service codes can be either two-digit numeric codes or one-digit alpha or numeric codes. Check with your individual payors for the best results when selecting place of service codes.

The place of service codes found in Box 7-1 are used for electronic transmission in the NSF format. The electronic clearinghouse then converts the codes into the format preferred by each payor.

Many payors have very specific rules about the authorized place(s) of service for each procedure code. If a procedure that can only be performed in select settings is billed with a place of service code for an unauthorized setting, the claim will be denied.

For example: Open-heart surgery typically can only be performed on hospital inpatients (21). This procedure is not an authorized office procedure (11). If the surgeon's bill is submitted with a place of service code 11, the claim will be denied.

A physician's hospital visits are not billed on the same claim form as the office visits for the same patient. When services are rendered in more than one place of service, a separate claim form is completed for each place of service.

TYPE OF SERVICE

The place of service and type of service codes work together to provide a clearer picture of what occurred. Reimbursement for the same service,

Box 7-1 Place of Service Codes

- ❏ 11-Office
- ❏ 12-Home
- ❏ 21-Hospital (inpatient)
- ❏ 22-Hospital (outpatient)
- ❏ 23-Emergency
- ❏ 24-ASC (Ambulatory Surgery Center)
- ❏ 25-Birthing Center
- ❏ 26-Military Facility
- ❏ 31-Skilled Nursing Facility
- ❏ 32-Nursing Facility
- ❏ 33-Custodial Care
- ❏ 34-Hospice
- ❏ 41-Ambulance (land)
- ❏ 42-Ambulance (air/water)
- ❏ 50-Federal Health Clinic
- ❏ 51-Psych. Facility (inpatient)

- ❏ 52-Psych. Facility (partial hospitalization)
- ❏ 53-Community Mental Health
- ❏ 54-Intermediate Care Facility
- ❏ 55-Residential Facility-Substance
- ❏ 56-Residential Facility-Psychiatric
- ❏ 61-Comp. Rehabilitation-Inpatient
- ❏ 62-Comp. Rehabilitation-Outpatient
- ❏ 65-End-Stage Renal Disease
- ❏ 71-Public Health Clinic (state or local)
- ❏ 72-Health Clinic (rural)
- ❏ 81-Independent Laboratory
- ❏ 99-Other Unlisted Facility
- ❏ 5*-Day Care Facility
- ❏ 6*-Night Care Psychiatric Facility
- ❏ W*-Walk-In Facility

procedure, or supply code may vary, depending on the information entered here. For example, valid types of service choices for durable medical equipment (DME) include used DME, rental DME, and purchased DME. Each of these has a different reimbursement value for the same supply code.

There is a wide range of type of service choices for consultation services. Valid choices include consultation, preadmission testing, second surgical opinion, third surgical opinion, surgery, ASC facility, medical care, anesthesia, and other medical. Reimbursement varies for different types and places of services for the same consultation codes, and the consultation code chosen must agree with the type of service code chosen.

Most payors require type of service codes. Although Medicare documents clearly state Medicare does not require type of service codes, these codes might be included in Medicare's black box edit

process. On the Noridian website for Arizona's Medicare Part B, the seventh reason listed under "Why Medicare claims are not paid the first time" is, "An invalid type of service compared to the provider specialty."

Valid national standard "type of service" code choices are found in Box 7-2.

Each line on a claim form could have the same place of service code but different type of service codes.

For example: In the course of one office visit, Mrs. Jones received a Level 4 E/M service, a chest x-ray, and a pneumonia vaccine.

Place of Service	Type of Service	Procedure
11	01	Level 4 E/M
11	04	Chest x-ray
11	19	Pneumonia vaccine

Legal Issues

Upcoding is billing for a higher level of service or a more extensive service than is supported by chart documentation. Upcoding includes circumstances when only a component part of a service is performed, but the comprehensive code is billed. Upcoding also includes using modifiers to report increased services that did not occur or failing to use modifiers to report reduced services.

Downcoding is billing for a lower level of service or a less extensive service than is supported by chart documentation. Downcoding includes circumstances when a comprehensive service is performed, but only a component part is billed. Downcoding also includes failing to use modifiers to report increased

services or using modifiers to report reduced services when the full service was actually performed.

Unbundling is often, but not always, an illegal billing practice. Illegal unbundling includes:

- ❏ Billing a comprehensive procedure as component parts to increase reimbursement
- ❏ Billing both a lesser procedure and a more extensive version of the same procedure performed on the same site at the same session
- ❏ Billing both a "with" and a "without" procedure on the same site at the same session, unless a comprehensive code lists both

Box 7-2 Type of Service Codes

- ❑ 01-Medical Care
- ❑ 02-Surgery
- ❑ 03-Consultation
- ❑ 04-Diagnostic X-ray
- ❑ 05-Diagnostic Laboratory
- ❑ 06-Radiation Therapy
- ❑ 07-Anesthesia
- ❑ 08-Surgical Assistance
- ❑ 09-Other Medical
- ❑ 10-Blood Charges
- ❑ 11-Used DME
- ❑ 12-DME Purchase
- ❑ 13-ASC Facility

- ❑ 14-Renal Supplies in Home
- ❑ 15-Alternate Method Dialysis
- ❑ 16-CDR Equipment
- ❑ 17-Pre-admission Testing
- ❑ 18-DME Rental
- ❑ 19-Pneumonia Vaccine
- ❑ 20-Second Surgical Opinion
- ❑ 21-Third Surgical Opinion
- ❑ H*-Hospice
- ❑ I*-Injections
- ❑ T*-Dental
- ❑ X*-Maternity
- ❑ 99-Other for (prescription drugs)

- ❑ Incorrectly sequencing procedures (sometimes)
- ❑ Incorrectly reporting lab services (sometimes)

There are times when the full service is not performed, and unbundling is the correct way to report the service. Unbundling is permissible when:

- ❑ Only one component is performed in a service that has both technical and professional components
- ❑ The description of the comprehensive service includes items that were not performed, and codes are available to report each component part

For example: If only three lab tests from a four-test panel are performed, each lab test should be listed individually unless another combination code is available that includes only the three tests actually performed.

Medicare rules sometimes differ. For Medicare, follow the rules in a current version of the CCI.

When component codes are not available to accurately report the lesser service by unbundling, the full comprehensive code is appended with modifier -52 to report the reduced service.

- ❑ A payor wants you to unbundle codes owing to a specific circumstance.

For example: In some states, Medicaid does not permit use of a global code to report a normal pregnancy and delivery with a global follow-up period. Instead, Medicaid wants each component visit and service to be billed separately at the time of service. This is because Medicaid eligibility is determined monthly. It is not

reasonable to use a code that encompasses a 10.5-month time period when eligibility can change many times during that period.

Fragmentation occurs when a service that is normally completed in one visit is broken apart to require two or more visits. Fragmentation is considered fraudulent anytime services are broken apart solely to generate charges for two visits, thereby increasing payment for the overall service or procedure. However, fragmentation is not always illegal.

There are times when fragmentation must occur. For example, when the patient is unable to tolerate completing the service in one visit, the service or procedure may be staged into two or more steps.

Procedures that are always staged have specific codes assigned to split the charges and correctly identify the service rendered at each stage. When "staged" codes do not exist and unbundling does not correctly identify the service rendered, modifiers are used to correctly report a fragmented service.

With surgical procedures, modifier -52 for reduced services is used in the first session, and modifier -58 for staged/related procedures during a postoperative period is used to report the completion of each stage. When the service or procedure is not surgical, each stage of the service is reported with modifier -52 for reduced services.

For example: Psychological testing is billed in hourly increments. Sometimes the condition and tolerance level of the patient is very limited. When a session lasts only 15 minutes, only 25% of the service has been delivered. The service is billed with a reduced services modifier (-52) and 25% of the usual fee is recorded on the charge line.

How to Help Physicians Meet Procedure Code Requirements

If your practice bills Medicare, the Correct Coding Initiative (CCI) manual and/or software will help you pass the thousands of Medicare edits contained in the CCI.

The *Surgical Cross-Coder,* published by Ingenix (Medicode/St. Anthony's), cross-references ICD-9-CM Volume 3 procedure codes (billed by hospitals) with CPT procedure codes (billed by physicians) so the codes match when they reach the payor.

The *Coder's Desk Reference,* published by Ingenix (Medicode/St. Anthony's), explains each CPT code in lay terms, gives lay terms for many medical abbreviations, includes an anesthesia crosswalk, gives tips for using modifiers, and gives coding tips.

A well-designed superbill guides the physician into fully describing each service so they may be coded correctly. When only a limited number of services is offered by the specialty, each available CPT code and HCPCS code may be listed on the superbill. If you choose to list procedure codes, you must list every procedure code in the scope of services offered by the practice to avoid being charged with pigeonholing.

When a wide range of services is offered by the practice, it becomes impractical to list every procedure code in the scope of services offered by the practice. Instead, properly worded fill-in-the-blank choices on the superbill can guide each physician into fully describing services. Please see Figure 3-11 in Chapter 3 for an example of a superbill that uses fill-in-the-blank choices.

Future Changes

HIPAA initiated sweeping changes in the entire medical industry, and medical coding is no exception. Many changes are on the horizon in the next few years.

NEW RULES

Since July 1, 2000, new vaccine product codes for specific routes of administration have been released twice a year for use as of July 1 and January 1 of each year. Only codes for new vaccines are released biannually in this manner. These codes are called "early release" codes.

In July 2000, a new modifier was also released. Modifier -27 denotes multiple outpatient E/M encounters on the same day. This modifier was designed to correlate with the new ambulatory payment classification (APC) requirements and is used in hospital outpatient settings.

PROPOSED FINAL RULE FOR CODE SETS

In June 2001, the Secretary of Health and Human Services released the final rule to establish standards for transactions and code sets, as required by the HIPAA. The implementation phase began when the final rule was released, and the initial date for mandatory compliance was October 16, 2002. This deadline was extended 1 year for small health plans, but by October 16, 2003, everyone should have come into compliance and all payors must accept all the code sets detailed by this rule.

All health plans will be required to receive and process all standard codes, even codes they do not cover and codes they do not reimburse. With very few exceptions, changes can be made to code sets only once a year. This will simplify claim submission for providers and improve data quality.

The code sets established under this rule as the official code sets are:

❒ ICD-9-CM *(International Classification of Diseases, Ninth Revision, Clinical Modification)*
❒ CPT-4, Level I *(Current Procedural Terminology, Fourth Edition)*
❒ HCPCS, Level II *(HCFA Common Procedure Coding System)*
❒ CDT-2 *(Current Dental Terminology, Second Edition)*

NDCs (National Drug Codes) were originally included but were temporarily dropped for everyone except pharmacies because software programs could not accommodate the 11-digit NDCs in a space designed to hold 5-digit CPT and HCPCS codes.

Modifications have been proposed for HCPCS Level II to eliminate some of the overlaps and duplications in two areas:

❒ *Dental codes:* The proposal eliminates dental codes from HCPCS Level II and makes the American Dental Association the sole source for the dental code set.
❒ *NDCs:* The proposal eliminates J-codes (medications) from HCPCS Level II and makes

the NDCs the national standard for all transactions requiring drug codes. Health plans, claims clearinghouses, medical facilities, physicians, and other providers will all be required to process the 11-digit NDCs in addition to the 5-digit codes currently processed.

Watch to see whether these proposals are adopted.

CPT-5

The AMA is in the process of developing a new edition, not just an annual update, of CPT. The new edition is called CPT-5. The AMA states the primary objective of CPT-5 is to maintain CPT as the authoritative source for correct procedural coding.

Advance information about CPT-5 states that it will preserve the core elements that everyone is familiar with in CPT. It will continue to use five-digit character codes. CPT-5 is expected to incorporate new procedures more quickly than CPT has in the past. It will be designed to interface more easily with electronic medical records and to streamline the reporting process. It is expected to eliminate ambiguous terms and to define better the differences between code choices for terms that are synonyms.

CPT-5 will contain three categories of codes. Category I codes are the traditional CPT codes first called Category I codes in the 2002 edition of CPT. Category II codes are completely new. They are designed to measure performance. Category III codes were introduced in the 2004 edition of CPT. These codes have four numeric digits and end in a letter (1234F). They will appear in a separate section of CPT following the Medicine section. Category III codes were introduced in the 2002 edition of CPT. These codes describe emerging technology. Services and procedures must demonstrate widespread use before they are assigned Category I codes. Category III codes allow a method to track these services and procedures. In addition, services and procedures that are in the FDA approval process or that have relevance for research will be assigned Category III codes. Category III codes have four numeric digits followed by a letter (1234T), and they currently appear in a separate section of CPT following the medicine section.

Additional information is available from the AMA website at www.ama-assn.org or by calling 312-464-5052.

STOP & REVIEW

Answer the following questions:

1. If a separately identifiable E/M service is performed on the same day as a procedure, may they both be billed? _____

2. If the patient comes in for an injection of tetanus immune globulin and no E/M service is provided, how is the injection billed? _____

3. When a liver profile is ordered, may other lab tests be added to the panel? _____

4. What codes are used to report new technology or advanced methods of performing a procedure?
   A. New technology codes
   B. Advanced method codes
   C. Unlisted service or procedure codes
   D. A and B, but not C

5. Each procedure must be linked to the diagnosis code for the service reported on that line.

   ____True   ____False

6. If your computer system has an incorrect default setting, is there anything you can do to fix the problem? If so, what? _____
   _____

7. If the reason code on an EOB states, "Payment is in the amount agreed to in the contract," you know you have received full payment from the insurance company.

   ____True   ____False

8. How does incorrect procedure coding influence reimbursement for your practice?
   A. Penalties can reduce the amount of payment.
   B. The practice will bear the expenses for rebilling the claims.
   C. Claims will avoid most penalties.
   D. A and B, but not C

9. Reimbursement can vary depending on where the service was performed.

   ____True   ____False

10. Payors never want you to unbundle a comprehensive code.

    ____True   ____False

Chapter Review

Always use current-year codebooks. CPT instructs that any qualified physician may report any of the codes in the CPT codebook. The listing of a service or procedure in a particular section of the codebook does not restrict the use of the codes in that section to any particular group or specialty. However, be aware that some payors use secret edits that seem to limit code choice based on a physician's credentials.

When more than one service or procedure code is reported for the same date of service, the order in which the codes are reported can influence the amount of reimbursement.

CCI edits are based on coding conventions defined in the AMA's CPT-4 codebook, coding guidelines developed by national medical societies, an analysis of standard medical and surgical coding practices, and an analysis of national and state coding policies and software edits. The stated purpose of the CCI is to control improper coding by promoting correct coding, defining comprehensive codes that describe multiple services commonly performed together, and preventing improper "unbundling" or "fragmentation" of services. The CCI defines when two codes can be billed on the same claim to completely identify a procedure, and it defines when specific code combinations cannot be billed on the same claim.

Modifiers indicate that the service or procedure described by a code has been altered or clarified by the additional information in the description of the modifier. Modifiers recorded in the codebooks for specific levels of CPT are not limited to that level. They may be used with codes from every level. Specific rules apply to the use of each modifier. Not every modifier may be used with every code.

Each procedure code must be linked to the principal diagnosis code for the service listed on that line. Payors use this information when they establish medical necessity. When improper code linkage is identified as a trend, many payors automatically impose a penalty on every claim from that physician. Medicare considers it to be an abusive practice when every procedure is linked to every diagnosis. Abuse that occurs repeatedly without correction can be reclassified as fraud.

The place of service and type of service codes work together to provide a clearer picture of what occurred. Reimbursement for the same service, procedure, or supply code may vary depending on the information entered here.

Upcoding is billing for a higher level of service or a more extensive service than is supported by chart documentation. Downcoding is billing for a lower level of service or a less extensive service than is supported by chart documentation.

Unbundling is often, but not always, an illegal billing practice. There are times when the full service is not performed, and unbundling is the correct way to report the service. Modifiers are often required when services must be unbundled.

Fragmentation occurs when a service that is normally completed in one visit is broken apart to require two or more visits. Fragmentation is considered fraudulent anytime services are broken apart solely to generate charges for two visits, thereby increasing payment for the overall service or procedure. However, fragmentation is not always illegal. For example, when the patient is unable to tolerate completing the service in one visit, the service may be staged into two or more steps. Modifiers are often required when services must be fragmented.

A well-designed superbill guides the physician into fully describing each service so they may be coded correctly. In addition, there are many publications and software tools available to help billers, coders, and providers report services correctly.

Answer the following questions:

1. How many levels of procedure codes are there?

_____

2. Who maintains and updates HCPCS codebooks?

_____

3. Who maintains and updates CPT codebooks?

_____

4. Which codebook would you look in first to find the code for a diagnostic procedure?

_____

5. Which codebook would you look in first to find the code for medical equipment or supplies?

_____

6. When sequencing procedure codes, how do you determine which code to list first?

_____

7. What is "CCI" an abbreviation for? _____

_____

8. All services essential to accomplishing a service or procedure are part of the _____ _____ for the service or procedure.

9. When a service includes a specified number of days of follow-up care, what is this timeframe of covered care called? _____

_____

10. What are starred procedures? _____
_____

11. May preprocedure and postprocedure work be billed separately when a full, comprehensive service is provided? Why or why not? _____
_____

12. If the preprocedure or postprocedure work is greater than normal, may the additional work be billed? Why or why not? _____
_____

13. What is the purpose of add-on codes? _____
_____

14. Why are single component codes included in CPT?
_____
_____

15. If a service is listed as a noncovered service for Medicare, may the physician provide the service and receive payment? If yes, what steps must be taken?
_____
_____
_____
_____
_____
_____
_____

16. A diagnostic proctosigmoidoscopy is followed during the same session using the same endoscope by a surgical proctosigmoidoscopy and removal of a single tumor using hot biopsy forceps. May both procedures be billed? Why or why not? _____
_____

17. A limited sonogram is followed by a complete sonogram during the same session. May both procedures be billed? Why or why not? _____
_____
_____

18. A CAT scan of the neck without contrast is followed by a CAT scan of the neck with contrast during the same session. May both procedures be billed? Why or why not? _____
_____
_____

19. Could CPT codes 53230 and 53235 both be performed on the same patient in the same session by the same physician? Why or why not? _____
_____
_____

20. When using the CCI, what does a "0" indicator mean? _____
_____
_____

Clinical Application Exercise

Samantha is a 25-year-old established patient seen in the office. The following entry is dated January 5, 2006:
S: C/O fever and sore throat × 1 day
O: Throat red with white spots on tonsils. Nasal congestion noted with clear drainage. Ears normal. Lungs clear.
A: Tonsillitis
P: Rx amoxicillin 500 mg P.O. QID × 10 days. RTC PRN.
Find the following information:

Diagnosis code(s): _____

Procedure code(s) with applicable modifiers: _____
_____

Procedure links to diagnosis: _____

Place of service code: _____

Type of service code: _____

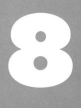

8

PRIVATE INDEMNITY AND MANAGED CARE MEDICAL PLANS

Objectives After completing this chapter, you should be able to:

- Distinguish the differences and similarities among the various private medical plans
- Relate facts unique to indemnity medical plans, such as: qualifications, patient expenses, coverage, circumstances in which they may interact with Medicare, and/or billing considerations
- Relate facts unique to HMO managed care medical plans, such as: qualifications, patient expenses, coverage, circumstances in which they may interact with Medicare, and/or billing considerations
- Relate facts unique to PPO managed care medical plans, such as: qualifications, patient expenses, coverage, circumstances in which they may interact with Medicare, and/or billing considerations
- Explain the meanings of various insurance clauses and how the clauses may affect patients and medical office employees

Key Terms

actuaries mathematicians who study trends and set insurance premiums, deductibles, and copays.

authorization number proof that prior approval was obtained for a specific service: treatment, test, or procedure. It does not guarantee coverage if the claim does not establish medical necessity.

Blue Cross and Blue Shield (BCBS) medical plans organized during the Great Depression as nonprofit, low-cost medical plans operating under special laws with less government red tape. Blue Cross covered hospital costs and Blue Shield covered physician costs. The plans have since merged, and many states dropped the nonprofit status to compete. They are no longer low cost.

capitation a method to pay physicians based on the number of patients assigned by the medical plan rather than actual costs incurred. The physician controls the expense of rendering care.

coinsurance the portion of covered medical care costs for which the patient has a financial responsibility. Often a deductible must be met first. *Copay* refers to either coinsurance or copayment.

coordination of benefits allows payors to reduce payments by the amount of coverage provided elsewhere so reimbursement is never greater than the actual charge.

copayment a cost-sharing agreement in which the patient pays a specified fee for specified services, and the medical plan pays the remainder of the cost. *Copay* can refer to either copayment or coinsurance.

deductible a specified amount of expense the patient must pay before the medical plan pays anything.

group medical plans medical insurance plans offered to groups, usually at a discounted rate or with special provisions. Employers are offered guarantee-issued coverage—employees cannot be excluded from the plan, and preexisting conditions are covered in accordance with the Health Insurance Portability and Accountability Act of 1996 (HIPAA) and subsequent related laws.

health insurance portability allows individuals to keep employer-group medical insurance plans when changing jobs.

HMO health maintenance organization; a managed care medical plan.

indemnity the purest form of commercial medical

insurance. The patient directs his or her own care and pays a deductible as well as a percentage of the costs.

individual medical plans insurance policies offered to individuals rather than groups. Individuals can be denied coverage. Under HIPAA, insurance portability is tied to employer-group plans in which an employee changes jobs.

medical necessity a medically sound reason for ordering a specific service.

MIB Medical Information Bureau; an organization formed by insurance companies in 1902 to share or pool subscriber information related to health and lifestyle in order to prevent fraud.

out-of-plan services rendered by providers or hospitals that do not have a contract agreement with the patient's medical plan.

participating physician (1) a physician who signed a contract with a medical plan and agreed to provide services to plan members; (2) a physician who signed a Medicare contract and agreed to provide services and accept the Medicare fee schedule for Medicare patients.

PP/PM per patient per month; the amount of money a physician receives each month for each assigned patient under a capitation payment system. Some payors call it per member, per month.

PPO preferred provider organization; a managed care medical plan.

preauthorization the process of obtaining prior approval before a service: treatment, test, or procedure. It does not guarantee coverage if the claim form does not establish medical necessity.

preexisting condition any condition with which a person has ever been diagnosed or for which a person has ever received medical treatment.

preferred provider a physician who has signed a contract with a PPO-type of medical plan (similar to an HMO-participating provider).

preventive medicine treatment rendered to prevent medical problems and reduce the incidence of costly medical care.

RBRVS resource-based relative value system; the prospective payment system used by Medicare to pay physicians. It considers the CPT code in relation to work, overhead expenses, and malpractice (risk). A geographical adjustment is then made to account for cost-of-living differences throughout the nation.

right of subrogation allows physicians to be reimbursed by medical plan payors for some or all of the patient charges until payor responsibility can be determined. This is considered a good faith payment. If a different payor is later found to be responsible, the medical plan that paid first is reimbursed for those expenses.

RVU relative value unit; a numeric value assigned to each procedure code in the RBRVS. This number represents the total of each of three parts (work, overhead, and malpractice). Each part is multiplied by the geographic practice site indicator (GPSI) and then added together to get a total adjusted RVU. The total adjusted RVU is multiplied by the conversion factor (the assigned per-RVU dollar value) to arrive at the RBRVS fee allowed for the service.

standards of care protocols tests and procedures are only considered covered services for specific predetermined diagnoses that are not usually disclosed to the physician because they are considered trade secrets. These are commonly called black-box edits.

UCR usual, customary, and reasonable; often the average payment rate that same-specialty providers have accepted in a given region.

Introduction

This chapter gives a broad overview of the major features for private medical plans. Private medical plans include private indemnity plans and private managed care plans. They are the types of policies that patients purchase through employers or organizations and the type they purchase through insurance agents.

The insurance industry separates private medical plans into two categories: commercial medical plans (indemnity) and service medical plans (managed care). Managed care plans include HMOs and PPOs, as well as some new types of policies that combine the features of HMOs and PPOs. Many managed care plans are private medical plans, but an increasing number of managed care plans are government medical plans. This chapter discusses the private managed care plans. Workers' compensation managed care plans are covered in Chapter 9. Medicare managed care plans are covered in Chapter 10. Chapter 11 covers Medicaid, TRICARE/CHAMPUS, and CHAMPVA managed care plans.

The lines of distinction between the various private medical plans are becoming more and more blurred each year as different plans are developed that combine the features of indemnity plans and the various managed care plans to offer a wide variety of choice in medical coverage.

With so many choices available, it is impossible to know everything about every medical plan on the market. Therefore it is important for you to understand the differences and the similarities between the basic features of indemnity and managed care medical insurance plans. Armed with a basic understanding of the industry, you will be able to determine when additional steps might be required, either to help patients obtain authorization for needed medical care or for the practice to receive payment for the care rendered.

Insurance agents offer **group medical plans** and **individual medical plans.** A person must belong to a group to qualify for a group plan. Employers are best known for offering group medical insurance plans. Sometimes organizations, associations, and unions also offer group medical plans.

The Health Insurance Portability and Accountability Act of 1996 (HIPAA) changed the insurance industry by requiring guaranteed-issue coverage for employer groups, with no exclusions for **pre-existing conditions** if there has been no lapse in coverage. This requirement significantly increased the cost of coverage for employer groups. Employers with fewer than 20 employees are defined as small groups. Employers with more than 100 employees are defined as large groups. The size of the group and the age range of the employees are considered in determining the cost of a group policy. Large groups are required by law to include at least one managed care plan in the group's menu of choices.

Individual medical plans may be acquired directly from an insurance agent. They once were the most expensive policies to obtain, but now they are actually a little less expensive than comparable employer group plans. This is because an individual with pre-existing conditions can still be disqualified from obtaining an individual medical policy.

Every state has its own method of oversight for the insurance industry, and they regulate the medical insurance plans available in their state. Therefore when you move from one state to another, your coverage may change even though you keep your existing policy.

The law holds medical plans accountable for specific actions, such as adherence to legal contract clauses and timely payment of clean claims, in much the same way it holds physicians and their employees accountable. Medical plans have also come under scrutiny since HIPAA was signed into law. A number of large, private medical plans were targeted for class action lawsuits under the RICO law (Racketeer-Influenced Corrupt Organization Act) in late 1999. Cost-containment measures were specifically cited in each of the lawsuits. These lawsuits are expected to require years of deliberations, but watch to see what changes, if any, they bring to medical insurance plans as well as to "national standard" medical billing and collections procedures.

Let's take a closer look at private medical insurance plans.

Indemnity Plan

The **indemnity** medical plan is the purest form of a commercial medical plan. This is the traditional policy in which a patient may choose any doctor or hospital. The medical plan pays a designated portion of the bill after a **deductible** is met.

> At one time the indemnity medical plan was an employee benefit at most major corporations. Now large employer groups are required to offer a menu that includes at least one managed care plan. Because indemnity plans are more expensive, employees tend to choose managed care options. As a result, indemnity plans now cover less than 20% of the market in the United States.

With most indemnity plans:

❏ Patients are expected to file their own claim forms. The patient fills out the top portion of the claim form, and the physician either fills out the bottom portion of the claim form or

gives the patient a copy of the superbill to attach to the claim form. (Chapter 4 contains detailed information about claim form requirements.)
❏ Patients may see any physician; they do not have to choose a "primary" physician.
❏ Patients do not need a written referral to see a specialist.
❏ Patients seldom need an authorization from the medical plan before getting tests or treatments the physician has ordered.
❏ Patients seldom need an authorization before admission to a hospital, and they may choose any hospital.
❏ Patients direct their own health care with very little interference from the medical insurance company.

Most indemnity plans cover hospitalization after a deductible has been met. A deductible is a specific amount of expense the patient must pay before the medical plan pays anything. Then the medical plan pays a percentage of costs the payor (the medical plan) decides are reasonable, and the patient pays the remainder of the costs. The patient's share of the cost for covered services is called **coinsurance.**

Hospitalization coverage does not include physician services. Some indemnity plans cover only inpatient physician services, but most plans cover inpatient and outpatient physician visits. Often a separate deductible applies to outpatient care.

Some indemnity plans cover "extras" such as emergency services, lab work, prescription drugs, home health care, maternity care, and wellness care. A few indemnity plans cover "luxury" items such as mental health, drug abuse, transplants, and experimental treatments.

Patients pay most of the medical costs "out-of-pocket" at the time of service and then file a claim with the medical plan for reimbursement. Many medical plans delay sending reimbursement for at least a few weeks and sometimes longer if the payor can find a valid reason for further delay. If the medical plan decides the cost of the service was too high, they will only send reimbursement for the amount the payor considers to be reasonable. Patient expenses are often higher than expected.

Individuals or groups who purchase indemnity plans choose:

☐ The level of coverage
☐ The amounts of the deductibles (inpatient and outpatient)
☐ The percentage of patient costs (**copayments** or coinsurance)

Pricing for indemnity plans varies widely depending on the level of coverage offered in the plan and the amount of costs the patient pays without reimbursement. The disadvantage with this level of customization is that there are no standards for coverage, and the wording of the policy can sometimes be misleading. Patients often believe they have a higher level of coverage than they actually have. Box 8-1 presents the pros and cons of indemnity plans for physicians.

BILLING CONSIDERATIONS

You may collect full payment from the patient at the time of service, and let the patient file the medical claim form. However, many medical offices choose

Box 8-1 Indemnity Pros and Cons for the Physician	
Advantages	**Disadvantages**
☐ Physicians and other providers are not required to sign contracts in order to provide services.	☐ Patient deductibles must be met before the medical plan pays anything.
☐ The scheduler may automatically schedule the appointment with any provider.	☐ Patients pay a larger portion of the costs.
☐ Authorizations are not required for office visits.	☐ Patients often delay seeking treatment when out-of-pocket expenses are high.
☐ Authorizations are seldom required for tests or treatments.	☐ Sometimes coverage is limited, and the patient assumes full financial responsibility for noncovered services.
☐ Authorizations are seldom required for hospitalizations.	☐ Preventive care is seldom covered.
☐ The patient may use any hospital.	☐ Patient statements must be prepared and mailed when patient balances are due.
☐ Authorizations are not required for referrals.	☐ The physicians have less leverage in disputes with the insurer because the physician only has an implied contract to provide services through the patient's medical plan.
☐ Medical practices are not required to submit claim forms, although they may choose to do so.	☐ Collecting past due amounts from patients is time consuming and tedious. It can easily cost more than the amount owed.
☐ Medical practices may ask the patient for payment in full at the time of service, or the practice may choose to extend credit to the patient or to accept assignment from the medical plan for payment of the plan's portion of the fee.	☐ The patient may receive the payment and the EOB, so you do not know if there were any errors causing penalties. Patient's can become annoyed when full payment is not received, even when the reduction was due to a deductible amount, and they may complain to friends and neighbors rather than discussing the problem with you. This is negative advertising.
☐ Medical practices may balance-bill patients for costs not reimbursed by the medical plan.	

to file indemnity claims for their patients in order to retain control over the quality of claim preparation. The rules for standard claim form preparation were covered in Chapter 4.

Regardless of who actually prepares the claim and submits it to the insurance company, the physician is responsible for the provider-supplied information required on the bottom half of the claim form. Even though the physician is not required to sign a direct contract with the medical plan, an implied contract still exists, and legal requirements must be met.

Use the national standard coding guidelines and coding conventions that you learned in Chapters 5 to 7 and follow the standard rules for claim form preparation that you learned in Chapter 4. Always use your physician's standard fee schedule for fees submitted on medical claims.

Monitor the payments received and the explanation of benefits (EOB) that accompanies payment. If full payment *is* received, then you know there are no plan-specific billing requirements to worry about.

If full payment *is not* received, call the medical plan using the telephone number listed on the patient's insurance card (a photocopy of the front and back of the insurance card should be located in the patient's medical record). Ask to speak with a claim adjustor. *Please make an effort to be very courteous every time you speak with a claim adjustor.* Supply the claim adjustor with the patient's insurance information and politely ask the adjustor if there are any plan-specific billing rules. Document the plan-specific billing rules in the patient's *financial* record (not the medical record) so that you do not have to call every time you submit a claim for this patient. In addition, document the claim adjustor's first and last name; his or her position, title or department, and telephone extension; and a summary of the call, including date and time. Then correct the claim using the plan-specific rules in addition to the national standard billing rules. Submit the claim and monitor the payment and EOB to be sure full payment is received.

If full payment *is not* received a second time, call the same adjustor again and politely request assistance. When you are able to ask for the same claim adjustor by name each time you call a medical plan, you are less likely to receive conflicting information. Most claim adjustors will appreciate your efforts to complete claims correctly and will be less critical when you heed their advice.

Do not give in to the temptation to be rude or to blame the claim adjustor for problems, even if you think the claim adjustor deserves the blame. An unhappy or angry claim adjustor can find many reasons to delay payments. The claim adjustor is much more likely to be of real assistance if you treat him or her with courtesy and respect. Remember, the claim adjustor is employed by the medical plan, and the medical plan wants to find valid reasons to delay, reduce, or deny payment.

Sometimes personalities do clash. If you are unable to establish a cordial relationship with one claim adjustor, try working with another claim adjustor until you find one with whom you can establish a good working relationship.

When a claim adjustor has been especially helpful, it is appropriate to send a note of thanks. Address the note to the director for the medical plan and remember to name the helpful claim adjustor. Medical plans receive a lot of negative publicity, and claim adjustors often spend the entire day, every day, dealing with irate people. It is nice to be thanked once in a while. The adjustor will be given a copy of your note, and you will be remembered in a good light.

Some billing employees add their favorite claim adjustors to the medical office's "Christmas and special occasions" list. Cards, and sometimes gifts, are sent to those on the list. This type of goodwill, combined with a sincere effort to file clean claims, paves the way for more favorable decisions when problems arise. This type of gratuity is allowed as long as the monetary value of the gift is nominal. The IRS allows expense deductions for business gifts less than $25.00 each in value, and the recipient is not required to report a nominal gift as "income." More importantly, a nominal gift of this nature is not considered a kickback. Because the office gift list is sometimes long, the typical medical office spends less than $7.00 per gift, well within the range allowed by the IRS.

When there is more than one payor, identifying the correct primary payor is very important. The primary payor is the one who is legally responsible for paying first. The secondary payor pays second, and the tertiary payor, if any, pays third. The one who pays first usually pays the largest portion of the charges, so insurance companies and government payors monitor this issue closely. A good understanding of primary payor/secondary payor rules is essential in a medical billing office.

The following primary payor/secondary payor rules apply for private indemnity plans:

❑ Private indemnity plans are usually the primary payor when there are two medical plans. An exception is when the indemnity plan is through a spouse's employer and the other medical plan is through the patient's employer. Then the medical plan through the patient's employer is the primary payor and the spouse's indemnity plan is the secondary payor.

❑ When a private indemnity plan and Medicare both cover a patient, the indemnity plan is the primary payor and Medicare is the secondary payor. *Note:* Medigap is not an indemnity plan. See Chapter 10 for instructions regarding Medigap.

❑ When a private indemnity plan and Medicaid both cover a patient, the indemnity plan is the primary payor and Medicaid is the secondary payor.

❑ When a private indemnity plan and TRI-CARE/CHAMPUS both cover a patient, the indemnity plan is the primary payor and TRI-CARE/CHAMPUS is the secondary payor.

❑ A private indemnity plan does not provide coverage for services covered by workers' compensation. However, if workers' compensation denies coverage, the normal primary payor/secondary payor rules for indemnity plans applies.

❑ A private indemnity plan does not provide coverage for service-connected care the patient is entitled to receive from the Department of Veterans Affairs (VA).

❑ Non–service-connected care a patient receives from the VA may be billed to private medical plans. When the VA bills an indemnity plan for non–service-connected care given to a veteran, the indemnity plan is the primary payor, and the VA is the secondary payor. See Chapter 11 for further information about the VA.

The insurance industry continuously tests to find the lowest payment rate physicians will accept. Although physicians and patients expect indemnity plans to pay for services using the physician's standard fee schedule, they seldom do so. Each payor tracks the standard fee submitted on claims by physicians across the nation. They also track the average payments accepted by individual physicians for each procedure code number. This is called fee profiling. Using this data, indemnity medical plans establish an unpublished rate that they call a usual, customary, and reasonable **(UCR)** rate.

When the UCR rate was first introduced, the insurance industry claimed it would represent the average fee charged by similar specialties in each geographic region. At that time, indemnity plans represented most of the medical insurance market, so standard fees submitted on claims were the prevailing fees used to find the UCR rate. "Usual" referred to the specific physician's standard fee. "Customary" referred to the average fee for physicians of the same specialty in the same geographic area. "Reasonable" referred to an average fee for physicians of the same specialty nationwide. All three pieces of information were considered when a payor set the UCR rate.

Today, managed care plans represent most of the medical market. Accordingly, *UCR rates today typically represent the average managed care payment rate that physicians have accepted in a given region* rather than the average rate charged by each physician. Because physicians are not allowed to discuss their fees with one another, it is more difficult to challenge a payor-assigned UCR rate unless it falls below the Medicare fee schedule. By law, you may not accept a higher fee as payment-in-full from a Medicare patient than the lowest fee you accept as payment-in-full for any other patient for the same service. Therefore you should not accept a UCR rate that is lower than the Medicare fee schedule.

When an indemnity plan pays 80% of medical costs, they pay 80% of the payor-assigned UCR rate, not 80% of the physician's fee schedule. The patient pays the full balance: 20% of the payor-assigned UCR rate plus the difference between the physician's fee and the UCR "allowed" amount.

For example: Dr. Anderson's fee for a procedure is $140.00. The patient, John Williams, pays this fee at the time of service and files a claim to Provident Indemnity for reimbursement. Provident Indemnity is responsible for 80% of the cost, but Provident Indemnity sets the UCR for the procedure at $100.00. Provident Indemnity reimburses John Williams for $80.00, and the EOB that accompanies the payment states that Dr. Anderson's charges are more than the usual, customary, and reasonable fee. John Williams' share of the cost is 20% of the UCR ($20.00) plus the difference between the physician's fee and the UCR ($40.00) for a total patient financial responsibility of $60.00. John expected Provident Indemnity to pay $112.00, and he expected his cost to be $28.00. John's share of the cost is more than double what he expected.

Indemnity plans do not sign contracts with physicians, and physicians rarely authorize discounts for indemnity plans. Your physician cannot control the indemnity plan's decision, and he or she has a right to full payment. Be prepared to explain to patients that the UCR is no longer based on a comparison of community-wide fees, and give the patient guidance if he or she chooses to appeal the decision.

Suggest the patient call other medical offices in the same specialty to compare pricing, and tell the patient to write down or document the fees quoted. This list should be included in the patient's official complaint or appeal to the indemnity plan. The indemnity plan will usually send additional reimbursement when patient research proves that actual fees in the community differ from the payor-assigned UCR rate. If the indemnity plan will not adjust the

Answer the following questions:

1. Is an indemnity plan a commercial plan or a service plan?

   _____

2. Is an indemnity plan a managed care plan?

   _____

3. Who files the claim form? _____

   _____

4. Are preauthorizations required for referrals?

   _____

5. Are preauthorizations required for hospitalizations?

   _____

6. Are there restrictions on which physicians the patient may see? _____

7. Are there any restrictions on which hospitals the patient may use? _____

8. Does the physician sign a contract with the medical plan? _____

9. Is payment determined by the medical plan fee schedule or the physician fee schedule?

   _____

10. Is the physician required to accept assignment of benefits? _____

   _____

UCR rate for that claim to reflect actual fees charged in your community, suggest the patient file a complaint with the state's insurance commissioner. A directory of State Insurance Commissioners can be found in the back of this book, and a current directory is also found at the official Medicare website www.medicare.gov.

Health Maintenance Organization (HMO)

Commercial insurers first began to offer private medical insurance in the 1940s, during World War II when Congress froze wages but declared medical insurance to be an allowable fringe benefit. In 1902, long before the first medical plan was offered, the insurance industry formed the Medical Information Bureau (MIB).

The stated purpose of the MIB is to prevent insurance fraud, but the actuaries also use the data to perform statistical studies. Because most individuals in the United States subscribe to at least one type of insurance (life, health, disability, liability), the pooled information gives a very good overall picture of health care in the United States. The concept of the HMO managed care plan was drawn from an analysis of data from the MIB. In 1973, Congress passed the Health Maintenance Organization Act, authorizing the formation of health maintenance organizations (HMOs)—the first managed care plan.

HMO policies were initially offered in 1975. However, HMOs did not really gain popularity until the mid-1980s.

The HMO is the purest form of a service medical plan (managed care). The insurance industry originally developed this type of plan to cut expenses so they could keep premiums low. HMOs use five major methods to reduce expenses.

- ❏ *Coverage for **preventive medicine:*** The insurance **actuaries** (mathematicians who study trends and set insurance premiums) established the MIB specifically to collect and track health and lifestyle information. Every MIB-member insurance plan is required to share health and lifestyle information about their subscribers with the MIB. Using data collected since 1902 for statistical studies, the actuaries learned that preventive medicine effectively reduces the incidence of more costly medical care.

- ❏ *Encouraging early treatment by limiting an individual's out-of-pocket expenses for medical care:* The insurance actuaries determined that it is less expensive to treat medical problems early, before little problems grow into bigger problems.

Because physicians collect the full fee from indemnity patients at the time of service, patients often delay seeking medical care until they can afford to pay for the visit, and small problems grow during the delay. At the end of each year, there are many indemnity patients who get every minor ailment taken care of before the next deductible period begins in January.

❏ *Improved employee utilization through efficient claim management:* The insurance actuaries determined that more timely receipt of claims would enable them to utilize their employees more effectively, reduce year-end over-time expenses, and enable better long-term planning.

Indemnity patients typically wait to submit insurance claims for reimbursement until they have enough claims to exceed the deductible. Many submit all their claims in one batch at the end of the year. HMOs assign health care providers the responsibility for filing claim forms and place time limits on the claim-filing process. This way, claims adjustors are busy at a steady pace throughout the year, and there is no backlog of claims at year-end.

❏ *Eliminating medically unnecessary tests and procedures:* HMOs require **preauthorization** before allowing most tests and procedures. Preauthorization is the process of obtaining approval from the payor based on **medical necessity** before tests and procedures are performed.

There have been several instances in which a patient won a malpractice judgment primarily because a jury agreed with the patient that the physician should have ordered either more tests or different tests. Therefore, insurance actuaries often suspect that some medical tests are performed routinely solely to limit the physician's legal liability and not for medical reasons. This is documented in a book titled *A History of the Actuarial Profession.* HMO physicians must justify or explain why the ordered tests are medically necessary, and payment is only sent for tests that meet the HMO's requirements for medical necessity. The diagnosis codes billed are usually used to determine medical necessity for a claim.

Medical necessity and preauthorization requirements cause the most friction between physicians and medical insurance carriers. Physicians take the position that they are the only ones qualified to determine if and when tests and procedures should be performed on their patients. From the time of Hippocrates to current times, physicians have vowed to keep patient information confidential. Physicians contend that revealing patient information to the insurance company in order to meet medical necessity requirements is a violation of patient-physician confidentiality.

The insurance industry pays the bills, so they take the position that they have a right to know medical information that proves whether tests and procedures are medically necessary. HMOs reserve the right to withhold payment if the medical-necessity information they are given is inadequate. Some HMOs employ nurses and physicians to confirm medical necessity and issue authorizations. Nurses typically handle routine authorizations, and physicians handle authorizations that are unusual or complex. Other HMOs use a computerized process based on recommendations of a physician employed by the HMO. For these payors, authorizations can sometimes be obtained over the Internet using a secure program.

❏ *Requiring **participating physicians** to sign contracts with predetermined fees.* Before the advent of HMOs, insurance companies did not have any control over the fees charged by physicians. The actuaries reasoned that regulation of physician fees was imperative if they were to be effective in controlling expenses.

HMOs use many methods to determine the fees they offer physicians in contracts:

❏ Plan-specific fee schedules with set prices listed for each service or procedure.

❏ *A set discount* listed as a percentage of the physician's standard fee schedule.

❏ *A resource-based relative value system (**RBRVS**).* RBRVS is a payment system that assigns a numeric relative value unit **(RVU)** to each service or procedure. The number of RVUs assigned each service, supply, and procedure depends on the amount of work performed, the expenses incurred (overhead), and the amount of risk (drives malpractice fees). In addition, there are other cost factors that vary by geographical location. To arrive at the fee, you multiply the number of RVUs assigned to an item by the geographic price indicator. This total is multiplied by the contract "conversion number" (a dollar value per RVU) to arrive at the contracted fee. RBRVS and RVUs are discussed further in Chapters 10, 12, and 14.

❏ ***Capitation.*** Under the capitation system, each physician is paid a set amount of money every month for each patient assigned to the physician's office, whether the patient seeks medical care or not. This is usually called per patient per month **(PP/PM),** but some payors call it per member, per month. The physician receives a guaranteed monthly income and controls the cost of services. The physician pays all expenses. Therefore a physician earns more money if the treatments he or she recommends are effective: if patients recover and then stay well. Chapter 4 covers how to use the claim form to report services under capitation plans.

Some physicians sign capitation contracts with PP/PM amounts that are not high enough to cover the average costs, and expenses are higher than revenue. Money is a powerful motivation. Some physicians who are paid under capitation contracts decide to ration care in an effort to keep expenses down.

HMO physician contracts have many other variables as well. Some limit the number of patients and others guarantee new patients. Some HMO contracts contain clauses that could influence physician decision-making, such as giving bonuses when few patients are sent to specialists or when inexpensive treatments are utilized. Fortunately, most HMO contracts do not try to influence physician decision-making.

Most HMO contracts list specific billing requirements, and many list specific scheduling requirements. Most HMO contracts require the use of current-year codebooks and require adherence to national standard coding guidelines and coding conventions (see Chapters 5, 6, and 7). Most physician contracts also allow for monetary penalties if contract requirements are not met.

Some HMOs also penalize physicians who give out too many referrals or who recommend expensive treatments. Most penalties are not clearly explained in contracts between physicians and medical plans. Many penalties are hidden when a contract has a section requiring the physician to comply with utilization review procedures and to be bound by the HMO's conclusions.

With an HMO, each patient must select a primary care physician (PCP) from the HMO's list of primary care physicians, or the patient may choose to have the HMO assign the PCP. The PCP directs the patient's medical care. Authorizations are required for referrals to specialists and for most tests and procedures. Physicians or their staff members are responsible for completing and submitting claim forms.

Patients pay a small fixed copayment amount for most outpatient services, a small fixed deductible amount for inpatient services, and a small fixed copayment for prescriptions (the copayment for brand names is sometimes higher than the copayment for generic medications). Patients have no other financial responsibility (out-of-pocket expenses) for covered services.

Balance-billing patients is usually a direct violation of physician-payor contract provisions. The difference between the physician's standard charge and the HMO "allowed" charge is a contracted discount, and it cannot be billed to the patient. However, patients may be billed only for noncovered services, although sometimes advance written notice must be given to the patient before the service is provided. See Chapters 3, 13, and 14 for more information about billing for noncovered services.

Many times patients do not know the extent to which durable medical equipment (e.g., wheelchairs, oxygen tanks, hospital beds) is covered by a medical plan. They often do not know the extent to which ancillary services (e.g., physical therapy, occupational therapy) are covered. Even if they ask these questions of an insurance agent, the agent usually cannot immediately find the answers; it takes a little research. Patients may contact member services at their medical plan (the phone number is on their insurance card) to learn specific levels of coverage for these items. Payors will readily answer these questions for patients, but they are reluctant to share this information with a medical office because services should be driven by medical necessity, not by levels of coverage.

In addition to standard closed HMOs, there are now new "open" HMOs and point-of-service plans (POS). These new HMOs allow coverage for out-of-network providers. The HMO pays less for **out-of-plan** (also called out-of-network) providers, and the patients pay all costs not covered by the HMO for out-of-plan physicians. With open HMOs, referrals are not required for out-of-plan physicians, but if medical necessity is not met, the plan will deny coverage, and the patient is responsible for payment in full. With POS HMOs, authorizations are still needed for out-of-plan physicians, but if medical necessity is not met on the resulting claim, the plan will deny coverage, and the patient is responsible for payment in full.

It is important to remember that patient insurance policies for HMOs are very different from physician contracts with HMOs, and patients are not told the provisions of the physician contracts. In addition, patients are often given only short descriptions of medical plans when they make purchase decisions. Medical care is presented to appear the same between plans, with the only difference being the cost of the care. The patient is asked to choose between paying a higher premium and higher out-of-pocket expenses for an indemnity plan (whose only advantage appears to be a choice of physicians and hospitals) or paying a lower premium and limiting out-of-pocket expenses for a managed care plan (HMO, PPO). See Table 8-1 for an example of how coverage choices are presented to patients.

TABLE 8-1
Patient's Insurance Plan Comparison Chart

Policy Provision	Indemnity	PPO	HMO
Hospital Inpatient	$700 deductible plus $150/day for first 5 days $4000/year max individual $8000/year max family	In-plan: $500 deductible Out-of-plan: plan pays 50%	$100 deductible
Office Visits	Plan pays 80%	In-plan: primary—copay $15 specialist—copay $25 Out-of-plan: plan pays 50%	In plan: primary—copay $10 specialist—copay $10 Out-of-plan: no coverage
Mental Health	Plan pays 50% Limit 5 inpatient days and 12 outpatient days per year	In-plan: copay $25, limit 15 days per year Out-of-plan: plan pays 50%, limit of 15 days per year	In-plan: copay $10, limit 20 days per year Out-of-plan: no coverage
Prescriptions	Not covered	Generic: copay $10 Brand: copay $20	Generic: copay $5 Brand: copay $15
Family Coverage Monthly Premium	$800	$600	$450

Box 8-2 HMO Pros and Cons for the Physician	
Advantages	**Disadvantages**
☐ Do not have to advertise for HMO patients. ☐ Guaranteed patients. ☐ Capitation provides guaranteed income. ☐ Known fee schedules. ☐ Services authorized are usually paid. ☐ Patients more apt to seek care early. ☐ Most preventive medicine is covered. ☐ Patient out-of-pocket expenses are small.	☐ Physicians must sign contracts. ☐ Must obtain authorization for tests and procedures. ☐ Must obtain authorization for referrals. ☐ Must obtain authorization for hospitalizations. ☐ Must wait for payment. ☐ Medical plan pays most of costs. ☐ Must submit claims. ☐ Payment often less than standard fee schedule. ☐ Capitation expenses could be higher than income some months.

Patients are promised high-quality medical care for low-cost premiums and limited out-of-pocket expenses. They do not view their medical plans as discounted medicine, and they expect to receive the same care regardless of the type of medical insurance they carry.

Patients have no control over the contracts offered to physicians and are not aware of physician-contract provisions. If the HMO's physician roster lists well-qualified physicians, patients are likely to sign an HMO contract.

Box 8-2 presents pros and cons of HMO plans for the physician.

BILLING CONSIDERATIONS

In order to receive full payment for services, contract requirements must be met. You cannot meet contract requirements unless you know what they are. In Figure 3-18 (Chapter 3), you were given an example of a managed care template that you can develop to track billing requirements for each payor.

Most HMO contracts state that services must be billed within a specified number of days after the service was rendered. If they are not billed in that time limit, the medical plan is not obligated to pay for the service, and the patient cannot be billed. The shortest time limit is only 10 days, and the longest is about 2 years. Most contracts give 30, 60, 90, or 180 days as the time limit in which the initial claim must be received by the payor. Prioritize billing so that claims for medical plans with the shortest billing window are always submitted first.

Many HMOs use **standards of care protocols.** Standards of care protocols are secret payor edits that link specific procedures to medical necessity, and medical necessity is determined by the diagnoses. Therefore many tests are only considered a covered service for specific diagnoses, and often the payor's computer is programmed to automatically determine when medical-necessity requirements are met on a claim form. Standards of care protocols are not published, but they are supposed to be based on medically sound standards. Accurately coding diagnoses and correctly linking diagnoses to procedures are very important. See Chapter 5 for details about diagnosis coding, and see Chapters 4, 7, and 14 for details about linking diagnoses to procedures.

Diagnoses are listed on lines 1 to 4 in *block No. 21, Diagnosis or Nature of Illness or Injury,* on the CMS-1500 medical claim form; procedures are listed in *block No. 24D, Procedures, Services, or Supplies;* and the two are linked in *block No. 24E, Diagnosis Code* (the most relevant diagnosis [or reason] for the procedure on the same line).

If preauthorization was required for the visit or the service, the **authorization number** should be placed in *block No. 23, Prior Authorization Number,* on the CMS-1500 medical claim form. A few payors do not require this information on the claim form and instead consider it adequate to have the information previously recorded in their computer system. Check your contracts carefully or call the claim adjustor to clarify this issue so you do not inadvertently trigger penalties by not following the payor's requirements.

When the HMO patient is referred to your office, the name of the referring physician must be placed in *block No. 17, Name of Referring Physician or Other Source,* and the ID number of the referring physician must be placed in *block No. 17a, ID Number of Referring Physician.* If either item is missing, the claim will be rejected when the payor's computer runs the claim edits.

Some medical plans specify which selection to mark in *block No. 1, Type of Insurance Plan.* Some add plan-specific billing and coding rules. Others require additional identifiers for certain medical plans included in the contract but not for others.

Most HMO plans require the physician to accept assignment, so *block No. 27, Accept Assignment,* should be marked "yes." By accepting assignment, the physician agrees to accept payment of the payor's portion from the payor, not the patient. The patient only pays the fixed copayment amounts. Some HMOs require the amount paid by the patient to be listed in *block No. 29, Amount Paid,* and others want that block left blank.

Note: It is helpful to maintain a notebook with a divider for each of your major payors. The first page in each section should list the physician-payor contract requirements for that payor. As you learn additional details about specific payor preferences, record it in the section for that payor. Document the date and time of the call, the name of the person you spoke with, and a summary of what you were told. This eliminates making repeat calls to obtain the same information. In addition, you may send a written summary of the call to the person you spoke with, and keep a copy in your notebook. Ask that person to promptly respond in writing if the information is not correct; otherwise, your office will begin to bill using this information effective 30 days from the receipt of the letter. Send the letter "return-receipt requested" and file the returned receipt with the copy of the letter. This gives you written documentation that will hold up in court if the payor later (after 30 days) claims the information was wrong.

When a physician is paid by capitation, claims must still be filed. Some physicians do not understand the importance of correctly listing the levels of service and the supplies used when capitated claims are filed, because they are not going to receive any additional reimbursement. By filing claims correctly, both the payor and the provider can track the actual expenses incurred. This process enables both the payor and the physician to determine if the capitation rates are too high or too low. Dollar signs and decimal points are always omitted on medical claim forms. When a capitation claim is filed, the charges are listed as "000" but appear as "0.00."

In addition to the monthly PP/PM capitated remittance the physician receives from the payor, the physician also collects copayments and deductibles from patients. The payor payment is based on the physician-payor contract; and the patient payment is based on the patient's medical policy (patient-payor contract).

If the HMO is a workers' compensation plan, a Medicare Advantage plan, a Medicaid plan, or any other government plan, additional requirements must be met. See Chapters 9, 10, and 11 for further discussion.

When there is more than one payor, identifying the correct primary payor is very important. The primary payor is the one legally responsible for paying first. The secondary payor pays second, and the tertiary payor, if any, pays third. The one who pays first usually pays the largest portion of the charges, so insurance companies and government payors monitor this issue closely. A good understanding of primary payor/secondary payor rules is essential in a medical billing office.

The following primary payor/secondary payor rules apply for private HMOs:

❑ Private HMO plans are usually the primary payor when there are two medical plans. An exception is when the HMO plan is through a spouse's employer, and the other medical plan is through the patient's employer. Then the medical plan through the patient's employer is the primary payor and the spouse's HMO plan is the secondary payor.

❑ When a private HMO and Medicare both cover a patient, the HMO is the primary payor and Medicare is the secondary payor.

❑ When a private HMO and Medicaid both cover a patient, the HMO is the primary payor and Medicaid is the secondary payor.

❑ When a private HMO and TRICARE/CHAMPUS both cover a patient, the HMO is the primary payor and TRICARE/CHAMPUS is the secondary payor.

❑ A private HMO does not provide coverage for services covered by workers' compensation. However, if workers' compensation denies coverage, the private HMO's normal primary payor/secondary payor rules apply.

❑ A private HMO does not provide coverage for any service-connected care a patient is entitled to receive from the VA.

❑ Non–service-connected care a patient receives from the VA may be billed to private medical plans, but an HMO is not obligated to pay for services from out-of-plan physicians. The VA sometimes contracts with HMOs to provide care to veterans who also are HMO plan members, but the VA does not treat any other HMO members. For these claims, the HMO is the primary payor and the VA is the secondary payor.

STOP & REVIEW

Answer the following questions:

1. Is an HMO plan a commercial plan or a service plan? _____
   _____

2. Is an HMO plan a managed care plan? _____

3. Who files the claim form? _____

4. Are preauthorizations required for referrals?
   _____

5. Are preauthorizations required for hospitalizations?
   _____

6. Are there restrictions on which physicians the patient may see? _____

7. Are there any restrictions on which hospitals the patient may use? _____

8. Does the physician sign a contract with the medical plan? _____

9. Is payment determined by the medical plan fee schedule or the physician fee schedule? _____
   _____

10. Is the physician required to accept assignment of benefits? _____
    _____

Preferred Provider Organization (PPO)

PPO stands for preferred provider organization. The insurance industry typically considers PPOs to be service (managed care) medical plans, but in truth, PPOs are a hybrid between commercial and service plans. Although not pure service plans, PPOs are managed care medical plans.

PPOs were developed in the early 1980s in response to patient complaints that, although patients liked the features of an HMO, they had trouble finding a plan that included *all* their various medical providers. The PPO plan was developed as a compromise. It has some features in common with HMOs and some features in common with indemnity plans.

Like an HMO, a PPO has a list of providers-physicians, hospitals, and other health care professionals who have signed contracts with the plan. These are the **preferred providers.** Unlike an HMO, the plan also routinely covers out-of-plan providers, but at a higher cost to the patient.

When the patient sees a **preferred provider** (one who signed a contract with the plan), the rules are much like those of an HMO.

❑ The patient may be required to choose a PCP.
❑ The patient pays a fixed copayment for the visit.
❑ The physician files the paperwork.

❏ Sometimes a referral is required for a patient to see a preferred specialist.

❏ Preauthorization is often required for tests.

❏ Preauthorization is often required for hospital stays at preferred facilities.

When the patient sees an **out-of-plan provider,** the rules are much like the rules for an indemnity plan.

❏ The patient pays the entire amount due at the time of the visit.

❏ The patient is responsible for filing the claim form.

❏ Referrals are not usually required to see out-of-plan specialists, but a few plans do require referrals.

❏ Often preauthorization is not required for tests.

❏ Often preauthorization is not required for hospital stays at out-of-plan facilities.

The patient's portion of the bill is typically higher when they use the out-of-plan options. Many PPOs only cover 50% to 60% of the UCR rate for out-of-plan services. Patient charges for out-of-plan services can go very high, very fast, especially with hospitalization at an out-of-plan hospital! Try to monitor the patient charges when your physician is an out-of-plan provider. If the expenses exceed the patient's ability to pay, collections could become a problem.

Most insurance carriers offer physicians one contract that includes all their insurance products. Many contracts allow the physician to select the products in which they want to participate under the contract. Choices usually include some of the following: HMO, PPO, workers' compensation, Medicare + Choice or Medicare Advantage products, Medicaid, TRICARE/CHAMPUS products, and other federal programs. The choices are different for each insurance company. Each type of program is listed separately, leading physicians to believe the terms differ, and provisions for government programs do differ significantly from provisions for private programs. However, if you do a side-by-side fee schedule comparison, you will see that often the fee schedules and methods of payment between the medical plan and the physician are identical for HMOs and PPOs, although the plans do differ for other contract considerations.

Insurers hope physicians will sign the contracts without making changes, because then the contract will favor the insurance company. Large insurance companies compare physician fees from their entire network. The lowest fees accepted by physicians in a given area become the base contract rate offered in new contracts, and often contracts that have an auto-matic rollover provision also are reduced to this rate. Physicians seldom take the time to read contracts closely and to negotiate for fee schedules and other contract provisions that would make the contracts reasonable and fair. Many physicians sign contracts as they are presented without negotiating the terms, and they allow new rates to take place automatically without comparing the new rates to the old rates during the negotiation period established by the contract.

PPOs require preferred providers to sign contracts with predetermined physician fees. The real difference for physicians between PPOs and HMOs is *not* in the physician's contracted fee schedule. The biggest difference for the physician between HMOs and PPOs is in the patient coverage provided by the medical plans. PPOs often have a larger choice of preferred physicians and patients can go out-of-plan at any time. Coverage is often better for ancillary services and medical equipment. The physician's office staff obtains better results when they request these services.

It is much easier for a physician to make referrals when the choices are less restricted. Unfortunately, a few physicians who sign contracts with PPOs take the increased freedom a little too far and thoughtlessly drive up patient expenses by not making an effort to use in-plan providers for referrals whenever possible. A few medical plans have unethical policies that reward physicians who keep the medical plan's costs down by intentionally sending patients to out-of-plan providers. Box 8-3 presents the pros and cons of PPO plans for the physician.

BILLING CONSIDERATIONS

PPO preferred providers follow the same billing considerations as they do for HMOs. Out-of-plan providers follow the same billing considerations as they do for indemnity plans.

If your provider is an out-of-plan provider, keep track of the amount the patient owes, especially if the payor's UCR rate is a lot lower than the physician's fee schedule. Patients are balance billed for anything the insurance does not pay, and the PPO often pays out-of-plan providers only 50% of the UCR rate. Patient expenses can be a lot higher than the patient expects. If patient costs exceed the patient's ability to pay, you will have a difficult time collecting the money owed.

If the PPO is a Medicare Advantage plan, a Medicaid plan, a workers' compensation plan, or any other government plan, additional requirements must be met (see Chapters 9, 10, and 11 for further discussion).

Box 8-3 PPO Pros and Cons for the Physician	
Advantages	**Disadvantages**
☐ Patients may see both in-plan and out-of-plan providers. ☐ Patient costs are limited for in-plan providers. ☐ Referrals are not needed for out-of-plan specialists. ☐ Authorizations are not needed for out-of-plan services. ☐ Out-of-plan providers do not have to sign contracts. ☐ Out-of-plan providers bill their own fee schedules. ☐ Preferred providers do not have to advertise for PPO patients. ☐ Preferred providers are guaranteed patients. ☐ Capitation provides guaranteed income for some preferred providers. ☐ Preferred providers have known fee schedules. ☐ Services authorized are usually paid. ☐ Patients are more apt to seek care early. ☐ Preventive medicine is covered. ☐ Patients may choose how much of their health care they want to direct. ☐ Out-of-plan providers may balance-bill patients for costs not paid by the medical plan.	☐ Patient out-of-pocket costs are not limited for out-of-plan providers. ☐ In-plan (participating, preferred) physicians must sign contracts. ☐ Referrals are needed for in-plan specialists. ☐ Authorizations are needed for in-plan tests and procedures. ☐ Authorizations are needed for in-plan hospitalizations. ☐ Preferred providers are paid at contract rates and must wait for payment. ☐ Preferred providers must submit claims. ☐ Payment is often less than standard fee schedules. ☐ Capitation expenses could be higher than income some months. ☐ Collecting past due amounts from patients is time consuming and tedious. It can easily cost more than the amount owed.

When there is more than one payor, identifying the correct primary payor is very important. The primary payor is the one who is legally responsible for paying first. The secondary payor pays second, and the tertiary payor, if any, pays third. The one who pays first usually pays the largest portion of the charges, so insurance companies and government payors monitor this issue closely. A good understanding of primary payor/secondary payor rules is essential in a medical billing office.

The following primary payor/secondary payor rules apply for private PPOs.

☐ Private PPO plans are usually the primary payor when there are two medical plans. An exception is when the PPO plan is through a spouse's employer, and the other medical plan is through the patient's employer. Then the medical plan through the patient's employer is the primary payor and the spouse's PPO plan is the secondary payor.

☐ When a private PPO plan and Medicare both cover a patient, the PPO plan is the primary payor and Medicare is the secondary payor.

☐ When a private PPO plan and Medicaid both cover a patient, the PPO plan is the primary payor and Medicaid is the secondary payor.

☐ When a private PPO plan and TRICARE/CHAMPUS both cover a patient, the PPO plan is the primary payor and TRICARE/CHAMPUS is the secondary payor.

☐ A private PPO plan does not provide coverage for services covered by workers' compensation. However, if workers' compensation denies coverage, the private PPO's normal primary payor/secondary payor rules apply.

☐ A private PPO does not provide coverage for service-connected care the patient is entitled to receive from the VA.

☐ Non–service-connected care a patient receives from the VA may be billed to private medical plans. When the VA bills a PPO for non–service-connected care given to a veteran, the PPO is the primary payor using the out-of-plan option, and the VA is the secondary payor.

STOP & REVIEW

Answer the following questions:

1. Is a PPO plan a commercial plan or a service plan? _____

2. Is a PPO plan a managed care plan? _____

3. Who files the claim form? _____

4. Are preauthorizations required for referrals? _____

5. Are preauthorizations required for hospitalizations? _____

6. Are there restrictions on which physicians the patient may see? _____

7. Are there any restrictions on which hospitals the patient may use? _____

8. Does the physician sign a contract with the medical plan? _____

9. Is payment determined by the medical plan fee schedule or the physician fee schedule? _____ _____

10. Is the physician required to accept assignment of benefits? _____ _____

Blue Cross and Blue Shield

Blue Cross and Blue Shield (BCBS) plans have been around since 1939. During the Great Depression, existing physician groups and hospital groups came together and created Blue Cross and Blue Shield to offer low-cost medical insurance. At that time, Blue Cross and Blue Shield were separate organizations. Special state laws and regulations were passed in each state to allow Blue Cross and Blue Shield to operate as nonprofit, low-cost medical plans with less government red tape.

The first physician-group health plan was organized in 1917 in Tacoma, Washington. The first hospital-group health plan was organized in 1929 in Dallas, Texas. Other physician and hospital groups soon organized as well.

Blue Cross was organized by hospital groups and was originally designed to cover hospital costs. Over the years, the program has evolved. Now it also covers some outpatient services, some skilled nursing facility services, and some home care.

Blue Shield was organized by physician groups and was originally designed to cover physician services. It too has evolved. Now it also covers some other outpatient (e.g., lab work, x-rays, physical therapy, occupational therapy), dental, and vision services.

Blue Cross and Blue Shield were the first health plans to require contracts with participating providers, and they still require contracts today. Because they were organized and operated by provider groups, the original contract provisions benefited both the medical plan and the providers.

Although Blue Cross and Blue Shield were originally developed as separate, nonprofit organizations, they have since merged into one organization in most states, and provider groups no longer own them. As other types of low-cost medical plans began to evolve, Blue Cross Blue Shield dropped the nonprofit status in some states to compete. BCBS plans are not always low-cost options today.

Unlike most medical plans, each BCBS organization is independently owned and operated, with local employees and a local board of directors. Collectively, BCBS offers hundreds of types of medical policies, encompassing every category of health insurance, including the traditional, separate Blue Cross and Blue Shield indemnity plans, indemnity plans that include both Blue Cross and Blue Shield, HMO plans, PPO plans, TRICARE/CHAMPUS plans, Medicare managed care plans, Medicare Advantage plans, and Medigap plans. Not every state offers every option. Some states offer only managed care options and the government plans.

A few states offer BCBS plans with "basic" coverage. These are catastrophic care plans. They have very high deductibles, such as $2,000.00 to $5,000.00 per person. Once the deductible is met, all medical care is covered.

In addition, a few states offer BCBS plans with "major medical" coverage. These plans are typically indemnity plans that cover both inpatient and outpatient care, with varying amounts of deductibles. BCBS indemnity plans differ somewhat from other private indemnity plans in that they require physician contracts and have preferred providers. However, the majority of physicians, hospitals, and other providers sign BCBS contracts, so finding preferred providers is seldom challenging.

BILLING CONSIDERATIONS

When filing claims to BCBS, a provider number must be listed in *block No. 24K, Reserved for Local Use,* on the claim form, and the group number (for a medical group or an incorporated solo physician) or the provider number (for a solo physician that is not incorporated) will be listed in *block No. 33, Physician's, Supplier's Billing Name, Address, Zip Code & Phone.* Occasionally, a specific state may have a different requirement. For example, in at least one state, BCBS requires a four-digit code to be added to the provider's EIN instead of placing a provider number in block No. 24K. Call your BCBS representative and ask about the requirements for your state. An Internet search for Blue Cross Blue Shield or BCBS with the postal abbreviation for your state (e.g., "BCBS OH" for Blue Cross Blue Shield of Ohio) can assist you in finding the telephone number.

Each BCBS plan is required to cover certain plans that cross state boundaries. Patients with three types of identification cards must be covered by every BCBS plan, and all participating physicians must see these patients: (1) Federal Employee BCBS ID card, (2) Reciprocity BCBS ID card, and (3) Central Certification BCBS ID card.

Please see the "Physician Advantages," "Physician Disadvantages," and/or "Billing Considerations" for the type of plan each policy most closely resembles: indemnity, HMO, PPO, TRICARE/CHAMPUS, Medigap, or Medicare Advantage.

STOP & REVIEW

Answer the following questions:

1. Is a Blue Cross Blue Shield plan a commercial plan or a service plan? _____

2. Is a Blue Cross Blue Shield plan a managed care plan? _____

3. Who files the claim form? _____

4. Are preauthorizations required for referrals? _____

5. Are preauthorizations required for hospitalizations? _____

6. Are there restrictions on which physicians the patient may see? _____

7. Are there any restrictions on which hospitals the patient may use? _____

8. Does the physician sign a contract with the medical plan? _____

9. Is payment determined by the medical plan fee schedule or the physician fee schedule? _____

10. Is the physician required to accept assignment of benefits? _____

Insurance Clauses

Insurance clauses in patient's medical policies influence many of the billing rules that medical offices must follow. When you learn what these clauses are and how they influence the delivery and reporting of medical care, you will be able to collect a better level of pertinent patient information, and you will be able to help patients understand their medical coverage.

HEALTH INSURANCE PORTABILITY

Current laws mandate that individuals may keep their medical insurance when they change jobs. This is called **health insurance portability.** What is not made clear by the news media is that people do not usually continue to pay the same price for this coverage as they did when they were employees. The volume discount only applies for a limited period (usually 18 months), but the former employer no longer pays any portion of the coverage. Many people discover after they have resigned from a job that the premium for continuing the exact same medical policy has increased dramatically. If a patient asks for your opinion, advise your patients to either ask their employer or call customer service at their medical plan to obtain this information before making a decision to leave an employer. The patient may want an opportunity to explore other options for health insurance coverage.

PREEXISTING CONDITIONS

Insurance companies usually define preexisting conditions as any conditions for which a person has *ever* received medical treatment. Even if a person has not seen a physician in a long time, a condition can be considered preexisting if it is usually chronic or long-term and if the person has ever been treated for it in the past. This is especially true if the person routinely takes prescription medication to control the condition. All disabilities that a person acquires before obtaining a medical policy are considered preexisting conditions for that policy.

HIPAA requires medical insurance companies to waive the waiting period for preexisting conditions as long as there has been no lapse in coverage. If there has been a lapse in coverage, the preexisting condition can be excluded from medical coverage for the number of months there was no coverage, up to a maximum of 2 years. Advise your patients to avoid incurring a lapse in medical coverage, and explain why this is important to them.

HIPAA clearly states that pregnancy may no longer be considered a preexisting condition. However, when a patient is pregnant, there are other factors you should consider and discuss with the patient. Babies are not automatically covered by insurance policies. Many women have individual policies with no provision for dependents. Other policies may cover an employee and spouse but no other dependents. When a dependent daughter is pregnant, the baby will become a grandchild. Dependent grandchildren are seldom covered by family medical policies. Ask about coverage for the baby as early in the pregnancy as possible.

HEALTH HISTORY

Many people in today's society do not give medical history the proper significance. Accuracy is very, very important. The **MIB** was formed in 1902 by insurance actuaries (mathematicians who analyze trends and set insurance policy prices). More than 700 member insurance companies support the MIB, and all member companies are required to supply the bureau with individually identifiable health and lifestyle information about the people they insure. The stated purpose of the MIB is to keep costs down by preventing insurance fraud. The medical directors of life, health, and disability insurance companies have ready access to the MIB's extensive database.

Any misrepresentation of health information by patients or by providers is considered fraud. The MIB has detailed health-history information in their database about everyone who has ever applied for any type of insurance from a member company and everyone who has received medical care that was paid for by a member company or that was paid for by a government plan that was administered by a member company.

People applying for medical insurance are asked to list preexisting conditions on the insurance application. The insurance company uses the MIB database to verify whether the information is accurate. When an insurance company notes a discrepancy, the insurance policy is sometimes, but not always, denied. Those that are not denied will be flagged to draw attention to the discrepancy. If the patient seeks medical care for the unlisted preexisting problem and files a claim for coverage, the insurance company may choose to take action. They may deny coverage for the condition; they could cancel the policy with no refund of premiums already paid; or they could file charges against the patient for insurance fraud.

MIB-member insurance companies give information from medical claims to the MIB, and they check medical claims for discrepancies with MIB data. Get an accurate health history from your patients, and update it frequently. Most procedures today are bundled and contain many components. Modifiers are supposed to be used to identify when the actual procedure performed varies from normal. If a bundled procedure includes removing something that has already been removed, modifier -52 indicates the reduced service. When an insurance company finds a medical claim discrepancy with MIB data, the insurance company may choose to take action. They could deny coverage for the service; they could apply steep penalties to the payment; or they could file charges against medical practice employees or the physician for insurance fraud. Claim accuracy is vitally important!

COORDINATION OF BENEFITS

Most medical insurance plans include a clause called **coordination of benefits.** This gives the insurance company the right to find out if any other medical, disability, liability, or casualty insurance policy covers medical care for the same illness or injury. It allows the insurance company to reduce its payments by the amount of coverage provided elsewhere.

At one time, most medical insurance policies guaranteed payment for covered illnesses and injuries, with no limitations to prevent duplicate coverage. It was an acceptable practice for a person to have more than one medical insurance policy and to collect benefits from each policy each time. Most people used the extra money to replace lost wages.

Unfortunately, a few unscrupulous people bought extra policies solely to profit from illnesses and injuries. As a result, very few such policies are still in existence today.

Today if a patient has two medical plans and one of the plans has coordination of benefits, the patient cannot collect more than the actual cost of care. For example: A patient has two policies. Policy A pays in addition to any other medical plan, and Policy B has coordination of benefits. Even if Policy B is primary and pays first, Policy B has the right to reduce payment by the amount the patient will receive from Policy A.

On the CMS-1500 claim form, in block No. 24J, COB, the COB stands for coordination of benefits. Although most payors use coordination of benefits, they do not usually require this block. It is usually left blank.

RIGHT OF SUBROGATION

In addition to coordination of benefits, many medical insurance plans also include a clause called the **right of subrogation.** This clause is designed to allow medical insurance plans to pay for the initial treatment of injuries as a courtesy until responsibility for payment can be determined through legal channels. If responsibility is later found to belong to another insurance plan or another person, the right of subrogation allows the medical insurance plan to be reimbursed for expenses already paid. If the injured person receives a monetary award from a lawsuit or from an out-of-court settlement, the right of subrogation allows the medical plan to be reimbursed for actual expenses up to the date of the award or settlement before any monies are paid to the sick or injured person. Awards and settlements do not usually include provisions for future medical costs, so the right of subrogation does not include costs that occur after the date of a legal settlement.

STOP & REVIEW

Answer the following questions:

1. A patient receives a settlement from a lawsuit for a personal injury. The medical insurance company wants to be reimbursed for expenses. Which insurance clause allows this?

   _____

2. A patient has two medical plans. Which insurance clause prevents the patient from collecting full payment twice?

   _____

3. How does an insurance company know that a patient has previously had an appendectomy?

   _____

4. Is pregnancy considered to be a preexisting condition?

   _____

5. Is the baby of a dependent daughter automatically covered under the family policy?

   _____

6. Any misrepresentation of health information by patients or by providers is considered

   _____.

7. What criteria are used to identify when the actual procedure performed varies from normal?

   _____

8. What clause gives the insurance company the right to find out if any other medical, disability, liability, or casualty insurance policy covers medical care for the same illness or injury?

   _____

9. What clause allows medical insurance plans to pay for the initial treatment of injuries as a courtesy until responsibility for payment can be determined through legal channels?

   _____

10. Any time an injury might be covered by another policy, the biller must determine which policy is responsible for paying first.

    ____True   ____False

Other Policies That Cover Health Care

Many liability insurance policies include a provision for bodily injury. Typically, auto insurance, homeowners insurance, and business liability insurance policies offer this coverage. Any time an injury might be covered by another policy, the biller must determine which policy is responsible for paying first. Failure to file a claim in the proper order of financial responsibility is considered insurance fraud. See Chapter 9 for further details about liability policies.

Chapter Review

Indemnity plans offer more customized coverage than any other medical plan. Unless the physician offers to accept assignment or authorizes payment arrangements before the visit, patients pay for care in full at the time of service. It is up to patients to seek reimbursement from their medical plan. Although the physician does not sign a direct contract, an implied contract still exists between the physician and the medical plan. The physician is still responsible for providing the physician-supplied information for the bottom half of the claim form.

An HMO, a managed care plan, is usually the most affordable type of insurance policy for patients to purchase, and it often covers more of the needed preventive services. It is also the most restrictive type of plan. Patients are often unaware of policy limitations, and they are usually unaware of physician-contract provisions.

A PPO, also a managed care plan, has features like both an HMO and an indemnity plan.

Insurance clauses explain coverage issues as well as what happens in special circumstances.

Answer the following questions:

1. Which type of medical plan allows a patient to see any physician and use any hospital in all circumstances?

   _____

2. Which type of medical plan does not allow out-of-plan providers?

   _____

3. Which type of medical plan contains costs while retaining flexibility and patient choice?

   _____

4. Which was first developed to cover hospital costs, Blue Cross or Blue Shield?

   _____

5. Which was first developed to cover physician costs, Blue Cross or Blue Shield?

   _____

6. Managed care plans usually cover preventive medicine.

   ____True   ____False

7. Indemnity plans cover a larger portion of the market than managed care.

   ____True   ____False

8. A patient with a PPO plan who uses out-of-plan services incurs the largest nonreimbursed expenses.

   ____True   ____False

9. A patient with an indemnity plan incurs the smallest out-of-pocket expenses.

   ____True   ____False

10. With which plan does a patient incur the largest hospital out-of-pocket expenses? _____

    _____

11. The right of subrogation means _____.

    _____

12. Coordination of benefits means _____.

    _____

13. How does a health plan know when a patient lies on an insurance application? _____

    _____

14. When a patient changes health plans with no lapse in coverage, how long are preexisting conditions excluded? _____

    _____

15. Blue Cross Blue Shield is still a nonprofit organization that offers only low-cost medical plans.

    ____True   ____False

16. What does health insurance portability mean?

    _____

17. HIPAA requires medical insurance companies to waive the waiting period for preexisting conditions as long as what occurs? _____

18. When an insurance company finds a medical claim discrepancy with MIB data, the insurance company may:
    A. Deny coverage for the service.
    B. Apply steep penalties to the payment.
    C. File charges against medical practice employees for insurance fraud.
    D. All of the above

19. At one time, most medical insurance policies guaranteed payment for covered illnesses and injuries, with no limitations to prevent duplicate coverage.

    ____True   ____False

20. Awards and settlements do not usually include provisions for future medical costs, so the right of subrogation does not include costs that occur after the date of a legal settlement.

    ____True   ____False

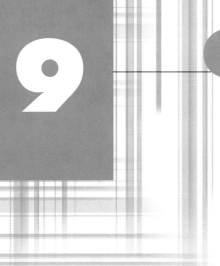

9 OTHER INSURANCE PLANS WITH MEDICAL COVERAGE AND DISABILITY PLANS

Objectives After completing this chapter, you should be able to:

- Relate facts unique to workers' compensation, such as qualifications, patient expenses, coverage, and/or billing considerations
- Relate facts unique to disability insurance, such as qualifications, patient expenses, coverage, and/or billing considerations
- Discuss the differences and similarities between workers' compensation and disability insurance
- Relate facts unique to auto and other liability policies that may cover medical care, such as coverage, circumstances in which they may interact with Medicare and other health plans, and/or billing considerations
- List at least one item that could put a medical billing employee at risk for a charge of fraud

Key Terms

authorization number proof that prior approval was obtained for a specific service: treatment, test or procedure. It does not guarantee coverage if the claim does not establish medical necessity.

deductible a specified amount of expense the patient must pay before the medical plan pays anything.

disability income policies policies to replace lost wages during an extended illness or injury.

IME independent medical exam; a second opinion requested and paid for by a third party. There must be a valid reason for conducting the exam. Valid reasons

include but are not limited to confirmation of level of impairment or injury or confirmation of medical condition for workers' compensation, disability insurance, liability lawsuit, other legal proceedings, etc.

MMI maximum medical improvement and impairment rating; measures long-term impairment, often as a percentage of total body function.

workers' compensation employer-owned combination medical insurance and disability income policy that covers employees' work-related illnesses, injuries, and deaths.

Introduction

This chapter addresses (1) types of insurance that are tied to medical conditions and (2) additional types of insurance that provide medical coverage.

Any time an illness or injury might be covered by a policy other than the patient's usual medical plan, the biller must determine which policy is responsible for paying first and whether the medical plan may also be billed. Claims must be filed in the proper order of financial responsibility, and they should only be filed to policies that actually bear financial responsibility or you could be at risk for charges of fraud.

These types of insurance plans include the following:

❑ Workers' compensation
❑ Disability insurance
❑ Liability insurance

Let's take a closer look at each of these types of insurance plans.

Workers' Compensation

Workers' compensation plans are governed by state law and regulated by each state to cover work-related illnesses, injuries, and deaths occurring in a business headquartered in that state or whose primary work site is located in that state. Yet because private insurance companies are among those who may sell policies, workers' compensation is not considered a true "government plan." In some states, all employers must use managed care networks.

Although the laws differ for every state, some elements are common to all states. This chapter focuses primarily on the elements that are common to all states.

Employers with more than four employees are required to provide workers' compensation benefits to their employees. Employers may buy coverage through state programs, private insurers, or by self insuring. The employer pays the entire premium.

Employees do not pay premiums for workers' compensation coverage. The size of an employee's benefit is based on the severity of the disability and the employee's wages.

Without admitting negligence, the employer is responsible for work-related disabilities that employees suffer. Disabled employees are entitled to benefits without having to sue for them. However, in return for the benefits, employees give up the right to sue.

Disabled employees are typically paid benefits to replace wages on a weekly or monthly basis, rather than in a lump sum. In addition, medical care is covered for the work-related condition as long as the case is considered to be active. If a worker is killed by an on-the-job industrial accident, the law provides for payment of burial expenses, up to an allowed amount, and compensation for the surviving spouse and other dependents at the time of the worker's death.

It is the employer's responsibility to provide workers' compensation coverage according to the laws of the state. It is the employee's responsibility to report injuries in a timely fashion. Employees are responsible for filing accident reports and for asking for medical treatment through the employer's workers' compensation plan.

Some employers or supervisors discourage employees from reporting work-related injuries because the employer's premiums are based on the company's history for work-related claims. Discouraging employees from reporting valid claims is unethical and violates the intent of the workers' compensation law. Unfortunately, if the employee does not file a report within the required time limits, the employee risks losing the protections offered by workers' compensation.

Workers' compensation also provides coverage for treatment of disabilities, including long-term or permanent disabilities, for as long as the case is considered to be active. A physician visit for a follow-up evaluation usually must be done at least once a year by an authorized workers' compensation provider in order for the case to remain active.

The disabled employee, not the employer, is responsible for scheduling the annual follow-up visit and for reminding the provider to obtain any necessary authorizations before the visit. It can be very difficult to reactivate a closed case, so it is a good policy to send reminder letters to workers' compensation patients who have on-going disabilities to remind them to schedule follow-up visits.

There are two main types of workers' compensation cases:

❏ Industrial illness
❏ Industrial accident

An industrial illness is an illness that occurs as the result of being exposed to chemicals or organisms in the course of employment. An industrial accident is an accident that occurs in the course of employment and results in an injury.

Worker's compensation considers two factors in determining disability:

❏ Partial disability versus total disability
❏ Temporary disability versus permanent disability

With partial disability, the person can perform some, but not all, functions of employment. A person with a partial disability usually can either work part-time or in a different capacity. With total disability, the person cannot perform enough functions to regain employment. Most states use some form of an impairment rating, often expressed as a percentage of impairment, to determine whether the disability is partial or total.

With temporary disability, the person is expected to regain the lost function. With permanent disability, the person is not expected to regain the lost function. Rehabilitation is often a major focus with workers' compensation to enable an ill or injured employee to regain as much function as possible.

Some workers' compensation policies are terminated when the patient becomes eligible for Medicare. In addition, if the ill or injured employee signs a settlement agreement, usually for a lump sum benefit, the case is then considered closed even though the illness or injury may persist. Once a workers' compensation case is closed in that fashion, private medical insurance pays for medical care and there is no further compensation for lost wages.

With workers' compensation, the physician relationship is between the insurance carrier and the physician. For legal purposes, there is no patient-physician relationship. No implied contract exists between the physician and the patient, and the physician is not legally obligated to the patient.

BILLING CONSIDERATIONS

Medical information recorded by a physician regarding treatment for a work-related injury is often made available to the patient's employer. Therefore physician documentation requirements are different than for other patient visits. Physicians must be careful to only record personal history details that are relevant to the treatment. They should only document information that is specific to the injury. Any

medical finding regarding other medical conditions, especially if the physician is treating the patient for other medical conditions, should be documented in a separate part of the chart. Dividers are often used to segregate workers' compensation chart notes and information from the rest of the chart. Some states require the use of a separate chart instead of a divider as an added measure of protection.

The rules for selecting evaluation and management (E/M) codes are also different for workers' compensation. Unlike other E/M coding, each new *injury* is billed as a "new" patient visit. Telephone conference E/M codes may be used with workers' compensation claims to bill for time spent talking with attorneys, the insurance company, etc. Usually, when using telephone conference codes, the plan of treatment cannot change and the physician cannot have seen the patient within 3 months nor anticipate seeing the patient within a month. The call must be documented, and the length of the call must be documented.

Authorizations are always required for workers' compensation claims. Make sure the authorization is from the proper source:

❏ Emergencies—authorization from employer
❏ Initial visit—authorization from insurance carrier or employer
❏ Subsequent visits—authorization from insurance carrier

Document who authorized the visit: record the name, position, and specifically, if he or she has the authority to give authorizations. For subsequent visits, get the carrier authorization in writing from the carrier. Document who the adjustor is, the claim number, the date of injury, and what the authorization allows the physician to do.

Specifics regarding authorization will vary by state. For example, in one state, every visit requires a separate authorization and every service performed during one visit requires a separate authorization. Except for emergencies and initial visits, the physician must be certified by the state to treat workers' compensation injuries. The provider must complete a 5-hour course to obtain certification. Surgical assistants cannot be physician's assistants (PAs), and anesthesia must be administered by an MD, not a PA, a nurse practitioner, or an advanced registered nurse practitioner.

MMI stands for maximum medical improvement and impairment rating. MMI is the point at which further improvement is no longer anticipated. The patient sometimes has a copayment responsibility once MMI is reached. Once again, requirements vary by state. For example, Florida requires use of the

Florida Impairment Rating Guide and the rating must be expressed as a percentage.

Most procedures, including minor procedures, have global follow-up days that are included in the procedure and may not be billed separately. Initial visit codes for a surgical procedure include wound cultures, supplies, application of initial dressings, and splints or casts. Unless your state specifies otherwise, national guidelines are followed.

On subsequent visits, supplies are billed using 99070, and the invoice for the supply must accompany the claim, or the entire claim may be returned unpaid. Documentation must include the supplies used, the reasons for the supplies used, the number or amount used, and the cost of supplies. Claims for an x-ray procedure with modifier -26 (professional component) will be returned if an x-ray report is not attached.

When an insurance carrier calls to schedule an independent medical exam **(IME),** find out the volume of records to be reviewed. When the volume is excessive, get a written agreement for a higher dollar amount and bill by adding 99080 (by report) to report the additional amount of work. Payment should be received within 45 days of submitting a clean claim. Figure 9-1 shows an example of an IME letter.

Office notes and the treatment plan for each visit are sent to the workers' compensation carrier in the same envelope with the claim, or, in some states, they may both be submitted electronically. The treatment plan is also sent to the industrial commissioner in most states.

CMS-1500 claim form requirements for workers' compensation claims:

❒ The injured employee's Social Security number is used for the "Insured's ID Number" (Block No. 1a) even though the employee is not the policyholder.

❒ List the employer as the policyholder (block No. 4 and all related blocks, but skip the fields for gender and date of birth).

❒ Accident field—check "yes" for "Employment" (block No. 10a).

❒ Date of injury required (block No. 14).

❒ A code for the external cause of the injury must be listed in the "diagnosis" section of the claim form (block No. 21).

❒ **Authorization number** required for each visit and each service (block No. 23). (Usually there is no compensation if there is no authorization.)

❒ Attach medical records and authorization, if available.

❒ Do not need signature in block No. 31 for a worker's compensation–certified physician—see the rules on the back of a current CMS-1500 claim form.

❒ Some states have additional requirements.

If the carrier does not pay a valid claim and you know the paperwork was prepared correctly, call the bureau of compliance for workers' compensation in your state and report that you have a workers' compensation carrier that is being "noncompliant." If you say the carrier is not paying the bill, you could easily be transferred from one department to another, and receive no help. If you specify "noncompliant," the specialist of the day will help you, even with coding disputes.

Some states post their workers' compensation fee schedule online. Many states want to avoid the cost of updating their software every year to include the annual code changes, so they require coding from the 1995 or 1996 CPT codebooks.

April 24, 20XX

\<attorney name\>
\<law firm name\>
\<law firm street address\>
\<law firm city and state\>

Litigation for \<client name\>

Dear \<attorney name\>:

Thank you for contacting me regarding your defense of \<client name\> on chemical exposure litigation. I understand that your client has decided to retain me on this case. As we discussed, I have background in this specific chemical from its discussion when I was a member of the American Conference of Governmental Industrial Hygienists' Chemical Threshold Limit Value Committee. I am sure you understand that I will be unable to determine my opinion until I have completed my review of the pertinent documents of the case.

As I may have mentioned, I am a physician who is Board Certified in Occupational Medicine. I am also a Certified Industrial Hygienist. My consultative practice primarily addresses the evaluation of individuals who may potentially be or previously have been exposed to hazardous substances.

After completing medical residency training, I worked at the OSHA national office in Washington. Following this, I became the full-time Medical Director for Lockheed Martin, the nation's largest defense contractor. I have served on national committees which determine safe exposure levels for chemicals in the workplace, and safe procedures for hazardous waste operations. I am also a member of the Scientific Review Panel for the Hazardous Substance Data Base operated by the National Institutes of Health.

I have participated in toxic tort litigation across the nation. In about two-thirds of these cases, the defense has retained my services.

I would like to review my usual financial arrangements:

1. My professional fee is $350 per hour. This rate applies to document review, literature search, preparation, phone calls, deposition, testimony, and travel (portal to portal). In general, no charge is made for routine office expenses (secretarial services, copying, online search fees). Travel and accommodations are billed at cost.

2. You may reserve time on my schedule for meetings, deposition, or testimony. These reservations should be made as early as possible, and those occurring with less than four weeks notice will frequently cause scheduling conflicts. Commitments canceled with notice of more than ten working days are without financial obligation. Cancellations with notice of six to ten working days incur a 50 percent cancellation fee, based on the billable time reserved. Those occurring with five ore less working days notice incur a cancellation fee of 100 percent of the billable time reserved. A minimum of eight hours will be billed for each day scheduled away from the office.

3. A retainer of $5000 is requested before work is started. The minimum fee for the case will be ten billable hours, or $3500. As the retainer is depleted, or when time is reserved, you may be requested to provide an additional retainer for application toward future billing. With the exception of the minimum of ten billable hours or actual invoices, whichever is larger, all retainers are fully refundable.

4. Invoices which are unpaid 30 days after mailing are subject to a 1.5 percent per month late fee.

5. Any controversy or claim arising out of or relating to this agreement, or the breach thereof, shall be settled by arbitration in accordance with the rules of the American Arbitration Association, and judgement upon the award rendered by the arbitrator(s) may be entered in any court having jurisdiction thereof.

6. This agreement shall be governed by the laws of the State of Florida. The venue for any legal action regarding this transaction shall be Orlando, Florida. The prevailing party shall be awarded reasonable legal and court costs.

After you have had an opportunity to review this, I would appreciate your signing one copy of this letter and returning it to indicate your acceptance of this arrangement.

If you would like to discuss any aspect of this, I welcome your call and look forward to working with you. I can be reached at 634-555-1212.

Sincerely,

Eric Anderson, MD, MPH, CIH, CSP

ACCEPTED BY:

_____ Date: _____
                Signature

_____
        Above Name Typed or Printed

SCH:cfa

FIGURE 9-1

A letter of agreement is a legal understanding between two or more parties. In this case, the agreement serves to verify the credentials of the physician performing an independent medical exam, clarify amount of work to be performed, and confirm the rate of payment for this work. (Courtesy the Center for Occupational and Environmental Health, Orlando, Fla.)

STOP & REVIEW Answer the following questions:

1. What does "MMI" stand for?

_____

2. What does "IME" stand for?

_____

3. Does the employee pay for workers' compensation insurance?

_____

4. Who is responsible for keeping a case active?

_____

5. Which employers are required to carry workers' compensation insurance?

_____

6. Are there any special documentation requirements? Explain your answer.

_____

_____

_____

_____

7. When is an authorization required?

_____

8. Who may issue an authorization for an initial visit?

_____

9. Who may issue an authorization for a subsequent visit?

_____

10. Who may issue an authorization for an emergency?

_____

Disability

Disability insurance is most often limited to income replacement coverage, but occasionally medical care is included. In addition, disability insurance is only tied to an illness or injury that is not covered by workers' compensation, such as one that occurs some place other than at work.

Disability income policies are designed to replace lost wages during an extended illness or injury. They are not considered medical plans and are not subject to coordination of benefits with medical plans. However, they usually include their own set of exclusions, limitations, and coordination of benefits clauses to prevent profiting from disability.

A disability income policy will not replace more income than actually was earned. The policy requires proof of income over a specified time period immediately before the onset of a disabling condition. Preexisting conditions are generally excluded from coverage to prevent people from waiting until they are already ill or disabled to sign up for a policy.

Some disability plans replace lost wages and provide medical care for the disabling condition. A few include other features such as paying someone else to perform household duties the disabled person is responsible for but can no longer perform. In some states, a person can add disability coverage to an automobile policy.

When a person incurs a qualifying illness, injury, or disability, specific plan requirements must be met within the time limits specified in the plan. Usually the first step includes submitting proof of the qualifying illness, injury, or disability. Most payors require a plan-specific form signed by the physician with a statement from the policyholder verifying what occurred. The policyholder also must provide proof of income for a specific time period, usually the preceding thirteen weeks.

Most disability policies have waiting periods before benefits begin. Short-term disability policies may begin immediately but generally only cover a 30- to 90-day period before benefits cease. Long-term disability policies generally have a 30- to 90-day waiting period before benefits begin, but then they usually continue for as long as the disability exists or until age 65 when Medicare benefits begin, whichever comes first.

Most policies require follow-up exams at specific intervals. Often it begins as weekly, progresses to biweekly, then monthly, quarterly, and finally annually. It is not unusual for a disability plan to require exams at least quarterly for 5 years or longer. Since medical necessity does not usually persist for quarterly exams for that entire period, the patient may have to pay for many of these visits out-of-pocket. (Remember, medical insurance does not pay for services that are not medically necessary.)

Often, there is paperwork that both the physician and the patient must complete for each required exam—as much as two pages each of very specific questions. The insurance company wants to know in minute detail exactly what the disability is, what the patient cannot now do that they could do before the disabling event, the likelihood of recovery, and the expected degree of recovery. Like workers' compensation, disability plans want to know when MMI has been reached, and they want an impairment rating for any permanent disabilities.

Because the physician is usually completing a form not required in any other circumstance, and the patient, not the physician, is the one who benefits financially, many physicians charge an additional fee for the additional work of completing paperwork.

In cases of long-term disability, many payors require periodic IMEs. This is the only time the disability insurance company pays for a disability exam. Because the disability plan does pay for those exams, there is no patient fee for that paperwork.

Some states offer state disability plans. Some of these plans only replace lost wages, but others replace lost wages and provide medical care for the disabling condition. Each state that offers a state disability plan has rules and coverage limits unique to that state. Like other types of disability plans, plan-specific forms must be completed both at the time of injury and at other set times.

Liability Insurance

AUTO INSURANCE

Most states require some form of liability insurance for every vehicle registered in the state, and residents are required to register vehicles. Automobile policies usually include coverage for bodily injury. Some states also require personal injury protection (PIP) as part of the mandatory automobile coverage.

When a patient is injured in an automobile accident, the automobile insurance policy for the person found to be at fault is usually the primary payor for the claim. If no one is found to be at fault, and the patient has an automobile policy with no-fault coverage, the patient's automobile policy is usually the primary payor for the claim. In some states that have PIP, the patient's automobile policy always pays first and the insurance for the person found to be at fault, if different than that of the patient, only pays when the patient's policy limits for medical care run out. The patient's *medical* plan is only considered to be the primary payor when no other policy provides coverage.

The receptionist must obtain additional documents when care is for treatment of injuries from an automobile accident: the patient's name, address, phone number, and driver's license; the name of the insured, the policy name, and the policy number for each involved automobile insurance company (usually there is more than one); and a copy of the police report. These documents are needed when determining the primary payor for the claim. Copies are kept with the billing information for every visit related to the accident, and additional copies of these documents should be submitted with the claim form.

Most medical management computer systems are set up to link every visit to the patient's *medical* insurance company. Visits due to automobile accidents must be flagged so the billing clerk can readily see that the claim requires special attention. The billing clerk must determine which payor is primary and often must manually change the information in the insurance section for every visit related to the automobile accident. If the wrong payor is billed as primary, the consequences can be severe for both the patient and the physician.

For example: An actual patient who was employed as an insurance agent was injured in an automobile accident. The patient knew that the automobile policy should be billed first and supplied all the proper information during registration for the medical office visit. The receptionist did not understand the significance of the automobile policy information and did not know what to do with it. She placed it in the patient's medical file, but she did not enter it into the computer system, and she did not discuss the situation with the biller.

The computer system automatically listed the patient's medical policy as the primary payor on the claim form. The billing clerk did not review the claim to verify the accuracy of information automatically entered by the computer system. The accident section (box No. 10b) was marked "yes" for an automobile accident, but the automobile policy was not listed anywhere on the claim form, and the claim was submitted to the patient's medical insurance plan.

Because the automobile policy was not billed as the primary payor and was not even listed on the claim form, the medical insurance company declared the claim to be fraudulent. The medical plan canceled the patient's insurance policy. Even though the patient is still employed as an insurance agent, the MIB database reveals that his previous policy was canceled due to fraud, and the patient is disqualified for medical insurance coverage from every MIB-member medical plan. The receptionist's "simple" error, compounded by the biller's lack of attention to detail, effectively rendered the patient uninsurable!

Some patients are not truthful about the cause of their automobile-related injuries. The patients do not usually intend to commit fraud; many just do not want the hassle of dealing with both auto and health insurers at a time when they are injured. Some are embarrassed, especially if they were at fault. Other patients do not realize that automobile insurance companies are legally responsible for payment of automobile-related medical claims. Some patients fear that medical care might be delayed if it is complicated by the automobile policy information.

Medical practices often find out that an injury was, in fact, an automobile injury when the patient receives a bill for the balance not covered by the medical plan; and the patient then wants the automobile insurance to pay the balance due. This situation creates extra work for the physician's office. The billing and collections department must return the first payment with an amended claim form showing the proper billing information. To protect the integrity of the practice, include the patient-supplied billing information showing that the patient misled the practice. Then the automobile policy must be billed. After maximum payment has been received from each possible automobile payor, the medical plan may be billed as the secondary or tertiary payor for any remaining balance.

When a patient misleads a medical provider about the cause of an injury, the patient has unwittingly committed a federal crime and could be subject to both jail time and fines of $5,000.00 to $10,000.00 per line item of charges billed incorrectly "due to false statements related to healthcare." Intent is no longer a requirement in this crime. Even honest billing mistakes can have this consequence for the person who makes the false statement or supplies the false information.

HOMEOWNER'S INSURANCE

Most homeowner's and most renter's property insurance includes liability coverage for injuries to visitors and injuries to hired workers not covered by workers' compensation. Insurance industry procedures are not as clear-cut when injuries occur on private property, because it is not as easy to determine fault. Some personal-injury liability lawsuits drag on for years.

Medical care cannot wait until liability is resolved. Medical practices traditionally have required patients to pay the full cost at the time of service and file their own claims. However, with managed care plans now providing more than 80% of the medical insurance coverage, this is no longer proper. If a hired worker is covered by workers' compensation, workers' compensation should be listed as the primary payor. Otherwise, the initial medical claim should list the liability insurance as the primary payor and the medical insurance as the secondary payor.

If the liability insurance does not send payment, if liability is doubtful, or if liability has not yet been determined, it is acceptable to submit a claim with the patient's medical insurance listed as primary payor. Additional paperwork will be required to document your efforts to determine the primary payor. Most medical policies contain a "Right of Subrogation" clause. If another party, such as the property insurance policy, is later determined to be responsible, the medical plan has the right to be reimbursed for the expenses they paid.

BUSINESS LIABILITY INSURANCE

Most business liability insurance covers injuries to visitors and injuries to hired workers who are not employees of the covered business and are not covered by workers' compensation. Insurance industry procedures also are not as clear-cut when injuries occur on business premises because it is not as easy to determine fault. Once again, personal-injury liability lawsuits can drag on for years.

Medical care cannot wait until legal responsibility is determined. When a hired worker is eligible for workers' compensation through his employer, workers' compensation should be listed as the primary payor. Otherwise, the initial medical claim should list the liability insurance as the primary payor and the medical insurance as the secondary payor.

If the liability insurance does not send payment, if liability is doubtful, or if liability has not yet been determined, it is acceptable to submit a claim with the patient's medical insurance listed as the primary payor. Additional paperwork is required to document the efforts made to determine the primary payor. Most health policies contain a "Right of Subrogation" clause. If the business liability insurance pays later, the health plan has a right to be reimbursed for the expenses they paid.

PROFESSIONAL LIABILITY INSURANCE

Professional liability insurance is very similar to business liability insurance, except that the *work performed* is the primary item covered rather than the *place of business*. A policy may cover one specific individual or it may cover all employees of a company. Malpractice insurance is the type of professional liability insurance purchased by most physicians.

Errors and Omissions insurance protects against accidental errors and omissions. If you are sued because of an error or omission at work, or if you incur a fine as the result of an audit, the insurance pays instead of you personally. Errors and Omissions insurance does not protect against intentional actions classified as fraud.

Errors and Omissions insurance is the type of professional liability coverage most often purchased by billers and coders not already covered by an employer's malpractice plan. Please be aware that if you have more than one employer and only one of them covers you for malpractice, you should consider purchasing your own policy to provide coverage when you are working for the employer that does not offer coverage.

Some individual professional liability policies also include a clause that provides coverage for accidental injuries occurring at the policyholder's home. Often this overlaps with homeowner's and renter's insurance. When this occurs, the homeowner's or renter's insurance is considered primary, the professional liability insurance is considered secondary, and the medical plan is considered tertiary (third). Otherwise, the rules are much the same as for the other liability plans.

BILLING CONSIDERATIONS WITH LIABILITY PLANS

Chapter 4 covers detailed instructions for filling out the CMS-1500 medical claim form. Any time a patient is treated for an injury, the appropriate choice(s) in the "accident" section of the CMS-1500 claim form, *block No. 10, Is Patient's Condition Related to: Employment, Auto Accident, Other Accident,* must be marked "yes."

Block No. 10a, Employment?, on the CMS-1500 claim form must be marked "yes" when the treatment rendered is due to an employment-related accident. When a hired worker is eligible for workers' compensation through his employer, workers' compensation would be listed as the primary payor. Anytime *block No. 10a, Employment?,* is marked "yes," the medical insurance company will immediately look for documentation that the claim was filed first with the appropriate workers' compensation insurance company. When the worker is not covered by workers' compensation insurance, the applicable liability plan should be billed as primary payor, and "no workers' compensation"

should be entered in *block No. 19, Reserved for Local Use.* The injured worker's medical insurance is only billed as primary payor when no other policy provides coverage.

Block No. 10b, Auto Accident?, on the CMS-1500 claim form must be marked "yes" and the two-digit state abbreviation for the location of the accident is entered when the treatment rendered is due to an automobile accident. Anytime *block No. 10b, Auto Accident?,* is marked "yes," the medical insurance company will immediately look for documentation that the claim was filed first with the appropriate automobile insurance company.

The automobile insurance for the person who is considered to be at fault in an automobile accident is usually, but not always, listed as the primary payor when injuries resulting from an automobile accident are billed. If no one is determined to be at fault, check the patient's policy to see if it contains "no-fault" provisions. If so, the patient's automobile insurance should be billed as the primary payor. In some states that require PIP, the patient's automobile policy is always the primary payor and the other auto plan, if that person was found to be at fault, is listed second. The patient's medical plan is only considered to be the primary payor when no other policy provides coverage. Some medical plans require you to file the claim with the automobile policy and get a written denial of benefits before the medical plan will pay. If you do not supply documentation proving that no other policy may be billed, the claim will automatically be denied.

When a medical claim is filed for an injury to a visitor on private property or a visitor on business property, "yes" would be marked under *"Other Accident?"* in *block No. 10c* on the CMS-1500 claim form. The liability policy should be billed as the primary payor. The patient's medical insurance is not billed unless no other policy provides coverage.

In addition, a code for the external cause of the injury must be listed in the "diagnosis" section of the claim form, *block No. 21, Diagnosis or Nature of Illness or Injury.* Codes in the diagnosis section must be listed in a specific order when injuries are reported. Chapter 5 covers diagnosis billing rules and coding conventions, including the injury rules. The date of injury must be listed in *block No. 14, Date of Current Illness or Injury or Pregnancy.*

When the injury was due to an auto accident in a state requiring PIP coverage, some states require the physician's medical license number to be placed in *block No. 31, Provider Signature and Date,* along with the physician's typed name and date.

When injuries could be covered by a liability plan, Medicare *requires* medical providers to always bill liability plans first. If payment is not received in 120 days, the provider may choose to wait longer for payment, or the provider may choose to request a "conditional primary payment" from Medicare.

Medicare structured the conditional primary payment provision to avoid imposing financial hardship on the patient. If a Medicare conditional payment is made, the provider may no longer bill the liability plan (Medicare considers this to be fraudulent double billing), no lien may be placed against the settlement, and the patient may only be billed for Medicare **deductibles** and coinsurance amounts. The provider does not have the option of later refunding Medicare and accepting a liability settlement.

In some instances, specific medical plans want to be billed as primary payor with the possible third party liability plan listed as secondary payor. The medical plan will then pay for the services initially, investigate the claim, and exercise the right of subrogation to collect from the third party payor when applicable. Additional paperwork may be required. Blue Cross Blue Shield and TRICARE often prefer this option. For fastest payment, call the medical plan first and ask how the plan wants to be billed. Get documentation in writing from the medical plan anytime they prefer to be billed as primary payor, and ask for a copy of the plan-specific billing rules. If the medical plan won't give you a written copy of their preferences, write them a letter summarizing the phone call and state that unless they respond in writing within 30 days to correct this information, you will consider it to be correct and will use it to bill. Send the letter "return receipt requested." Unless they send a correction in the time limit, the information stands. This is your proof that you tried in good faith to establish the primary payor.

STOP & REVIEW

Answer the following questions:

1. There are no other billing considerations when filling out a claim form for an injury claim.

____True ____False

2. Billing a medical plan as primary payor when a claim is submitted for an automobile injury is considered fraudulent.

____True ____False

3. A hired worker who is not covered by workers' compensation is injured repairing Sam's home. What insurance policy is billed as the primary payor for the claim?

_____

4. An employee is injured at work. Is the business owner's liability policy billed as the primary payor?

_____

5. A patient is injured in an automobile accident. No one was found to be at fault, and her policy has a no-fault accident provision. What insurance company is billed as the primary payor?

_____

6. What type of insurance plans replace income when an injury prevents a person from working?

_____

7. Most homeowner's and most renter's property insurances do not include liability coverage for injuries to visitors or to hired workers not covered by workers' compensation.

____True ____False

8. Most business liability insurance covers injuries to visitors or to hired workers who are not employees of the covered business and who are not covered by workers' compensation.

____True ____False

9. A disability income policy will not replace more income than actually was earned.

____True ____False

10. Professional liability insurance is very similar to business liability insurance, except that the *place of business* is the primary item covered rather than the *work performed*.

____True ____False

Chapter Review

When a patient is treated for an injury, the biller must determine which plan should be billed as the primary payor the first time a claim is submitted for the injury. In many instances, the patient's medical plan is not the primary payor.

Answer the following questions:

1. A patient was injured by slipping on a wet floor while shopping in a grocery store. What insurance plan is billed as primary the first time the claim is submitted?

   _____

2. A patient was injured in an automobile accident. The patient was the passenger in the car. The driver of the other car was charged with reckless driving. What insurance plan is billed as primary payor for the claim?

   _____

3. The patient was injured when she slipped and fell in the bathtub at home. What insurance plan is billed as the primary payor for the claim?

   _____

4. A burglar is injured while breaking into your house. What insurance plan is billed as primary payor for the claim?

   _____

5. Is it fraudulent to bill a medical plan as the primary payor on an initial automobile injury claim?

   _____

6. May a medical plan be billed as the secondary payor after a liability plan has paid a claim if there are remaining unpaid expenses?

   _____

7. A business hired a repairperson to repair a leaky faucet. The repairperson slipped on the wet floor and fractured his coccyx. The repairperson is self-employed and is not covered by workers' compensation. What insurance plan is billed as primary payor for the claim?

   _____

8. An employee of a large company was burned in a grease fire. What insurance plan is billed as primary payor for the claim?

   _____

9. What insurance plan covers both medical care and lost wages?

   _____

10. Who pays the premium for the insurance plan in question 9?

    _____

11. In workers' compensation, the size of an employee's benefit is based on the severity of the disability and what else?

    _____

12. Does the employer admit negligence when taking the responsibility for work-related disabilities that employees suffer?

    _____

13. If an employee has accepted medical care for a work-related injury and has accepted monetary reimbursement for lost wages, does the employee have the option of suing the company?

    _____

14. Do employees pay premiums for workers' compensation coverage?

    _____

15. Whose responsibility is it to report a work-related injury?

    _____

16. Disability insurance cannot exclude preexisting conditions from coverage under the policy.

    ____True   ____False

17. Medical practices often find out that an injury was, in fact, an automobile injury when the patient receives a bill for the balance not covered by the medical plan, and the patient then wants the automobile insurance to pay the balance due. What steps do you take when this occurs?

    _____

18. Some personal injury liability lawsuits drag on for years.

    ____True   ____False

19. Errors and Omissions insurance does not protect against intentional actions classified as fraud.

    ____True   ____False

20. Some medical plans require you to file the claim with the automobile policy and get a written denial of benefits before the medical plan will pay.

    ____True   ____False

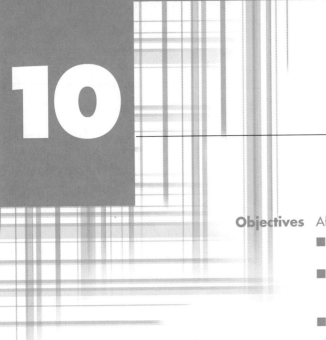

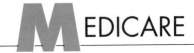

10

MEDICARE

Objectives After completing this chapter, you should be able to:

- Distinguish the differences and similarities among the various government medical plans
- Relate facts unique to traditional Medicare, such as: eligibility, patient expenses, Part A coverage, Part B coverage, and/or billing considerations
- Relate facts unique to Medicare supplemental policies, such as: eligibility, patient expenses, coverage, relationship to traditional Medicare, and/or billing considerations
- Relate facts unique to Medicare Part C, such as: eligibility, patient expenses, relationship to traditional Medicare, and/or billing considerations

Key Terms

benefit period the time period in which an additional hospitalization for a Medicare patient is considered to be part of a previous hospitalization for the purpose of calculating the Medicare Part A patient financial responsibility. Readmission within 60 days of discharge is considered to extend an existing benefit period. When there have been 60 consecutive days without inpatient status, a new benefit period begins. There is no limit on how many benefit periods a person may have.

capitation a method to pay physicians based on the number of patients assigned by the medical plan rather than actual costs incurred. The physician controls the expense of rendering care.

carrier the insurer or medical plan chosen to administer the portions of a government medical plan specific to one state. For Medicare, the private insurer chosen to administer Part B claims.

deductible a specified amount of expense the patient must pay before the medical plan pays anything.

end-stage renal disease (ESRD) end-stage renal disease is kidney failure.

fee for service (FFS) the physician is paid a fee for each service provided; private fee-for-service medical plans are an option under Medicare Part C.

fiscal intermediary (FI) the insurer or medical plan chosen to administer Medicare Part A and some Medicare Part B claims for the government, or the insurer or medical plan chosen to administer other government programs (e.g., Medicaid, CHAMPUS, TRICARE).

Kyle provision legislation included in the 1997 Balanced Budget Act that allows providers who opt out of the Medicare program (minimum 2-year opt-out) to enter into private contracts with Medicare recipients for services that would normally be covered by Medicare. Special rules apply.

lifetime reserve an extra 60 days of hospital coverage that a Medicare recipient may use only once. When the days are gone, Medicare coverage for hospitalization beyond 90 days ceases.

Medicare the federal medical program that provides hospital and medical expense protection for the elderly (age 65 or older), anyone who suffers from chronic kidney disease (any age), and those who receive Social Security disability benefits.

Medicare Advantage the current name for Medicare Part C, formerly Medicare + Choice; options Medicare beneficiaries may choose instead of traditional Medicare. Enrollees must have Medicare Part A and Part B, and they cannot have end-stage renal disease (kidney failure).

Medicare Part A a Medicare program that provides coverage for hospital and hospitalization-related expenses.

Medicare Part B a Medicare program that provides coverage for physician services, ambulances, diagnostic tests, medical equipment and supplies, and ancillary services.

Medicare Part C also called Medicare + Choice and Medicare Advantage; a Medicare program that gives

Medicare recipients the option of replacing traditional Medicare with a plan that covers Part A and Part B services in one plan. In order to qualify, the enrollee must have both Part A and Part B coverage, and the enrollee cannot have end-stage renal disease (kidney failure).

Medicare Part D was created by the Medicare Modernization Act of 2003. It is a voluntary program designed to provide a prescription drug benefit.

Medicare provider number a Medicare-assigned number that identifies the exact physician in a practice who provided the service reported on line 24 of the CMS-1500 claim form. This number is placed in block No. 24K for a group practice and for a single-physician practice that is incorporated. It is placed in block No. 33 for a single-physician practice not incorporated. This will be replaced by the National Provider Identifier (NPI) when the NPI becomes available. Providers began obtaining NPIs in June 2005, but the implementation date to begin using the NPI is expected to be at least 1 year later.

Medicare Select Medicare supplemental policies similar to Medigap except they only provide coverage when preferred providers are used, and they cost less than unrestricted Medigap plans.

Medicare UPIN a unique provider identification number issued by Medicare to identify each individual physician who is authorized to give referrals for Medicare patients. On a claim form, the UPIN distinguishes between the referring physician and the rendering physician. This number will be replaced with the National Provider Identifier (NPI) when the NPI becomes available.

Medigap Medicare supplemental policies designed to cover some or all the costs not covered by traditional Medicare. Enrollees must have both Medicare Part A and Medicare Part B.

MSA medical savings account; a medical plan option under Medicare Part C.

nonparticipating provider a provider who signs a Medicare contract but does not accept assignment of benefits.

participating provider a provider who signs a Medicare contract and who accepts assignment of benefits. Also, a provider who signs a Medicaid or an HMO managed care contract.

POS point of service; an option that allows HMO patients limited coverage for out-of-plan providers.

PSO provider-sponsored organization; a new medical plan created by Medicare Part C.

working aged any person age 65 or older who continues to work.

Introduction

The amount of time Congress spends analyzing medical issues is roughly proportional to the slice of the federal budget consumed by Medicare, and every year Medicare's slice grows larger. Politicians have strong incentives to consider issues from both the payor perspective (the government is the largest third-party payor) and the voter perspective. They strive to balance a fine line between controlling payor costs for government medical plans and appeasing voters. Polls show that Medicare recipients are more active than any other voter group. They follow legislation, write to politicians, and, most importantly, they vote.

Medicare's rules are legislated by Congress and not by individual states, so other payors seldom face legal challenges when they adopt rules or reimbursement strategies already in use by Medicare. Therefore other government and private medical programs often adopt fee structures and reimbursement rules that are set first for Medicare. For that reason, even if your practice does not participate in Medicare, it is wise to learn Medicare's rules and to keep informed of changes as they occur.

Medicare is the federal program with the most participants, but there are other government medical plans, and they are not all alike. Each plan has a distinctly different set of internal rules and regulations. This chapter covers Medicare. You will find the rules for the other government medical plans in Chapter 11.

Medicare

Medicare is a federal medical program that provides hospital and medical expense protection for the elderly (age 65 and older), for anyone who suffers from chronic kidney disease (any age), and for those who receive Social Security disability benefits.

Medicare is a federal medical program that became law in 1965 and took effect in 1966.

Medicare now consists of four parts:

❑ **Medicare Part A** covers specific hospital and hospitalization-related benefits. All workers finance Medicare Part A through a portion of the Federal Insurance Contributions Act (FICA) tax deducted from paychecks, and if they have worked at least 40 quarters, they are automatically eligible for Part A benefits with no monthly premiums once they qualify for Social Security benefits. Part A has **deductibles** and copayments. *Note:* Workers who have worked fewer than 40 quarters must pay monthly premiums for Medicare Part A. In 2005, the premiums are as follows: with 30 to 39 quarters, the cost is $206.00 monthly; with fewer than 30 quarters, the cost is $375.00 monthly.

❑ **Medicare Part B** is a voluntary program that covers many other medical costs, such as physician fees, lab tests, x-rays, supplies, and ancillary services, such as physical therapy and occupational therapy. It is financed by a combination of tax revenues (which cover most of the cost) and monthly premiums paid by enrollees. In 2005 the premium is $78.20 monthly. Part B also has deductibles and copayments.

❑ **Medicare Part C**, currently called **Medicare Advantage** and formerly known as Medicare + Choice, allows beneficiaries to select managed care programs or other choices to provide both Part A and Part B coverage in one plan. Some of the plans offer more services than traditional Medicare. The recipient must continue to pay at least the same premium or a higher premium than with traditional Medicare. People who have **end-stage renal disease (ESRD)** (kidney failure) are excluded from eligibility for the Part C option. The 1997 Balanced Budget Act created Medicare Part C, and the first of these plans became available in 1998.

❑ **Medicare Part D** was created by the Medicare Modernization Act of 2003. It is a voluntary program designed to provide a prescription drug benefit. The first of these plans will become available in 2006.

Medicare has 10 administrative regions, each of which serves a specific geographical area. Each state is assigned to one of these regions. Each region chooses at least one insurance company to administer Medicare for that region. This company is called the **fiscal intermediary (FI)**. According to the CMS glossary, an FI is a private company that has a contract with Medicare to administer Part A and some Part B bills. Sometimes one FI administers Part A claims, and another FI administers the payment of Part B claims for durable medical equipment and supplies.

Each state appoints an insurance company to serve as a Medicare **carrier** for the state. The CMS glossary defines a carrier as a private company that has a contract with Medicare to pay Part B bills. The carrier for each state administers payment for the physician portion of Part B claims.

Each FI and each carrier function just like a regular insurance company, except they must follow federal regulations for Medicare instead of their own policies for Medicare clients.

Someone who is new to the United States and has never worked here, *after* they have lived here for at least 5 years and *if* they would otherwise be qualified, may purchase Medicare. If they purchase Part A, they must also purchase Part B. If they sign up late, they must also pay the same late penalties any citizen would pay for signing up late.

For example: Maria was age 66 when she arrived in the United States, and she could not enroll in Medicare until 2005 when she had lived here for 5 years. Maria pays a late penalty because she could have enrolled at age 65 if the residency requirement had been met by then. In 2005, when Maria reached age 71, the cost to buy Medicare Part A ($375.00) with a late penalty of 10% is a total of $412.50 per month. For Part B, the premium ($78.20) with a late penalty of 10% multiplied by the number of years late (7), is $132.94 per month. Maria has to buy both Part A and Part B, so the total monthly cost for Maria is $545.44 per month. Medicare supplements, such as Medigap, are not included in the Medicare monthly premium. If Maria wants a supplement, that is an additional cost.

AN OVERVIEW OF MEDICARE PART A

Medicare Part A provides only hospital and hospitalization-related coverage. It covers inpatient hospitalization *and* skilled-facility and/or home care following a hospitalization. Covered services include a semiprivate room, nursing services, and other inpatient hospital services. Medicare Part A does not cover in-hospital physician visits.

The coinsurance amounts (e.g., deductibles and copayments) for Part A services are rather steep, and these amounts usually increase each year when the Social Security cost-of-living increases take effect. The Medicare deductible and copayment amounts listed in this chapter were valid in the year 2005 and may have changed. You can find current premium and coinsurance rates at the Medicare website, www.medicare.com.

In 2005, after an initial deductible amount of $912.00, the first 60 days of hospitalization are covered for any one illness or injury. Readmission for any reason within 60 days of discharge is considered to be the same incident, or **benefit period,** for tracking the number of days of hospitalization. For the sixty-first day through the ninetieth day of hospitalization, the patient incurs a daily copayment of $228.00 per day. After 90 days, the patient is responsible for all hospital charges.

> A benefit period starts on the first day of hospitalization and ends when the patient has been out of the hospital for 60 consecutive days or has not been an inpatient anywhere (such as a short-term skilled nursing facility) for 60 consecutive days. The hospital deductible is paid only once during a benefit period, and the "number of days hospitalized" for the daily copayment calculations include all hospitalized days that fall within the benefit period.

There is a **lifetime reserve** of an extra 60 days with a copayment of $456.00 per day that the patient can use for hospitalizations longer than 90 days. However, once that is gone, Medicare coverage for hospitalization beyond 90 days ceases.

> A patient may not want to use his or her reserve days for an extended hospital stay if there is any other insurance that could cover those costs. These days could then be saved for a time when extra coverage is not available.

Following a hospitalization, Medicare will cover all expenses for the first 20 days in a skilled nursing facility. For days 21 through 100, the patient must make a daily copayment of $114.00 per day. After 100 days, Medicare coverage ceases.

Medicare Part A also covers post-hospital home health services, but only if Medicare considers the services to be reasonable. Only a limited amount of inpatient psychiatric care is covered. For a full and complete listing of Medicare's current rules and levels of coverage, contact the Social Security Administration or go to the Medicare website at www.medicare.gov.

AN OVERVIEW OF MEDICARE PART B

Medicare Part B is available to Medicare Part A recipients for a monthly premium that is withheld from the enrollee's Social Security check. The Medicare base rate is $78.20 per month. Beginning in 2007, those with an annual income of $80,000 for a single person or $160,000 for a couple will pay higher annual premiums. If a person does not enroll during the first 6 months that he or she is eligible, a higher amount is charged as a penalty when enrollment does occur. The late penalty is 10% multiplied by the number of years since enrollment was first available. This amount is added to every monthly premium.

Late penalties are designed to discourage people from waiting until they are sick to enroll.

For example: Victoria enrolled in Medicare Part B 5 years late. Therefore Victoria pays an additional $39.10 per month (10% or $7.82 x 5 years = $39.10), for a total of $117.30 per month, to receive the same coverage most beneficiaries receive at $78.20 per month.

The patient's premium is much lower than the cost of the average insurance premium because tax revenues cover a large share of the cost of the program. After the patient's deductible has been met, Part B covers 80% of the *covered* services that Medicare considers reasonable. The patient is responsible for paying an annual deductible for Part B ($110.00 in 2005) plus 20% of the Part B *covered* services that Medicare considers reasonable.

> ❏ Medicare Part B pays 80% of Medicare's "allowed amount" for covered services that Medicare considers reasonable, not 80% of the physician's fee schedule.
> ❏ In addition, covered services must be medically necessary for Medicare to consider them reasonable. Medicare does not pay for services that do not meet medical necessity requirements.

Covered Medicare services include:

❏ Physician services—both inpatient and outpatient
❏ Diagnostic tests
❏ Ambulance services
❏ Medical equipment and supplies
❏ Ancillary services, such as physical therapy and occupational therapy

Medicare coverage varies for different types of services. The Medicare deductible and copayment amounts listed in this book were valid in 2005 and may have changed. For a full and complete listing of Medicare's current rules and levels of coverage, contact the Social Security Administration or visit the Medicare website at www.medicare.gov.

The Medicare contract also governs the percentage of cost sharing for Part B services in special circumstances.

For example, for outpatient mental health services, Medicare pays 50% of the "allowed" amount and the patient pays 50%. For inpatient mental health services, Medicare pays 80% of the "allowed" amount for physician services and the patient pays 20%.

MEDICARE MODERNIZATION ACT OF 2003

The Medicare Modernization Act (MMA) is a proposed regulation that creates Medicare Part D. The final rule is expected to be released in late 2005 with a target date for the prescription drug *benefit* plan to begin on January 1, 2006. Prescription drug cards were an interim measure that was passed until the new regulation could take effect. Medicare recipients could purchase a prescription drug discount card at an annual cost of $30.00 from May 2004 through December 2005. Until this law, Medicare did not cover prescription drugs.

The prescription drug discount card cost $30 per year and resulted in a savings of 11% to 18% of the cost of brand name prescription drugs and 30% to 60% or more on generic prescription drugs.

Those with monthly incomes below $1,048 for a single person or $1,406 for a married couple did not have to pay for the card and some qualified for a credit of $600 per year on the card to help pay for prescription drugs in 2004 and 2005. If a portion of the credit was not used in 2004, it rolled over into 2005. Some also qualified for larger discounts. People who received prescription drug benefits from Medicaid were not eligible for the prescription drug discount cards.

Under the proposed regulation, effective January 1, 2006, everyone with Medicare may choose to enroll in Part D plans that cover prescription drugs. The various payor participants who offer the Part D plans will negotiate discounts with the pharmaceutical companies just as they always have for managed care plans.

The enrollee will choose a Part D plan and Medicare will cover 75% of the cost of the new premium, with the beneficiary paying 25% of the cost of the premium. Depending on the plan chosen, the beneficiary portion of the premium is expected to be around $35.00 a month in 2006. There is a $250 deductible, and then Medicare will pay $75% of drug costs up to $2,250. Between $2,250 and $3,600, there is no coverage from Medicare. However, after $3,600, Medicare pays 95% of drug costs.

In the proposed regulation, Medicare covers the premiums and deductibles, and there are only nominal copays with no gaps in coverage for those "dual eligible" low income beneficiaries who qualify for both Medicare and Medicaid. The copays are expected to be as little as $1.00 to $3.00 per prescription. Nursing home residents who are "dual eligible" will have no copays.

In addition, Medicare pays most of the costs for those with limited assets who have annual incomes less than 135% of the federal poverty level (below $12,124 for a single person or $16,363 for a married couple). Those who qualify do not have to pay premiums, deductibles, and there is no gap in coverage. However, they are expected to have small copays of a few dollars per prescription. Medicare will cover 95% of their drug costs on average.

For those with assets up to $10,000 ($20,000 if married) and incomes less than 150% of the federal poverty level ($13,942.00 for a single person or $18,875.00 for a married couple), the Medicare benefit will provide 15% copays with a sliding scale premium and no gaps in coverage, covering 85% of their drug costs on average.

PARTICIPATING/NONPARTICIPATING PHYSICIANS

Each physician who applies for a Medicare provider number signs a Medicare contract and designates whether he or she wants to be a **participating** ("par") **provider**. Participating physicians are listed in the Medicare Provider Directory. In addition, they may not charge Medicare patients more than the amount "allowed" by Medicare, and they are required to submit electronic claims to Medicare for their patients. They are given priority in claims processing over nonparticipating providers. Participating providers must accept "assignment of benefits," and Medicare sends payment directly to the provider. The "allowed" amount is determined by the Medicare fee schedule and by medical necessity requirements. *After the patient's deductible has been met,* Medicare pays 80% of the allowed amount and the patient pays 20% of the allowed amount. FIs receive bonuses for recruitment of new par providers to the Medicare program.

Those who designate they do not want to participate in Medicare are called **nonparticipating** ("nonpar") **providers.** They *may not* accept assignment of benefits for Medicare, so payment is sent to the patient, and it may be difficult to collect. Nonparticipating physicians also must submit claim forms electronically to Medicare for their patients. The Medicare fee schedule for nonpar providers is 5% less than the Medicare fee schedule for par providers.

Nonpar providers may charge Medicare patients up to 15% above the current-year Medicare nonparticipating physician fee schedule. This is called the limiting charge. Medicare pays 80% of the nonpar physician allowed amount for each claim, and the patient pays 20% to 35% of the allowed amount. The physician may collect up to a total of 115% of the allowed amount.

The lower nonpar provider fee schedule and the rule allowing an additional 15% to be charged to the patient are designed to discourage Medicare patients from seeing nonpar providers.

For example: Gerald, a Medicare patient who has already met his deductible for the year, saw a nonpar physician who billed him for the maximum amount allowed by law: Medicare's allowed amount for nonpar providers plus 15%, for a total of $92.00. Medicare's nonpar allowed amount for the visit was $80.00. Medicare paid $64.00 (80%). Gerald paid $28.00: $16.00 (20%) + $12.00 (15%) = $28.00 (35%).

If Gerald had seen a par provider, the allowed amount for the visit would have been $84 (5% more than nonpar). Medicare would have paid $67.20 (80%). Gerald would have paid $16.80 (20%). Gerald paid an additional $11.20 to see the nonpar provider.

When there is a private medical plan in addition to Medicare, the private plan must be billed first. The private plan is usually, but not always, through the patient's employer or a spouse's employer. Sometimes a private medical plan is part of a retirement package. Medicare will only consider coverage for charges that are not paid by the private plan.

Medigap is a supplement to Medicare. Although private insurance companies sell Medigap supplements, be careful not to confuse a Medigap supplement with a full-fledged private medical insurance plan.

BILLING CONSIDERATIONS

The Centers for Medicare and Medicaid Services (CMS) falls under the authority of the Department of Health and Human Services (HHS). The CMS sets very specific billing requirements that must be followed for Medicare. A good rule of thumb is Medicare pays the least and Medicare pays last. The only exception is Medicaid, which truly pays least and pays last.

Medicare payment is the *lesser* of (1) the current-year Medicare fee schedule or (2) *the lowest amount the provider accepts for the service*. When a physician signs a managed care contract that sets fees lower

than the Medicare fee schedule, the lower fees automatically become the new fee schedule for Medicare for that physician. *Except with Medicaid, Medigap, and Medicare supplemental policies, Medicare is always the second payor when two medical plans may be billed.*

Medicare *requires* beneficiaries to pay the specified copayment and deductible amounts. If you do not try to collect the patient's portion of the bill, the federal government could charge you with fraud. Remember to document your collection efforts.

When a procedure is officially listed as a Medicare noncovered service, the patient must sign an Advance Beneficiary Notice (ABN) *before* the procedure is performed that clearly states that (1) Medicare will not pay for the service and (2) the patient agrees to pay for the service. If the ABN is not signed, the provider cannot legally collect payment from the patient for the service. A similar ABN also should be signed if you are unsure whether Medicare will cover a service. That way if Medicare does not pay, you can legally collect from the patient. Examples of Medicare ABNs are found in Chapter 3.

Medicare requires every physician who provides care to Medicare patients to sign a contract. The Medicare unique provider identification number (UPIN) identifies each individual physician authorized to *issue referrals* for Medicare patients. The **Medicare provider number** identifies each individual physician authorized to *render care* to Medicare patients. These numbers are not issued until the contract has been signed.

In the contract, each physician is asked to choose whether he or she wants to be paid as a participating provider or as a nonparticipating provider. The Medicare fee schedule is higher for participating providers, who collect 80% from Medicare and 20% from the patient. Nonparticipating providers use a fee schedule that is 95% of the fee schedule for participating physicians to collect 80% from Medicare and 20% to 35% from the patient, for a possible 115% of the nonparticipating physician fee-schedule amount.

Physician's assistants (PAs) and nurse practitioners (NPs) must be credentialed with Medicare and must sign their own contracts in order to render services to Medicare patients. The Medicare fee schedule for credentialed PAs and NPs is 85% of the fee schedule for participating physicians.

At one time, PAs and NPs were not credentialed and a modifier was used to identify when a PA or NP rendered the care. Those modifiers were deleted after credentialing for PAs and NPs was fully implemented. However, if you perform retrospective audits or work old claims from that time period, you may see them.

The referring physician's **Medicare UPIN** is listed in *block No. 17a, ID Number of Referring Physician,* on the medical claim form. The rendering physician's Medicare provider number is listed in *block No. 24K, Reserved for Local Use,* except when the rendering provider is a solo physician who is not incorporated and the provider number is placed in *block No. 33* instead. The Medicare practice ID number (PIN) (for groups and incorporated solo physicians) or the Medicare provider number (for solo physicians who are not incorporated) is listed in *block No. 33, Physician's, Supplier's Name, Address, Zip Code, & Phone No.*

If the patient signs the assignment of benefits, *block No. 13,* the physician must mark "yes" in *block No. 27, Accept Assignment of Benefits,* or the payment on the claim will be sent to the patient, and you might have a difficult time collecting it.

Like many medical plans, Medicare has developed a standard set of edits each claim must pass before payment is issued. Initially, Medicare's edits were all published in the Correct Coding Initiative (CCI), and they were updated quarterly. In 1999 and 2000, Medicare used unpublished "black box" edits in addition to standard CCI edits. Medicare's black box edits were used to evaluate the way diagnosis codes were linked with procedure codes to establish medical necessity for each service or procedure. Black box edits are intended to prevent fraud by making it difficult to circumvent cost-containment measures. Medicare adopted this policy because some providers had been altering diagnoses solely to meet the medical necessity guidelines published in the CCI and in "code-linkage" reference books. If you perform retrospective audits or work old claims from that period, you may encounter claims that were denied because of black box edits.

The unpublished edits did not prove successful in reducing Medicare's expenditures, and they made the process more complex for medical collections employees who wanted to determine the cause of penalties and who wanted to collect full payment for valid claims. It was very difficult to meet requirements that were not known. In 2001, Medicare abandoned the black box edit system and returned to their previous system. Code-linkage guides, now called "cross coders," are once again available, by specialty, to help physicians meet medical necessity requirements and bill correctly.

A few other points to remember for Medicare are:

- ☐ Do not schedule a patient's appointment as a routine physical if the patient has any type of complaint that must be addressed during the appointment. Medicare does not cover routine physical examinations, but it does cover examinations performed during a visit for specific symptoms or specific health problems.
- ☐ When an appointment is scheduled for a routine physical and a new problem is discovered during the visit, be sure the physician includes the diagnosis for the new problem on the superbill and documents the new problem in the patient's medical record. On the claim form, diagnoses for routine physical exams cannot be used on the same claim as a diagnosis for a problem, so only the diagnosis for the problem is listed. The appointment is billed as a routine appointment.
- ☐ When an appointment is scheduled for one specific problem, and the physician discovers an additional problem during the appointment, be sure the physician includes the diagnosis codes for both the original problem and the new problem on the superbill and documents both problems in the patient's medical record. Otherwise, treatment for the new problem might not be covered.

Medical coding rules specific to Medicare are covered in more detail in Chapters 5, 6, and 7. Claim preparation issues specific to Medicare are included in Chapter 4; hospital and other facility billing for Medicare is covered in Chapter 12; collections idiosyncrasies specific to Medicare are covered in Chapter 13; and problem solving for Medicare is covered in Chapter 14. In addition, Medicare coverage issues are explained in detail in a supplemental section of the Level II *Healthcare Common Procedural Coding System* (HCPCS) codebook, and an excellent online Medicare training program is available at www.cms.hhs.gov/medlearn/.

STOP & REVIEW

Answer the following questions:

For questions 1 to 4, the choices are: (A) fiscal intermediary, (B) carrier, (C) both

1. Which one pays Medicare Part B claims for physician services? _____

2. Which one must follow Medicare's rules?

   _____

3. Which one pays for medical supplies and prescribed equipment? _____

4. Which one pays Medicare Part A claims?

   _____

For questions 5 to 9, the choices are: (A) participating, (B) nonparticipating, (C) both

5. Which physician has a higher Medicare fee schedule? _____

6. Which physicians must file claims for their Medicare patients? _____

7. Which physician may collect more from the patient? _____

8. Which physician must sign a Medicare contract?

   _____

9. Which physician is issued a Medicare provider number? _____

10. Does Medicare cover diagnostic tests?

    _____

Medicare Supplemental Policies

Out-of-pocket expenses with Medicare can be very costly. Many seniors buy a supplemental policy if they do not have any other medical coverage. Although Medigap plans are the best-known Medicare supplements, they are not the only Medicare supplements.

Medicare calls senior citizens who continue to work working aged. Many working aged are covered by an employer's group medical plan or have a medical policy as part of their retirement benefits. Others are covered by a spouse's policy. These policies are not supplements. They are always considered primary, and they pay before Medicare.

MEDIGAP

Medigap policies are supplemental policies designed to cover some or all the costs that Medicare does not cover. They are purchased from private insurance companies, and coverage varies. Many include additional features not covered by Medicare. A person must be enrolled in Medicare Part B to participate.

For many years, private insurance companies offering Medigap plans were unregulated, and they often did not provide the promised coverage. Now, federal and state laws establish minimum requirements for Medigap policies.

In most states, insurance companies may only offer one or more of 10 standardized Medigap plans. The Medigap plans are labeled as plans A through J. Plan A has the least amount of coverage and is the least expensive; Plan J has the largest amount of coverage and is the most expensive. Plans H, I, and J are the plans that previously offered prescription drug benefits. These plans will be phased out by 2006 for new enrollees, but those who already have the plans may keep them as long as they do not enroll in a prescription drug benefit plan.

Minnesota, Wisconsin, and Massachusetts were exempted from the federal Medigap law because different rules were already in effect before this law was passed.

When an enrollee signs up for a Medigap policy during the first 6 months after Medicare Part B coverage begins, the insurance company is not allowed to reject the application, and they are not allowed to exclude preexisting conditions, although some exceptions apply for a limited period if there was a break in coverage. If the enrollee waits until later to apply for coverage, he or she runs the risk of rejection or exclusion of preexisting conditions. In addition, if the enrollee chooses to change the level of Medigap coverage at a later date, he or she runs the risk of rejection or exclusion of preexisting conditions.

Federal guidelines state that Medicare participating providers must file claims to Medigap plans as well as Medicare. You can find the list of Medigap carriers for your state online at your state Medicare carrier's website. If you cannot find your state carrier's website, a link is available at www.medicare.com.

MEDICARE SELECT

Medicare Select is another type of Medicare supplemental policy. Like Medigap, a person must be enrolled in Medicare Part B to participate. The types of Medicare Select plans are almost identical to the types of Medigap plans, with one important difference: except in the case of an emergency, enrollees must use specific doctors and specific hospitals to get the full benefits from the supplemental portion of the plan.

When enrollees use *preferred providers,* Medicare pays the Medicare portion of the bill and the Medicare Select insurer pays the rest of the bill. If the enrollee uses an out-of-plan provider for nonemergency services, Medicare will still pay their portion of the plan, but the Medicare Select insurer is not responsible for any additional benefits. In this respect, Medicare Select is very much like a PPO (preferred provider organization) managed care plan.

Medicare Select policies generally have lower premiums than standard Medigap policies because of the additional restrictions. Congress designed Medicare Select as an experimental program. Medicare Select is still available, but it is subject to change. If Congress should terminate Medicare Select, the current policyholders will be able to keep their policies as long as the insurer offers it, or they may choose another plan. If the insurer discontinues Medicare Select, the replacement policy would have to offer similar benefits.

BILLING CONSIDERATIONS

Only participating Medicare providers may become participating Medigap providers. Only *participating* Medigap providers may list a Medigap plan on a claim form sent to Medicare, and they are *required* to list both Medicare and Medigap on the claim form. Specific information must be listed in blocks No. 9 through 9d, the sections for the "other" insured, and block No. 11d, where you indicate that there is another insurance plan. In addition, the Medigap plan may only be listed on the claim form if the patient signs the "assignment of benefits" and authorizes the "release of information" for both Medicare and Medigap (blocks No. 12 and No. 13). Chapter 4 provides specific block-by-block medical claim form requirements.

Medicare is listed as the primary insurance plan on the claim form, and the Medicare supplement is listed as the secondary policy. Many supplemental plans are registered with Medicare. After paying the claim, Medicare automatically forwards billing information to supplemental plans that are registered with them. These are called crossover claims. You can find a list of the supplemental plans registered with Medicare online at the Medicare carrier's website for your state. The Medicare remittance notice (MRN) that accompanies payment from Medicare will indicate whether the claim was forwarded. If it was not automatically forwarded, you must include a photocopy of the Medicare MRN with the claim form when you submit a claim to the supplemental plan.

Answer the following questions:

Questions 1 to 3 are about people who continue to work past age 65 (working aged) and are covered by an employer group medical plan.

1. For those who pay premiums to purchase Medicare Part B, which plan is primary: Medicare or the employer's medical plan?

2. Is the employer plan a Medigap plan?

3. It is always a good idea to purchase a Medigap plan.

____True   ____False

4. Which states are exempt from offering Medigap plans and why?

5. What is the difference between Medigap and Medicare Select?

6. Who may list Medigap plans on claim forms sent to Medicare?

7. Where can you look to find out if Medicare did indeed forward the Medigap claim?

8. When Medicare does not forward Medigap claims, what must be sent with the Medigap claim when you file it?

9. Which Medigap plan costs the least and covers the least?

10. Which Medigap plan costs the most and covers the most?

Medicare Part C

The 1997 Balanced Budget Act created Medicare Part C, now known as Medicare Advantage and formerly called the Medicare + Choice program. It allows beneficiaries to select a medical plan that provides both Part A and Part B coverage in one comprehensive plan.

Medicare beneficiaries may choose between remaining in traditional Medicare and enrolling in a Medicare Advantage program. An enrollee must participate in both Medicare Part A and Part B to be qualified to join Part C. People who have end-stage renal disease are excluded from the Part C option.

Generally, enrollees may only join a plan that serves the geographic area in which they live. A Medicare Advantage plan may not deny enrollment based on health status or other factors described by the Health Insurance Portability and Accountability Act of 1996 (HIPAA).

Medicare Advantage replaces the previous Medicare HMO "risk" and "cost" programs with a wider variety of choices, some of which are based on the original Medicare HMO "risk" and "cost" plans. If you perform retrospective audits or work with old collections, you may run into some of these former plans.

With Medicare Part C, eligible Medicare recipients may choose between HMOs with or without a point of service **(POS)** option, PPOs, provider-sponsored organizations **(PSOs),** medical savings accounts (MSAs), private **fee-for-service (FFS)** Medicare, and several new types of medical plans.

Medicare Advantage plans are required to cover all standard Medicare Part A and Part B benefits. Since January 1, 2003, medical plans have been allowed to offer a benefit reducing the amount the recipient pays for Part B premiums. However, with most plans, the recipient must continue to pay at least the same premium as with traditional Medicare Part B. Many plans also offer supplemental benefits for which they may or may not charge an additional premium. Enrollees are not allowed to opt out of supplemental benefits.

Medicare Advantage insurers receive payment two ways: (1) Medicare pays them a set **capitation** rate (a monthly per-person reimbursement rate) and (2) they receive any additional premium amount added to the standard Part B premium for supplemental benefits. The rules are different for medical savings accounts. Except for the medical savings account option, plans are required to pass on any "savings" they achieve (when their costs are less than the Medicare payment) by providing additional benefits.

During the first few years, enrollees could change plans monthly, if desired. In 2003, enrollees could make one change every 6 months. Since January 1, 2004, an enrollee may make one change once a year during the open enrollment period. The annual open enrollment is from November 15 through December 31 each year, taking effect the following January first. In addition, individual plans have the option of offering additional enrollment periods. Beginning in 2002, those newly eligible for Medicare may choose to reenroll in traditional Medicare fee-for-service throughout the first 12 months of Medicare Advantage membership.

The rules for Medicare supplements did not change when Medicare Advantage was created. Enrollees may not disenroll and reenroll in a Medigap plan or change Medigap plans without risk. Once a Medicare beneficiary drops a Medigap plan or another Medicare supplement, he or she risks exclusion of preexisting conditions and/or disqualification from rejoining the plan at a later date.

This is true even when a Medicare Advantage option is no longer available in a specific geographic area. Unfortunately, many senior citizens in one state learned this lesson the hard way in 1999. Medicare decreased the capitation rate for less-populated counties in that state, and soon afterward, every Medicare + Choice (Medicare Advantage) plan pulled out of those counties. Thousands of senior citizens were involuntarily placed back in the traditional Medicare program. Many were not able to reenroll in previously held supplemental plans.

In 2004, payments for rural providers increased significantly and Medicare began phasing in a system to pay Medicare plans by the level of risk (diagnosis) instead of by capitation. In addition, two new Medicare Advantage plans were introduced in 2004 to add *regional* HMO and *regional* PPO options.

The first Medicare + Choice (Medicare Advantage) plans became available in 1998. Let's take a closer look at each of the options available in 2005.

MEDICARE ADVANTAGE HMOs— MANAGED CARE

Medicare through a health maintenance organization (HMO) is set up quite differently from a traditional Medicare plan. The enrollee continues to pay the Part B premium to Medicare, but he or she is not responsible for Medicare's deductibles and coinsurance. Instead, the enrollee is responsible for the HMO deductibles and copayments. Premiums and copayments vary from plan to plan and can be changed each year. The additional premiums for Medicare Advantage HMO plans are generally lower than the premiums for Medicare supplemental policies.

HMOs are managed care medical plans. Many Medicare HMO rules are much like the rules for private HMOs. (See Chapter 8 for details about private HMOs.) Each plan has its own network of hospitals, physicians, home health agencies, nursing facilities, and other professionals. The patient selects a primary care physician (PCP) from the list of plan physicians. The primary care physician manages the patient's medical care.

A Medicare Part C HMO plan based on the original Medicare-through-an-HMO "cost" plan works much like Medicare Select, and current Medicare reports still call this option a cost plan. When the patient sees in-plan providers, the Part C HMO provides coverage. The Part C HMO does not provide any coverage for out-of-plan services, but with this type of Medicare HMO, traditional Medicare provides coverage for out-of-plan providers. The patient pays traditional Medicare deductibles and copayments for out-of-plan providers. People who travel frequently like this flexibility.

A Medicare Part C HMO plan based on the original Medicare-through-an-HMO "risk" plan is still called a risk plan in current Medicare reports. The risk plans have a *lock-in* requirement. This means the patient must receive all his or her medical care, except for emergencies, through the Medicare Advantage HMO plan. If the patient sees an out-of-plan provider, the patient is responsible for the entire bill. Neither the Medicare Advantage HMO plan nor Medicare will pay any portion of it.

When a patient signs up for a *point of service* (POS) option with any of the Medicare Advantage HMO plans, the plan is responsible for a percentage of out-of-plan, nonemergency charges. In return for this flexibility, the patient pays a portion of the cost, typically 20%. This option makes the Medicare Advantage HMO function much like a PPO.

To enroll in a Medicare Advantage HMO plan, the patient:

❑ Must live in the plan's service area
❑ Cannot be receiving care from a Medicare-certified hospice
❑ Cannot have permanent kidney failure at the time of enrollment
❑ Must continue to pay Medicare Part B premiums

MEDICARE ADVANTAGE PPOs— MANAGED CARE

Medicare through a PPO is set up quite differently from a traditional Medicare plan. The enrollee continues to pay the Part B premium to Medicare, but the patient is not responsible for Medicare's deductibles and coinsurance. Instead, he or she is responsible for the PPO deductibles and copayments. Premiums and copayments vary from plan to plan and can be changed each year.

PPOs are managed care medical plans. The Medicare PPO rules are much like private PPOs. (See Chapter 8 for details about private PPOs.) The patient may either choose to limit costs by using plan-selected providers or may pay a little more and choose non-PPO providers.

When a patient signs up for a POS option with any of the Medicare Advantage PPO plans, the plan is responsible for a higher percentage of out-of-plan, nonemergency charges. The patient's portion of the cost is typically similar to in-plan services.

To enroll in a Medicare Advantage PPO plan, the patient:

- ❏ Must live in the plan's service area
- ❏ Cannot be receiving care from a Medicare-certified hospice
- ❏ Cannot have permanent kidney failure at the time of enrollment
- ❏ Must continue to pay Medicare Part B premiums

MEDICARE ADVANTAGE MANAGED FEE-FOR-SERVICE PLAN

A Medicare Advantage managed fee-for-service (FFS) plan allows the enrollee access to any doctor and any hospital, and, like traditional Medicare, the enrollee is responsible for deductible and coinsurance amounts. Physicians and other providers are paid for each service, such as an office visit or a test. Costs are controlled by managing patient care through an authorization process and medical necessity requirements. This type of plan uses preferred provider networks.

Private fee-for-service plans are not bound by Medicare rates and CMS does not review their premiums. Contract providers might be paid at higher rates than the traditional Medicare fee schedule, increasing the costs to enrollees who choose this plan. A Medicare Advantage FFS plan might also choose to offer supplemental plans (similar to Medigap) for an additional charge to cover the patient's out-of-pocket costs.

To enroll in a Medicare Advantage FFS plan, the patient:

- ❏ Must live in the plan's service area
- ❏ Cannot be receiving care from a Medicare-certified hospice
- ❏ Cannot have permanent kidney failure at the time of enrollment
- ❏ Must continue to pay Medicare Part B premiums

MEDICARE ADVANTAGE NEW MANAGED CARE MEDICAL PLANS

Medicare Advantage created two new qualified medical insurers. These options were created primarily to enable areas that are underserved by HMOs and PPOs to develop Medicare Advantage options: primarily rural areas and low-cost urban areas. Minimum enrollment requirements are not as high for these plans.

- ❏ One new qualified insurer is called a provider-sponsored organization (PSO). PSOs allow hospitals, hospital organizations, and physician organizations to contract directly with Medicare to offer Part C medical plans.
- ❏ The second new qualified insurer is called a religious fraternal benefit plan. These plans also may contract directly with Medicare to offer Part C medical plans. Religious fraternal benefit plans may choose to restrict enrollment to members of their organizations, but they are not required to restrict membership.

The original Medicare HMO legislation required that HMOs become state licensed and meet federal requirements in order to contract with Medicare.

Until federal solvency standards are established, PSOs must meet state HMO licensing requirements. PSOs may apply for a federal waiver for up to 3 years to meet state licensing requirements. The waiver is applicable only to a single state.

To enroll in one of these new Medicare Advantage managed care plans, the patient:

- ❏ Must live in the plan's service area
- ❏ Cannot be receiving care from a Medicare-certified hospice
- ❏ Cannot have permanent kidney failure at the time of enrollment
- ❏ Must continue to pay Medicare Part B premiums
- ❏ Must meet membership requirements for a religious fraternal benefit plan

MEDICARE ADVANTAGE MEDICAL SAVINGS ACCOUNT

Originally, the Medicare Advantage MSA option was offered on a trial basis to only a limited number of enrollees (390,000), with an enrollment deadline of December 31, 2004. Under the Medicare Modernization Act of 2003, it became a permanent program option and the limit on the number of enrollees and the deadline for enrollment were removed.

The main concept governing an MSA is for the enrollee to be the account holder and to make direct contributions. Each enrollee must purchase a catastrophic health plan with deductible and out-of-pocket expenses of not more than $6,000.00 per year. If the enrollee incurs Medicare-covered expenses above the annual out-of-pocket expense amount, the catastrophic plan pays the remaining expenses. CMS does not review the premiums.

Premiums are paid into the enrollee's MSA. The MSA must provide reimbursement for items and services covered under Medicare Part A and Part B after the enrollee reaches the MSA deductible. This means funds are withdrawn from the MSA to reimburse the enrollee. Payments and cost sharing must equal payments and cost sharing authorized under Medicare Part A and Part B.

For example: An MSA enrollee pays a monthly premium of $250.00. This includes the Part B premium of $45.50 and the monthly premium of $50.00 per month for a catastrophic health plan for coverage after $4,000.00 of Medicare-covered out-of-pocket expenses.

This MSA covers only expenses covered by Medicare. The MSA has a $100.00 deductible and then reimburses the patient for 80% of Medicare-covered medical expenses until the total Medicare-covered medical expenses reach $4,000.00. At that time, the catastrophic plan begins to pay 100% of the Medicare-covered expenses.

MSA plans cannot offer supplemental benefits to cover the MSA deductible, but they may include supplemental benefits for additional services at an additional charge if they so choose.

If the premium for the catastrophic plan is less than the Medicare Advantage capitation rate that Medicare pays to Part C medical plans, the difference between the premium and the capitation rate is deposited in each enrollee's MSA. The money placed in the MSA is not considered taxable income as long as it remains in the account or is withdrawn solely for qualified medical expenses. Any funds that are left over are carried forward into the next year and, in some instances, are available to the enrollee. MSA plans are not required to pass on savings in the form of benefits.

For example: An MSA enrollee pays a monthly premium of $250.00. This includes the Part B premium of $45.50 and the monthly premium of $50.00 per month for a catastrophic health plan for coverage after $4,000.00 of Medicare-covered out-of-pocket expenses.

If the Medicare capitation rate is more than $50.00 per month per enrollee in a Medicare Advantage plan, the difference is deposited in the enrollee's MSA.

If the Medicare capitation rate is less than $50.00 per month per enrollee in a Medicare Advantage plan, Medicare does not contribute to the funds in the MSA.

To enroll in a Medicare Advantage MSA plan, the patient:

☐ Cannot be receiving care from a Medicare-certified hospice
☐ Cannot have permanent kidney failure at the time of enrollment
☐ Cannot be prohibited from participation
☐ Must continue to pay Medicare Part B premiums

MEDICARE ADVANTAGE SPECIAL NEEDS PLAN

The Medicare Modernization Act of 2003 also created a new plan option for special needs beneficiaries. Specialized Medicare Advantage plans can limit enrollment to special needs subgroups of the Medicare population. Two groups are specifically mentioned in the legislation: the institutionalized and those who also have Medicaid coverage. The CMS can establish other groups for those with severe or disabling chronic conditions. Payment will be on the same basis as payment for other nonspecialized Medicare Advantage plans. Initially, enrollment must take place before January 1, 2009. Many of the other details are expected to be released with the final rule for the MMA.

MEDICARE ADVANTAGE BILLING CONSIDERATIONS

Physician payment varies depending on individual contract agreements with the medical plans offering Medicare Advantage. It is up to each medical plan whether claims are sent to the medical plan or to Medicare. Read your contract provisions carefully. When claims are sent to Medicare, Medicare forwards the claims to the appropriate Medicare Advantage plan. The Medicare Advantage medical plans set their own physician fee schedules, and many cover additional services. Physicians are paid by the Medicare Advantage plan.

With Medicare Advantage, Medicare pays the Advantage medical plans on a capitated basis. The Medicare payment rate structures are phased in over a number of years. As the rate structures have changed, some Medicare Advantage plans have had to reduce supplemental benefits or increase premiums. Others have closed their doors.

Urgently needed and emergency services received outside a Medicare Advantage plan are covered by each plan. Congress adopted the prudent lay person standard to define emergency medical care, and severe pain is specifically listed as a symptom that indicates an emergency situation.

Medicare Part C legislation in the 1997 Balanced Budget Act also provides procedures for grievances, hearings, and appeals. Appeals are covered in more detail in Chapter 13. Providers are protected from civil liability caused by a medical plan's denial of medically necessary care. For the first time, the federal statute states that federal standards for Medicare Advantage supersede state standards.

Physicians and other providers who sign a contract establishing a payment rate for a private FFS Medicare Advantage plan may bill up to 115% of the rate determined by the private FFS plan. Noncontract providers are to be paid at the Medicare FFS rate. Private FFS rates should be higher than the Medicare rate. Private FFS contracts are expected to have complex and confusing language. It is wise to have these contracts reviewed and interpreted by a qualified medical attorney before the physician signs the contract.

Kyle Provision

The **Kyle provision,** named after the original Senate sponsor for the legislation, allows physicians who opt out of the Medicare program to enter into private contracts with Medicare recipients for health services that normally would be covered by Medicare. The physician-patient contract must clearly state that Medicare will not be billed for these services. The patient and the patient's heirs must agree not to submit claims to Medicare for the services. The physician must agree not to bill Medicare for the services. (See Chapter 3 for an example of this agreement.) The physician also must sign an affidavit with Medicare promising not to submit *any* claims to Medicare for a period of 2 years after signing the contract with the patient. Physicians who enter into private contracts under the Kyle provision do not have to follow Medicare fee guidelines and may individually determine the fees charged. The 2-year opt-out requirement has been challenged, but the challenge was dismissed in court.

The Kyle provision only applies to services normally covered by Medicare. Under the Kyle provision, a physician who participates with Medicare may obtain waivers for noncovered services and set the fees for those services without entering into a private contract. Also, a Medicare recipient who does not want Medicare to have a record of a particular office visit or course of treatment may avoid submitting a claim to Medicare by simply refusing to sign the "Release of Records" and "Assignment of Benefits" forms that authorize a physician or provider to submit a claim, *and* privately paying the full amount of the visit. A private contract is not required and the physician may only charge the Medicare rate.

The Medicare Modernization Act of 2003 also changed the scope of the Kyle provision. Before enactment of the MMA, only doctors of medicine (MDs) and doctors of osteopathy (DOs) could opt out of Medicare. The MMA added dentists, podiatrists, and optometrists to the list of providers who may opt out.

This is a very important issue with significant impact for medical offices. Develop a plan of action to keep informed of changes as they occur. The professional organizations discussed in Chapter 2 are very useful for tracking changes to legislation and discussing the impact for medical employees. Government Internet websites and the Internet websites for professional organizations also are good resources to track legislation.

Answer the following questions:

1. What legislation created Medicare Part C?

_____

2. Are any Medicare beneficiaries excluded from participation in Medicare Part C and, if so, who is excluded?

_____

3. How do participants pay for Medicare Part C coverage?

_____

4. How does Medicare reimburse payors for providing Medicare Part A and Medicare Part B covered services?

_____

5. What is the name of the provision that allows a physician to completely opt out of the Medicare program?

_____

6. Are Medicare Advantage programs considered to be Medicare supplemental policies? Why or why not?

_____

_____

7. How does POS coverage add to a Medicare Advantage HMO?

_____

8. Which Medicare Advantage options are new medical plans?

_____

9. What are the restrictions for joining a Medicare Advantage managed care plan?
   A. Must live in the plan's service area
   B. Must not use hospice services
   C. Must not have ESRD (kidney failure)
   D. All of the above
   E. None of the above

10. The MSA option is currently offered on a trial basis to a limited number of enrollees.

   ____True   ____False

Chapter Review

Medicare is a federal medical program that provides hospital and medical expense protection for the elderly, for anyone who suffers from chronic kidney disease, and for those who receive Social Security disability benefits.

Medicare Part A covers hospital costs and hospitalization-related costs. Medicare Part B covers physicians and outpatient services. The premium for Part B is deducted from the beneficiary's Social Security check. Both Medicare Part A and Medicare Part B have copayments and deductibles. Medicare supplemental policies, purchased separately, are designed to cover costs that Medicare does not cover.

Medicare Part C (Medicare Advantage) gives seniors many more options for medical care. Medicare Part C covers both Medicare Part A and Medicare Part B in one program. To qualify, seniors must be enrolled in Medicare Part B, they cannot have ESRD, and they must continue to pay Part B premiums.

Answer the following questions:

1. Are physician services covered if a patient only has Medicare Part A?

_____

2. Do Medicare Part A or Medicare Part B offer coverage for prescription medications?

_____

3. Medicare Advantage plans are not required to cover prescription medications, but they may choose to do so.

   ____True   ____False

For questions 4 to 7, tell which part(s) of Medicare cover each listed item or service. The choices are:
(A) Medicare Part A, (B) Medicare Part B, (C) Medicare Part C

4. Hospital _____

5. Skilled nursing following a hospitalization

_____

6. Physician services _____

7. Both hospitalization and physician services

_____

8. Does Medicare coverage include prescription medical equipment and supplies? _____

9. What is the difference between POS and PSO?

_____

_____

10. Is a Medicare participating provider required to become a preferred provider for Medicare Select or Medicare Advantage managed care plans?

_____

List the primary plan and the secondary plan, if any, for the combinations listed in questions 11 to 19.

11. Medicare and Medigap.

Primary: _____   Secondary: _____

12. Medicare and Medicare Select.

Primary: _____   Secondary: _____

13. Medicare and Medicare Advantage.

Primary: _____   Secondary: _____

14. Medicare and employer plan.

Primary: _____   Secondary: _____

15. Medicare and Part C PSO.

Primary: _____   Secondary: _____

16. Medicare and Part C religious fraternal benefit plan.

Primary: _____   Secondary: _____

17. Medicare and Part C HMO.

Primary: _____   Secondary: _____

18. Medicare and Part C MSA.

Primary: _____   Secondary: _____

19. Medicare and Part C PPO.

Primary: _____   Secondary: _____

20. Medigap plans must offer specific choices for plans A to J, but Medicare Advantage plans may choose what additional benefits they want to offer and the choice may change from time to time.

____True   ____False

11

MEDICAL PLANS

Objectives After completing this chapter, you should be able to:

- Relate facts unique to Medicaid, such as qualifications, patient expenses, coverage, circumstances in which it may interact with Medicare, and/or billing considerations
- Discuss the Indian Health Service
- Relate facts unique to TRICARE/CHAMPUS, such as eligibility, patient expenses, coverage, circumstances in which it may interact with Medicare, and/or billing considerations
- Relate facts unique to CHAMPVA and the VA, such as eligibility, patient expenses, coverage, how Medicare influences coverage, and/or billing considerations

Key Terms

AFDC Aid to Families with Dependent Children; a government assistance program for those with qualifying low incomes.

authorization number proof that prior approval was obtained for a specific service: treatment, test, or procedure. It does not guarantee coverage if the claim does not establish medical necessity.

categorically needy the state is *required* to give these people Medicaid coverage if the state is to be eligible for federal funds.

CHAMPUS Civilian Health and Medical Program of the Uniformed Services; the law that established an entitlement program to provide medical coverage for families of military service members.

CHAMPVA Civilian Health and Medical Program of Veterans Affairs; the law that established an entitlement program to provide medical coverage for dependents of veterans totally disabled with a service-connected disability and dependents of veterans who died while on active duty and in the line of duty.

deductible a specified amount of expense the patient must pay before the medical plan pays anything.

DEERS Defense Enrollment Eligibility Reporting System; the military organization that determines eligibility and issues military ID cards for CHAMPUS.

FPL federal poverty line.

MedCHAMP a program for CHAMPUS-eligible persons

younger than age 65 who qualify for both Medicare and CHAMPUS. Medicare is the primary payor, and CHAMPUS is the secondary payor.

Medicaid a government medical program developed to provide coverage for qualified low-income applicants.

Medical Care Cost Recovery Program (MCCRP) a program developed to enable the Department of Veterans Affairs (VA) to bill third-party payors for non–service-connected care rendered by the VA to veterans, and to collect copayments from veterans with less than a 50% service-connected disability rating for non–service-connected care rendered, based on ability to pay.

medically needy this option allows states to extend Medicaid eligibility to additional people as defined by the state—usually people who can meet ordinary expenses but cannot afford medical care.

nonparticipating provider for Medicaid, a provider who signs a Medicaid contract but does not accept assignment of benefits.

non–service-connected a medical problem that did not develop during military service and is not related to or caused by military service.

preauthorization the process of obtaining prior approval before a service: treatment, test, or procedure. It does not guarantee coverage if the claim form does not establish medical necessity.

service-connected a medical problem that arose while the person was serving on active duty or that was caused by active duty military service, or a problem that was incurred during reserve duty with a military unit.

SSI Supplemental Security Income; a Social Security program that provides additional income to qualified beneficiaries.

TANF Temporary Assistance for Needy Families.

TRICARE a program with three levels of coverage established to administer CHAMPUS.

Introduction

Medicare is the largest government medical plan, but it is not the only government medical plan. This chapter addresses the other significant government medical plans: Medicaid, Indian Health Service, CHAMPUS/TRICARE, the VA, and CHAMPVA.

Medicaid

Medicaid is a government health program for qualified low-income and very-low-income applicants. The program is administered by each state, but the federal government provides matching funds and establishes regulations that are tied to those funds. Therefore Medicaid is a state program with federal oversight.

Medicaid became law in 1965 and took effect in 1966.

Eligibility is complex. Income guidelines are intended to keep this program only for those with low and very low incomes. All types of income and all types of assets are considered for the income requirements. A child's eligibility is based upon his or her parents' income and assets.

Originally, Medicaid was developed as a medical care program tied to federally funded programs that provided cash income assistance for the very poor, with a focus on dependent children and their mothers, the disabled, and the elderly. Over the years, however, Medicaid eligibility has been expanded. Legislation in the late 1980s extended Medicaid coverage to a greater number of low-income pregnant women, children from low-income families, and to some low-income Medicare beneficiaries who are not eligible for any cash assistance programs. To be eligible for federal funds, states are *required* to provide Medicaid coverage for certain people, some of whom receive federal cash income assistance. The following **categorically needy** groups qualify for federal Medicaid matching funds:

❑ People are generally eligible for Medicaid if they meet the requirements for the Aid to

Families with Dependent Children **(AFDC)** program that were in effect in their state on July 16, 1996. AFDC was a program administered and funded jointly by federal and state governments to provide financial assistance to low-income families with dependent children. Public Law 104-193, the welfare reform bill, repealed AFDC and replaced it with Temporary Assistance for Needy Families **(TANF).** (Although most persons covered by TANF meet the AFDC requirements and still receive Medicaid, the law does not require Medicaid coverage for everyone in the TANF program.)

❑ Children younger than age 6 whose family income is at or below 133% of the federal poverty level **(FPL)**

❑ Pregnant women whose family income is below 133% of the FPL. Services are limited to those related to pregnancy, complications of pregnancy, delivery, and postpartum care.

❑ Supplemental Security Income **(SSI)** recipients in most states (a few states use more restrictive requirements that predate SSI). SSI benefits are available to low-income individuals of any age who have a disability. SSI is part of the Social Security program. Individuals must meet both disability and financial criteria. A child's financial criteria are based on his or her parents' resources (assets such as bank accounts, stock, houses, cars, and other valuables) and income.

❑ Recipients of adoption or foster care assistance under Title IV of the Social Security Act

❑ Special protected groups (i.e., certain qualified individuals who lose eligibility for cash assistance due to earnings from work or from increased Social Security benefits, but who may keep Medicaid for a period)

❒ All children in families with incomes at or below the FPL
❒ Certain Medicare beneficiaries

States also have the option of providing Medicaid coverage for other categorically related groups. The broadest of the *optional* groups for which states may receive federal Medicaid matching funds include the following:

❒ Infants up to age 1 and pregnant women not covered under the mandatory rules whose family income is no more than 185% of the FPL (The percentage amount is set by each state.)
❒ Children younger than age 21 who meet the AFDC income and resources requirements that were in effect in their state on July 16, 1996 (The child need not have been born before July 16, 1996—the date indicates the date the AFDC program was repealed.)
❒ Eligible institutionalized people who have less than a designated income level (The amount is set by each state—up to 300% of the SSI federal benefit rate.)
❒ People who would be eligible if they were institutionalized but who are receiving care under home and community-based service waivers
❒ Certain aged, blind, or disabled adults who have incomes above those requiring mandatory coverage but below the FPL
❒ Recipients of state supplementary income payments
❒ Certain working-and-disabled persons with family income less than 250% of the FPL who would qualify for SSI if they did not work
❒ TB-infected people who would be financially eligible for Medicaid at the SSI income level if they were within a Medicaid-covered category. Coverage is limited to TB-related ambulatory services and TB drugs.
❒ Optional targeted low-income children included within the State Children's Health Insurance Program (SCHIP) established by the Balanced Budget Act (BBA) of 1997 (Public Law 105-33)
❒ Medically needy beneficiaries who can meet ordinary expenses but cannot afford medical care

The medically needy option allows states to extend Medicaid eligibility to additional people as defined by the state. Usually these people would be eligible for Medicaid under one of the mandatory or optional groups, except that their income and/or resources are above the eligibility level set by their state. These people may qualify whenever they incur medical expenses that reduce their income to or below their state's medically needy income level. Medicaid benefit provisions for the *medically needy* are not as extensive as for the *categorically needy*, and may be quite limited.

Federal matching funds are available for medically needy programs if the state meets the federal requirements: Children younger than age 19 and pregnant women who are medically needy must be covered; and prenatal and delivery care for pregnant women, as well as ambulatory care for children, must be provided. A state may choose to provide medically needy eligibility to certain additional groups and may elect to provide certain additional services within its medically needy program.

Currently, 38 states have elected to have a medically needy program. The remaining states use the special income level option to extend Medicaid to low-income people in medical institutional settings.

The Personal Responsibility and Work Opportunity Reconciliation Act of 1996 (Public Law 104-193)—known as the welfare reform bill—made several changes regarding eligibility for SSI coverage that affected the Medicaid program:

❒ Now legal resident aliens and other qualified aliens who entered the United States on or after August 22, 1996, are ineligible for Medicaid for 5 years. It is a state's option to offer Medicaid coverage for aliens entering before that date and to offer coverage for those eligible after the 5-year ban. Medicaid can only continue for aliens who lose SSI benefits because of the new restrictions if the person is eligible for Medicaid for some other reason. Emergency services, however, are always covered.
❒ Public Law 104-193 also affected a number of disabled children, who lost SSI as a result of the changes. However, Public Law 105-33, the BBA, reinstituted their eligibility for Medicaid.
❒ In addition, Public Law 104-193 repealed the federal entitlement program known as Aid to Families with Dependent Children (AFDC) and replaced it with Temporary Assistance for Needy Families (TANF). TANF provides states with grants to be spent on time-limited cash assistance. It generally limits a family's lifetime cash welfare benefits to a maximum of 5 years and permits states to impose a wide range of other requirements as well—especially those related to employment. However, the impact on Medicaid eligibility is not significant. Under

welfare reform, persons who would have been eligible for AFDC under the AFDC requirements in effect on July 16 1996, generally will still be eligible for Medicaid. Although most persons covered by TANF will receive Medicaid, the law does not require it.

Title XXI of the Social Security Act, known as the State Children's Health Insurance Program (SCHIP), is a new program created by the Balanced Budget Act of 1997. In addition to allowing states to design or expand an existing state insurance program, SCHIP provides more federal funds for states to expand Medicaid eligibility to include a greater number of children who are currently uninsured. With certain exceptions, these are low-income children who would not have qualified for Medicaid before this plan went into effect.

Funds from SCHIP also may be used to provide medical assistance to children during a "presumptive" eligibility period for Medicaid. Medicaid coverage may begin as early as the third month before an application is submitted—*if* the person would have been eligible for Medicaid during that period, had they applied sooner. This is one of several options from which states may select to provide health care coverage for more children. The BBA allows states to provide 12 months of continuous Medicaid coverage (without reevaluation) for eligible children under the age of 19. Medicaid coverage generally stops at the end of the month in which a person no longer meets the eligibility criteria.

The Ticket to Work and Work Incentives Improvement Act of 1999 (Public Law 106-170) provides or continues Medicaid coverage to certain disabled beneficiaries who work despite their disability. Those with higher incomes may pay a sliding scale premium based on income.

In addition to the above guidelines for people the state is required to cover, each state may establish its own eligibility requirements. They also may determine which services are covered and the amount of reimbursement given for covered services. As long as the federal guidelines are covered within their program, states are free to run their own programs. Most states have additional "state-only" programs that provide medical assistance for specified low-income people who do not qualify for programs with mandated or optional Medicaid coverage tied to federal reimbursement. Federal funds are *not* provided for state-only programs. To find state-specific Medicaid information, go to the website www.cms.gov and click on the link to Medicaid. From there, follow the directions to each state-specific website.

THE MEDICAID-MEDICARE RELATIONSHIP

Medicare beneficiaries who have low incomes and limited resources also may receive help from the Medicaid program. Because Social Security payments vary based on the income history of each person and because some people have additional sources of income, not everyone who receives Medicare will meet the income requirements to also receive Medicaid.

For those who are eligible for some type of Medicaid coverage, the Medicare health care coverage is supplemented by services that are available under their state's Medicaid program. Services will vary according to which program the person qualifies for, but could include, for example, nursing facility care beyond the 100-day limit covered by Medicare, prescription drugs, eyeglasses, and hearing aids. The Medicare program pays for any services that are covered by Medicare before any payments are made by the Medicaid program. Medicaid is always the "payor of last resort."

Some Medicare beneficiaries receive help with Medicare premiums and cost-sharing payments through their state Medicaid program. Qualified Medicare Beneficiaries (QMBs, pronounced "kwimbees") and Specified Low-Income Medicare Beneficiaries (SLMBs, pronounced "slim-bees") are the best-known categories. These programs have the most participants.

QMBs are those Medicare beneficiaries who have resources (assets such as bank accounts, stock, houses, cars, and other valuables) at or below twice the standard allowed under the SSI program, and incomes at or below 100% of the FPL. For QMBs, Medicaid pays the Hospital Insurance (Medicare Part A) and Supplementary Medical Insurance (Medicare Part B) premiums and the Medicare coinsurance and **deductibles,** subject to limits that states may impose on payment rates.

SLMBs are Medicare beneficiaries with resources (assets) like the QMBs, but with incomes less than 120% of the FPL. For SLMBs, the Medicaid program pays only the Medicare Part B premiums.

A third category of Medicare beneficiaries who may receive help from Medicaid are disabled-and-working individuals. According to the Medicare law, disabled-and-working individuals who previously qualified for Medicare because of disability, but who lost entitlement because of their return to work (despite the disability), are allowed to purchase Medicare Part A and Part B coverage. If these persons have incomes below 200% of the FPL but do not meet any other Medicaid assistance category, they may qualify to have Medicaid pay their Part A premiums as Qualified Disabled and Working Individuals (QDWIs).

MEDICAID SERVICES

Title XIX of the Social Security Act allows considerable flexibility within the states' Medicaid programs. However, if federal matching funds are received, some federal requirements are mandatory. A state's Medicaid program must offer medical assistance for certain basic services to most *categorically needy* populations. These services generally include the following:

- ❒ Inpatient hospital services
- ❒ Outpatient hospital services
- ❒ Prenatal care
- ❒ Vaccines for children
- ❒ Physician services
- ❒ Nursing facility services for persons age 21 or older
- ❒ Family planning services and supplies
- ❒ Rural health clinic services
- ❒ Home health care for persons eligible for skilled-nursing services
- ❒ Laboratory and x-ray services
- ❒ Pediatric and family nurse practitioner services
- ❒ Nurse-midwife services
- ❒ Federally qualified health center (FQHC) services and ambulatory services of an FQHC that would be available in other settings
- ❒ Early periodic screening and diagnostic testing (EPSDT) services for children younger than age 21. The EPSDT program is a Medicaid preventive- medicine program. (Some states require an EPSDT exam every year for children younger than age 10 who are enrolled in Medicaid.)

States may also receive federal matching funds to provide certain *optional* services. Following are the most common of the 34 currently approved optional Medicaid services:

- ❒ Diagnostic services
- ❒ Clinic services
- ❒ Intermediate care facilities for the mentally retarded
- ❒ Prescribed drugs and prosthetic devices
- ❒ Optometrist services and eyeglasses
- ❒ Nursing facility services for children younger than age 21
- ❒ Transportation services
- ❒ Rehabilitation and physical therapy services
- ❒ Home and community-based care to certain persons with chronic impairments

The Balanced Budget Act of 1997 also included a state option known as Programs of All-inclusive Care for the Elderly (PACE). PACE provides an alternative to institutional care for persons age 55 or older who require a *nursing facility* level of care. The PACE team manages *all* health, medical, and social services and gathers together other services as needed to provide preventive, rehabilitative, curative, and supportive care. This care can be provided in day health centers, homes, hospitals, and nursing homes. It helps the person maintain independence, dignity, and quality of life.

PACE functions within the Medicare program as well. The individuals enrolled in PACE receive benefits solely through the PACE program. PACE providers receive payment only through the PACE agreement and must make available all items and services covered under both Titles XVIII and XIX, without limitations and without charging any deductibles, copayments, or other cost sharing.

Long-term care is an important provision of Medicaid that is utilized more each year as the baby-boomer population ages. Historically, the Medicaid program has paid for almost 45% of the costs for persons using a nursing facility or home health services. In addition, Medicaid has paid a much larger percentage for people who used more than 4 months of long-term care. Because the percentage of our population that is elderly or disabled is increasing faster than that of the younger groups, the need for long-term care is expected to increase.

Sometimes it is legal to transfer assets to meet the income requirements for Medicaid. This transfer of assets must take place at least 3 to 5 years before receiving benefits. This rule is designed to limit the number of people who are eligible to participate in the program. There are specific instances in which a transfer of assets is allowed without time limits or penalties. Please check with Medicaid to obtain the most current rules.

States may not charge premiums for Medicaid except in rare instances, but they may charge small deductibles and small copayments. Please obtain and read a current set of rules for your state's Medicaid program to see if any of these costs would apply in your state. Many states now offer a variety of types of health plans, including HMOs, in their Medicaid programs.

Each state chooses an insurance company to administer Medicaid for that state. This company is called the fiscal intermediary (FI) for that state. The FI functions just like a regular insurance company, except it must follow the state and federal regulations for Medicaid instead of their own policies for their Medicaid clients.

BILLING CONSIDERATIONS

Medicaid eligibility can change monthly. Some states issue new ID cards each month, and some states use an ID card similar to a credit card for instant eligibility verification. Eligibility must be effective on the date care is rendered, or payment will be denied.

Medicare is always primary when both Medicare and Medicaid may be billed. However, Medicaid only pays the portion of the fee that does not exceed Medicaid's allowable payment. When the portion of the bill paid by Medicare exceeds the Medicaid allowable, no Medicaid payment is issued.

Medicaid never covers services that are available from any other plan, including Medicare. However, within a particular Medicaid program's limitations, Medicaid might cover a variety of noncovered services, such as hearing aids.

A Medicaid physician who sees patients covered by both Medicare and Medicaid must participate in both in order to receive payment from both. If the physician only participates in Medicaid, he or she must enroll in Medicare in order to receive payment from Medicare, or the physician will lose the money Medicare would have paid.

Several blocks on the claim form are set aside for Medicaid use. *Block No. 10d, Reserved for Local Use, block No. 22, Medicaid Resubmission Code, and block No. 24H, EPSDT Family Plan* on the claim form are not used by any other payor. The patient's Medicaid number, preceded by MCD, is placed in *block No. 10d, Reserved for Local Use.* The Medicaid resubmission code and original reference number are placed in *block No. 22, Medicaid Resubmission Code.* EPSDT claims will have a "Y" entered in *block No. 24H, EPSDT Family Plan.*

To reduce patient fraud, some states use electronic ID cards. These cards are swiped in the same manner as a credit card is swiped during patient registration to obtain instant eligibility verification. In some states, Medicaid requires direct deposit for provider payments.

Each state also has state-specific requirements that must be met. For example: In one state, the physician enrollment packet includes notarized fingerprinting and a background check. Claims sent to Medicaid in that state must be sent on paper because they require original "wet ink" signatures in the signature boxes. When the claims arrive at Medicaid, they are scanned into the system. Correction fluid smears when it is scanned, so errors may only be corrected using correction tape. Medicaid in that state requires special codes that must be entered in *block No. 19, Reserved for Local Use,* to identify the type of claim; the applicable codes are found in the Medicaid workbook. Also, Medicaid in that state requires the entire diagnosis code number, not the line number from *block No. 21, Diagnosis or Nature of Illness or Injury,* to be entered in *block No. 24E, Diagnosis Code,* to link the diagnosis to the procedure.

In many states, Medicaid does not allow the use of global (bundled) codes when billing for pregnancies. Each individual service is billed separately (unbundled). This is because eligibility can change many times during a 9-month pregnancy.

The most common error on Medicaid claims is a missing provider number in *block No. 24K, Reserved for Local Use,* and a missing referring physician Medicaid ID number in *block No. 17a, ID Number of the Referring Physician.* The provider's Medicaid ID number can be 6 to 10 digits long, depending on the state.

Many states do not update the Medicaid computer systems very often, so they require the use of codebooks from previous years. For example, many states require the use of codebooks from 1995 or 1996 to code Medicaid claims, although the Medicaid fee schedule does keep up with the times by changing every year. Check with your state's Medicaid FI for billing rules specific to your state. See Appendix B or go to the CMS website for Medicaid to find contact information and the FI for each state.

STOP & REVIEW

Answer the following questions:

1. Medicaid is a federal program.
____True   ____False

2. Which of the following people must be covered to meet federal guidelines? (Circle all that apply.)
A. All disabled people
B. Those receiving SSI
C. Those receiving welfare
D. Those receiving AFDC

3. States may charge Medicaid premiums.
____True   ____False

4. Level of coverage may vary by state.
____True   ____False

5. Sometimes it is legal to transfer assets to meet income requirements.
____True   ____False

6. If a patient has both Medicaid and Medicare, what expenses does Medicaid pay?

A. Part B premium
B. Most or all of the copayments
C. Most or all of the deductibles
D. All of the above

7. If a patient has both Medicaid and Medicare, which is the primary payor and which is the secondary payor?

_____

8. The claim form has some blocks that are used exclusively by Medicaid.
____True   ____False

9. Electronic ID cards for instant eligibility verification are an antifraud measure used by at least one state.
____True   ____False

10. States never use HMOs to run their Medicaid programs.
____True   ____False

Indian Health Service

Since 1787, the United States has had an unusual relationship with Indian Tribal governments. Today, an Indian tribe is defined as an Indian or Alaska Native tribe, band, nation, pueblo village, or community that the Secretary of the Interior acknowledges to exist as an Indian tribe in compliance with the Federally Recognized Indian Tribe List Act of 1995. The United States recognizes Indian tribes as domestic dependent nations under its protection. In treaties, Indian tribes are guaranteed the right of self-government.

The Indian Health Service (IHS) is an agency of the Department of Health and Human Services. The IHS is responsible for providing federal health services to members of federally recognized Indian tribes. The goal of the IHS is to ensure that comprehensive, culturally acceptable personal and public health services are available and accessible to all American Indian and Alaska Native people.

To meet this goal, the IHS does the following:

❑ Assists Indian tribes in developing their health programs through activities such as health management training, technical assistance, and human resource development
❑ Assists Indian tribes in coordinating health planning, in obtaining and using health resources available through federal, state, and local programs, and in operating comprehensive health care services and health programs
❑ Provides comprehensive health care services, including hospital and ambulatory medical care, preventive and rehabilitative services, and development of community sanitation facilities
❑ Serves as the principal federal advocate in the heath field for Indians to make certain comprehensive health services are there for American Indian and Alaska Native people

IHS services are provided both directly and through tribally contracted and operated health programs. More than 9,000 private providers render care under the IHS annually. The federal system consists of 5 residential treatment centers, 49 health stations, 61 health centers, and 36 hospitals. In addition, there are 34 urban Indian health projects that provide a variety of health and referral services. Through Public Law 93-638 self-determination contracts, American Indian tribes and Alaska Native corporations administer another 28 residential treatment centers, 76 health stations, 158 health centers, 13 hospitals, and 170 Alaska village clinics.

Effective January 1, 2005, section 630 of the Medicare Modernization Act allows for 100%

reimbursement of the reasonable cost of ambulance services that meet the 35-mile rule when provided by IHS/tribal hospitals that manage and operate hospital-based ambulances, including critical access hospitals.

Trailblazer Health, LLC, is the FI for IHS hospitals and skilled nursing facilities nationwide.

TRICARE/CHAMPUS

CHAMPUS stands for Civilian Health and Medical Program of the Uniformed Services. CHAMPUS is the name of a law originally designed to enhance medical coverage for the *families* of military service members and military retirees and their families. CHAMPUS is an entitlement program: It is a right granted by Congress to eligible persons.

CHAMPUS is valid for all seven of the uniformed services: the Army, Navy, Marine Corps, Air Force, Coast Guard, Public Health Service, and National Oceanic and Atmospheric Administration.

CHAMPUS now provides medical benefits to:

❒ Active duty service members and their families
❒ Unremarried surviving family members of deceased active duty service members
❒ Military retirees and their families
❒ Unremarried surviving family members of deceased retired military members
❒ Families of reservists ordered to active duty for more than 30 days
❒ Families of reservists who die on active duty
❒ Some former spouses of active or retired military members if certain conditions have been met
❒ Unmarried children until the age of 21, unless they are in school full time—then until the age of 23—or unless they are severely handicapped and the condition existed before the child's twenty-first birthday (or twenty-third birthday if a full-time student)
❒ Captives
❒ Former captives and their families
❒ Certain NATO-eligible foreigners are eligible for some outpatient services.

CHAMPUS now covers both active duty service members and retirees. Military retirement can come from longevity (time in the military), or it can come from a disability. CHAMPUS does not provide benefits to veterans other than those who retire from the military. Eligible veterans (both CHAMPUS and non-CHAMPUS eligible) may receive care from the Department of Veterans Affairs (VA).

The military service member is the "sponsor" for each CHAMPUS-eligible person. Participants *and* their military sponsor, even if retired, must be enrolled in the Defense Enrollment Eligibility Reporting System **(DEERS)** to receive care in a service hospital or to receive reimbursement from CHAMPUS for civilian health care. DEERS is a worldwide Department of Defense computer network used to establish CHAMPUS eligibility and to accomplish other military purposes.

All CHAMPUS-eligible persons have a military-issued ID card. The military ID card cannot be expired, and it must say "yes" under the word "Civilian" in the medical block on the back of the card. Before providing services, check for these requirements and make a photocopy of both sides of the military ID card. Reservist ID cards usually do not meet these requirements. Reservists typically purchase private medical plans for themselves and their families, usually through their civilian employers.

Note: A new law effective October 1, 2004, provides special CHAMPUS benefits to reservists serving more than 30 days on active duty, so you will begin to see some reservists and their families with military ID cards that say "yes" under the word "Civilian" in the medical block on the back of the card.

TRICARE is the name of the current program that meets the CHAMPUS law. TRICARE provides three options for medical coverage:

1. TRICARE Standard—an indemnity option identical to the original CHAMPUS program
2. TRICARE Extra—similar to a PPO
3. TRICARE Prime—similar to an HMO

Only one of the three TRICARE programs issues an additional ID card—TRICARE Prime, the HMO option. The TRICARE Prime ID card does not establish CHAMPUS eligibility; only the military ID establishes whether the beneficiary is CHAMPUS eligible.

Active duty service members are required to enroll in TRICARE Prime. They are sent to civilian physicians when the service requested is not available locally from a military physician. The authorization is printed on a CHAMPUS form. However, civilian medical bills for active duty service members are paid from active duty funds, not CHAMPUS funds.

TRICARE is essentially a new way to administer CHAMPUS benefits. TRICARE is most often referred to as TRICARE/CHAMPUS or CHAMPUS/TRICARE to avoid confusion for those who do not understand their health care benefits. Remember, TRICARE simply refers to the three options for health care under the CHAMPUS entitlement. TRICARE is not affiliated with CHAMPVA, and a patient can never be eligible for both CHAMPUS and CHAMPVA at the same time.

People younger than age 65 no longer lose CHAMPUS eligibility when Medicare coverage becomes available to them due to disability or end-stage renal disease. When CHAMPUS-eligible persons younger than age 65 participate in both Medicare Part A and Medicare Part B, they are covered under both Medicare and CHAMPUS. These beneficiaries are sometimes called **MedCHAMP.**

The computer systems for Medicare and DEERS are linked to identify when a patient has both CHAMPUS and Medicare. Medicare is the primary payor and CHAMPUS is the secondary payor for these claims. If the patient loses Medicare eligibility and still qualifies for CHAMPUS, he or she may return to the regular CHAMPUS program.

People age 65 and older also no longer lose CHAMPUS eligibility when Medicare coverage becomes available to them. When they enroll in Medicare Part A and Part B, they are automatically enrolled in a program called TRICARE for Life. The automatic enrollment feature prevents any break in coverage. TRICARE for Life provides Medicare supplemental coverage that is very similar to Medigap. However, to become eligible for TRICARE for Life, each participant must purchase Medicare Part B coverage. TRICARE for Life is covered in more detail later in the chapter.

CHAMPUS was established to supplement care received in military clinics or hospitals. It does not duplicate those benefits. Copayments, deductibles, and other fees listed in this chapter for TRICARE were valid in the last quarter of 2004 for the fiscal year 2005 and may have since changed. Deductibles are based on the federal government's fiscal year— October 1 through September 30. See Table 11-1 for a comparison of the costs and features of each TRICARE option.

The active duty or retired military member is referred to as the sponsor. Copayments and deductibles for all three TRICARE options are based on the military rank of the sponsor. A numbering convention was established to designate various levels of rank for all branches of service. Using the numbering system limits confusion about the out-of-pocket expenses that are based on rank, especially as the names for the military ranks differ with each branch of service. The letter "E" stands for "Enlisted." The letter "O" stands for "Officer." The number "1" indicates the lowest level of service and salary. Higher numbers indicate higher levels and higher salaries according to rank and longevity. For example, "E-4" indicates a level 4 enlisted person and "O-2" indicates a level 2 officer. Officers are a type of manager and outrank enlisted personnel.

Many civilians do not know that a petty officer is the same as a noncommissioned officer (NCO). Both refer to mid-to-high level enlisted personnel in different branches of the military.

Likewise, many civilians do not know that the term "captain" varies by branch of service. In the Army, Air Force, and Marine Corps, O-3 indicates a captain and O-6 indicates a colonel. In the Navy, O-3 indicates a lieutenant and O-6 indicates a captain. Regardless of the name given the rank, O-3 represents the same pay grade and same level of importance, and O-6 represents the same pay grade and same level of importance, in every military branch.

The National Defense Authorization Act for fiscal year 2005 made permanent several of the temporary TRICARE benefits first authorized for fiscal year 2004. Reservists with delayed effective date orders to serve on active duty for more than 30 days are authorized for TRICARE eligibility for themselves and their families for up to 90 days before the effective date on the orders. The TRICARE standard and extra deductibles are waived for these reservists and their families, and TRICARE is authorized to pay **nonparticipating providers** up to 115% of the TRICARE maximum allowable charge to enhance continuity of care with their civilian providers. There is now a 180-day transitional TRICARE benefit after the reservists are no longer serving on active duty. The legislation also requires each reservist to receive a comprehensive examination before ending active duty.

In addition, reservists who serve 90 continuous days or more are now given the opportunity to purchase TRICARE for themselves and their families when they end active duty. Each reservist who signs an agreement to continue to serve in the reserves for 1 year or more after the active duty period ends may purchase 1 year of TRICARE for every 90 days of consecutive active duty service served. However, the reservist must continue to serve in the reserves during the effective dates for the purchased TRICARE coverage.

Military authorization legislation changes annually, so watch the TRICARE website each fall for updates: www.tricare.osd.mil.

TABLE 11-1
TRICARE Comparison Charts

The charts below provide cost shares for families using TRICARE. Current updates can be found at www.tricare.osd.mil.

Active Duty Family Members

	TRICARE Prime	TRICARE Extra	TRICARE Standard
Annual Deductible	None	$150/individual or $300/family for E-5 and above; $50/$100 for E-4 and below	$150/individual or $300/family for E-5 and above; $50/$100 E-4 and below
Annual Enrollment Fee	None	None	None
Civilian Outpatient Visit	No cost	15% of negotiated fee	20% of allowed charges for covered service
Civilian Inpatient Admission	No cost	Greater of $25 or $13.90/day	Greater of $25 or $13.90/day
Civilian Inpatient Mental Health	No cost	$20/day	$20/day
Civilian Inpatient Skilled Nursing Facility Care	$0 per diem charge per admission No separate copayment/cost share for separately billed professional charges	$11/day ($25 minimum) Charge per admission	$11/day ($25 minimum) Charge per admission

Retirees, Their Family Members, and Others

	TRICARE Prime	TRICARE Extra	TRICARE Standard
Annual Deductible	None	$150/individual or $300/family	$150/individual or $300/family
Annual Enrollment Fee	$230/individual $460/family	None	None
Civilian Copays		20% of negotiated fee	25% of allowed charges for covered service
Outpatient Emergency Care Mental Health Visit	$12 $30 $25 $17 for group visit		
Civilian Inpatient Cost Share	$11/day ($25 minimum) Charge per admission	Lesser of $250/day or 25% of negotiated charges plus 20% of negotiated professional fees	Lesser of $512/day or 25% of billed charges plus 25% of allowed professional fees
Civilian Inpatient Skilled Nursing Facility Care	$11/day ($25 minimum) Charge per admission	Lesser of $250 per diem copayment or 20% cost share of total charges, whichever is less, institutional charges, plus 20% cost share of separately billed professional charges	25% cost share of allowed charges for institutional services, plus 25% cost share of allowable for separately billed professional charges
Civilian Inpatient Mental Health	$40 per day	20% of institutional and negotiated professional fees	Lesser of $169/day or 25% of allowable fees

Courtesy of TRICARE.

TRICARE STANDARD

TRICARE Standard is the indemnity or "fee-for-service" option. TRICARE Standard has an annual outpatient deductible of $50.00 per individual and $100.00 per family for active duty level E-4 and below (the lowest paid military members) and $150.00 per individual and $300.00 per family for all others, plus a copayment amount of 20% for active duty families

and 25% for all others. The deductible starts all over again every October 1, the beginning of the federal government's fiscal year.

There is not a separate deductible for inpatient care. However, there is an inpatient daily fee of $13.90 ($25.00 minimum per hospitalization) for active duty families. This amount covers the cost-share amount for both the hospital bill and the physician's bill for active duty families. For all others, there is an inpatient daily fee of the lesser of $512.00 per day or 25% of bill charges, plus 25% of all separately billed physician charges.

An active duty family will not pay more than $1,000.00 per fiscal year. A retiree and family will not pay more than $3,000.00 per fiscal year in total out-of-pocket expenses. This is called a catastrophic cap. The cap applies to the allowable charges for covered services: annual deductibles, pharmacy copays, and other cost shares based on the TRICARE-allowable charge. Cost-share amounts usually increase slightly every year beginning on October 1.

TRICARE Standard does not cover all health care, and there is a standard list of items that require **preauthorization.** Special rules and limits apply. The patient pays for noncovered items. In addition, there are separate rules for mental health coverage.

A physician does not have to sign a contract with TRICARE to provide services under TRICARE Standard, but the physician must submit his or her credentials for the government to review. Beginning September 1, 2004, all Medicare-certified providers who are recognized as a provider class under TRICARE are considered TRICARE-authorized providers. TRICARE will not cover or pay for any service provided by a physician who has not submitted his or her credentials for review. The patient is then responsible for the bill in full until the provider submits his or her credentials for review. If the provider is then approved, the approval will be retroactive back to the date the provider received his or her license. This allows previously denied claims to be reprocessed and paid. Please consult a current TRICARE handbook for specific coverage and limitation rules.

TRICARE EXTRA

The PPO option is called TRICARE Extra. TRICARE Extra has an annual outpatient deductible that is the same as TRICARE Standard. The copayment amount is 15% for active duty families and 20% for all others when a network provider is seen. When a patient sees an out-of-network provider, coverage reverts to TRICARE Standard coverage.

There is an inpatient daily fee of $13.90 ($25.00 minimum per hospitalization) for active duty families. This amount covers the cost-share amount for both the hospital bill and the physician's bill for active duty families. For all others there is an inpatient daily fee of the lesser of $250.00 per day or 25% of negotiated charges plus 20% of all separately negotiated physician charges. This is applicable for all inpatient care in network hospitals. Out-of-network hospital bills revert to TRICARE Standard

coverage. The catastrophic cap for out-of-pocket expenses is the same as TRICARE Standard.

TRICARE Extra does not cover all health care, and there is a list of items that require preauthorization. Special rules and limits apply. In order for the patient to be responsible for any noncovered services performed by network providers, the patient must sign a statement agreeing to pay each noncovered service before it is performed. The government does not consider a blanket statement satisfactory. There are separate rules for mental health coverage.

Network physicians must be credentialed with regular CHAMPUS, sign a contract with TRICARE, and negotiate any discounted fees.

Eligible beneficiaries do not have to sign up for TRICARE Extra and can flow freely between TRICARE Extra and TRICARE Standard.

TRICARE PRIME

The HMO option is TRICARE Prime. Participants who choose TRICARE Prime must enroll for a minimum of 12 months and must use network providers. TRICARE Prime has no annual outpatient deductible and no copayment amounts for active duty service members and their families. All care except mental health must be rendered or approved by the primary care manager—the primary care physician. Active duty former spouses and retirees and their families pay annual (or quarterly) enrollment fees of $230.00 for an individual or $460.00 for a family.

The inpatient daily fee is at no cost for active duty families, and a fixed rate of $11.00 per day for all others. This amount covers everything, including separately billed professional fees. In addition, under TRICARE Prime, those other than active duty families have a $12.00 copay for office visits, a $25.00 copay for mental health ($17.00 for group visit) and a $30.00 copay for emergency care.

The total out-of-pocket expense for active duty families is $1,000.00 per fiscal year. This is called a catastrophic cap. The cap applies to the allowable charges for covered services: annual deductibles, pharmacy copays, and other cost shares based on the TRICARE-allowable charge. This amount does not apply to the point-of-service (POS) option. POS is any care received that the primary care physician has not authorized.

Retirees and their families will not pay more than $3,000.00 per enrollment year if they do not use the POS option. In addition to the items the cap applies to for active duty families, it also applies to the Prime enrollment fee. POS has a deductible of $300.00 per person and $600.00 per family plus a 50% copay for all Prime beneficiaries. In addition, out-of-network providers may charge up to 15% above the allowed charge and the beneficiary must pay this entire additional charge.

TRICARE Prime does not cover all health care, and there is a list of items that require preauthorization. This is the same list that applies to TRICARE Standard and Extra. Special rules and limits apply. The patient pays for noncovered services, but only if they agree in writing to pay for it before the noncovered service is rendered. There are separate rules for mental health coverage.

Network physicians sign a contract with TRICARE and negotiate the rate of discounted fees. Referrals are required if the beneficiary is to see any provider other than the primary care physician. If a referral is not given, the bill is paid as POS.

The POS deductibles and copays do not count toward the annual limit on out-of-pocket expenses. There is no limit on out-of-pocket expenses for POS costs.

By law, TRICARE is always the secondary payor except for Medicaid, Indian Health Plan, and TRICARE supplemental policies. Many organizations and military service-related associations offer policies that supplement TRICARE coverage. Each policy has its own eligibility requirements and rules for coverage. TRICARE supplement policies are secondary to TRICARE.

The government appoints a company to act as the FI to administer CHAMPUS/TRICARE. The FI functions like most insurance companies, except they must follow the Department of Defense regulations for CHAMPUS/TRICARE instead of their own policies for their CHAMPUS/TRICARE clients.

See the TRICARE website at www.tricare.osd.mil or call your TRICARE representative for more extensive details about CHAMPUS eligibility and program benefits.

CHAMPVA

CHAMPVA is a law established to provide medical benefits to eligible survivors and dependents of veterans who are, or who were before their death, permanently and totally disabled with a **service-connected** condition. "CHAMPVA" stands for Civilian Health and Medical Program of Veterans Affairs.

CHAMPVA is valid for all seven of the uniformed services: the Army, Navy, Marine Corps, Air Force, Coast Guard, Public Health Service, and National Oceanic and Atmospheric Administration.

Unlike children with CHAMPUS benefits whose coverage lasts to age 21 if unmarried, CHAMPVA children are covered until the age of 18, unless they are in school (then until the age of 23) or unless they are severely handicapped and the condition existed and was documented by CHAMPVA before CHAMPVA benefits ended. Children with CHAMPVA benefits must also be unmarried.

CHAMPVA is not part of the TRICARE program. CHAMPVA does not cover anyone who is eligible for CHAMPUS, and CHAMPVA does not cover veterans. Eligible veterans receive care from the Department of Veterans Affairs.

CHAMPVA is a program in which the VA shares the cost of medical care. CHAMPVA beneficiaries are not eligible for services in a military treatment facility.

Eligible CHAMPVA participants are responsible for an outpatient deductible of $50.00 per person and $100.00 per family. This deductible starts over every January 1, at the beginning of the calendar year.

After the deductible is met, CHAMPVA pays 75% of allowable costs, and the patient pays 25% of allowable costs. There is a $7,500.00 cap to the total family out-of-pocket expenses. The cap is per calendar year, and it only applies to covered services. There are no limits to costs for noncovered expenses.

CHAMPVA covers most health care that is considered medically necessary. Special rules and limitations apply. Participants *and* their military sponsors, if living, do not have to be enrolled in DEERS as CHAMPUS beneficiaries do.

Unlike CHAMPUS, when eligible participants become eligible for Medicare, CHAMPVA coverage ceases. Except for Medicaid, all other health plans pay first.

CHAMPVA serves as its own FI, processing its own claims and making payments for services rendered.

BILLING CONSIDERATIONS

The military sponsor serves as the "insured" for TRICARE/CHAMPUS and CHAMPVA claims. The patient's name and street address are listed under "Patient Information" on the medical claim form (blocks No. 2 and No. 5) and the military sponsor's ID number, name, and home address are listed under "Insured Information" on the medical claim form (blocks No. 1a, No. 4, and No. 7). When the military sponsor is away from home on an active duty assignment, the sponsor's home address is listed under "Insured," or the family's home address can be used if the sponsor's military address is unknown.

Military addresses sometimes use APO or FPO box numbers or codes. In some instances, a patient's address will also be an APO or FPO box number or code. An address listed this way will include:

☐ Sponsor's name and rank, APO box/code (FPO box/code), city, state, and zip code

or

☐ Sponsor's name and rank, APO box/code (FPO box/code), and zip code

APO/FPO boxes are not the same as post office boxes. A post office box is a locked box in a post office building and the recipient uses a key or combination to unlock the box and pick up mail.

An APO/FPO box or code number is a military mail clearinghouse. The mail recipients are not located in the same city as the APO/FPO address. The military mail clearinghouse sorts the mail and sends it to the recipient wherever the recipient is located.

APO/FPO addresses allow military personnel to receive mail even when their location changes frequently. Mail can be sent to military personnel overseas without charging the sender for overseas postage. APO/FPO addresses allow the military to keep the recipient's location a secret.

When a CHAMPUS-eligible person who lives overseas travels to the United States for health care, the patient's overseas home address (APO/FPO address) is used on the claim. If the patient is not enrolled in TRICARE Prime, the claim is sent to the TRICARE claim address for the CHAMPUS region in which the care is rendered. If the patient is enrolled in TRICARE Prime, the claim is sent to the contractor that processes all overseas claims—WPS in Madison, Wisconsin.

When CHAMPUS-eligible persons who live in the United States travel within the United States, claims are sent to the region for the patient's home address. (There are 15 CHAMPUS regions worldwide—12 of them are in the United States.)

Although TRICARE/CHAMPUS and CHAMPVA are separate programs, they both use the CHAMPUS maximum-allowable-charge (CMAC) fee schedule. TRICARE preferred-physician contracts include negotiated fee schedules that may not exceed the maximum-allowable-charge fee schedule. When a physician chooses to sign a contract for a fee that is less than the maximum allowable charge, the physician agrees to take a discount off the CMAC fee schedule.

Remember, all providers must be at least Standard CHAMPUS credentialed or approved by the government in order for TRICARE to pay a claim. Physician's assistants (PAs) and nurse practitioners (NPs) must also be credentialed with TRICARE if they provide services to TRICARE patients. PAs and NPs are always paid a reduced fee as compared to a payment to a physician.

Physicians must file the claim only if they are accepting "Assignment of Benefits." The physician may accept assignment on a claim-by-claim basis. When the physician accepts assignment, he or she is agreeing to accept the CMAC along with the patient's deductible and cost share as payment-in-full and may not balance-bill the beneficiary for the remainder of the bill.

Credentialed physicians who are not contracted by TRICARE (nonnetwork) may balance-bill patients for no more than 15% above the allowable amount (CMAC). Only the allowed amounts are applied toward the deductible and cost share/copayments.

For CHAMPUS/TRICARE, the deductible period coincides with the federal government's fiscal year—October 1 to September 30 of the following year. Only CHAMPVA uses the calendar year.

Whenever a CHAMPUS/TRICARE patient is admitted as an inpatient, or whenever one of the procedures on the preauthorization list is done on an outpatient basis, prior authorization must be obtained by the provider. Each approved authorization is given an **authorization number.** This authorization number is placed on the claim form by the physician's billing office, and it is also entered into the government contractor's claims processing system. When the claim is processed, the system will search for an authorization number that matches the patient and procedure listed on the claim form. If an authorization is not obtained before the admission or before the outpatient procedure being performed, a penalty will be applied to the provider's payment—50% penalty for network providers (who should know better) and 10% penalty for nonnetwork providers. Preauthorization is always required for these services even when CHAMPUS/TRICARE is the second or third payor.

Congress mandates by law how third-party liability issues are to be handled for CHAMPUS patients. When a claim is filed with ICD-9-CM codes 800 to 999 (injury and poisoning codes), the system will not process it unless there is a third-party liability form on file with the claims processor. Many times, an injury has occurred and there is a possibility of a third-party payor. For this reason, a third-party liability form is mailed to the patient for completion and return to the claims processor. Until the form is completed and returned, the claim cannot be processed, and no payment can be made. The whole bill is now the responsibility of the patient.

When the provider knows there is another payor, that is, PIP coverage with the auto insurance, PIP should be billed first and CHAMPUS second. If other third-party coverage is unknown, bill CHAMPUS first and let the government do the third-party research. The government will then investigate and determine liability. CHAMPUS will pay the claim and the government will exercise the right of subrogation to collect from the third-party payor.

All claims must be filed within 1 year of the date of service for outpatient care and 1 year from the date of discharge from the hospital for inpatient care.

All corrected claims must be sent on paper, and the words "corrected claim" should appear on both the top and bottom of the claim form. These claims go to a different P.O. box than first-time submissions.

If the patient lives near any military hospital with inpatient capabilities, care should be rendered at the military hospital. Any time care is rendered at a civilian hospital, including when the patient travels, the patient must obtain a nonavailability statement (NAS) authorizing care in the civilian hospital. An NAS is only required for inpatient care for patients who live near a military hospital. The need for an NAS is based on the patient's home zip code, as is indicated on the claim form. An NAS is not required when:

- ☐ The admission is an emergency
- ☐ The patient has other health insurance (not a supplement)
- ☐ The patient is enrolled in TRICARE Prime
- ☐ The patient lives more than 40 miles from a military treatment facility

The government has mandated that CHAMPUS subject claims to edits very similar to the edits and audits used by Medicare. Because this rule is new, it is greatly emphasized. Every procedure code will be cross-referenced with the diagnosis codes, gender codes, etc., to determine the appropriateness of the care and to establish medical necessity.

A "good faith payment" is a payment made by the government when the patient's military ID card indicates he or she is eligible, but in reality, the patient is not eligible for CHAMPUS benefits. This sometimes proves to be an act of fraud by the patient. *If* the provider has a copy of the military ID card (front and back) *and* it indicates the beneficiary was eligible for CHAMPUS benefits at the time services were rendered, *and* the provider can show a reasonable attempt has been made to collect from the patient without success, the government will make a good faith payment to the provider for the services rendered. The card must not be expired and it must say "yes" in the medical block under the word "civilian." A TRICARE Prime card is not adequate to establish eligibility and will not work to obtain a good faith payment. Only the military ID can be used to establish eligibility.

A copy of the military ID should always be kept in the patient's medical record. For children younger than age 10, use a copy of the custodial parent's card. If that parent does not have a military ID, then the children must each have an ID card of their own regardless of the children's age. The patient who does not have a current military ID card should be considered a "self-pay." If the card is questionable, call DEERS at 800-538-9552. This is the government's worldwide computer network used to establish CHAMPUS eligibility.

Answer the following questions:

1. Does the TRICARE program include CHAMPVA?

2. Does the TRICARE program include CHAMPUS?

3. Which level of TRICARE is like an HMO?

4. Which level of TRICARE is like traditional CHAMPUS?

5. Which level of TRICARE requires enrollment?

6. Who pays for the visit if the physician is not credentialed through TRICARE?

7. Are all TRICARE preferred providers credentialed?

8. Are all TRICARE credentialed providers part of the preferred-provider program?

9. What happens when TRICARE/CHAMPUS or CHAMPVA participants become eligible for Medicare?

10. What does "DEERS" stand for?

VA

"VA" stands for the Department of Veterans Affairs. The VA provides comprehensive health care to veterans with *service-connected* disabilities, as well as to veterans who meet certain eligibility requirements and need care for **non–service-connected** health problems. A service-connected disability is a disability that first occurs while the service member is serving on active duty, including temporary active duty. The disability does not have to be work related.

Eligibility for VA services is determined by the discharge status of the veteran as indicated on his or her discharge papers (DD 214):

❑ Honorable and general discharges qualify the veteran to receive veterans' benefits, including health care.

❑ Dishonorable discharges and some "bad conduct" discharges disqualify the veteran from receiving veterans' benefits, including health care.

❑ The remaining bad conduct discharges and "other than honorable" discharges are determined on a case-by-case basis by the VA.

In addition, most veterans whose first term of active duty began after September 1980 must have completed 24 continuous months of active duty before they become eligible for veterans benefits, including health care. The exceptions to this rule include reservist and National Guard members called to active duty and service members with service-connected conditions or disabilities.

The Veterans' Health Care Eligibility Reform Act of 1996 (Public Law 104-262) mandated that the VA create a national enrollment system to manage the delivery of health care services. The law mandated that the enrollment system be effective October 1, 1998. After that date, veterans must be enrolled to receive care. Veterans may apply for enrollment at any time during the year. The following veterans need not enroll:

❑ Veterans who need treatment for a VA-rated service-connected disability

❑ Veterans with a VA-rated service-connected disability of 50% or greater

❑ Veterans who were released from active duty within the previous 12 months for a disability incurred or aggravated in the line of duty

The provisions of the law include:

❑ Eliminating the distinction between outpatient care and hospital care

❑ Permitting VA to provide health care services in the most clinically appropriate setting

❑ Giving VA the authority to furnish health promotion and disease prevention services and primary care

❑ Allowing greater flexibility in applying state-of-the-art health care techniques and more efficient use of VA resources

Priority groups were established to allow VA to best allocate resources. Although the same services are now available to all enrolled veterans, the priority groups establish the VA's priorities for available services. There are currently eight priority groups, and group 1 is given the highest priority for care.

❑ Priority Group 1: veterans with service-connected disabilities rated 50% or more disabling

❑ Priority Group 2: veterans with service-connected disabilities rated 30% to 40% disabling

❑ Priority Group 3: veterans who are former POWs, veterans awarded the Purple Heart, veterans whose discharge was for a disability incurred or aggravated in the line of duty, veterans with service-connected disabilities rated 10% to 20% disabling, and veterans awarded special eligibility classification under Title 38, U.S.C., Section 1151

❑ Priority Group 4: veterans who are receiving aid and attendance or housebound benefits, and veterans who have been determined by VA to be catastrophically disabled

❑ Priority Group 5: veterans receiving VA pensions, veterans eligible for Medicaid benefits, non–service-connected veterans, and noncompensable service-connected veterans rated 0% disabled whose annual income and net worth are *below* the established VA Means Test thresholds

❑ Priority Group 6: compensable 0% service-connected veterans, World War I veterans, Mexican Border War veterans, veterans seeking care solely for disorders associated with specific types of service-connected hazard exposure while serving in specific places on specific dates or date ranges

❑ Priority Group 7: veterans who agree to pay specified copayments with income and/or net worth *above* the VA Means Test threshold and income *below* the HUD geographic index for their locality. This group has subpriority groups a, c, e, and g.

❑ Priority Group 8: veterans who agree to pay specified copayments with income and/or net worth *above* the VA Means Test threshold and *above* the HUD geographic index. This group also has subpriority groups a, c, e, and g.

When a veteran in Priority Group 7 or 8 projects substantially lower income than the previous year, a hardship determination may be requested to see if he or she qualifies for Priority Group 5, which has a higher priority of care as well as no copayment requirements. Circumstances that could warrant a hardship determination might be loss of employment, bankruptcy, or significant out-of-pocket medical expenses.

State Veterans Affairs offices are an excellent resource to help a veteran in applying for a change in eligibility status. For example, the counselors there guide veterans through the process of applying for an increase in disability percentage for service-connected problems that have progressed or grown worse, and the counselors help in obtaining other veterans' benefits. Veterans should bring with them on the first visit to a Veterans Affairs office a copy of their discharge papers (DD214) and any other documentation that supports their request.

Contact the VA for a complete list of available benefits, including the eligibility requirements, coverage, and allowed charges for each service. The VA website is www.va.gov.

BILLING CONSIDERATIONS

The Consolidated Omnibus Budget Reconciliation Act of 1986 (COBRA) gave the VA the authority to seek reimbursement from insurance companies for non–service-connected care of veterans. The VA established the **Medical Care Cost Recovery Program (MCCRP)** in 1991 in response to the 1986 law. The VA pays secondary to private heath plans for non–service-connected care.

Veterans with a less than 50% service-connected disability who can afford to pay copayments must do so when they receive non–service-connected care from a VA facility. However, the copayments are not collected at the time of service. Instead, bills are mailed to these veterans on a monthly basis. There are four basic types of copayment charges (as of fiscal 2005):

❑ Medication: The charge is $7.00 for each 30-day supply or less of medication provided on an outpatient basis for non–service-connected conditions.
❑ Outpatient: The charge for primary care visits for non–service-connected care is $15.00, and the charge for specialty care visits for non–service-connected care is $50.00.
❑ Inpatient: Congress determined the appropriate inpatient copayment for non–service-connected care should be at the current inpatient Medicare deductible rate ($912.00 in 2005) for the first 90 days that the veteran remains in the hospital plus a $10.00 per diem charge.
❑ Long-Term Care: VA charges for non–service-connected long-term care services vary by the type of service provided and the individual veteran's ability to pay.

Originally, the VA could only charge medical plans for actual costs and did not take administrative costs into consideration. Various laws since then have revised the program. The Balanced Budget Act of 1997 gave the VA the authority for reasonable charge recovery. MCCRP charges are now based on amounts that third parties (private insurance companies) pay for the same services furnished by private (civilian) medical providers in the same geographic area. The claims are sent out on UB-92 claim forms (see Chapter 12) and follow the standard billing rules for each type of medical plan billed. The VA does not bill Medicare and Medicaid.

The VA sends claims electronically through a national clearinghouse (currently WebMD). All of the money collected is placed in the operating budget for the VA to improve health care for veterans.

Answer the following questions:

1. All veterans may receive medical care at VA facilities.

____True   ____False

2. Veterans do not ever pay any of the costs for care received at a VA facility.

____True   ____False

3. What is the name of the program that allows the VA to bill third-party payors?

_____

4. What is a service-connected disability?

_____

_____

5. What is a DD214?

_____

6. Does the VA bill Medicare?

_____

7. Does the VA bill Medicaid?

_____

8. After what percentage disability is all medical care covered with no copayments or deductibles?

_____

9. Once a disability percentage is established, may it ever be changed, and if so, what steps are taken?

_____

_____

_____

10. Who does Priority Group 1 cover?
    A. Veterans with a 50% or greater service-connected disability
    B. Veterans with non–service-connected disabilities
    C. POWs
    D. Veterans with a hardship determination

Chapter Review

Government medical plans include Medicare, Medicaid, Indian Health Service, TRICARE/CHAMPUS, CHAMPVA, and the VA. Each has different rules and different eligibilities, and most now offer variations of managed care programs. The billing considerations are different for each of the government programs.

Medicaid is a state program with federal oversight intended to provide medical care for those with very low incomes. As long as states meet federal guidelines, they may run the programs as they choose.

Indian Health Service provides medical coverage to each Indian or Alaska Native tribe, band, nation, pueblo village, or community that the Secretary of the Interior acknowledges to exist as an Indian tribe in compliance with the Federally Recognized Indian Tribe List Act of 1995.

TRICARE is the name of a program that administers CHAMPUS benefits and provides medical care to active duty and retired service members and their families.

CHAMPVA provides care to dependents of disabled veterans with 100% service-connected disabilities before and after the veteran's death and dependents of deceased active duty service members.

The VA provides medical care for eligible veterans. Treatment for service-connected injuries and disabilities is given priority preference.

For questions 1 to 5, match the program in list A with the description in list B.

LIST A
1. Medicaid
2. VA
3. TRICARE/CHAMPUS
4. Indian Health Service
5. CHAMPVA

LIST B
A. Designed for active duty and retired service members and their families
B. Covers each Indian or Alaska Native tribe, band, nation, pueblo village, or community that the Secretary of the Interior acknowledges to exist as an Indian tribe in compliance with the Federally Recognized Indian Tribe List Act of 1995
C. Designed for families of those killed on active duty and families of those with 100% service-connected disability
D. Designed for people with very low income
E. Covers most military veterans

6. Medicaid is administered by each state, but the federal government provides matching funds and establishes regulations that are tied to those funds. Therefore Medicaid is a state program with federal oversight.

____True   ____False

7. With Medicaid, a child's eligibility is based upon his or her parents' income and assets.

____True   ____False

8. SSI benefits are available to low-income individuals of any age who have a disability. Do SSI recipients meet eligibility requirements for Medicaid, and if so, are they medically needy or categorically needy?

_____

9. The Ticket to Work and Work Incentives Improvement Act of 1999 (Public Law 106-170) provides or continues Medicaid coverage to certain disabled beneficiaries who work despite their disability.

____True   ____False

10. Under Medicaid for the categorically needy, is prenatal care a required basic benefit or an optional service?

_____

11. All CHAMPUS-eligible persons have a military-issued ID card. The military ID card cannot be expired, and it must say "yes" under the word "civilian" in the medical block on the back of the card.

____True   ____False

12. Who is the "sponsor" for each CHAMPUS-eligible person?

_____

13. What is the name of the current program that meets the CHAMPUS law?

_____

14. Do people age 65 and older lose CHAMPUS eligibility when Medicare coverage becomes available to them?

_____

15. Does a physician have to sign a contract with TRICARE to provide services under TRICARE Standard?

_____

16. Do eligible beneficiaries have to sign up for TRICARE Extra?

_____

17. Participants who choose TRICARE Prime must enroll for a minimum of 12 months and must use network providers.

____True   ____False

18. Is CHAMPVA part of the TRICARE program?

_____

19. With the VA, are there any copayment charges for service-connected care?

_____

20. What should veterans bring with them on the first visit to a Veterans Affairs office?

_____

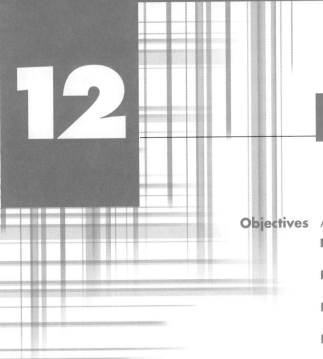

12

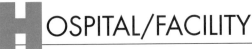

HOSPITAL/FACILITY

BILLING RULES

Objectives   After completing this chapter, you should be able to:

- Explain diagnosis related groups (DRGs) for hospital inpatient facility reimbursement
- Discuss the importance of complications and comorbidities in the DRG process
- Describe ambulatory payment classifications (APCs) for hospital outpatient facility reimbursement
- Explain how inpatient and outpatient hospital facility billing differs from billing for physician services performed in an inpatient or outpatient hospital setting
- List at least two of the billing requirements for nursing facilities
- Explain when to use ICD-9-CM Volume 3 and when to use CPT-4 to code hospital inpatient procedures
- Find the codes for inpatient hospital procedures using ICD-9-CM Volume 3, and find codes for the same procedures using CPT-4
- Identify when to use the morphology codes in Appendix A of ICD-9-CM Volume 1
- Describe how to complete a UB-92 claim form for facility reimbursement
- Discuss the purpose of revenue codes

Key Terms

ambulatory payment classification (APC) the prospective payment system used by Medicare to determine payment for hospital outpatient services. It is based on the procedure codes billed. Also called OPPS.

complications and comorbidities (CC) those additional conditions that increase the length of stay by at least 1 day in at least 75% of patients.

diagnosis related group (DRG) the prospective payment system used by Medicare to determine payment for hospital inpatient services. It is based on the diagnosis codes billed.

facility fee a charge representing the expenses incurred by a facility when providing a service.

length of stay (LOS) the actual length of time a patient spends as an inpatient in the hospital.

major diagnostic category (MDC) each category groups patients who are medically related by diagnosis, treatment similarity, and statistically similar length of hospital stay. The more than 10,000 available ICD-9-

CM diagnosis codes are divided into 25 major diagnostic categories.

outpatient prospective payment system (OPPS) the prospective payment system used by Medicare to determine payment for hospital outpatient services. It is based on the procedure codes billed. Also called APC.

peer review organization (PRO) PROs consist of physicians and other health care professionals (nurses, data technicians, etc.) who review the care given to Medicare patients. Hospitals must enter into a contract with a PRO in order to receive DRG payments. The federal government pays PROs, but they are separate from Medicare and have their own functions. The newest title for this organization is quality improvement organization, or QIO.

quality improvement organization (QIO) the new title for PRO. QIOs consist of physicians and other health care professionals (nurses, data technicians, etc.) who review the care given to Medicare patients. Hospitals must enter into a contract with a QIO in order to receive DRG payments. The federal government pays QIOs, but they are separate from Medicare and have their own functions.

relative value unit (RVU) a numeric value assigned to each procedure code in the RBRVS. This number represents the total of each of three parts (work, overhead, and malpractice). Each part is multiplied by the geographic practice site indicator (GPSI) and then added together to get a total adjusted RVU. The total adjusted RVU is multiplied by the conversion factor (the assigned per-

RVU dollar value) to arrive at the RBRVS fee allowed for the service.

resource-based relative value system (RBRVS) the prospective payment system used by Medicare to pay physicians. It considers the CPT code in relation to work, overhead expenses, and malpractice (risk). A geographical adjustment is then made to account for cost-of-living differences throughout the nation.

Uniform Bill 1992 (UB-92) the claim form used in facility billing.

Introduction

Hospitals and facilities such as surgicenters and nursing homes bill for something called facility fees. **Facility fees** are the expenses incurred by the facility when providing a service. Often referred to as overhead costs, facility fees include some of the following:

❑ The cost of the building space used, such as a patient room, an exam room, or an operating room

❑ The cost of any supplies and/or equipment purchased by the facility and used to provide the service(s) billed

❑ The cost of salaries for facility employees who participated in providing the service(s) billed

❑ The portion of each utility bill that represents costs incurred when performing the service(s) billed

Facility fees are submitted on a different claim form than the fees for physician services. Hospitals and facility services are sent out on a **Uniform Bill** claim form, most commonly referred to as the **UB-92,** but also called a CMS-1450 claim form. Physician services are sent out on a CMS-1500 claim form with the name and address of the facility listed in block No. 32. The payor then divides the total fee for the service between the physician and the facility, usually in a 60/40 split, with 60% going to the physician for his work and malpractice costs and 40% going to the facility for the facility's overhead and malpractice costs.

In this chapter, you will learn the differences between the billing rules for physician services performed in a facility and the billing rules for hospitals and facilities, and you will learn how to complete a UB-92 claim for the facility fees.

Physician Reimbursement

You must first understand a bit about how Medicare and many other payors use the **resource-based relative value system (RBRVS)**, also referred to as the resource-based relative-value scale, to calculate physician fees. Then it is easier to understand how fees are split when a physician performs services in a facility, with the facility absorbing the overhead costs of the service and part of the malpractice risk for the service.

The California Medical Committee on Fees originally developed the resource-based relative value system in 1956. They named it the California Relative Value Studies (CRVS). The purpose was to help physicians determine a fair market value (price) for their services. The studies were updated periodically from 1957 through 1974. In 1975, the Federal Trade Commission decided that the CRVS

might constitute a price-fixing scheme. Consequently, the CRVS has not been updated since 1974.

Since then, workers' compensation (in many states) and many other payors have adopted their own relative value systems based on the original California studies.

In 1992, the Health Care Financing Administration (HCFA, now called the Centers for Medicare and Medicaid Services [CMS]) commissioned a **relative value unit (RVU)** study for Medicare. The study was performed by Harvard University's Public Health Department and was named the Resource-Based Relative Value Study (RBRVS). RBRVS is the basis for today's Medicare physician fee schedule, and it has been adopted by many other payors that use relative values to determine fee schedules.

The RBRVS fee schedule considers the CPT code in relation to three additional factors:

1. Work: the amount of work performed to deliver the service
2. Overhead: costs associated with the process (staff, rent, equipment, supplies)
3. Malpractice: the amount of inherent risk in the performance of the procedure

The diagnosis code order and the code specificity for every listed diagnosis are considered in the determination of both the amount of work performed and the amount of inherent risk. Geographic considerations are used to determine the overhead portion of the RBRVS fee.

A specific number of RVUs are assigned to each of the three factors considered in the procedure code. A payor contract will specify the dollar value, or conversion factor (CF), of each RVU. The number of RVUs for each factor is multiplied first by the geographic practice site indicator (GPSI) (a fixed number for each location), the three parts are added together, and the sum is then multiplied by the conversion factor (dollar value per unit) to determine the fee for each procedure.

Although the GPSI is a fixed number for each location, sometimes the GPSI is the same for each factor of the procedures for that location, and sometimes it is different for each factor of the procedures for that location. For example: In one location the work GPSI is 1.0, the overhead GPSI is .99, and the malpractice GPSI is 1.3. However, in another location the work GPSI is .99, the overhead GPSI is .99, and the malpractice GPSI is .99. Therefore it is standard in the industry to multiply the GPSI for each factor separately and then add them together before multiplying the sum by the conversion factor: [(work RVU = work GPSI) + (overhead RVU = overhead GPSI) + (malpractice RVU = malpractice GPSI)] = CF = $ fee.

For example: A procedure is assigned .7 work RVUs, .3 overhead RVUs, and .8 malpractice RVUs for a total of 1.8 RVUs. The GPSI is .99 for each factor and the conversion factor in the contract is 43.2.

❏ You will multiply the work RVU of .7 times the work GPSI of .99, which equals .693.
❏ Then multiply the overhead RVU of .3 times the overhead GPSI of .99, which equals .297.
❏ Then multiply the malpractice RVU .8 times the malpractice GPSI of .99, which equals .792.
❏ Next, you add them together to get what is called an adjusted RVU of 1.782.
❏ Then you multiply the adjusted RVU of 1.782 by the conversion factor of 43.2 to get 76.982.
❏ Round the total to the nearest cent to arrive at a fee of $76.98.

Occasionally a contract will specify different conversion factors for different types of service. For example, surgical procedures might have a higher conversion factor than medical procedures. Additional information about using RVUs to find the fee is included in Chapter 14.

Sometimes the only difference between physician fee schedules for the various plans is the RVU conversion number, but be aware that there is more than one version of RBRVS. One physician office often must work with multiple contracts, each of which uses a specific version of RBRVS. Medicare's version only includes services that are covered services for Medicare. Other versions of RBRVS usually cover a greater number of services. You must be careful to always use the correct version of RBRVS for each payor.

When the physician performs his or her services in a facility, such as for a hospital inpatient, the physician receives the work portion plus a portion for the physician's malpractice costs. The facility then receives the overhead portion plus a portion for the facility's malpractice costs. The physician sends a bill on the CMS-1500 and lists the facility in block No. 32. The physician's fee is calculated using the version of RBRVS specified in the contract.

The facility sends a bill on the UB-92 claim form. Each numbered block on the UB-92 is called a field locator (FL). The facility sends a bill on the UB-92 claim form with the name of the attending physician and the physician's ID number in FL 82, and physicians other than the attending physician are listed with their ID numbers in FL 83. The facility's fee portion of the total fee for the service is calculated using diagnosis related groups (DRGs) for inpatients and ambulatory payment classifications (APCs) for outpatients. DRGs, APCs, and details about specific field locators (FLs) on the UB-92 claim form are discussed later in this chapter.

Answer the following questions:

1. What is the billing term used when a hospital incurs overhead costs?

   _____

2. Who divides the payment allowed between the hospital and the physician? _____

3. Who developed the CRVS? _____

   _____

4. Who decided that the CRVS might constitute a price-fixing scheme? _____

5. What system does Medicare use to reimburse physicians? _____

6. Who developed RBRVS? _____

Use the following to answer questions 7 through 9: The RBRVS fee schedule considers the CPT code in addition to what three additional factors?

7. _____

8. _____

9. _____

10. Is there more than one version of RBRVS? _____

   _____

Diagnosis Related Groups (DRGs)—Inpatient Hospital Reimbursement

Diagnosis related groups (DRGs) are an inpatient classification system that was developed at Yale University and tested from 1977 to 1979. Originally, it was developed for utilization review and it considered medical necessity and length of stay when determining whether the cost of the services provided were appropriate for each patient.

Medicare took a look at the DRG system and decided it could easily be adapted for payors to use when making payment decisions. Paying by DRGs would put the burden of limiting medical costs on the hospital and not the payor. Medicare adopted DRGs under the prospective payment system (PPS) for payment of all hospitalizations and other specific hospital-related expenses, effective October 1, 1983. Since that time, any time the hospital expenses on behalf of a patient exceed Medicare's DRG payment, the hospital loses money. As a result, hospitals are now very motivated to contain costs as much as possible.

In the DRG system, the more than 10,000 available ICD-9-CM diagnosis codes are grouped into 25 **major diagnostic categories (MDCs)** and are assigned a three-digit code from 001 to 475. Each category groups patients who are medically related by diagnosis, treatment similarity, and statistically similar length of hospital stay. Each MDC is then subdivided into DRG groups based on the historical data for the nationwide average payment amounts per hospitalization. Similar payment amounts within an MDC are grouped into one DRG and are then assigned a fixed payment value.

Hospitals use DRG grouper software to evaluate all the pertinent factors, starting with discharge diagnosis, and assign a DRG for each hospitalization. Six variables are included in the calculations to determine DRG classification:

1. Principal diagnosis
2. Secondary diagnoses
3. Surgical procedures
4. Complications and comorbidities (CC)
5. Age and gender
6. Discharge status

The principal diagnosis is the diagnosis that *after study* is found to be chiefly responsible for the hospitalization. The principal diagnosis cannot be determined until the time of discharge. Usually the physician lists it first among the diagnoses listed in the discharge summary.

Secondary diagnoses are other diagnoses that affect this hospitalization. They do not include diagnoses that do not affect this hospitalization. If the patient is given treatment, including medication or increased monitoring, the diagnosis has affected the hospitalization and is included. If the physician had to consider the diagnosis when making treatment decisions, the diagnosis is included. Only the physician can make that determination. If the diagnosis was relevant the last time the patient was admitted, but the condition resolved and does not affect this hospitalization, the diagnosis is not included.

Surgical procedures that cause the hospital to incur significant expense are each listed on the claim form and are considered when the DRG is chosen. Minor surgical procedures that do not cause the hospital to incur significant expense, such as suturing a small, simple laceration, are not listed on the claim form and are not considered when the DRG is chosen. The physician may bill for the minor surgical procedures that require the expertise of a physician, but the facility does not because it does not significantly increase the facility fees.

Complications and comorbidities (CC) are defined as conditions that increase the length of stay by at least 1 day in at least 75% of the patients nationwide. This section allows the hospital to identify which of the secondary diagnoses and other specific circumstances usually cause a significant increase in facility fees. The versions of the ICD-9-CM codebook used by hospitals (Volumes 1, 2, and 3) often list acceptable CC and excluded CC under the code number and description for diagnoses that are considered acceptable to be principal diagnoses. This makes the determination of which additional diagnoses to enter into the DRG grouper software a little more straightforward so the correct overall DRG can be assigned.

Age is important because patients of extreme age (very young and very old) often have significantly increased average costs. Therefore age can provide medical necessity for a higher DRG payment group. Gender is important because many procedures and many diagnoses are gender specific. The gender for the diagnosis and/or procedure must match the gender of the patient to meet medical necessity requirements.

Discharge status tells the circumstances of the patient upon discharge—where the patient went and whether additional skilled care was required. Some examples of discharge status include: own home with no home health care, own home with home health care, home of friend or relative with assistance from friend or relative, independent living facility, assisted living facility, nursing facility, hospice, county morgue, and funeral home.

The DRG reimbursement rate for Medicare is a fixed dollar amount based on the average of all patients in a specific DRG category in the base year. Reimbursement is adjusted periodically for inflation, economic factors, and bad debt. Other payors may have a higher DRG payment rate than Medicare, but with the possible exception of Medicaid, they cannot have a lower DRG payment rate than Medicare. The DRG payment rates for specific other payors are negotiated in the contracts between each payor and the facility.

Hospitals must enter into a contract with a **quality improvement organization (QIO**, formerly **peer review organization, PRO**) in order to receive DRG payments. QIOs consist of physicians and other health care professionals (nurses, data technicians, etc.) who review the care given to Medicare patients. The federal government pays QIOs, but they are separate from Medicare and have their own functions.

QIOs investigate patient complaints for care provided in the following settings:

❑ Inpatient hospitals
❑ Hospital outpatient departments
❑ Emergency room
❑ Skilled nursing facilities
❑ Ambulatory surgery centers
❑ Certain health maintenance organizations (HMOs)

QIOs determine:

❑ If the services provided were necessary
❑ If the services provided were appropriate
❑ If the quality of care given was sufficient
❑ If care was given in the proper setting

A hospital may request a QIO review when it receives a Medicare remittance notice (MRN) that states noncoverage was determined for a claim and no payment will be sent. A QIO review is required before an appeal can be filed. The only communication from a QIO follows a review. When a Medicare patient's care is still denied following the QIO process, the hospital, physician, or patient may appeal the denial.

When a physician submits a claim (using a CMS-1500 medical claim form) for services rendered to an inpatient, the primary diagnosis listed on the physician's claim should fall within the DRG category billed by the hospital (on a UB-92 medical claim form).

Answer the following questions:

1. What is DRG an abbreviation for?

_____

2. What are QIO and PRO abbreviations for? _____

_____

3. Who bills using a CMS-1500 claim form?

_____

4. Who bills using a UB-92 claim form?

_____

5. Who developed DRGs?

_____

For Questions 6 to 8, name three of the variables assessed when assigning a DRG:

6. _____

7. _____

8. _____

For questions 9 and 10, name two of the things that QIOs determine:

9. _____

10. _____

Ambulatory Payment Classifications (APCs)—Outpatient Hospital Reimbursement

The Omnibus Reconciliation Act (OBRA) of 1986 instructed the Health Care Financing Administration (HCFA), now called the Centers for Medicare and Medicaid Services (CMS), to develop an **outpatient prospective payment system (OPPS)** for payment of the facility fees for hospital-based outpatient care and for payment of the facility fees for ambulatory surgery center procedures. Effective July 1, 1987, OBRA also required all outpatient claims to be submitted with CPT codes to standardize the reporting of procedures performed by hospital outpatient departments. The revisions were supposed to assist in controlling outpatient payments to hospitals, but originally they did not cover every outpatient service.

HCFA (now the CMS) contracted with 3M Health Information Systems (3M HIS) to develop an OPPS that was based on the amount of resources used. The system 3M HIS developed was called ambulatory payment groups (APGs). APG payments are based on the number and type of procedures performed rather than the diagnosis. This system was developed and tested over a 10-year period, but implementation was repeatedly delayed. The APG system ultimately was scrapped by HCFA in 1999, as APG did not adequately address the newest "hot topic": medical necessity. During the years of APG testing, a number of other payors began using the APG system in anticipation that it would become a national standard.

A new system called **ambulatory payment classification (APC)** was released in 1999. APC was designed to consider diagnoses and procedures, as well as the appropriateness of each service and medical necessity. Codes are assigned by combining two factors: (1) The level of CPT service, and (2) MDC similar, but not identical, to those used for DRG classifications.

The final rule for the OPPS was issued on April 1, 2000, with a compliance deadline (implementation date) only 90 days later on July 1, 2000. In the final rule, Medicare dropped the requirement added in 1999 to include diagnosis codes in the APC classification. In the final rule, APCs are based on procedure codes only and the number of APC classifications was increased to 451 classifications.

Currently, physicians report services they perform in a hospital outpatient facility using a CMS-1500 claim form with the name and address of the hospital listed in block No. 32. The procedures listed by the physician on the CMS-1500 as having been performed in the hospital outpatient department must match procedures reported by the hospital on the UB-92 claim form.

Hospitals report the facility fees for outpatient services on a UB-92 claim form, with the name of the physician and the physician's ID number in field locator 82 (FL 82). When more than one physician is seen on a single date of service, other physicians are listed with their ID numbers in FL 83.

Although each physician will send separate CMS-1500 claim forms, the facility can report their facility fees for multiple encounters for one date of service on one UB-92 claim form. Only one APC is assigned for the facility for the date of service.

Unlike DRGs, the APC for an episode of care is not listed on the UB-92 claim form. The facility's fee for the day is calculated using APC grouper software and is used internally by the hospital to estimate correct payment and to check for accuracy when payment is received from the payor.

Initially, APC has been used only in hospital outpatient departments. Soon, however, CMS plans to require also an OPPS similar to hospital outpatient APCs for ambulatory surgery centers, and eventually also for nursing facilities, and physician billing.

Nursing Facility Services

The term *nursing facility* includes:

- ❑ Skilled nursing centers
- ❑ Intermediate care centers
- ❑ Long-term care centers
- ❑ Psychiatric residential treatment centers

When a hospital discharge is performed on the same date as admission to a nursing facility, both the hospital discharge and the nursing facility admission are coded, and separate claims are sent by each facility.

People in nursing facilities are called residents, not patients. Nursing facilities are required by law to provide a variety of periodic evaluations or assessments of each resident.

Physician services rendered in nursing facilities are governed by rules similar to inpatient settings, and there are three levels of service. Physician services are classified in two main categories: comprehensive nursing facility assessments and subsequent nursing facility care. See the evaluation and management section of the CPT codebook for complete descriptions of these services. Nursing facility discharge codes are time based, so time must be documented in the medical record.

Physician services rendered in a nursing facility are reported on the CMS-1500 claim form with the name and address of the facility listed in block No. 32. Physicians send their claims at the time service is rendered.

Nursing facilities send claims monthly at the end of the month, or upon discharge. The facility fees are reported by the nursing facility on the UB-92 claim form with the name and ID number of the attending physician listed in field locator 82 (FL 82), and the name and ID of any other physicians who provided services at the nursing facility during that month listed in FL 83.

STOP & REVIEW

Answer the following questions:

1. What is APC an abbreviation for?

_____

2. What company spent 10 years developing the APGs that were ultimately discarded by Medicare?

_____

3. What claim form do physicians use to report services provided in a hospital outpatient department? _____

4. What claim form do hospitals use to report facility fees for outpatient services?

_____

5. Does MDC mean the same thing for both hospital inpatient billing and hospital outpatient billing?

_____

6. Do nursing homes currently use APCs? _____

7. Do surgicenters currently use APCs? _____

8. What is the name for people who receive treatment at a nursing facility?

_____

9. Which claim form do physicians use to report services provided in a nursing facility?

_____

10. Which claim form do nursing facilities use to report their facility fees?

_____

Utilization Review

The utilization review (UR) team, usually a group of RNs, LPNs, and/or certified coders trained in DRGs and hospital reimbursement issues, work to help the hospital remain profitable. CC are those complicating factors and underlying diseases that have been determined in at least 75% of the cases to increase a patient's length of stay by at least 1 day.

The UR team has a computer system that tells them the average number of hospital days for each DRG classification. They use this information to analyze the expected **length of stay (LOS)** for each patient. They encourage doctors to either document why it is medically necessary for a patient to stay longer than the average, or to send the patient home if the physician cannot document medical necessity for a longer stay.

Many hospitals have a punishment system in place, often fines, for physicians who do not work with the utilization review team to safeguard the profitability of the hospital. Some hospitals go so far as to remove repeat offenders from their roster of physicians on staff at the hospital.

Facility Coding for Inpatient Services

Medicare pays hospitals based on the DRG code assigned each inpatient hospital stay. The DRG system requires the use of ICD-9-CM Volumes 1 and 2 to locate the codes for diagnoses (please see Chapter 5) and ICD-9-CM Volume 3 to locate the codes for procedures. Only the hospital's inpatient facility fee is billed on the UB-92 claim form using ICD-9-CM diagnosis and procedure codes. The facility fee is paid by Medicare using the DRG system to determine payment amount.

Many of the other payors also use the DRG payment system for inpatient charges. However, please be aware that there are few payers that want CPT codes for inpatient hospital charges for procedures. If you want the hospital to receive the correct payment, you must use the codebook preferred by each payor.

When you are doing hospital coding, your most important task is to identify the principal diagnosis. The principal diagnosis is not always the same as the admitting diagnosis. The admitting diagnosis is the reason the person was admitted to the hospital, whereas the principal diagnosis is the diagnosis that, *after study,* is determined to be chiefly responsible for the hospitalization.

For example: Mary was admitted through the emergency room with a diagnosis of acute abdominal pain. Tests performed the next day showed she was suffering from acute appendicitis. Her surgeon performed an emergency appendectomy. The rest of her hospital stay was uneventful, and Mary was discharged 2 days after the surgery.

The admitting diagnosis is acute abdominal pain. The principal diagnosis is appendicitis. In addition, the hospital will list the ICD-9-CM, Volume 3, procedure code for the appendectomy.

Once you have identified the admitting diagnosis and the principal diagnosis, you look for any other valid diagnoses. You code the additional established diagnoses that affect this hospital stay. Then you code any differential, or "rule-out" diagnoses. Lastly, you code any symptoms not already included in a diagnosis.

Please remember that the only time you may code the differential, or "rule-out" diagnoses is for hospital inpatients. In every other instance, you may only code the symptoms. The diagnosis coding guidelines that govern this issue, including code order, are found in the ICD-9-CM codebook just before the main index in Volume 2. Also remember that coding guidelines can and often do change from year to year. The guidelines may have changed since this text was written. Current-year coding guidelines always take precedence, so any time there is a discrepancy with the information in this textbook, please follow the guidelines.

If the case you are coding is for a patient with either a benign or a malignant neoplasm, you might need to code an additional morphology code. These codes are found in Appendix A of the ICD-9-CM Volume 1, Tabular List. Not every hospital chooses to participate in using morphology codes. However, if your hospital does use the morphology codes, you will be required to use them for every neoplasm case. Although the morphology codes are not found in the neoplasm table in ICD-9-CM, they can be found by looking up the main term for the specific neoplasm in the alphabetic index in Section 1 of ICD-9-CM Volume 2.

The patient is diagnosed with a squamous cell carcinoma in situ of the middle lobe of her right lung. You find the diagnosis code by going to the neoplasm table and looking up lung, middle lobe, then read across to the column for "in situ" to find code 231.2. You find the morphology code by going to the main index and looking up carcinoma, squamous cell, to find code M8070/3. Remember to confirm your codes in the tabular list.

Like physician offices, hospitals also use E-codes to show the external causes of accidents and poisonings. There is a special box on the UB-92 claim form for the first E-code, and any additional E-codes are listed after the other additional diagnoses.

Volume 3 of ICD-9-CM, for inpatient hospital procedures, begins with an alphabetical index and is followed by the tabular list. Volume 3 uses the same index usage rules as the Volume 2 index in ICD-9-CM. Please note that these are not the same rules as the CPT index.

Look up the procedure in the alphabetical index, then confirm the code in the tabular list. The main term is usually the name of the procedure. Because Volume 3 of ICD-9-CM is used to report the hospital's facility fees for the procedures rather than the skill of the physician, the code descriptions in ICD-9-CM volume 3 are not identical to those in CPT.

> *Note:* Unlike Volumes 1 and 2 of ICD-9-CM, both the index and the tabular list are in the same volume in Volume 3 of ICD-9-CM.

When you do physician billing for inpatient procedures, you want to be sure your CPT code matches the description of the ICD-9-CM Volume 3 code billed by the hospital. Some codebook publishers also publish "Crosswalk" books to aid in this task. A surgical crosswalk will tell you both the CPT code and the matching Volume 3 of ICD-9-CM code for each surgical procedure. Codebook publishers (e.g., Ingenix, PMIC, AMA) often publish this type of coding reference book.

Completing the UB-92 Claim Form

The data fields on the UB-92 claim forms, called field locators (FLs), are numbered from FL 1 to FL 86 (Figure 12-1). The UB-92 claim form does not clearly separate patient and insured information from physician and supplier information the way the CMS-1500 claim form does. Yet the patient and insured information is still supplied by the patient, and the provider of the services still supplies the remaining information.

Every medical claim is a legal document. It is the patient's responsibility to provide the most current and accurate demographic and insurance information for every claim that is filed on their behalf. It is the facility's responsibility to supply accurate information about the services rendered, the necessary supplies, and any other associated costs. Knowingly supplying false or inaccurate information on a medical claim form is considered fraud, a federal crime, and is punishable by fines, prison or both.

It is the biller's responsibility to compare the patient information gathered during check-in with the information already on file and to compare billed charges with the documentation in the medical record. When a discrepancy is noted, the biller must verify which information is correct and update the file from which the claim is printed. In most hospitals, the billing and coding are performed in different departments. The biller may not change codes and may not change the code order from that submitted by the coding department. However, the biller can ask the coding department to reevaluate the codes if the biller finds a discrepancy between the codes and the information in the medical record.

The primary payor is the medical plan that is responsible for paying when there is only one payor and the medical plan that pays first when there is coverage from more than one payor.

If you want to file clean claims and receive correct payments the first time, you must learn to look at each claim through the payor's eyes. Follow optical character recognition (OCR) and electronic data interchange (EDI) guidelines as listed in Chapter 4. Use only alphanumeric characters with no punctuation.

When a claim arrives at the payor, the claim editing and claim auditing processes begin immediately. Any time there is a discrepancy, there is no obligation for payment and the claim will be either rejected or penalized, or both. The payor wants to know:

❑ Was the claim sent to the correct address as listed on the patient's insurance card? Each payor has different billing addresses for different policies.
❑ Is the "insured" for the primary plan listed on the claim form covered under that plan?
❑ Is the patient covered by the plan?
❑ Is the insurance policy current?
❑ Is the correct payor identified as primary payor? If not, there is no obligation for payment until the primary payor has paid and correct information is submitted.

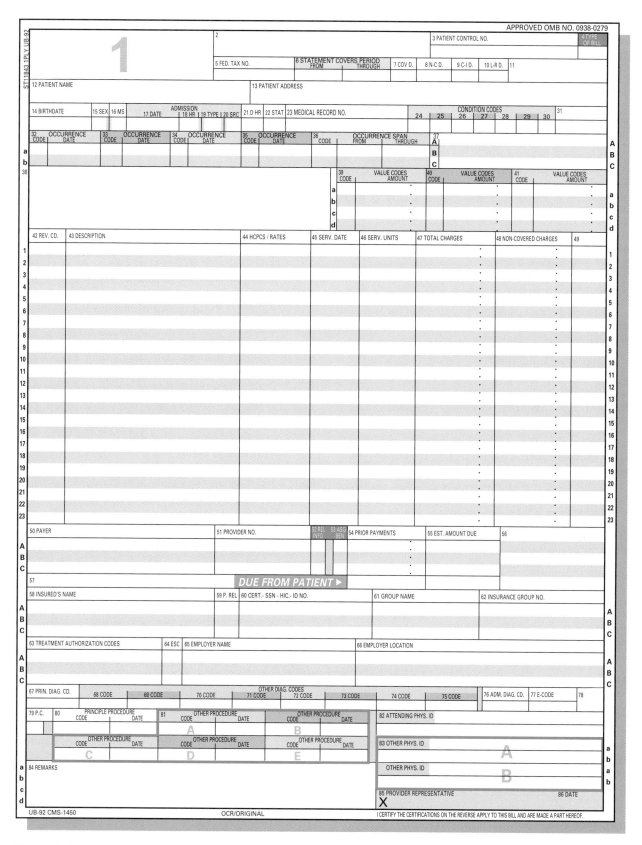

FIGURE 12-1
UB-92 claim form.

Answer the following questions:

1. What is the name of the team, usually a group of RNs trained in DRGs and hospital reimbursement issues, that works to help the hospital remain profitable? _____

2. What are those complicating factors and underlying diseases that have been determined in at least 75% of cases to increase a patient's length of stay by at least 1 day called?

_____

3. What is LOS an abbreviation for?

_____

4. Medicare pays hospitals based on what number that is assigned each inpatient hospital stay?

_____

5. Who supplies the patient and insurance information? _____

6. Who supplies the remaining information?

_____

7. Knowingly supplying false or inaccurate information on a medical claim form is considered _____ and is punishable by fines, prison, or both.

❏ Does the demographic information for both the patient and the insured match payor records?

❏ Were the services rendered appropriate for the age and gender of the patient?

❏ Were the services rendered appropriate for the nature of the presenting illness?

❏ Are any required modifiers present, and are they reported correctly? Note that modifiers are not a part of ICD-9-CM Volume 3 for inpatient hospital claims. Only CPT and HCPCS codes require modifiers. The front cover of the CPT codebook usually lists the modifiers approved for use in outpatient facilities.

❏ Are the type of service and place of service codes appropriate for the service rendered?

❏ Does the facility accept assignment of benefits? If not, all authorized payments will be sent to the patient.

PROVIDER AND PATIENT INFORMATION (FL 1 TO FL 23) (FIGURE 12-2)

FL 1—Provider Name, Address, and Telephone Number

FL 1 is for the name of the facility submitting the bill and the address where payment is to be sent. FL 1 is a required field. The data in this field are matched to the provider number in FL 51 to verify the provider's identity. FL 1 allows four lines of text with a maximum of 25 characters per line.

Abbreviations accepted by the post office may be used. The 2-digit state abbreviation should be entered in capital letters. The country code can be found in the front of the telephone book.

Line a: Enter the name of the facility.
Line b: Enter the street address or post office box number of the facility.
Line c: Enter the city, state, and 9-digit zip code of the facility.
Line d: Enter the telephone number(s) of the facility as follows: area code first, telephone number, fax number, country code.

FL 2—Unlabeled Field

FL 2 allows 2 lines of text with 29 characters on the upper line and 30 characters on the lower line.

States have traditionally used this field to report financial class codes, the patient's race, and other patient information.

Effective October 16, 2003, this field is reserved for national assignment. This means the CMS will define FL 2 at a later date and it should be left blank until then.

FL 3—Patient Control Number

Enter the patient control number in FL 3. The patient control number is a unique number assigned by the facility to identify individual patient accounts, case records, and medical records. It is used when posting payments and to find records when payors request additional information.

The patient control number is used to identify where to post payments received. Third party payors are required to reference this number on payment checks and vouchers, explanation of benefits (EOB) forms, and Medicare's remittance advice or remittance notice (RA/MRN) forms. The patient control number further identifies the patient and distinguishes between patients who have the same name.

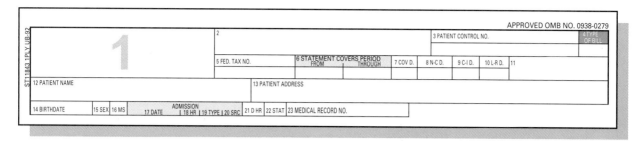

FIGURE 12-2
FL 1 to Fl 23 from UB-92 claim form.

FL 3 is a required field for all payors. FL 3 allows for 20 characters, with no spaces between digits. The data in FL 3 must be left justified.

FL 4—Type of Bill

FL 4 is a required field for all payors. The 3-digit number entered here provides the payor with specific information for billing and payment purposes. The type of bill code and the provider number in FL 51 must be consistent with the type of service rendered. The outpatient code editor uses this field to determine which outpatient claims to edit and estimate for an APC payment under the OPPS.

- ☐ The first digit identifies the type of facility (hospital, ambulatory surgery center, nursing facility, home health agency [HHA], etc.).
- ☐ The second digit classifies the type of care being billed. Each type of facility is authorized to use specific second-digit codes. Hospitals may use 1, 2, 3, 4, 8; skilled nursing facilities (SNFs) may use 1, 2, 3; HHAs may use 2 or 3. Each digit has a specific use. For example, the second digit: 1 is used for inpatient (Medicare Part A); 2 is used for inpatient (Medicare Part B, HHA with Part B plan of treatment); 3 is used for outpatient (HHA with Part A plan of treatment and durable medical equipment [DME] under Part A).
- ☐ The third digit indicates the sequence of a bill for a specific episode of care. A facility may bill Medicare after 60 days and every 60 days thereafter, or it may submit the entire claim upon discharge. Psychiatric units, cancer units, and children's hospitals must bill monthly, upon discharge, when the need for care changes, and when benefits are exhausted. Specific digits tell the circumstances, such as whether discharge has occurred, whether the patient is still an inpatient, and whether the bill is for services in the middle of a long stay. The third digit is cross-referenced with many other fields on the claim form, and the information must be

consistent with the information provided elsewhere.

There are many other considerations for FL 4 that deal with payment issues for specific circumstances. Most hospital billing computer-systems have drop-down boxes to guide you in the selection of each digit for FL 4.

There are also outside resources available to guide you in selections for FL 4. For example, the *UB-92 Editor* published by Ingenix with quarterly updates for 1 year, gives more than 60 pages of detailed guidance about selections for each digit in FL 4 and how to avoid conflicts with the cross-referenced items in other fields.

FL 5—Federal Tax Number

FL 5 has two lines. The upper line is four characters long and is used to report the facility's affiliated subsidiaries using a federal tax subidentification number. The lower line is 10 characters long, and is used to report the facility's tax identification number (TIN) or the employer identification number (EIN) as XX-XXXXXXX.

FL 6—Statement Covers Period

Enter the beginning and ending dates for the services reported on the bill using the 8-digit format with a 2-digit month, a 2-digit day, and a 4-digit year: MMDDYYYY for OCR claims sent on paper and YYYYMMDD for EDI claims sent electronically. The dates cannot be earlier than the date of admission or start of care date listed in FL 17.

Do not report dates of services before the entitlement date for the medical plan billed. A medical plan will not pay for services that occurred before a person was entitled to receive coverage from that plan for those services.

For services rendered on a single date, both the "from" and "through" dates will be the same.

When a patient is discharged or dies before the end of a normal billing cycle, the "Through" date is the date of discharge or the date of death.

FL 6 is cross-referenced with FL 4, FLs 7 to 8, FL 22, FLs 24 to 30, FLs 39 to 41, and FLs 45 and 46. The information entered here must be consistent with the information entered in each of these fields.

FL 7—Covered Days

The number of inpatient days expected to be covered by the primary payor is entered here. The number of covered days should equal the number of accommodation units (FL 46) reported with the room and board (FL 42).

The date of discharge or death is not counted as a covered day unless admission and discharge occurred on the same day.

FL 7 allows three numeric characters. The number of covered days must not exceed 150 days for hospitals and 100 days for skilled nursing facilities.

For Medicare patients, the number of covered days, including any lifetime reserve days, entered here for the billing period, are also applied to the Medicare cost report. Please see Chapter 10 to learn more about Medicare's lifetime reserve days.

FL 7 is cross-referenced with FL 4, FL 6, FLs 8 to 10, FLs 24 to 30, FL 42, FL 46, and FL 50. The information entered here must be consistent with the information entered in each of these fields.

FL 8—Noncovered Days

The number of inpatient days *not* expected to be covered by the primary payor is entered here. FL 8 allows four numeric characters.

FL 8 is required in Medicare billing, both for Medicare as primary payor and for Medicare as secondary payor. Enter the total number of noncovered days for the billing period that are not considered Medicare patient days on the Medicare cost report. These are days under Part A utilization that will not be charged to the Beneficiary according to Medicare Publication 100-04, Chapter 25, Section 60. However, when the facility notifies the patient in writing that a Medicare service is a noncovered service using an Advance Beneficiary Notice (ABN) (see Figures 3-8, 3-9, and 3-10 in Chapter 3), the patient is responsible for any charges incurred after the date notified. This notice must include the patient's name, address, Medicare number, a specific reason for noncoverage, whether the patient requested a demand bill, the provider's signature, the date of determination, the patient's signature, and the date the patient received the notice.

The day of discharge or death is not counted as a noncovered day.

The number of noncovered days in FL 8 added to the number of covered days in FL 7 must equal the number of days covered by the billing period for this claim.

FL 8 is cross-referenced with FL 4, FLs 6 to 8, FLs 24 to 30, FLs 32 to 35, FLs 39 to 42, FL 46, FL 50, and FL 84. The information entered here must be consistent with the information entered in each of these fields.

FL 9—Coinsurance Days

FL 9 reports the inpatient days for a Medicare patient occurring after the sixtieth day and before the ninety-first day of the Medicare benefit period. Remember, a benefit period does not end until the Medicare patient has not been an inpatient anywhere for 60 consecutive days. See Chapter 10 for more details about Medicare.

FL 9 allows three numeric characters. For certain entries in FL 4, the number in this field should not exceed 30 days.

FL 9 is cross-referenced with FL 4, FL 7, FLs 32 to 35, FLs 39 to 41, and FL 50. The information entered here must be consistent with the information entered in each of these fields.

FL 10—Lifetime Reserve Days

Report here the total number of Medicare lifetime reserve days only if the patient chooses to use them. After the ninetieth day of inpatient services, a patient may elect to use lifetime reserve days if the Medicare patient still has lifetime reserve days available for use. Only 60 lifetime reserve days are available for use during the Medicare patient's lifetime, so the number entered here may not exceed 60. See Chapter 10 for more information about Medicare's lifetime reserve days.

Fl 10 is cross-referenced with FL 4, FL 7, FL 9, FLs 32 to 35, FLs 39 to 41, and FL 50. The information entered here must be consistent with the information entered in each of these fields.

FL 11—Unlabeled Field

As of October 16, 2003, FL 11 is reserved for national assignment. FL 11 allows 12 characters in the upper line and 13 characters in the lower line. This means CMS will define FL 11 at a later date and it should be left blank until then.

FL 12—Patient Name

FL 12 is a required field. Enter the name as last name, first name, middle initial (when applicable). The patient's name must be spelled exactly as it appears on the insurance card. FL 12 allows 30 alphanumeric characters.

The name entered in FL 12 is the name of the patient—the person who received the treatment(s) or service(s) listed on the claim form. Only one patient name may be entered on each claim form. When you are filing a batch of claims for patients who have similar names, be very careful to verify that each piece of information is completed for the correct person.

The name entered in FL 12 should be the patient's legal name. However, if the patient has changed names, such as occurs when a woman marries, do not change the name in the facility records until the insurance card lists the new legal name. The name in the medical record must match the name on the claim form. If the claim is filed using the new name before the insurance company changes their records, the payor will not recognize the patient, and the claim will be denied. Be very careful with record keeping during the interval between the time a patient's name legally changes and the time the payor recognizes the new name. However, be sure to list the correct information in FL 16, marital status.

Also, call the payor to see if coverage changed when the patient married. A dependent daughter who marries is no longer covered under a parent's policy. Knowingly supplying false or inaccurate information is considered a federal crime and is punishable by fines, imprisonment, or both.

FL 12 is cross-referenced with FL 4. The information entered here must be consistent with the information entered in that field.

FL 13—Patient Address
FL 13 is a required field. Enter the full mailing address of the patient, including the postal zip code. FL 13 allows 50 alphanumeric characters. Approved postal abbreviations may be used, but do not use any other abbreviations.

If the patient resides in a skilled nursing facility (SNF), only list the SNF address if the SNF is the legal representative of the patient.

FL 13 is cross-referenced with FL 1 and FL 4. The information entered here must be consistent with the information entered in each of these fields.

FL 14—Birth Date
FL 14 is a required field. Enter the patient's birth date using an 8-digit date. For paper claims, use OCR standards and report the date as MMDDYYYY. For electronic claims, use EDI standards and report the date as YYYYMMDD.

Some diagnosis codes and some procedure codes are age specific. The age of the patient must be consistent with the codes selected. If the patient's age is greater than 124 years, the claim will be reviewed for an error.

FL 14 is cross-referenced with FL 4, FL 6, FLs 19 to 20, FLs 39 to 41, and FLs 67 to 75. The information entered here must be consistent with the information entered in each of these fields.

FL 15—Patient Sex
FL 15 is a required field. Enter the gender of the patient as recorded at the time of registration or at the start of care. Enter M for male and F for female.

Some diagnoses and some procedures are gender specific. The information entered here must be consistent with the codes selected.

FL 15 is cross-referenced with FL 4, FL 44, FLs 67 to 75, and FLs 80 to 81. The information entered here must be consistent with the information entered in each of these fields.

FL 16—Marital Status
FL 16 is not required as of April 1, 2004. If you choose to report this information, enter the patient's marital status on the date of admission or at the start of care as follows:

S	Single
M	Married
P	Life partner (domestic partner, or significant other)
D	Divorced
W	Widowed
X	Legally separated
U	Unknown

FL 17—Admission Date/Start of Care Date
FL 17 is a required field. Use an eight-digit date to report the admission date or the start of care date. For paper claims, use OCR standards and report the date as MMDDYYYY. For electronic claims, use EDI standards and report the date as YYYYMMDD.

Any procedure performed and reported in FLs 80 to 81 must have occurred during the period covered by the claim.

FL 17 is cross-referenced with FL 4, FL 6, FLs 24 to 30, FL 36, FLs 39 to 41, FL 67, and FLs 80 to 81. The information entered here must be consistent with the information entered in each of these fields.

FL 18—Admission Hour
FL 18 contains the hour of the day during which the patient was admitted for inpatient care or initiated outpatient care. Hours are entered in military time (24-hour clock) using two numeric characters as follows:

00	12:00 midnight - 12:59 AM
01	01:00 - 01:59 AM
02	02:00 - 02:59 AM
03	03:00 - 03:59 AM
04	04:00 - 04:59 AM
05	05:00 - 05:59 AM
06	06:00 - 06:59 AM
07	07:00 - 07:59 AM

08	08:00 - 08:59 AM
09	09:00 - 09:59 AM
10	10:00 - 10:59 AM
11	11:00 - 11:59 AM
12	12:00 (noon) - 12:59 PM
13	01:00 - 01:59 PM
14	02:00 - 02:59 PM
15	03:00 - 03:59 PM
16	04:00 - 04:59 PM
17	05:00 - 05:59 PM
18	06:00 - 06:59 PM
19	07:00 - 07:59 PM
20	08:00 - 08:59 PM
21	09:00 - 09:59 PM
22	10:00 - 10:59 PM
23	11:00 - 11:59 PM
99	hour unknown (This code was discontinued effective October 16, 2003.)

FL 19—Admission Type

The single digit code in FL 19 tells the priority (the urgency) of the admission or of the care received. Most payors, including Medicare, require completion of FL 19 for inpatient care. FL 19 is not usually used for outpatient claims. When in doubt, check your payor contract or call the payor to verify whether and when to use this field. The code choices are as follows:

1 Emergency	This code is used for severe, life-threatening, or potentially disabling conditions. Usually the patients are admitted through the emergency department.
2 Urgent	This code is used for patients who require immediate treatment. Often they are admitted to the first available bed for the type of care required.
3 Elective	This code is used for patients whose condition allows treatment to be scheduled.
4 Newborn	This code is used for babies born in the facility.
5 Trauma center	This code is used for care given in a trauma center designated by state or local government.
6-8	These codes are reserved for national assignment.
9 Information not available	This code is seldom used. It indicates the facility was unable to classify the type of admission.

Fl 19 is cross-referenced with FL 4, FL 20, FL 42, and FL 47. The information entered here must be consistent with the information entered in each of these fields.

FL 20—Admission Source

The code in FL 20 tells the source of the admission or other service. Most payors, including Medicare, require FL 20 for all inpatients and certain outpatients. When in doubt, check your payor contract or call the payor to verify whether and when to use this field. In addition, when the type of admission code in FL 19 is 4 for newborn, the meaning of the code in FL 20 changes.

The code choices (except when the code in FL 19 is 4) are as follows:

1	Physician referral
2	Clinic referral
3	HMO referral
4	Transfer from another hospital
5	Transfer from an SNF
6	Transfer from another health care facility
7	Emergency department
8	Court/Law enforcement
9	Information not available
A	Transfer from a critical access hospital
B	Transfer from another HHA
C	Readmission to same HHA
D-Z	Reserved for national assignment

When the code in FL 19 is 4, the code choices are as follows:

1	Home delivery
2	Premature delivery
3	Sick baby
4	Extramural birth
5-8	Reserved for national assignment
9	Information not available

FL 20 is cross-referenced with FL 4, FL 19, FL 42, and FL 57. The information entered here must be consistent with the information entered in each of these fields.

FL 21—Discharge Hour

This field is required on inpatient claims. Enter the hour of the day during which the patient was discharged from inpatient care. Hours are entered in military time (24-hour clock) using two numeric characters, as in FL 18.

FL 21 is cross-referenced with FL 18. The information entered here must be consistent with the information entered in that field.

FL 22—Patient Status

FL 22 is required by most payors for facility claims

(inpatient, outpatient hospital, SNF, hospice, and HHA). The code entered in FL 22 describes the patient's disposition on the last date of service billed on the claim form. Medicare and many other payors use this field to monitor benefit periods.

The code choices are:

01	Discharged to home or self care (routine discharge)
02	Discharged/transferred to another short-term general hospital for inpatient care
03	Discharged/transferred to SNF with Medicare certification
04	Discharged/transferred to an intermediate care facility (ICF)
05	Discharged/transferred to another type of institution
06	Discharged/transferred to home under care of organized home health service organization.
07	Left against medical advice or discontinued care
08	Discharged/transferred to home under care of home IV therapy provider
09	Admitted as an inpatient to this hospital
10-19	Reserved for national assignment
20	Expired (or did not recover—Christian Science patient)
21-29	Reserved for national assignment
30	Still a patient
31-39	Reserved for national assignment
40	Expired at home
41	Expired in a medical facility, such as a hospital, SNF, ICF, or freestanding hospice
42	Expired, place unknown
43	Discharged/transferred to a federal hospital (effective October 1, 2003)
44-49	Reserved for national assignment
50	Discharged to hospice—home
51	Discharged to hospice—medical facility
52-60	Reserved for national assignment
61	Discharged/transferred within this institution to a hospice-based Medicare approved swing bed
62	Discharged/transferred to an inpatient rehabilitation facility (IRF), including rehabilitation distinct part units of a hospital
63	Discharged/transferred to a Medicare certified long-term care hospital (LTCH)
64	Discharged/transferred to a nursing facility certified under Medicaid but not certified under Medicare
65	Discharged/transferred to a psychiatric hospital or psychiatric distinct part unit of a hospital
66-70	Reserved for national assignment
71-72	Reserved for national assignment (discontinued effective October 1, 2002)
73-99	Reserved for national assignment

FL 22 is cross-referenced with FL 4, FLs 6 to 8, FLs 24 to 30, FL 36, FL 44, FLs 47 to 48, and FL 67. The information entered here must be consistent with the information entered in each of these fields.

FL 23—Medical Record Number

FL 23 is a required field, 17 alphanumeric characters long. Enter the number assigned by the facility to identify the patient's medical record.

The entry in FL 23 is used to provide an audit trail for the medical record. It is not the same as the control number in FL 3, which identifies the patient's financial record.

FL 23 is cross-referenced with FL 3. The information entered here must be consistent with, but not the same as, the information entered in that field.

CONDITION, OCCURRENCE, AND VALUE CODES (FL 24 TO FL 41) (FIGURE 12-3)

FLs 24 to 30—Condition Codes
The codes in FLs 24 to 30 identify conditions that

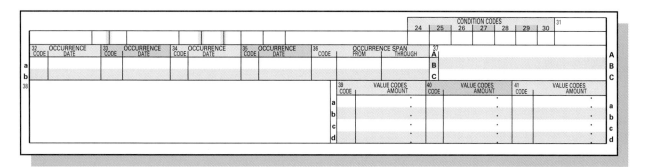

FIGURE 12-3
FL 24 to FL 41 from UB-92 claim form.

TABLE 12-1
Condition Codes

Insurance Codes	
01	Military service related
02	Condition is employment related
03	Patient covered by insurance not reflected here
04	Information only bill (The facility does not expect to receive payment from this claim.)
05	Lien has been filed
06	ESRD patient in first 18 months of entitlement covered by employer group health insurance
07	Treatment of nonterminal condition for hospice patient
08	Beneficiary would not provide information concerning other insurance
09	Neither patient nor spouse is employed
10	Patient and/or spouse are employed but no employer group health plan coverage exists
11	Disables beneficiary, but no large group health plan coverage
12-16	Codes are for payor use only

Special Conditions	
17	Patient is homeless
18	Maiden name retained
19	Child retains mother's name
20	Beneficiary requested billing
21	Billing for denial notice
22	Patient on multiple drug regimen
23	Home care giver available
24	Home IV patient also receiving HHA services
25	Patient is a non-U.S. resident
26	VA-eligible patient chooses to receive services in Medicare-certified facility
27	Patient referred to a sole community hospital for a diagnostic laboratory test
28	Patient and/or spouse's employer group health plan is secondary to Medicare
29	Disabled beneficiary and/or family member's large group health plan is secondary to Medicare
30	Nonresearch services provided to patients enrolled in a qualified clinical trial

Student Status	
31	Patient is student (full-time day)
32	Patient is student (cooperative/work study program)
33	Patient is student (full-time night)
34	Patient is student (part time)
35	Reserved for national assignment

Accommodations	
36	General care patient in a special unit
37	Ward accommodation at patient's request
38	Semi-private room not available
39	Private room medically necessary
40	Same-day transfer
41	Partial hospitalization
42	Continuing care not related to inpatient admission
43	Continuing care not provided within prescribed postdischarge window
44	Inpatient admission changed to outpatient
45	Reserved for national assignment

CHAMPUS Information	
46	Nonavailability statement on file
47	Reserved for CHAMPUS
48	Psychiatric residential treatment centers for children and adolescents
49-54	Reserved for national assignment

SNF Information	
55	SNF bed not available
56	Medical appropriateness
57	SNF readmission
58	Terminated Medicare + Choice organization enrollee
59	Reserved for national assignment

Prospective Payment	
60	Day outlier
61	Cost outlier

TABLE 12-1
Condition Codes—cont'd

Prospective Payment—cont'd

62	Payor code
63	Incarcerated beneficiaries
64-65	Payor only code
66	Provider does not wish cost outlier payment
67	Beneficiary elects not to use lifetime reserve days
68	Beneficiary elects to use lifetime reserve days
69	IME/DGME/N&AH payment only

Renal Dialysis Setting

70	Self-administered Epoietin (EPO)
71	Full care in unit
72	Self-care in unit
73	Self-care training
74	Home
75	Home—100% reimbursed
76	Back-up in-facility dialysis

Other Codes

77	Provider accepts or is obligated/required due to a contractual arrangement or law to accept payment by primary payor as payment in full
78	New coverage not implemented by HMO
79	CORF (comprehensive outpatient rehabilitation facility) services provided off-site
80-99	Reserved for national assignment

Special Program Indicator Codes

A0	CHAMPUS external partnership program
A1	EPSDT/CHAP
A2	Physically handicapped children's program
A3	Special federal funding
A4	Family planning
A5	Disability
A6	Vaccines/Medicare 100% payment
A7	Induced abortion—danger to life (code discontinued on October 1, 2002)
A8	Induced abortion—victim rape/incest (code discontinued on October 1, 2002)
A9	Second opinion surgery
AA	Abortion performed due to rape (effective October 1, 2002)
AB	Abortion performed due to incest (effective October 1, 2002)
AC	Abortion performed due to serious fetal genetic defect, deformity, or abnormality (effective October 1, 2002)
AD	Abortion performed due to a life-endangering physical condition caused by, arising from, or exacerbated by the pregnancy itself (effective October 1, 2002)
AE	Abortion performed due to physical health of mother that is not life endangering (effective October 1, 2002)
AF	Abortion performed due to emotional/psychological health of the mother (effective October 1, 2002)
AG	Abortion performed due to social or economic reasons (effective October 1, 2002)
AH	Elective abortion (effective October 1, 2002)
AI	Sterilization (effective October 1, 2002)
AJ	Payor responsible for copayment (effective April 1, 2003)
AK	Air ambulance required effective October 16, 2003)
AL	Specialized treatment/bed unavailable (effective October 16, 2003)
AM	Nonemergency medically necessary stretcher transport required (effective October 16, 2003)
AN	Preadmission screening not required (effective January 1, 2004)
AO-AZ	Reserved for national assignment
B0	Medicare coordinated care demonstration program
B2	Critical access hospital ambulance attestation
B3	Pregnancy indicator (effective October 16, 2003)
B4-BZ	Reserved for national assignment

Q10-PRO Approval Indicator Services

C0	Reserved for national assignment
C1	Approved as billed
C2	Automatic approval as billed based on focused review
C3	Partial approval
C4	Admission/services denied
C5	Postpayment review applicable
C6	Admission preauthorization

Continued.

TABLE 12-1
Condition Codes—cont'd

Q10-PRO Approval Indicator Services—cont'd	
C7	Extended authorization
C8-CZ	Reserved for national assignment
Claim Change Reasons	
D0	Changes to service dates
D1	Changes to charges
D3	Second or subsequent interim PPS bill
D4	Changes in ICD-9-CM diagnosis and/or procedure codes
D5	Cancel to correct HICN (health insurance card number) or provider identification number
D6	Cancel only to repay a duplicate or OIG overpayment
D7	Change to make Medicare the secondary payor
D8	Change to make Medicare the primary payor
D9	Any other change
E0	Change in patient status
E1-E9	Reserved for national assignment
G0	Distinct medical visit
G1-G9	Reserved for national assignment
H0	Delayed filing, statement of intent submitted
H1-LZ	Reserved for national assignment
M0-MZ	Reserved for national assignment
N0-WZ	Reserved for national assignment
X0-ZZ	Reserved for national assignment

could affect how the payor processes the claim. The codes help both primary and secondary payors determine patient eligibility, benefits, and amount of available insurance coverage.

FLs 24 to 30 allow for as many as seven condition codes to be listed, as applicable, in alphanumeric sequence. Enter information as required by each payor plan or contract.

See Table 12-1 for a listing of condition codes.

FLs 24 to 30 are cross-referenced with FL 4, FL 6, FLs 32 to 35, FL 37, FLs 39 to 42, FL 36, FLs 44 to 47, FL 51, FL 60, FLs 67 to 75, FLs 80 to 81, and FL 84. The information entered here must be consistent with the information entered in each of these fields.

FL 31—Unlabeled Field

FL 31 is reserved for national use effective October 16, 2003. FL 31 allows five characters in the upper line and six characters in the lower line.

FLs 32 to 35—Occurrence Codes and Dates

Valid occurrence codes are 01 to 69 and A0 to L9. Occurrence codes are used to determine liability, coordination of benefits, and to administer subrogation clauses (see Chapter 8). A specific occurrence code may be used only once on a claim. Some of the occurrence codes are accident-related codes and some are medical condition codes. Some of the occurrence codes are insurance-related codes and some are service-related codes.

Each FL in this section has line a and line b. In total, as many as seven occurrence codes and the associated date for each may be entered in FLs 32 to 35. They are completed in alphanumeric sequence but there must be an entry in each "a" field before the "b" field spaces may be used (e.g., use FL 32a, then FL 33a, then FL 34a…). If more than seven occurrence codes are needed on a bill, use FL 36 to report the overflow, leaving the "through" date blank.

Enter the date of the occurrence as an eight-digit date: YYYYMMDD. May 1, 2005, would be listed as 20050501. The date used with an occurrence code must fall within the date range of the claim as listed in FL 6.

See Table 12-2 for valid occurrence codes.

Occurrence Codes

FLs 32 to 35 are cross-referenced with FL 6, FLs 32 to 36, and FL 84. The information entered here must be consistent with the information entered in each of these fields.

FL 36—Occurrence Span Codes and Dates

Valid occurrence span codes are 70 to 99 and M0 to Z9. Occurrence span codes and dates identify an event that relates to payment of the claim. These codes identify occurrences that happen over a span of time. For each of the three lines, report the occurrence code with the beginning (from) date and the ending (through) date for the occurrence span code on that line. See Table 12-3 for valid occurrence span codes.

Enter each date of the occurrence span as an eight-digit date: YYYYMMDD. May 1, 2005, would be listed as 20050501. The dates used with an occurrence span code must fall within the date range

TABLE 12-2
Occurrence Codes

Accident-related Codes	
01	Accident/Medical coverage
02	No-fault insurance involved—including auto accident/other
03	Accident—tort liability
04	Accident—employment-related
05	Accident/no medical or liability coverage
06	Crime victim
07-08	Reserved for national assignment

Medical Condition Codes	
09	Start of infertility treatment cycle
10	Last menstrual period
11	Onset of symptoms/illness
12	Date of onset for a chronically dependent individual (CDI)
13-15	Reserved for national assignment

Insurance-related Codes	
16	Date of last therapy
17	Date outpatient occupational therapy plan established or last reviewed
18	Date of retirement of patient/beneficiary
19	Date of retirement of spouse
20	Guarantee of payment began
21	UR notice received
22	Date active care ended
23	Date of cancellation of hospice election period
24	Date insurance denied
25	Date benefits terminated by primary payor
26	Date SNF bed became available
27	Date of hospice certification or recertification
28	Date comprehensive outpatient rehabilitation plan established or last reviewed
29	Date outpatient physical therapy plan established or last reviewed
30	Date outpatient speech pathology plan established or last reviewed
31	Date beneficiary notified of intent to bill (accommodations)
32	Date beneficiary notified of intent to bill (procedures or treatments)
33	First day of the Medicare coordination period for ESRD beneficiaries covered by an EGHP
34	Date of election of extended care services
35	Date treatment started for physical therapy
36	Date of inpatient hospital discharge for covered transplant patient
37	Date of inpatient hospital discharge for noncovered transplant patient
38	Date treatment started for home IV therapy
39	Date discharged on a continuous course of IV therapy

Service-related Codes	
40	Scheduled date of admission
41	Date of first test for preadmission testing
42	Date of discharge
43	Scheduled date of cancelled surgery
44	Date treatment started for occupational therapy
45	Date treatment started for speech therapy
46	Date treatment started for cardiac rehabilitation
47	Date cost outlier status begins
48-49	Payor codes
50-69	Reserved for national assignment
70-99	Reserved for occurrence span codes
A0	Reserved for national assignment
A1	Birth date—insured A
A2	Effective date—insured A policy
A3	Benefits exhausted
A4	Split bill date (effective October 16, 2003)
A5-AZ	Reserved for national assignment
B0	Reserved for national assignment
B1	Birth date—insured B
B2	Effective date—insured B policy
B3	Benefits exhausted

Continued.

TABLE 12-2
Occurrence Codes—cont'd

Service-related Codes—cont'd	
B4-BZ	Reserved for national assignment
C0	Reserved for national assignment
C1	Birth date—insured C
C2	Effective date—insured C policy
C3	Benefits exhausted
C4-CZ	Reserved for national assignment
D0-DZ	Reserved for national assignment
E0	Reserved for national assignment
E1	Birth date—insured D
E2	Effective date—insured D policy
E3	Benefits exhausted
E4-E4	Reserved for national assignment
F0	Reserved for national assignment
F1	Birth date—insured E
F2	Effective date—insured E policy
F3	Benefits exhausted
F4-FZ	Reserved for national assignment
G0	Reserved for national assignment
G1	Birth date—insured F
G2	Effective date—insured F policy
G3	Benefits exhausted
G4-GZ	Reserved for national assignment
H0-IZ	Reserved for national assignment
J0-LZ	Reserved for national assignment
M0-ZZ	Reserved for national assignment

TABLE 12-3
Occurrence Span Codes

70	Qualifying stay dates (for SNF use only)
70	Nonutilization dates (for payor use on hospital bills only)
71	Prior stay dates
72	First/last visit
73	Benefit eligibility period
74	Noncovered level of care/LOA
75	SNF level of care
76	Patient liability
77	Provider liability period
78	SNF prior stay dates
79	Payor code
80-89	Reserved for national assignment
M0	PRO/UR approved stay dates
M1	Provider liability—no utilization
M2	Dates of inpatient respite care
M3	ICF level of care
M4	Residential level of care
M5-WZ	Reserved for national assignment
X0-ZZ	Reserved for national assignment

of the claim as listed in FL 6. If more than one occurrence span code is reported, the codes must be listed in numeric sequence.

FL 36 is cross-referenced with FL 6, FLs 32 to 35, and FL 84. The information entered here must be consistent with the information entered in each of these fields.

FL 37—Internal Control Number or Documentation Control Number

FL 37 is used when sending adjustment claims. Enter the internal control number (ICN) or the documentation control number (DCN) assigned to the original bill by the payor or the fiscal intermediary (FI) for the payor. Some payors do not require this information.

FL 37 allows 23 alphanumeric characters on each of the three lines.

FL 37 is cross-referenced with FL 4. The information entered here must be consistent with the information entered in that field.

FL 38—Responsible Party Name and Addresses

Enter the name and address of the person who has accepted financial responsibility for paying the bill. In most cases, this will be either the patient or the legal guardian of the patient.

Sometimes when a claim is being submitted to a secondary payor, the secondary payor wants the name and address of the primary payor to be entered here. Check your payor contract.

Hospice wants the name, address, and provider number of a transferring hospice, if any, to be reported here.

FL 38 has 5 lines and allows 40 alphanumeric characters per line. You may use standard post office abbreviations for the address.

TABLE 12-4
Value Codes

01	Most common semi-private room rate
02	Hospital has no semi-private rooms
03	Reserved for national assignment
04	Inpatient professional component charges that are combined bill
05	Professional component included in charges and also billed separately to carrier
06	Medicare blood deductible
07	Reserved for national assignment
08	Medicare lifetime reserve amount in the first calendar year
09	Medicare coinsurance amount in the first calendar year in the billing period
10	Lifetime reserve amount in the second calendar year
11	Coinsurance amount for the second calendar year
12	Working aged beneficiary/spouse with EGHP
13	ESRD beneficiary in a Medicare coordination period with an EGHP
14	No-fault, including auto/other
15	Workers' compensation
16	Public health service (PHS) or other federal agency
17	Outlier amount
18	Disproportionate share amount
19	Indirect medical education amount
20	Total PPS capital payment amount
21	Catastrophic
22	Surplus
23	Recurring monthly income
24	Medicaid rate code
25	Offset to the patient-payment amount—prescription drugs
26	Offset to the patient-payment amount—hearing and ear services
27	Offset to the patient-payment amount—vision and eye services
28	Offset to the patient-payment amount—dental services
29	Offset to the patient-payment amount—chiropractic services
30	Preadmission testing
31	Patient liability amount
32	Multiple patient ambulance transport
33	Offset to the patient-payment amount—podiatric services
34	Offset to the patient-payment amount—other medical services
35	Offset to the patient-payment amount—health insurance premiums
36	Reserved for national assignment
37	Pints of blood furnished
38	Blood deductible pints
39	Pints of blood replaced
40	New coverage not implemented by HMO (for inpatient claims only)
41	Black lung
42	Veterans Affairs
43	Disabled beneficiary under age 65 with LGHP
44	Amount provider agreed to accept from the primary insurer when this amount is less than total charges, but greater than the primary insurer's payment
45	Accident hour
46	Number of grace days
47	Any liability insurance
48	Hemoglobin reading
49	Hematocrit reading
50	Physical therapy visits
51	Occupational therapy visits
52	Speech therapy visits
53	Cardiac rehabilitation visits
54	Newborn birth weight in grams
55	Eligibility threshold for charity care
56	Skilled nurse—home visit hours (HHA only)
57	Home health aide—home visit hours (HHA only)
58	Arterial blood gases (PO_2/PA_2)
59	Oxygen saturation (O_2 sat/Oximetry)
60	HHA branch MSA
61	Location where service is furnished (HHA and hospice)
62	HHA visits—Part A (effective October 1, 2000)
63	HHA visits—Part B (effective October 1, 2000)

Continued.

TABLE 12-4
Value Codes—cont'd

64	HHA reimbursement—Part A (effective October 1, 2000)
65	HHA reimbursement—Part B (effective October 1, 2000)
66	Medicaid spend-down amount
67	Peritoneal dialysis
68	EPO—drug
69	State charity care percent
70-72	Payor codes
73	Payor code; drug deductible
74	Payor code; drug coinsurance
75-76	Payor codes
77	Payor code; new technology add-on payment (effective April 1, 2003)
78-79	Payor codes
80-99	Reserved for national assignment
A1	Deductible payor A
A2	Coinsurance payor A
A3	Estimated responsibility payor A
A4	Covered self-administrable drugs—emergency
A5	Covered self-administrable drugs—not self administrable in form and situation furnished to patient
A6	Covered self-administrable drugs—diagnostic study and other
A7	Copayment payor A
A8-A9	Reserved for national assignment
AA	Regulatory surcharges, assessments, allowances or health care–related taxes payor A (effective October 16, 2003)
AB	Other assessments or allowances (e.g., medical education) payor A (effective October 16, 2003)
AC-AZ	Reserved for national assignment
B0	Reserved for national assignment
B1	Deductible payor B
B2	Coinsurance payor B
B3	Estimated responsibility payor B
B4-B6	Reserved for national assignment
B7	Copayment payor B
B8-B9	Reserved for national assignment
BA	Regulatory charges, assessments, allowances or health care–related taxes payor B
BB	Other assessment or allowances (e.g., medical education) payor B (effective October 16, 2003)
BC-C0	Reserved for national assignment
C1	Deductible payor C
C2	Coinsurance payor C
C3	Estimated responsibility payor C
C4-C6	Reserved for national assignment
C7	Copayment payor C
C8-C9	Reserved for national assignment
CA	Regulatory charges, assessments, allowances or health care–related taxes payor C
CB	Other assessment or allowances (e.g., medical education) payor C (effective October 16, 2003)
CC-CZ	Reserved for national assignment
D0-D2	Reserved for national assignment
D3	Estimated responsibility patient
D4-DZ	Reserved for national assignment
E0	Reserved for national assignment
E1	Deductible payor D
E2	Coinsurance payor D
E3	Estimated responsibility payor D
E4-E6	Reserved for national assignment
E7	Copayment payor D
E8-E9	Reserved for national assignment
EA	Regulatory charges, assessments, allowances or health care–related taxes payor D
EB	Other assessment or allowances (e.g., medical education) payor D (effective October 16, 2003)
EC-EZ	Reserved for national assignment
F0	Reserved for national assignment
F1	Deductible payor E
F2	Coinsurance payor E
F3	Estimated responsibility payor E
F4-F6	Reserved for national assignment
F7	Copayment payor E
F8-F9	Reserved for national assignment

TABLE 12-4
Value Codes—cont'd

FA	Regulatory charges, assessments, allowances or health care–related taxes payor E
FB	Other assessment or allowances (e.g., medical education) payor E (effective October 16, 2003)
FC-FZ	Reserved for national assignment
G0	Reserved for national assignment
G1	Deductible payor F
G2	Coinsurance payor F
G3	Estimated responsibility payor F
G4-G6	Reserved for national assignment
G7	Copayment payor F
G8-G9	Reserved for national assignment
GA	Regulatory charges, assessments, allowances or health care–related taxes payor F
GB	Other assessment or allowances (e.g., medical education) payor F (effective October 16, 2003)
GC-GZ	Reserved for national assignment
HO-WZ	Reserved for national assignment
X0-ZZ	Reserved for national assignment

FL 38 is cross-referenced with FL 1, FL 58, and FL 84. The information entered here must be consistent with the information entered in each of these fields.

FLs 39 to 41—Value Codes and Amounts

Enter value codes and the related dollar amounts identifying monetary data required for processing claims. The information entered in FLs 39 to 41 is required for benefit determination. It enables you to report data elements that are used routinely but that do not warrant a separate FL assignment. When more than one value code applies, report the codes in alphanumeric order. Each FL has line a and line b. Use FLs 39a to 41a before using FLs 39b to 41b. See Table 12-4 for valid value codes.

The value code dollar amounts may use up to eight characters. Do not report negative numbers except in FL 41. A nondollar amount, when applicable, is reported using two zeros (00).

FLs 39 to 41 are cross-referenced with FL 4, FLs 24 to 30, FLs 39 to 41, FL 42, and FL 47. The information entered here must be consistent with the information entered in each of these fields.

Answer the following questions:

1. The codes in which FL(s) identify conditions that could affect how the payor processes the claim? These codes help both primary and secondary payors determine patient eligibility, benefits, and amount of available insurance coverage.

2. Information in which FL(s) identifies an event that relates to payment of the claim? These codes identify occurrences that happen over a span of time.

3. The information entered in which FL(s) is required for benefit determination? It enables you to report data elements that are used routinely but that do not warrant a separate FL assignment.

REVENUE DESCRIPTIONS, CODES, AND CHARGES (FL 42 TO FL 49) (FIGURE 12-4)

There are 23 lines available on the claim form for each FL in this section of the claim. You may submit up to nine claim pages (450 lines) at a time.

FL 42—Revenue Code

Revenue codes are four-digit codes defined by the national uniform billing committee (NUBC). (Before April 1, 2002, the revenue codes had three digits.) Each code represents a specific service, accommodation, or billing calculation.

These codes affect reimbursement, especially for outpatient claims. A revenue code must be assigned for each line item billed in FL 47, and each code must be valid for the type of claim being billed. The revenue code reported here also must match the description or abbreviation in FL 43.

There are three basic types of revenue codes: payment, accommodation, and ancillary services. Each

42 REV. CD.	43 DESCRIPTION	44 HCPCS / RATES	45 SERV. DATE	46 SERV. UNITS	47 TOTAL CHARGES	48 NON-COVERED CHARGES	49	
1								1
2								2
3								3
4								4
5								5
6								6
7								7
8								8
9								9
10								10
11								11
12								12
13								13
14								14
15								15
16								16
17								17
18								18
19								19
20								20
21								21
22								22
23								23

FIGURE 12-4
FL 42 to FL 49 from UB-92 claim form.

type of revenue code is divided into categories and subcategories of charges.

Under the payment type of revenue codes, for example, category 002X identifies which health insurance prospective payment system (PPS) is used for the claim. Subcategory code 0022 identifies an SNF PPS. Subcategory code 0023 identifies a home health PPS. Subcategory code 0024 identifies an inpatient rehabilitation facility PPS.

In the accommodation revenue codes, one category identifies if the bill is for room and board or room and board plus ancillary services for a specified number of days (listed in FL 46 as units). Other categories identify a private room (regular vs. deluxe) with subcategory codes to identify the type of floor or unit (e.g., general, medical, surgical, GYN, OB, pediatric) for a specified number of days (listed in FL 46 as units). Other categories identify semi-private rooms (two patients vs. three or four patients per room) for a specified number of days and wards (five or more patients per room) for a specified number of days. Each has subcategories to identify the type of floor. Even the newborn nursery has a revenue category with multiple subcategory codes. There also are categories to indicate special care services like intensive care or coronary care. And there is a category to indicate special circumstances, such as when the patient has to leave for a few days and then returns to finish treatment. This is called a leave of absence (LOA) and might occur if there is a death in the patient's family. There are zero charges for the days the patient is away.

All the rest of the revenue codes are for ancillary services that are billed separately. The majority of revenue codes fall under this type of revenue code. Examples of the wide variety of categories found here include incremental nursing rates, pharmacy, IV therapy, med/surg supplies and devices, durable medical equipment (several categories), laboratory (several categories), radiology (several categories), operating room services, anesthesia, blood services (several categories), respiratory, and many more.

The codes are found in the chargemaster for each department in the facility. The individual assigned to update the chargemaster should attend continuing education courses on a regular basis to be sure that only valid revenue codes are available for use on claims. Billing guidelines for revenue codes are extensive. Each is valid only for certain types of bills (TOB) in FL 4. Most of the rules governing use of revenue codes are programmed into the billing programs that hospitals and facilities use to generate claims.

The revenue codes are listed on the claim in revenue code order (from low number to high number) by date of service, when applicable. If the services encompassed in a code are performed more than once, the code may be repeated.

Payors compare revenue codes with diagnosis and procedure codes to identify excluded services.

FL 42 is cross-referenced with FL 4, FL 44, FL 47, and FLs 67 to 75. The information entered here must be consistent with the information entered in each of these fields.

FL 43—Revenue Description

In FL 43, enter the narrative description or the standard abbreviation for the revenue code report in FL 42 on the same line. There are 23 lines available for use in this field. Complete this field for each line in use.

FL 43 is cross-referenced with FL 44 and FL 84. The information entered here must be consistent with the information entered in each of these fields.

FL 44—HCPCS/Rates

Each of the 23 lines in FL 44 will contain one of the following:

❑ For inpatients: the accommodation rate. This is often referred to as the bed charge for the hospital bed, but it encompasses all the associated overhead costs: nursing care, other staff members whose services benefit the patient, supplies, electricity, water, and more.

❑ For outpatient claims: a Level I CPT code or a Level II HCPCS code. These codes may identify ancillary services or many other types of supplies and services as required under the rules for ambulatory payment classifications (APCs), the OPPS for hospital outpatient services.

❑ For SNFs: the health insurance prospective payment system (HIPPS) rate code. This code consists of the RUG III code from the minimum data set (MDS) grouper software and the 2-digit modifier that identifies the type of assessment completed by the physician for the service identified in the RUG III code. *Note:* The physician sends a CMS-1500 claim form using E/M codes from the CPT codebook to bill the physician aspect of the service. The RUG III code and modifier are used to bill the facility's overhead costs associated with providing the service.

❑ For home health care: the home health rate group (HHRG) code. This is a HIPPS code under the rules for the home health prospective payment system (HHPPS). When you enter the services performed into the computer system, a software program should help you find the associated HHRG code.

❑ For hospital-based ambulance services: Enter the level II HCPCS code and the 2-digit modifier to show the pick-up origin and the destination.

Certain entries in FL 44 have specific requirements that must be met. Most facilities use billing software with the requirements for the specific type of facility programmed into the software. There should be a help screen to assist you in choosing the correct entry.

FL 44 is cross-referenced with FL 4, FL 22, and FL 42. The information entered here must be consistent with the information entered in each of these fields.

FL 45—Service Date

FL 45 is a required field. Enter the date on which the service reported on this line was provided. Enter the correct date for the items entered on each of the 23 possible lines. Enter the eight-digit date as YYYYMMDD. May 1, 2005, would be listed as 20050501.

Each line item date of service reported on the claim must fall within the dates reported in FL 6.

Many therapeutic services are performed daily. Each service provided is reported on a separate line with the specific date for each occurrence. If the service is provided more than once on the same date, it is reported on one line with number of visits reflected in the number of units billed in FL 46. The number of units for each date reflects the number of units per occurrence plus the services provided during additional visits on that date.

FL 45 is cross-referenced with FL 4, FL 6, FL 42, and FLs 44 to 46. The information entered here must be consistent with the information entered in each of these fields.

FL 46—Service Units

Enter the number of services rendered per revenue code category or subcategory to or for the patient. This number might represent the number of accommodation days, the number of visits, the number of pints of blood, the flow rate of oxygen, the number of units, the number of treatments, or the number of miles traveled.

When the number of service units for a particular item is based on time, the time it took to render the service must be documented in the medical record.

FL 46 allows up to seven positions in each line. FL 46 allows a decimal to be entered, but be aware that when a decimal is entered, many payors will round the number to the nearest whole number.

FL 46 is cross-referenced with FL 4, FLs 6 to 7, FL 42, FLs 42 to 46, and FL 48. The information entered here must be consistent with the information entered in each of these fields.

FL 47—Total Charges

FL 47 is a required field. Enter the total charge pertaining to the revenue code category or subcategory listed on the same line.

The UB-92 claim form is a summary form. The total charge is a summary amount representing the sum of all charges for services that fall within the listed revenue code category or subcategory for the date of service listed on that line. The total charge includes charges for both covered and noncovered services. Each UB-92 claim form is accompanied by an itemized list of charges that details every charge summarized by the total charge on each line in FL 47.

FL 47 allows up to 10 digits on each of the four lines. Not counting the dollar sign and commas, 7 digits are for dollars and 2 digits are for cents with a space to the right of the cents to indicate a credit amount. For example, $7,395,514.89_.

FL 47 is cross-referenced with FL 4, FL 6, FL 42, FL 44, and FLs 46 to 48. The information entered here must be consistent with the information entered in each of these fields.

FL 48—Noncovered Charges
In FL 48, enter the total charges for noncovered services, if any, for the primary payor included in the revenue code listed on the same line for the date of service listed on the same line

Medicare and many other payors want a claim to be submitted for every hospital stay, including those for which no payment is made or expected. A Medicare benefit period begins the first inpatient day and ends when the patient has not been an inpatient anywhere for 60 consecutive days. FL 48 enables Medicare and other payors to track this information.

FL 48 allows up to 10 digits on each of the four lines. Not counting the dollar sign and commas, 7 digits are for dollars and 2 digits are for cents with a space to the right of the cents to indicate a credit amount. For example, $1,284,718.91_.

FL 48 is cross-referenced with FL 4, FL 8, and FLs 46 to 47. The information entered here must be consistent with the information entered in each of these fields.

FL 49—Unlabeled Field
FL 49 is reserved for national assignment effective October 1, 2003. FL 49 allows four characters in each of the 23 lines.

PAYOR, INSURED, AND EMPLOYER INFORMATION (FL 50 TO FL 66) (FIGURE 12-5)

FL 50—Payor Identification
In FL 50, enter the name of the payor and, if required, the payor identification number. FL 50 is a required field. Twenty-five alphanumeric characters are allowed on each of the three lines.

- ❏ 50 A is for the primary payor.
- ❏ 50 B is for the secondary payor, if applicable.
- ❏ 50 C is for the tertiary (third) payor, if applicable.

FL 50 is cross-referenced with FLs 24 to 30, FLs 32 to 35, FLs 39 to 41, FLs 52 to 55, FLs 59 to 60, FLs 67 to 75, and FL 84. The information entered here must be consistent with the information entered in each of these fields.

FL 51—Provider Number
In FL 51, enter on lines A, B, and C the provider numbers assigned by the payors listed in FL 50.

- ❏ 51 A is for the provider number assigned by the primary payor.
- ❏ 51 B is for the provider number assigned by the secondary payor, if applicable.
- ❏ 51 C is for the provider number assigned by the tertiary payor, if applicable.

FL 51 allows 13 alphanumeric characters on each of the three lines.

When the National Provider Identifier (NPI) from the Centers for Medicare and Medicaid Services (CMS) becomes available, that number will be entered here for Medicare and any other payor who chooses to use that number as the provider number.

FL 51 is cross-referenced with FL 4, FL 22, and FL 50. The information entered here must be consistent with the information entered in each of these fields.

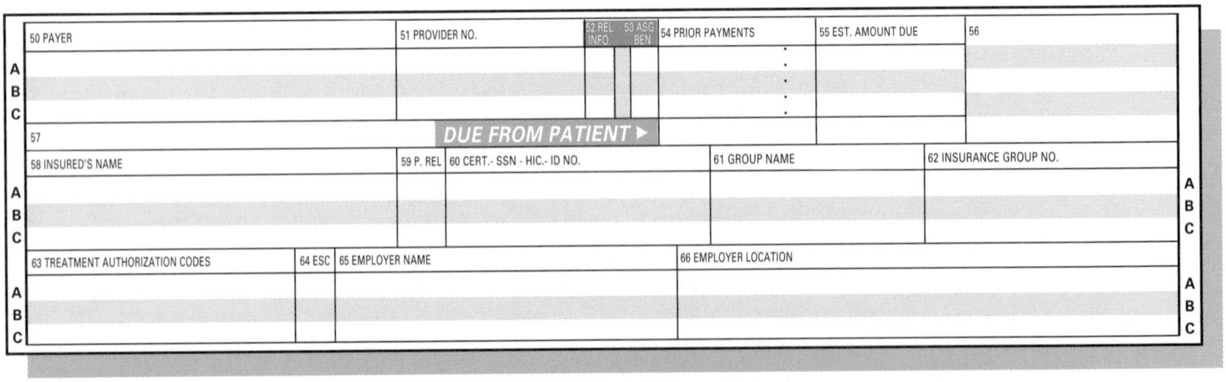

FIGURE 12-5
FL 50 to FL 66 from the UB-92 claim form.

FL 52—Release of Information Certification Indicator

FL 52 is a required field. The information entered in FL 52 tells whether or not the provider has on file a signed statement from the patient (or the legal guardian of the patient) permitting the provider to release billing information to each of the payor(s) listed in FL 50 on lines A, B, and C.

Valid choices are:

- ❐ Y   Yes
- ❐ R   Restricted or modified release
- ❐ N   No release

FL 52 is cross-referenced with FL 50. The information entered here must be consistent with the information entered in that field.

FL 53—Assignment of Benefits

The information entered in FL 53 tells whether the provider has on file a signed statement from the patient (or the legal guardian of the patient) permitting each of the payor(s) listed in FL 50 on lines A, B, and C to send payment for services directly to the provider.

Valid choices for each line are:

- ❐ Y   Yes
- ❐ N   No

FL 53 is cross-referenced with FL 50. The information entered here must be consistent with the information entered in that field.

FL 54—Prior Payments—Payors and Patient

In FL 54, enter the amount of payment the facility has already received (before sending the claim) toward payment of this bill from each of the payors listed in FL 50 on lines A, B, and C and from the patient. Secondary and tertiary payors require completion of this field. Some primary payors also require completion of FL 54.

FL 54 allows up to 10 digits on each of the four lines. Not counting the dollar sign and commas, 7 digits are for dollars and 2 digits are for cents with a space to the right of the cents to indicate a credit amount. For example, $1,326,294.63_.

- ❐ 54 A is for the prior payment made by the primary payor.
- ❐ 54 B is for the prior payment made by the secondary payor.
- ❐ 54 C is for the prior payment made by the tertiary payor.
- ❐ The last line is for the prior payment made by the patient.

FL 54 is cross-referenced with FL 50. The information entered here must be consistent with the information entered in that field.

FL 55—Estimated Amount Due

In FL 55, enter the amount still due from each of the payors listed in FL 50 on lines A, B, and C and from the patient.

FL 55 allows up to 10 digits on each of the four lines. Not counting the dollar sign and commas, 7 digits are for dollars and 2 digits are for cents with a space to the right of the cents to indicate a credit amount. For example, $1,284,718.91_.

- ❐ 55 A is for the amount due from the primary payor.
- ❐ 55 B is for the amount due from the secondary payor.
- ❐ 55 C is for the amount due from the tertiary payor.
- ❐ The last line is for the amount due from the patient.

FL 55 is cross-referenced with FL 50. The information entered here must be consistent with the information entered in that field.

FL 56—Unlabeled Field

FL 56 is reserved for national assignment effective October 16, 2003. FL 56 allows 14 characters in each of the 5 lines.

FL 57—Unlabeled Field

FL 57 is reserved for national assignment effective October 16, 2003. FL 57 allows 27 characters.

FL 58—Insured's Name

FL 58 has three lines to allow information to be entered for each of the payors listed in FL 50. The field allows 25 alphanumeric characters on each of the three lines.

The insured is the policyholder, the person whose name is listed in the medical plan's files as the owner of the policy. Some medical plans call the insured the "subscriber," and Medicare calls the insured the "beneficiary." The *employee* is the "insured" for an individual or a family medical plan obtained through an employer, and the *employer* is the "insured" for workers' compensation.

- ❐ 58 A is for the insured's name spelled as listed on the insurance card for the primary payor.
- ❐ 58 B is for the insured's name spelled as listed on the insurance card for the secondary payor, if applicable.

❏ 58 C is for the insured's name spelled as listed on the insurance card for the tertiary payor, if applicable.

Unless otherwise indicated by a particular payor, enter the information as: last name, first name, middle initial (if any).

Use a comma to separate the last name from the first name. A hyphen with no spaces may be used between hyphenated names (e.g., Smith-Jones). Leave a space between the first name and the middle initial. Leave a space between the last name and any suffixes (e.g., Brown III, or Brown Jr.). Do not use titles (e.g., Sir, Dr., Mr., Mrs., Ms.).

FL 58 is cross-referenced with FL 4 and FL 50. The information entered here must be consistent with the information entered in each of these fields.

FL 59—Patient Relation to Insured

On each line in FL 59 enter the code that indicates the relationship of the patient to the insured individual(s) identified in FL 58 on lines A, B, and C.

The information in FL 59 is left justified. FL 59 allows alphanumeric characters.

If you are working with old claims, valid choices before October 16, 2003, were:

01	Patient is insured
02	Spouse
03	Natural child/insured has financial responsibility
04	Natural child/insured does not have financial responsibility
05	Stepchild
06	Foster child
07	Ward of the court
08	Employee
09	Unknown
10	Handicapped dependent
11	Organ donor
12	Cadaver donor
13	Grandchild
14	Niece/Nephew
15	Injured plaintiff
16	Sponsored dependent
17	Minor dependent of minor dependent
18	Parent
19	Grandparent
20	Life partner
21-99	Reserved for national assignment

Valid choices since October 16, 2003, are:

01	Spouse
04	Grandfather or grandmother
05	Grandson or granddaughter
07	Nephew or niece
10	Foster child
15	Ward
17	Stepson or stepdaughter
18	Self
19	Child
20	Employee
21	Unknown
22	Handicapped dependent
23	Sponsored dependent
24	Dependent of a minor dependent
29	Significant other
32	Mother
33	Father
36	Emancipated minor
39	Organ donor
40	Cadaver donor
41	Injured plaintiff
43	Child where insured has no financial responsibility
53	Life partner
G8	Other relationship

FL 59 is cross-referenced with FL 58. The information entered here must be consistent with the information entered in that field.

FL 60—Certificate—Social Security Number—Health Insurance Claim Identification Number

In FL 60, enter the insured's identification number assigned by each payor. This number is found on the patient's insurance card.

FL 60 allows 19 alphanumeric characters in each of the three lines.

❏ 60A: Enter the identification number for the insured in FL 58 A with the primary payor in FL 50 A.

❏ 60 B: Enter the identification number for the insured in FL 58 B with the primary payor in FL 50 B.

❏ 60 C: Enter the identification number for the insured in FL 58 C with the primary payor in FL 50 C.

FL 60 is cross-referenced with FL 4 and FL 12. The information entered here must be consistent with the information entered in each of these fields.

FL 61—Group Name

On each line in FL 61, enter the name of the group or plan through which the health insurance coverage is provided to the insured in FL 58 on the same line. Unless otherwise stated in a payor contract, provide this information only when group coverage applies. FL 61 allows for 14 alphanumeric characters.

❑ 61 A: Enter the name of the group or plan, when applicable, for the insured in FL 58A with the primary payor in FL 50 A.

❑ 61 B: Enter the name of the group or plan, when applicable, for the insured in FL 58 B with the primary payor in FL 50 B.

❑ 61C: Enter the name of the group or plan, when applicable, for the insured in FL 58 C with the primary payor in FL 50 C.

FL 62—Insurance Group Number

In FL 62, enter the group number, control number, or code assigned by the payor to each group under which the individual is covered. FL 62 allows 17 alphanumeric characters for each line.

❑ 62 A: Enter the group number assigned by the payor in FL 50 A for the group plan, if any.

❑ 62 B: Enter the group number assigned by the payor in FL 50 B for the group plan, if any.

❑ 62 C: Enter the group number assigned by the payor in FL 50 C for the group plan, if any.

FL 63—Treatment Authorization Codes

In FL 63, enter the authorization number or other indicator, if any, that shows prior approval for services was obtained from the payor in FL 50 on lines A, B, and C. FL 63 allows 18 alphanumeric characters in each of the three lines.

Unless otherwise indicated in a contract, only the authorization from the primary payor (FL 50 A) is listed here on line 63 A. Secondary and tertiary treatment authorization codes are traditionally reported in FL 84.

FL 63 is cross-referenced with FL 50 and FL 84. The information entered here must be consistent with the information entered in each of these fields.

FL 64—Employment Status Code of the Insured

FL 64 is no longer used for claims, effective April 1, 2004.

If you are working with older claims, the valid choices for the insured listed on each line were:

1	Employed full time
2	Employed part time
3	Not employed
4	Self-employed
5	Retired
6	On active military duty
7-8	Reserved for national assignment
9	Unknown

FL 64 is cross-referenced with FL 58. The information entered here must be consistent with the information entered in this field.

FL 65—Employer Name of the Insured

In FL 65, enter the name of the employer, if any, who provides the health care coverage for each insured listed in FL 58 on lines A, B, and C.

❑ 65 A: Enter the name of the employer who provides the coverage for the insured listed in FL 58 A.

❑ 65 B: Enter the name of the employer who provides the coverage for the insured listed in FL 58 B.

❑ 65 C: Enter the name of the employer who provides the coverage for the insured listed in FL 58 C.

FL 65 is cross-referenced with FL 58. The information entered here must be consistent with the information entered in this field.

FL 66—Employer Location of the Insured

In FL 66, enter the specific location of the employer, if any, of the insured individual in FL 58. The location can be a specific city, plant, or other location. FL 66 is especially significant when an employer operates from more than one location.

FL 66 allows 35 alphanumeric characters in each of the three lines.

❑ 66 A: Enter the location of the employer, if any, listed in FL 65 A for the insured listed in FL 58 A.

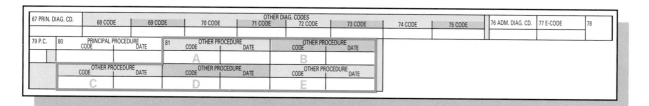

FIGURE 12-6
FL 67 to FL 81 from the UB-92 claim form.

☐ 66 B: Enter the location of the employer, if any, listed in FL 65 B for the insured listed in FL 58 B.

☐ 66 C: Enter the location of the employer, if any, listed in FL 65 C for the insured listed in FL 58 C.

FL 66 is cross-referenced with FL 58. The information entered here must be consistent with the information entered in this field.

DIAGNOSIS AND PROCEDURE CODES (FL 67 TO FL 81) (FIGURE 12-6)

FLs 67 to 81 are used to report clinical information. The information reported here must match documentation in the medical record as closely as possible.

For most inpatient facility claims, codes from ICD-9-CM Volumes 1 and 2 are used to report diagnoses and codes from ICD-9-CM Volume 3 are used to report inpatient procedures. No modifiers are used when reporting inpatient procedures. For example, with inpatient claims, you list the code twice to indicate a bilateral procedure. You do not use a modifier.

For outpatient facility claims, codes from ICD-9-CM Volumes 1 and 2 are used to report diagnoses, and codes from CPT-4 Level I and HCPCS Level II are used to report outpatient procedures and, when applicable, supplies or transportation. Only specific modifiers from Level I CPT and Level II HCPCS may be used with outpatient procedure, supply, and transportation codes. A complete list of these modifiers is found on the inside front cover of a current-year CPT-4 codebook. For example, with outpatient claims you list modifier -50 after the procedure code to indicate a bilateral procedure.

FLs 67 to 77 allow for six alphanumeric characters. FLs 67 to 77 have room to include the decimal, but check with each payor for their preferences. Some payors do not want the decimal to be reported on the claim form because their computer system is programmed to automatically insert the decimal, and having two decimals would make the code invalid. Remember, the CMS-1500 claim form has the decimal in dropout red, so the decimal is not typed in on those claim forms and is instead always added in by the payor's computer system.

Valid ICD-9-CM codes have either three numbers or an uppercase letter and two numbers followed by a decimal point and up to two additional numbers. This gives a total of four to six characters, including the decimal point.

When ICD-10-CM is implemented, expect FLs 67 to 77 to be reprogrammed to allow eight case-sensitive alphanumeric digits. ICD-10-CM codes are expected to begin with an upper case letter followed by two numbers, a decimal point, up to three additional numbers and, when applicable, an additional lower case letter. This gives a total of four to eight alphanumeric characters, including the decimal point.

FL 67—Principal Diagnosis Code

In FL 67, enter the full diagnosis code, including all applicable additional digits, for the principal diagnosis. Always code to the highest degree of specificity that matches medical record documentation.

Follow the coding guidelines in the ICD-9-CM codebook governing how to select the principal diagnosis. For inpatients, the principal diagnosis is the condition determined after study to be chiefly responsible for causing the hospitalization. For outpatients, the principal diagnosis is based on test results.

FL 67 is a required field only when the first 2 digits of the 3-digit codes for the type of bill (TOB) in FL 4 are 11, 12, 13, 14, or 18.

FL 67 is cross-referenced with FL 4, FL 6, FLs 14 to 15, FL 42, FL 44, FLs 68 to 75, FL 77, FLs 80 to 81, and FL 84. The information entered here must be consistent with the information entered in each of these fields.

FLs 68 to 75—Other Diagnosis Codes

In FLs 68 to 75, enter the full diagnosis code, including all applicable additional digits, for all other conditions that the patient has. For inpatients, report other conditions the patient has at the time of admission, that develop after admission, or that affect treatment received and/or the length of stay. Do not include a diagnosis that no longer affects the patient or that has no bearing on this admission. For outpatients, report other conditions the patient has in addition to the principal diagnosis. Always code to the highest degree of specificity that matches medical record documentation.

Follow the coding guidelines in the ICD-9-CM codebook governing additional diagnoses. For inpatients, there are often specific CC that cannot be reported with a specific principal diagnosis. Some versions of ICD-9-CM for hospitals list these exclusions with the code descriptions in the Volume 1 tabular list. Report additional diagnosis in the order of priority given by the provider in medical record documentation unless the codebook rules specify a different order.

FLs 68 to 75 are cross-referenced with FL 4, FLs 67 to 75, FL 77, FLs 80 to 81, and FL 84. The information entered here must be consistent with the information entered in each of these fields.

FL 76—Admitting Diagnosis/Reason for Visit

In FL 76, enter the full diagnosis code, including all applicable additional digits, for the reason for the admission or the reason the patient registered for outpatient services. Only report one code in this field.

For *inpatients,* this code describes the reason for admission. The condition might describe a significant abnormal finding, patient distress, a poisoning, an injury, a possible diagnosis based on significant findings, follow-up for a diagnosis previously established, or another reason or condition (such as pregnancy and labor).

For *outpatients,* the code should be the patient's stated reason for seeking care. The condition might be follow-up for a diagnosis previously established, a significant abnormal finding, patient distress, a poisoning, an injury, or another reason or condition (such as pregnancy).

FL 76 is cross-referenced with FL 4 and FL 42. The information entered here must be consistent with the information entered in each of these fields.

FL 77—External Cause of Injury (E-Code)

In FL 77, enter the full E-code, including all applicable additional digits, for the external cause of: injury, poisoning, and/or adverse effects of treatment. List only one code here. Additional E-codes, if any, may be listed following the "other" diagnosis codes in FLs 67 to 75 if there is space available.

All valid code choices in ICD-9-CM begin with the letter E. When ICD-10-CM is released, the valid code choices will begin with a different letter.

Hospital guidelines say the E-code for the principal diagnosis, if any, should be listed first, followed by E-codes for additional diagnoses, if any, in the same order as the corresponding diagnosis codes. Some E-codes tell "how" and others tell "where" an event occurred. Payors usually want to know "where" more than they want to know "how" an event occurred. This is because "where" often determines which payor is to be listed as the primary payor for the claim. When adequate space is available, list both the "how" and the "where" for each applicable diagnosis code in the order dictated by codebook guidelines. When space for E-codes is limited, guidelines direct you to list the "how" code(s) first.

FL 77 allows for six alphanumeric characters.

FL 78—Unlabeled Field

FL 78 is reserved for national assignment effective October 16, 2003. FL 78 allows two characters in the upper line and three characters in the lower line.

FL 79—Procedure Coding Method Used

FL 79 is not used for claims reporting effective April 1, 2004.

If you are working with old claims with a date-of-service before that date, the field was used to identify whether the procedure codes reported on the claim were taken from ICD-9-CM, CPT-4, or another source. The valid choices were:

1-3 Reserved for state assignment (e.g., workers' compensation's local codes, Medicaid's local codes, and HCPCS level III local codes for Medicare) (discontinued effective April 1, 2004)
4 CPT-4 (HCPCS Level I) (discontinued effective April 1, 2004)
5 HCPCS (HCPCS Level II) (discontinued effective April 1, 2004)
6-8 Reserved for national assignment
9 ICD-9-CM (Volume 3) (discontinued effective April 1, 2004)

FL 80—Principal Procedure Code and Date

FL 80 is primarily used to report procedures performed on inpatients. For outpatients, procedures are reported in FL 44. Outpatients with a 3-digit TOB in FL 4 with the first 2 digits of 13 or 14 may list an ICD-9-CM code here and a CPT or HCPCS code in FL 44.

In FL 80, enter the full ICD-9-CM Volume 3 procedure code, including any additional digits, for the principal procedure performed during the period covered by the claim, if any. When a code is entered here, also enter the date on which the procedure was performed.

The principal procedure is one performed for treatment, not for diagnosis, exploration, or to take care of a complication. If more than one procedure meets this definition, the one most related to the principal diagnosis is designated as the principal procedure. If more than one is related to the principal diagnosis, the most resource-intensive or the most complex procedure is designated as the principal procedure.

> *Note:* Operating room charges are listed in FLs 42 to 43. For open biopsies, the size of the incision must be reported in FL 84.

FL 80 allows seven alphanumeric characters for the procedure and eight numeric characters for the date. For claims with a date of service before April 1, 2004, the code structure must be consistent with the code source reported in FL 79. The date is reported as a 4-digit year, a 2-digit month, and a 2-digit day (YYYYMMDD). April 1, 2004, would be reported as 20040401.

At some point in the future, ICD-10 PCS might replace ICD-9-CM Volume 3. When this occurs, the code structure and coding guidelines approved for ICD-10 PCS will replace the current requirements.

FL 80 is cross-referenced with FL 4, FL 6, FL 17, FL 42, FL 44, FL 67, and FL 81. The information entered here must be consistent with the information entered in each of these fields.

FL 81—Other Procedure Codes and Dates

FL 81 is primarily used to report procedures performed on inpatients. For outpatients, procedures are reported in FL 44. Outpatients with a 3-digit TOB in FL 4 with the first 2 digits of 13 may list an ICD-9-CM code here and a CPT or HCPCS code in FL 44.

FL 81 allows you to report the ICD-9-CM codes for up to five additional significant procedures performed during the billing period, other than the significant procedure reported in FL 80. With each listed procedure, list the date it was performed. Report the other procedures that are the most significant to this episode of care. Be sure to include any therapeutic procedures that are closely related to the principal diagnosis. Enter the codes in FL 81 in descending order of importance. Do not repeat codes unless they are bilateral procedures.

FL 81 allows seven alphanumeric characters for the procedure and eight numeric characters for the date. For claims with a date of service before April 1, 2004, the code structure must be consistent with the code source reported in FL 79. The date is reported as a 4-digit year, a 2-digit month, and a 2-digit day (YYYYMMDD). April 1, 2004, would be reported as 20040401.

At some point in the future, ICD-10 PCS might replace ICD-9-CM Volume 3. When this occurs, the code structure and coding guidelines approved for ICD-10 PCS will replace the current requirements.

FL 81 is cross-referenced with FL 4, FL 6, FL 17, FL 42, FL 44, FL 80, and FL 84. The information entered here must be consistent with the information entered in each of these fields.

PHYSICIAN INFORMATION (FL 82 TO FL 83) (FIGURE 12-7)

FL 82—Attending Physician ID

In FL 82, enter the name and license number of the physician who has primary responsibility for the patient's medical care and treatment.

FL 82 has two lines. The upper line allows for 23 characters. It is used most often to list the name and the state physician license number or a payor-specific ID number for the attending physician (inpatient). When the CMS implements the NPI number, it will be listed on the first line for inpatients for the payors that use it.

The second line allows 32 alphanumeric characters and is primarily used to meet UPIN requirements for outpatients and for skilled nursing facilities. When the CMS implements the NPI number, it will be listed on the second line for outpatients and SNFs for the payors that use it.

On either line, enter the number first followed by two spaces and then the name, last name first.

In the "name" section, do not use any special characters. Do not use a comma between the first name and the last name. Do not use a hyphen, an apostrophe, or any other special characters in names that include them.

If the patient is self-referred (as often happens in the ER), enter the code SLF000 and do not enter a physician's name. Other surrogate UPINs that may be used when needed are:

INT000	Each intern
OTH000	Other situations in which no UPIN is assigned
PHS000	PHS physician
RES000	Each resident
RET000	Retired physician
SLF000	Self-referred patients (This code cannot be used when a referral is required.)
VAD000	Veterans Affairs physicians

FL 83—Other Physician ID

In FL 83, enter the name and license number of the physicians other than the attending physician who have responsibility for any of the patient's medical care and treatment.

This field has two lines. The upper line allows for 25 characters. It is used most often to list the name

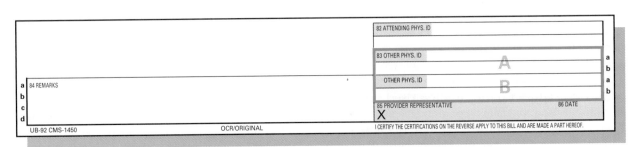

FIGURE 12-7
FL 82 to FL 86 from the UB-92 claim form.

and the state physician license or a payor-specific ID number for each other physician. When the CMS implements the NPI number, it will be listed on the first line for the payors that use it.

The second line allows 32 alphanumeric characters and is primarily used to meet UPIN requirements. When the CMS implements the NPI number, it will be listed on the second line for the payors that use it. On either line, enter the number first followed by two spaces and then the name, last name first.

Line 1 and line 2 may be used to report two different physicians, or just one line may be used.

In the "name" section, do not use any special characters. Do not use a comma between the first name and the last name. Do not use a hyphen, an apostrophe, or any other special characters in names that include them.

There are special requirements for FL 83 in specific circumstances. The help screen in the computer program should alert you to these issues as they arise. For example, FL 83 must be completed when there is a principal procedure identified in FL 80. The name of the physician who performed the principal procedure is entered here. If the attending physician performed the principal procedure, the information for the attending physician is also listed here.

FL 83 is cross-referenced with FL 4, FL 42, FL 44, FL 67, and FLs 80 to 82. The information entered here must be consistent with the information entered in each of these fields.

REMARKS, PROVIDER SIGNATURE, AND DATE (FL 84 TO FL 86)

FL 84—Remarks

FL 84 is used for any information required by a specific payor that is not listed anywhere else on the claim form. FL 84 allows 48 alphanumeric characters on each of four lines. See your payor-specific contracts for guidance on using FL 84.

Any required information that does not belong somewhere else is entered on FL 84. For example, a notation of "noncovered service" or "primary payor denied coverage" might be valid notations for an item not covered by the primary payor, but covered by the secondary payor. The information entered here often speeds up claim processing and reimbursement.

FL 84 is cross-referenced with FL 4, FLs 24 to 30, FLs 32 to 36, FLs 39 to 41, FL 50, FLs 64 to 66, FLs 68 to 75 and FL 81. The information entered here must be consistent with the information entered in each of these fields.

FL 85—Provider Representative Signature

When needed, enter the authorized signature on the claim in FL 85 to indicate the information entered on the front of the claim meets the requirements listed on the back of the claim. This field allows 22 alphanumeric characters. Stamped and facsimile signatures are acceptable to some payors.

No signature is required for a general hospital stay unless the physician's certification or recertification was required during the stay.

FL 85 is cross-referenced with FL 4. The information entered here must be consistent with the information entered in that field.

FL 86—Date Bill Submitted

In FL 86, enter the date the claim is submitted. The field allows 10 numeric characters on one line. The 8-digit date is reported as a 4-digit year, a 2-digit month, and a 2-digit day (YYYYMMDD). April 1, 2004, would be reported as 20040401. The two extra spaces allow a larger space to accommodate a handwritten date on paper claims.

FL 86 is cross-referenced with FL 4 and FL 85. The information entered here must be consistent with the information entered in each of these fields.

Legal Issues

Some hospitals do not want their coders to know anything about hospital billing rules. They say they want to avoid even the appearance of coding for increased reimbursement.

Realistically, coders and billers work in different departments within the hospital. Even though you learn both billing and coding in school, you will only practice one or the other on the job. Therefore it is highly unlikely that a coder would ever learn the contract-specific issues that one would have to know

to violate the law and code solely for increased reimbursement.

Some hospitals try to "cook the books" by directing coders to upcode certain services. Upcoding makes a patient seem more ill than he or she actually is. Downcoding makes a patient seem less ill than he or she actually is. Upcoding and downcoding are just as fraudulent for the hospital as they are for the physician's office.

Hospitals usually capture their charges from each department by using a computer program called a chargemaster. Typically, each department is responsible for updating the chargemaster for that department. If even one department fails to update its chargemaster, services can be reported incorrectly, leading to charges of either fraud or abuse.

STOP & REVIEW

Answer the following questions:

1. A _____ code must be assigned for each line item billed in FL 47, and each code must be valid for the type of claim being billed.

2. Many therapeutic services are performed daily. Each service provided is reported on a separate line with the specific date for each occurrence.

   ____True   ____False

3. The total charge in FL 47 includes charges for both covered and noncovered services.

   ____True   ____False

4. In FL 50, what payor is listed on line A?

   _____

5. In FL 50, what payor is listed on line B?

   _____

6. In FL 50, what payor is listed on line C?

   _____

7. For inpatients, the principal diagnosis is the same as the admitting diagnosis.

   ____True   ____False

8. The principal procedure in FL 80 is one performed for treatment, not for diagnosis, exploration, or to take care of a complication.

   ____True   ____False

9. The _____ physician has primary responsibility for the patient's medical care and treatment and is listed in FL 82.

10. Upcoding and downcoding are just as fraudulent for the hospital as they are for the physician's office.

    ____True   ____False

Chapter Review

Medicare pays physicians and facilities under a payment system called the prospective payment system. For physicians, the Medicare prospective payment system is called the resource-based relative value system (RBRVS). For hospital inpatients, the Medicare prospective payment system is called diagnosis related group (DRG). For hospital outpatients, the Medicare prospective payment system is called ambulatory payment classification (APC). Nursing facilities and home health agencies are also paid using a prospective payment system.

The facility fees for hospital inpatients, hospital outpatients, and nursing facilities and the fees for home health agencies (HHAs) are billed using a UB-92 claim form. The fields on the UB-92 claim form are numbered using field locator (FL) numbers. Each field has very specific requirements.

Upcoding and downcoding are just as fraudulent for facilities as they are for a physician's office.

Answer the following questions:

1. The resource-based relative value system (RBRVS) considers the CPT code in relation to what three additional factors?

   _____

   _____

   _____

2. In the DRG system, the more than 10,000 available ICD-9-CM diagnosis codes are grouped into 25 major diagnostic categories (MDCs).

   ____True   ____False

3. Each MDC is then subdivided into DRG groups based on the historical data for the nationwide average payment amounts per hospitalization. Similar payment amounts within an MDC are grouped into one DRG and are then assigned a fixed payment value.

   ____True   ____False

4. APC was designed to consider diagnoses and procedures, as well as the appropriateness of each service and medical necessity.

   ____True   ____False

5. The APC for an episode of care is not listed on the UB-92 claim form.

_____True   _____False

6. What are people who use nursing facilities called?

_____

7. What claim form is used by a nursing facility?

_____

8. What team, usually a group of RNs trained in DRGs and hospital reimbursement issues, works to help the hospital remain profitable?
A. PRO
B. UR
C. CC
D. LOS

9. Hospitals bill their inpatient services using:
A. RBRVS
B. DRG
C. APC
D. APG

10. Hospitals bill their outpatient services using:
A. RBRVS
B. DRG
C. APC
D. APG

11. When coding for hospital inpatients, may you code rule-out or suspected conditions as if they exist?

Yes _____   No _____

12. When coding for hospital outpatients, may you code rule-out or suspected conditions as if they exist?

Yes _____   No _____

13. Which diagnosis is the reason the patient is admitted to the hospital?

_____

14. Which diagnosis is the reason, after study, determined to be chiefly responsible for occasioning the admission to the hospital?

_____

15. What is the name of the most important therapeutic procedure performed on an inpatient?

_____

16. When the diagnosis codes billed make the patient seem more ill than he or she actually was, what improper coding practice occurred?

_____

17. When the diagnosis codes billed make the patient seem less ill than he or she actually was, what improper coding practice occurred?

_____

18. A revenue code must be assigned for each line item billed in FL 23.

True _____   False _____

19. What FL is used to report the dates of service for the entire UB-92 claim?

_____

20. What FL is used to report the name of the attending physician?

_____

13 REIMBURSEMENT SUCCESS

Objectives After completing this chapter, you should be able to:

■ Organize and track financial documentation for the medical office
■ Make decisions that result in correct payments from payors and patients
■ Read and interpret an EOB/EOMB/MRN
■ Compare payments received with fee schedules
■ Determine when to rebill a service provided and when to file an appeal
■ Gather the documents needed for a retrospective payment audit

Key Terms

adjustment codes codes used by payors to explain why a claim or a service is paid differently than it was billed.

aging reports reports used to report the status of claims to the physician and to identify individual transactions that require follow-up.

bad debt write-off a write-off that records payments owed, but not collectable. It does not represent a discount.

case number a payor-assigned number that must appear on each page of each document sent with an appeal.

concurrent payment audit an audit that occurs at the time payments are posted to evaluate the correctness of payments received on the day of the audit.

electronic payment posting the payor automatically posts a payment to your practice management system after making an automatic deposit into the practice bank account.

electronic remittance voucher an electronic EOB (explanation of benefits) that is sent when the payor sends an electronic payment that is automatically deposited in the practice bank account.

explanatory notes these give additional information about items referenced by footnotes or symbols on an EOB.

financial hardship discount a discount given when a patient is in financial difficulty and cannot meet the patient financial obligation. A hardship waiver must be on file before this discount is given. The physician collects the payor's portion of the charge and writes off the patient portion of the charge.

financial policy statement a patient-signed document that protects the physician's right to collect money earned.

insurance write-off the insurance discount given to a payor in a contract.

ledger card an old-fashioned patient accounting method that does not allow you to track payments by transaction.

line item posting an accounting method by which every payment is posted to the exact transaction for which the payment is received.

patient discount a discount often offered to self-pay patients if they pay their bills on time. It must not cause the total fee to become lower than the Medicare fee schedule for the service.

patient eligibility the process of contacting each payor and verifying that the patient is covered by the policy, the policy information is correct, and the policy has not expired. Sometimes additional information is needed to determine the primary payor for the claim.

professional courtesy the physician sees a patient at no charge.

reimbursement decision tree a tool to help you decide what your next action is when you receive an EOB from a payor.

retrospective payment audit an audit that tracks and evaluates patient financial records for a specific number of completed transactions. It verifies the correctness of payments received from every source and the correctness and appropriateness of the write-offs for each transaction.

Introduction

The reimbursement process follows the lifecycle of the medical insurance claim. It begins when the patient first requests an appointment, and it ends when full payment is received and the paperwork is complete.

The single greatest obstacle to correct reimbursement is fragmentation in the billing process. Fragmentation occurs when medical office employees do not work together as one team. Employee errors can occur repeatedly when employees do not share information and therefore do not learn from past mistakes.

The greatest reimbursement success occurs when employees do work together as one team to oversee the claim cycle from start to finish. In a team environment, a billing problem is everyone's problem. Team meetings allow the sharing of information. The team works together to identify the causes of problems and to devise methods to prevent recurrences. The entire team is responsible for failures and for successes, and everyone shares in the accomplishment of getting the office paid.

Billing and collections directly influence one another. Even in the best team environment, billing and collections should not be separated into different positions. When you receive and post payments for every claim you personally send, you read the information codes on every explanation of benefits (EOB) form that accompanies the payments. You will quickly learn billing preferences for each payor, and you can adjust your internal procedures to match payor-specific requirements. Important trends are often missed when different people perform these functions and they do not share information.

Even in large practices, the billing department can be structured so every billing employee performs both the billing and collections functions for specific claims. In one setup, each employee is assigned to work with smaller teams organized around specific providers. In another setup, each employee is assigned to work with smaller teams organized around specific payors. In yet another setup, each employee is assigned a range of patient last names, using the alphabet to divide patients evenly between the billing employees.

In this chapter you will learn how to verify **patient eligibility,** interpret payment documents, determine what steps to take next in a variety of situations, appeal claims, and follow through and complete the claim cycle for both simple and complex claims.

The Reimbursement Process

The lifecycle of a medical claim was first introduced in Chapter 3 to give you an overview of the claim process and to lay the groundwork for the remainder of the process. A single-payor "clean" claim was used as an example in Figure 3-1 in Chapter 3.

Let's begin our discussion of the reimbursement process in this chapter by taking another look at the lifecycle of the medical claim, but this time we'll expand the discussion to include other payors and to include the additional cycles that occur when a claim is not error free (Figure 13-1).

SCHEDULER

The medical claim cycle begins when the patient requests an appointment. In addition to scheduling the appointment with an authorized provider for the patient's medical plan, the scheduler begins to gather or verify patient-supplied claim information and sometimes information for preauthorization when needed for the appointment. Your work as a scheduler does not end at the conclusion of the telephone call.

In most offices, it is a standard policy to contact each payor and verify that the billing information is correct and the policy or patient eligibility has not expired. This is called verifying patient eligibility. It is done so a clean claim can be sent to the correct payor when the patient incurs billable charges.

Some payors are beginning to offer secure websites and "participating" providers are given free software or passwords that enable employees to verify eligibility and preauthorizations instantly over the Internet. Not every payor offers this capability, and payors that offer it in some regions might not offer it in every region. In addition, there are now sites, such as WebMD, that allow an office to access multiple payors from one site. There may be a monthly membership fee for this service.

When a procedure is scheduled and/or when you work for a specialist, you must ask the payor about preauthorization requirements for the *provider*. Next,

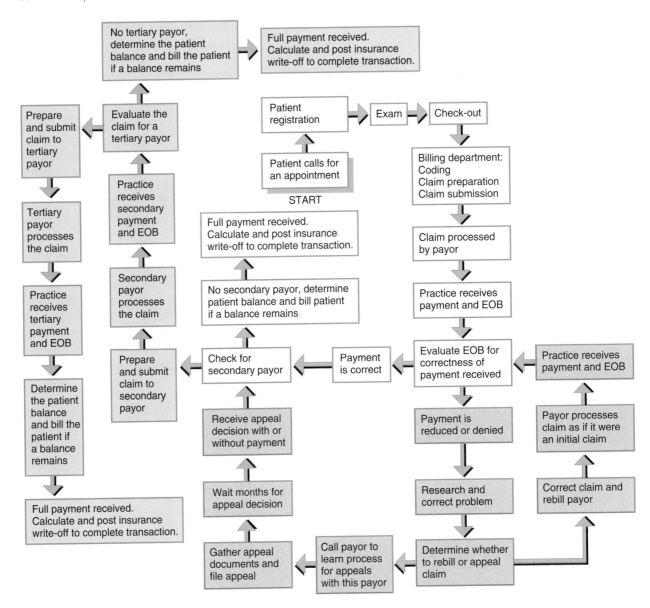

FIGURE 13-1
This expanded lifecycle of the medical claim includes secondary and tertiary payors, and it includes rejected and penalized claims. The single-payor, clean-claim portion of the lifecycle has a white background, the extra twists for additional payors have a colored background, and the extra cycles for claims that are not clean (rejected or penalized claims) have a gray background.

you must determine whether you need to obtain preauthorization for the *procedure* or for the *location* of the service. You could need as many as three different authorizations from *each payor*, and there will be times when you need to call the referring provider to initiate or confirm each authorization. This process often takes a few days, and occasionally it takes a few weeks. Therefore you should begin to verify preauthorizations as soon as possible after the appointment is scheduled. *Every preauthorization must be verified before the patient receives services if you want the resulting claim to be considered for payment.*

When preauthorization is not obtained before performing a service that requires preauthorization, the payor does not have to pay the claim. The payor's computerized edit and audit process is sometimes programmed to automatically deny payment. However, many payors make it a policy to penalize the payment, thereby paying a smaller amount instead of issuing a direct denial.

Obtaining a preauthorization only means the claim will be *considered* for payment; the preauthorization does not *guarantee* payment. The payor will also look at the diagnosis codes billed on the resulting claim for the service to see if they explain why the service was needed. This process is called meeting medical necessity. Payors do not pay for services that are not medically necessary.

RECEPTIONIST

As patients arrive for their appointments, the receptionist gathers patient-supplied billing information for new patients and confirms this information for existing patients. The receptionist checks for the completion of any required preauthorizations. The receptionist obtains patient signatures for release of information and assignment of benefits and makes photocopies of both sides of the insurance card and driver's license for every patient.

When the medical plan is a TRICARE/CHAMPUS program, the receptionist also makes a photocopy of both sides of the military ID card with a "Yes" under "Civilian" to authorize civilian benefits. The military ID must not be expired. In addition, a nonavailability slip is required for inpatient hospital services when the patient lives within 40 miles of a military hospital. A nonavailability slip is issued only if treatment is not available in the military treatment facility near the patient's home or if the patient is away from home. See Chapter 11 for further details about TRICARE/CHAMPUS requirements.

If you cannot obtain a legible photocopy of one or more of the IDs, you must handwrite the information from the insurance card, driver's license, or military ID onto the photocopy in a clear space near the applicable ID.

It is the responsibility of the receptionist to verify patient eligibility and to determine all possible payors. When the information already on file is inadequate to verify eligibility before the appointment, the receptionist must gather additional information during check-in. See Figure 13-2 for a tool you may use to assist in determining eligibility. It is up to office policy whether you ask the questions verbally or whether you ask the patient to complete the form.

Insurance Eligibility Questionnaire

To help our office determine who is responsible for coverage of your medical expenses, please answer each of the following questions and further explain each "yes" response.

1. Is your illness or injury due to:

    A work-related accident or condition? ___Yes ___ No

    A condition covered under the Federal Black Lung Program? ___ Yes ___ No

    An automobile accident? ___ Yes ___ No

    An accident other than an automobile accident? ___ Yes ___ No

    The fault of another party? ___ Yes ___ No

    What were the circumstances of the condition/injury? _____

    _____

    _____

    _____

2. Are you eligible for coverage under the Veterans Administration? ___ Yes ___ No

3. Are you eligible for coverage under the United Mine Workers of America (UMWA)?

    ___ Yes ___ No

4. Are you employed? ___ Yes ___ No

    Do you have coverage under an Employer Group Health Insurance? ___ Yes ___ No

5. Is your spouse employed? ___ Yes ___ No

    Do you have coverage under your spouse's Employer Group Health Insurance?

    ___ Yes ___ No

6. Are you a dependent covered under a parent's/guardian's Employer Group Health

    Insurance? ___ Yes ___ No

7. Do you have any other medical plan coverage, including supplemental plans?

    ___ Yes ___ No

    Please give details _____

    _____

    _____

    _____

FIGURE 13-2
Insurance eligibility questionnaire. (Courtesy Medical Compliance Management, Inc., Orlando, Fla.)

The eligibility questionnaire provides enough information to determine the primary payor. However, as Medicare has complex rules, you may want also to develop a decision chart to help you determine whether Medicare is the primary or the secondary payor in a wide variety of special circumstances. See Figure 13-3 for an example of a Medicare decision chart. As Medicare requirements change, revise your chart to illustrate the new requirements.

Most payor contracts also define coverage restrictions for various situations. For example, many payors do not cover care for service-connected disabilities that are covered by the VA, and they do not cover care for work-related injuries that are covered by workers' compensation. Therefore you might want to create a similar decision chart to relate information from your payor contracts for each of your major payors. This tool can be used together with the managed-care chart introduced in Chapter 3 (see Figure 3-15) to meet payor-specific billing and collection requirements for each patient.

As a receptionist, you are responsible for entering new information into the computer correctly and,

Medicare Decision Chart for Primary/Secondary Payor

Patient Situation or Program Combination		Medicare Primary	Medicare Secondary	No Coverage
Medicare eligible with:	No other insurance	Yes		
	Medigap coverage	Yes		
	Medicaid coverage	Yes		
	Employer group health plan (EGHP)* coverage		Yes	
End stage renal disease in the 30 month coordination period†			Yes	
Disability:	Not working or unemployed	Yes		
	Employed with large group health plan (LGHP)‡ coverage		Yes	
Condition or injury due to accident where there is:	No fault coverage (auto)		Yes	
	Liability coverage (home, commercial, malpractice, auto)		Yes	
	Workers' compensation (If a claim or a portion of a claim is denied by workers' comp, a claim can be filed with Medicare as primary.)	Special circumstances		Usually
Veterans Administration (VA) Benefits— no coverage for injuries or conditions covered by the VA				Always
Medicare is not secondary to the Black Lung program. However, if a Medicare eligible patient has a condition not related to Black Lung, a claim can be filed with Medicare as primary.		Special circumstances		Usually
United Mine Workers of America (UMWA) – services covered by UMWA are never covered by Medicare.				Always

* An employer group health plan (EGHP) is a health insurance plan sponsored by either a patient's or the spouse of a patient's employer when: a single employer of 20 or more employees is the sponsor and/or contributor to the EGHP, or two or more employers are sponsors or contributors and at least one of them has 20 or more employees.

† The entitlement of Medicare benefits for an ESRD patient begins with a 30-month coordination period. During that period, Medicare is the secondary payor to the patient's private insurance or private funds. Medicare remains the secondary payor during that entire 30-month period even if the beneficiary becomes eligible for Medicare coverage due to age or disability status.

‡ A large group health plan (LGHP) is a health insurance plan that is formed by or contributed to by an employer or an employer organization having 100 or more employees, or a plan having at least one member with at least 100 employees.

FIGURE 13-3
A Medicare decision chart is used to determine whether Medicare is the primary or secondary payor in a wide variety of special circumstances. As Medicare requirements change, revise the chart to illustrate the new requirements. (Courtesy Medical Compliance Management, Inc., Orlando, Fla.)

when necessary, correcting inaccurate information. You must double-check all patient identifiers, including birthdays. You also must double-check the preauthorization requirements. If an authorization was denied or if you have any reason to suspect the payor might not cover the service, you should disclose this to the patient and get a written statement confirming payment responsibility in the event the payor denies payment. Examples of a variety of Medicare Advance Beneficiary Notices (ABNs) and consent forms are found in Chapter 3, Figure 3-6 through Figure 3-9. You may use these examples to create similar forms for use with other payors.

PROVIDER

During the appointment, in addition to providing medical care, the authorized physician is responsible for (1) documenting the details of the encounter in the patient's medical record in a manner that meets legal requirements (see Chapter 6) and (2) approving the charges and instructions listed on the superbill for the billing department.

CLINICAL SUPPORT PERSONNEL

At the end of the appointment, clinical support personnel review the physician's instructions with the patient, and they review the billing instructions. They compare the medical record documentation to the charges to be sure nothing was overlooked and to verify that documentation meets legal requirements for the items listed on the superbill. See Chapter 6 for documentation requirements with evaluation and management services.

When documentation does not match the superbill, the clinical support personnel may discuss it with the physician immediately, so a correction can be made while the physician still remembers all the relevant details. Sometimes the medical record documentation will be revised, and other times the superbill will be corrected.

CHECKOUT PERSONNEL

The checkout personnel schedule a follow-up appointment, if needed, and verify that the patient's financial responsibility for the appointment has been met or appropriate payment arrangements have been made. When finished, the patient leaves the office.

In many offices, checkout is an additional duty of the receptionist.

BILLERS AND CODERS

Next, the billing department is given the superbill. Billing and coding personnel once again verify both the patient-supplied billing information and the provider-supplied billing information as they code the services and prepare the claim. See Chapter 4 for detailed claim preparation instructions.

The primary payor is the insurance company to be billed first when more than one insurance company can be billed, and the secondary payor is the insurance company that is billed for any remaining unpaid bills after the primary payor has sent payment. When a third payor exists, the payor that is billed third is called the tertiary payor. The tertiary payor pays any remaining unpaid bills after the secondary payor has sent payment. The biller is usually held accountable for making the final determination about which payor is primary. Failure to identify the correct primary payor is considered a violation of most provider contracts or agreements and is usually considered a breach of trust.

Each employee in the reimbursement chain is part of the reimbursement team and must perform his or her job correctly. The quality and accuracy of billing information and clinical documentation, as it flows through each department and is entered on the claim form, has the single greatest impact on the profit margin for the claim.

When complete, the medical claim is submitted to the payor either electronically or by mail. Payment is received a little faster with electronic submission of claims, usually in about 10 days, and electronic submission eliminates the potential for data entry errors when the claim reaches the payor. Paper claims that meet optical character recognition requirements and can be scanned into the payor's computer are usually processed and paid in about a 3-week cycle. Paper claims that cannot be scanned are usually processed and paid in about an 8-week cycle.

The patient is not billed unless a "patient responsibility" balance remains after all identified payors have sent the correct reimbursement for the claim.

CLEARINGHOUSE

When an electronic medical claim is sent through a clearinghouse, the clearinghouse puts the claim through a series of edits before sending the claim to the payor. There is usually a per-claim charge each time a claim is sent to a clearinghouse. If the claim has errors and is rejected by the clearinghouse, it is sent back to the medical practice. An opportunity exists for the medical practice to correct the claim *before* it reaches the payor.

PAYOR

Once the claim reaches the payor, a record of the transaction is established by the payor, and the stage is set for the remainder of the claim cycle. When an initial claim reaches the payor, it is automatically subjected to a series of claim edits and claim audits established by the medical plan. Claim edits verify the completeness and accuracy of information entered on the claim form. Claim audits check for duplication of services or billing that is in excess of normal.

"Excess of normal" means the payor compared the nature of the presenting illness and the linked diagnosis to each service provided and found a higher level of visits than normal, more visits than normal, or a more complex procedure than normal.

If the claim is clean and passes the payor edits for obvious mistakes, then the payor audit process begins. For physician and outpatient claims, the physician's diagnoses are linked to the procedures billed, and this information is used to determine whether medical necessity was met so the payor can authorize payment. For inpatient hospital claims, the principal diagnosis and DRG group billed are compared to the services provided to determine whether medical necessity was met so the payor can authorize payment. Sometimes the payor requests a copy of the medical record documentation for the visit. Then the nature of the presenting illness and the physician's findings may also be considered. If the claim is still clean and it passes all the payor audits as well, a payment amount is determined and payment is sent to the physician, either electronically or by mail.

If the claim is "dirty" and does *not* pass all of the payor edits and audits, one of the following events is likely to occur: (1) the claim is either rejected or denied and no payment is sent, or (2) the claim is processed and penalties are applied, reducing the amount of payment that is sent.

COLLECTIONS: POSTING PAYMENTS AND ADJUSTMENTS

An EOB is sent either electronically or by mail to the physician for every claim received by the payor. When payment is authorized, the payment is either deposited electronically into the physician's bank account or it is enclosed with the EOB. The remarks on the EOB and the amount paid are the first indications of whether follow-up procedures are required for the claim.

When the full payment amount due from the payor is received and verified, a collections employee posts the payment. If secondary insurance is responsible for an additional amount or if the patient has an outstanding balance for his or her portion, the account for this transaction (claim) remains open. When no further payment is expected, the account is closed, and a record of the transaction remains on file for the time specified in the payor contract or the time specified in state or federal laws, whichever is *longer.* The longest period is usually 7 years, so most practices choose to keep all their records, both medical records and financial records, for at least 7 years.

> Some organizations are lobbying to have the laws changed so patient medical records and patient financial records, including insurance records, are kept for the life of the patient or 7 years, whichever is longer.

When no payment is received or when only partial payment is received, a collections employee posts the payment (if any), but the account for the transaction remains open for further action. In most cases, the next action is to correct the claim information and either rebill the claim or file an appeal.

Note: When the primary payor did not send payment because the service is not covered by the plan, a secondary payor may be billed or the patient may be billed for any remaining "patient responsibility" amount.

REBILLING

Payment is not sent with rejected claims and "unprocessable" claims. Usually these claims do not provide enough correct information to pass the payor edits, and the payor will not even consider the claim for payment. These claims may be corrected and rebilled within periods established by the payor contract. The time period for a payor to receive a clean claim may be as short as 30 days or as long as 2 years from the date of service. Most payors allow rebilled claims to be submitted either electronically or on paper. Since October 16, 2003, Medicare has required claims to be sent electronically.

PENALTIES AND APPEALS

Payor contracts usually allow the payor to reduce the payment owed for dirty claims. These are claims that provide enough correct information to process the claim, but the claims do not pass all the edits and audits, so the claims are not clean. This reduction in payment is called a penalty. Partial payment is usually sent with penalized claims, although occasionally a penalized claim receives zero payment, and once in a while, the provider owes money due to the penalty.

Penalized claims cannot be rebilled; they must be appealed. Appeals also must occur within the period established by the payor contract. The time period may be as short as 60 days from the date of the EOB or it may be as long as 2 years from the date of the EOB. Appeals obtain better results when they are submitted by mail with supporting documentation.

Rebilling claims and filing appeals are discussed in more detail later in this chapter.

CORRECTED CLAIMS

Whether filing an appeal or resubmitting a rejected claim, corrected claims always have *at least one change* somewhere on the claim form. Sometimes the change is accompanied by a stamped message: "resubmission" or "corrected claim." When a claim is resubmitted with *no* changes, it is called a duplicate claim. Payors interpret duplicate claims as a fraudulent attempt to collect twice on the same claim. Payment is not sent for duplicate claims.

When a corrected claim is received by a payor, whether rebilled or appealed, the claim is immediately flagged for closer scrutiny. Even if the claim is now clean and can pass the payor's standard claim edits and claim audits, claim adjusters are not authorized to make payment decisions on repeat claims, and the claim is sent to a review department.

CLAIM REVIEW

Most payor contracts have many loopholes (legal or not) that state the payor may deny or reduce payment for a wide variety of reasons. A claim review employee closely scrutinizes the claim, and every box on the claim form represents a potential reason to deny or reduce payment. Payor contract provisions often give the payor complete control and authority over claim review.

Claim review is normally performed by hand—it is not automated or computerized—and repeat claims are not subject to the payment time limits that apply to initial claims. The review process and payment decision for a repeat claim can take anywhere from 6 weeks to 6 months. Most of that time the claim just sits in a "claim review" inbox, also called a pending or suspense file, waiting to be processed. Contested claims often must go through this process at least twice before other alternatives, such as arbitration, are available.

BILLING SECONDARY AND TERTIARY PAYORS

Once every effort has been made to collect payment from the primary payor, and no further payment is expected, the secondary payor, if applicable, is billed. A copy of the EOB or MRN received from the primary payor must accompany secondary claims. Medicare sometimes, but not always, automatically forwards information to Medigap payors that are registered in the Medicare system. See Chapter 10 for further details about Medicare and Medigap.

Once every effort has been made to collect payment from the secondary payor, and no further payment is expected, the tertiary payor, if applicable, is billed. A copy of the EOB or MRN received from both the primary and secondary payors must accompany tertiary claims.

BILLING PATIENTS, POSTING WRITE-OFFS, AND CLOSING TRANSACTIONS

After all insurance payments are received, collections employees check to see whether the patient is responsible for any of the remaining balance. Secondary and tertiary insurance payments reduce the patient responsibility amount before they reduce any physician write-off amounts from the primary payor.

More than 80% of all medical care is now subject to managed care rules and contract provisions. Most managed care contracts do not allow a provider to bill patients for anything except a deductible or copayment amount, and many payor contracts specifically stipulate that penalty amounts are not a patient responsibility. In addition, services that are deemed as "noncovered" services usually may be billed to the patient only if the patient signed a specific "Noncovered Service Payment Agreement" (or Advance Beneficiary Notice, ABN) *before* the service was rendered. See Figure 3-6 in Chapter 3 for an example of a Medicare noncovered service ABN.

When all expected payments from all sources, including the patient, have been received, remaining balances are typically written off, and the account for the transaction (claim) is closed. These write-offs also are called claim adjustments, and they are discussed in more detail later in this chapter. A record of the transaction remains on file for the time specified in the payor contract or the time specified in state or federal laws, whichever is longer.

Explanation of Benefits

While completing and submitting clean claims is very, very important, it is only the first segment of the reimbursement process. The next segment begins when a response is received from the primary payor.

Payors respond in writing to every claim sent. A document commonly called an EOB accompanies each payment and each denial of payment. The purpose of the EOB is to explain the payor's payment decision. Medicare calls this document a Medicare remittance notice (MRN), although some billers call it Medicare's remittance advice (RA).

The explanation of Medicare benefits (EOMB) is the old name for the patient statement sent to Medicare beneficiaries. The new name for Medicare's patient statement is the Medicare summary notice (MSN).

Most payors send a separate EOB for each claim. Medicare batches the claims for each practice ID number and sends one check with a multipatient, often multipage MRN. Dividing lines separate each patient, and the payment considerations for each patient are broken down individually for each line item procedure. Medicare sometimes separates line items from a single claim into separate payment batches when some of the items are approved immediately and other items are sent to review. The MRN then identifies each item billed on the claim, and remarks codes are used to tell you which items have been sent to review. Even though Medicare's MRN represents a batch of patients, it still supplies the same information for each patient and each procedure as the individual EOBs sent by other payors.

HOW TO EVALUATE AN EOB

When you receive an EOB or MRN, read every item pertaining to each transaction, including each explanatory note. Often footnotes or symbols are placed next to specific items on the EOB. The footnotes or symbols indicate that you should look for **explanatory notes** for additional information pertaining to that item. The footnotes and symbols are used to tie together the items in the EOB with the applicable explanatory notes that are usually located at the bottom of the page. Medicare's explanatory notes are placed on the last page, after the last reported transaction.

Most footnotes are error codes or claim **adjustment codes,** but some convey other types of information. Error codes are sometimes very vague. "Incomplete data" or "missing data" can occur in any

part of the claim form. Often when information changes in one block on the CMS-1500 claim form, it influences information in other blocks. Because the payor does not know the missing information, the payor cannot tell you in precise detail how to correct the claim. The vague phrases are intended to guide you into re-evaluating the entire claim.

You are expected to know whether a correction in one block influences information in other blocks, and you are expected to make every adjustment related to the first correction before evaluating the rest of the claim for accuracy.

Sometimes error codes are cleverly worded. "Payment is in the amount agreed to in the contract" rarely means that payment is in the amount published in the payor fee schedule. Usually this phrase means the physician agreed to accept decisions made by the payor's utilization review (UR) or quality assurance (QA) personnel, and the UR or QA personnel applied a penalty to the claim, reducing the amount of payment. Payor research has shown that few payment decisions are challenged when payments that have been reduced by penalties or by downcoded levels of services are explained in this manner. The statement is not false, but it can be misleading.

Adjustment codes are used by payors to explain why a claim's line item is paid differently than it was billed. Many payors use these codes for internal purposes and report vague phrases on the EOB. Individual payors may assign different numbers or symbols to these codes, and the wording may vary from payor to payor.

Table 13-1 shows a small sampling of the Health Care Claim Adjustment Reason Codes. The full list has more than 180 codes. A government committee with multi-payor representation maintains this list for the Secretary of the Department of Health and Human Services to meet the code set requirements of the Health Insurance Portability and Accountability Act of 1996 (HIPAA). The full list of codes can be found at www.wpc-edi.com under "HIPAA, Code Lists."

Figure 13-4 is an example of a generic EOB. Although each payor reports the information in a slightly different manner, the basic elements of an EOB are similar.

A patient identifier is present on every EOB. Most often, the patient name is used, but a few payors use the patient account number from block No. 26 on the CMS-1500 claim form, and some use the patient-specific insured's ID number from block No. 1a of the claim form.

TABLE 13-1
Health Care Claim Adjustment Reason Codes

Item	Description
1	Deductible amount.
2	Coinsurance amount.
3	Co-payment amount.
4	The procedure code is inconsistent with the modifier used or a required modifier is missing.
5	The procedure code/bill type is inconsistent with the place of service.
6	The procedure code is inconsistent with the patient's age.
7	The procedure code is inconsistent with the patient's gender.
11	The diagnosis is inconsistent with the procedure.
13	The date of death precedes the date of service.
14	The date of birth follows the date of service.
15	Claim/service denied because the authorization number is missing, invalid, or does not apply to the billed service.
16	Claim/service lacks information which is needed for adjudication.
17	Claim/service denied because requested information was not provided or was insufficient/incomplete.
18	Duplicate claim/service.
19	Claim denied because this is a work-related injury/illness and thus the liability of a workers' compensation carrier.
20	Claim denied because this illness/injury is covered by the liability carrier.
21	Claim denied because this illness/injury is covered by the no-fault carrier.
29	The time limit for filing has expired.
31	Claim denied as patient cannot be identified as our insured.
45	Charges exceed your contracted/legislated fee amount.
46	This (these) service(s) is (are) not covered.
47	This (these) diagnosis(es) is (are) not covered.
48	This (these) procedures(s) is (are) not covered.
49	These are noncovered services because this is a routine exam or screening procedure done in conjunction with a routine exam.
50	These are noncovered services because this is not deemed a "medical necessity" by the payor.
57	Claim/service denied/reduced because the payor deems the information submitted does not support this level of service, this many services, this length of service, or this dosage.
110	Billing date predates the date of service.
138	Claim service denied. Appeal procedures not followed or time limits not met.
A2	Contractual adjustment.
B2	Noncovered visits.
B4	Late filing penalty.
B5	Claim/service denied/reduced because coverage/program guidelines were not met or were exceeded.
B12	Services not documented in patient's medical records.

Source: U.S. Department of Health and Human Services.

EOB

Name	Date Svc	Proc	Mod	Charge	Allowed	Co-ins	Ded	CO	Payment
Busey, Carl	10072000	99214		180.00	150.00	30.00	40.00	30.00	80.00

Patient Responsibility: $70.00   CO Contractual obligation. Do not bill patient for this amount.

FIGURE 13-4

A generic explanation of benefits (EOB). Although each payor reports the information in a slightly different manner, the basic elements of any EOB are similar.

The date of service from block No. 24A and the procedure code from block No. 24D are usually used together to identify each exact transaction reported on the EOB. A few payors use only the date of service.

Many payors tell you both the amount you charged for the visit and the payor-specific "allowed" amount for the claim. However, a few payors only include the allowed amount and expect you to have a record of the original charge.

Most payors provide a breakdown of the charges you may bill to the patient. This breakdown includes, but is not limited to, deductibles, copayments, coinsurance, noncovered items, and the total amount you may bill the patient. This total is provided for record-keeping purposes. It is not a mandate to send a bill to the patient. Many times a secondary payor is responsible for at least a portion of the "patient responsibility" amount from the primary payor.

The EOB also specifies the dollar amount of the contractual write-off. You may not bill the patient for an insurance discount agreed to in a payor-physician contract. However, do not be misled into believing a penalty is a contractual discount. Check the payor fee schedule and your summary of contract billing requirements to see what the allowed amount and the contractual discount for each transaction should be according to the actual contract.

If the allowed amount on the claim is less than the amount agreed to in the contract, a penalty has probably been applied to the claim. Penalties are most often applied when something on the claim

was incorrect or when the service did not meet medical necessity requirements. When you find an error, you may correct it and appeal the decision. If the diagnosis codes billed did not accurately portray the encounter, you may appeal the claim and send supporting documentation that shows the actual diagnoses and complexity of decision-making.

Finally, the amount of payment is listed on every EOB. The payment represents the payor's share of the allowed amount. The payor payment plus the "patient responsibility" total should equal the allowed amount for that payor.

Many times footnotes, codes, and symbols are present in many locations on the EOB. The legend for the footnotes, codes, and symbols is listed at the bottom of the EOB in a section commonly called "explanatory notes." The explanatory notes convey the calculation considerations and/or other relevant information for each referenced item.

Sometimes footnotes or symbols convey other important information. Medicare often uses line level and claim level remark codes. Table 13-2 is a select

TABLE 13-2
Medicare Remark Codes

Item	Description
M1	X-ray not taken within the past 12 months or near enough to the start of treatment.
M2	Not paid separately when the patient is an inpatient.
M12	Diagnostic tests performed by a physician must indicate whether purchased services are included on the claim.
M13	No more than one initial office visit may be covered per specialty per medical group. Visit may be rebilled with an established visit code.
M14	No separate payment for an injection administered during an office visit, and no payment for a full office visit if the patient only received an injection.
M15	Separately billed services/tests have been bundled as they are considered components of the same procedure. Separate payment is not allowed.
M24	Claim must indicate the number of doses per vial.
M25	Payment has been (denied for the/made only for a less extensive) service because the information furnished does not substantiate the need for the (more extensive) service. If you believe the service should have been covered as billed, or if you did not know and could not reasonably have been expected to know that we would not pay for this (more extensive) service, or if you notified the patient in writing in advance that we would not pay for this (more extensive) service and he/she agrees in writing to pay, ask us to review your claim within six months of receiving this notice. If you do not request review, we will, upon application from the patient, reimburse him/her for the amount you have collected from him/her (for the/in excess of any deductible and coinsurance amounts applicable to the less extensive) service. We will recover the reimbursement from you as an overpayment.
M29	Claim lacks the operative report.
M30	Claim lacks the pathology report.
M31	Claim lacks the radiology report.
M33	Claim lacks the UPIN of the ordering/referring or performing physician or practitioner, or the UPIN is invalid. (Substitute NPI for UPIN when effective.)
M37	Service not covered when patient is under the age of 35.
M39	The patient is not liable for payment for this service as the advance notice of noncoverage you provided the patient did not comply with program requirements.
M41	We do not pay for this as the patient has no legal obligation to pay for this.
M52	Incomplete/invalid "from" date(s) of servive.
M58	Please resubmit the claim with the missing/correct information so that it may be processed.
M62	Incomplete/invalid treatment authorization code.
M68	Incomplete/invalid attending or referring physician identification.
M81	Patient's diagnosis code(s) is truncated, incorrect, or missing; you are required to code to the highest level of specificity.

TABLE 13-2
Medicare Remark Codes—cont'd

Item	Description
MA01	Initial Part B determination, carrier or intermediary:
	If you do not agree with what we approved for these services, you may appeal our decision. To make sure that we are fair to you, we require another individual that did not process your initial claim to conduct the review. However, in order to be eligible for review, you must write to us within 6 months of the date of this notice, unless you have a good reason for being late. (Carrier or intermediary may add additional remarks.)
MA03	Hearing:
	If you do not agree with the approved amounts and $100.00 or more is in dispute (less deductible and coinsurance), you may ask for a hearing. You must request a hearing within 6 months of the date of this notice. To meet the $100.00, you may combine amounts on other claims that have been reviewed/reconsidered. This includes open reviews if you received a revised decision. You must appeal the claim on time. At the hearing, you may present any new evidence that may affect our decision.
MA04	Secondary payment cannot be considered without the identity of or payment information from the primary payor. The information was either not reported or was illegible.
MA07	The claim information has also been forwarded to Medicaid for review.
MA13	You may be subject to penalties if you bill the patient for amounts not reported with the PR (patient responsibility) group code.
MA15	Your claim has been separated to expedite handling. You will receive a separate notice for other services reported.
MA29	Incomplete/invalid provider name, city, state, and zip code.
MA36	Incomplete/invalid patient's name.
MA38	Incomplete/invalid patient's birthdate.
MA39	Incomplete/invalid patient's sex.
MA44	No appeal rights on this claim. Every adjudicative decision based on law.
MA48	Incomplete/invalid name and/or address of responsible party or primary payor.
MA58	Incomplete release of information indicator.
MA60	Incomplete/invalid patient's relationship to insured.
MA83	Did not indicate whether we are the primary or secondary payor. Refer to item 11 in the CMS-1500 instructions for assistance.
MA87	Our records indicate that a primary payor exists (other than ourselves); however, you did not complete or enter accurately the correct insured's name.
MA100	Did not complete or enter accurately the date of current illness, injury or pregnancy.
N1	You may appeal this decision in writing within the required time limits following receipt of this notice.
N3	Required/consent form not on file.
N11	Denial reversed because of medical review.
N13	Payment based on professional/technical component modifier(s).
N15	Services for newborn must be billed separately.
N19	Procedure code incidental to primary procedure.
N24	Electronic funds transfer (EFT) banking information incomplete/invalid.

Source: U.S. Department of Health and Human Services, Centers for Medicare and Medicaid Services.

sampling of the Medicare line level and claim level remark codes. The complete list of Medicare line level remark codes has 122 codes, each of which begins with "M," followed by numbers 1 to 122. The complete list of Medicare claim level remark codes has 131 codes, each of which begins with "MA," followed by numbers 1 to 131. Medicare also has 26 generic claim or line level remark codes, each of which begins with "N," followed by the numbers 1 to 26.

The Centers for Medicare and Medicaid Services (CMS) maintains the Medicare remark codes for the secretary of the Department of Health and Human Services to meet the code set requirements of HIPAA. The full list of codes can be found at www.wpc-edi.com under "HIPAA, Code Lists."

The best clues to penalties and other payment reductions are found in the explanatory notes and remarks on the EOB. However, the only way to truly know if your payment was reduced is to compare the EOB to a copy of the original claim *and* to compare the EOB allowed amount to the payor fee schedule.

❑ Was the service or procedure code listed on the EOB for payment the same as the service or procedure code billed?
❑ Does the allowed amount reported on the EOB match the payor fee schedule for that service?

The information present on the EOB is vital in determining your next action.

Answer the following questions:

1. Billing and collections are separate functions and should always be assigned to different people.

_____True   _____False

2. Who bears the greatest responsibility for determining and/or verifying patient eligibility for services paid by the patient's medical plan?
   A. The biller
   B. The receptionist
   C. The scheduler
   D. None of the above

3. A Medicare-eligible patient is seen for a problem covered by the Black Lung program. Do you bill Medicare as a secondary payor for this claim?

_____Yes   _____No

4. A Medicare-eligible patient is seen for a work-related injury that is not covered by workers' compensation. Who is the primary payor for this claim?

_____

5. A 70-year-old patient is covered by United Mine Workers of America. Can you bill Medicare, and if so, is Medicare primary or secondary?

_____

6. Who is responsible for making the final determination about which payor is primary?

_____

7. When do you write off the insurance discount?
   A. Before the first bill is sent
   B. After the primary payor sends payment for the claim
   C. After the secondary payor sends payment for the claim
   D. After all possible payors have sent payment for the claim, and no further payment is due

8. What is the purpose of an EOB?

_____

9. Where can you find the best clues to penalties and other payment reductions?

_____

10. How do you determine whether a payor's payment is reduced?

_____

Collection Actions

A **reimbursement decision tree** may be helpful as you decide what your next action is when you receive an EOB from a payor. The statistics from the EOB in Figure 13-4 are used in the reimbursement decision tree shown in Figure 13-5.

When the allowed amount on an EOB does not match the payor fee schedule for the service, you should investigate and determine whether further action should be taken with the primary payor before considering other options. Most of the time further action is advisable, but occasionally it is not.

When a claim is returned as unprocessable, the claim can usually be corrected and rebilled. However, when the payor processes a claim and payment is either penalized or denied, the payor's decision must be evaluated to determine whether the claim may be rebilled or appealed. Begin by reading the EOB, including every footnote and every remark code.

When a claim is denied because it was submitted to the wrong primary payor, you should reevaluate the patient eligibility information and confirm with

both the patient and the payor(s) who the primary payor really is. Once you correct the primary payor information in your practice management computer system, you may resubmit the claim to the correct primary payor. This is considered a new claim, not a rebilled claim.

When payment is denied because you billed a true noncovered service (as opposed to a service that is normally covered, but is not covered this time due to medical necessity issues), do not take further action with the primary payor. Evaluate the claim to see if it can be billed to a secondary payor and/or a tertiary payor. Many secondary and tertiary payors cover items that are not covered by the primary payor. If you cannot bill another payor, you must determine whether the patient may be billed for the service. Each payor has a specific policy regarding payment for noncovered services, so you must check the EOB and your payor contract to determine whether you may bill the patient. If you cannot find the information, call the payor and ask.

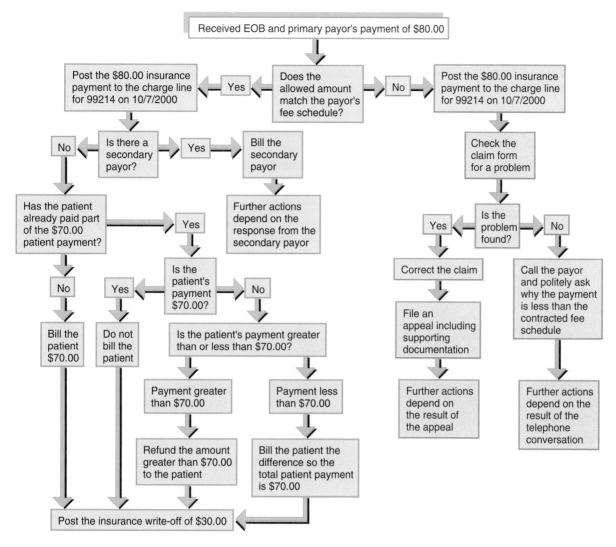

FIGURE 13-5
Reimbursement decision tree. When correct payment was received from the primary payor, the decision tree segments have a colored background. When an incorrect payment was received from the primary payor (usually penalized or rejected claims), the decision tree segments have a gray background.

Medicare requires the patient to sign a "Non-covered Service ABN" (see Figure 3-8 in Chapter 3) specific to the exact service before the noncovered service occurs if the patient is going to be billed for the service. HCPCS modifiers "-GY" and "-GA" must be placed on the claim next to the service to indicate that the service is a noncovered service and a signed ABN (waiver) is on file. If you did not have the Medicare patient sign an ABN before the noncovered service occurred, you cannot bill the patient for the service.

When a partial service was delivered and was reported correctly with a reduced services modifier (-52), a reduced payment is expected from the primary payor. Check to see if the correct percentage of payment is received. If so, proceed to the next step. Evaluate the claim to see if the balance can be billed to a secondary payor and/or a tertiary payor. If there is no additional payor, determine whether the patient may be billed for the remaining balance.

When a claim for a covered service is processed by the correct primary payor, and payment is penalized (reduced or denied) because of a problem or error that you can correct or for a reason that you disagree with, such as "lack of medical necessity," you may usually appeal the payor's decision.

REBILLING

Most payors have specific preferences for receiving corrected claims. You may find it helpful to call each of your major payors and ask what format they prefer. Then make a chart showing each payor's preferences, and post the chart where everyone may easily reference it. Many payors have claim submission time limits that begin with the date of service. You will want to resubmit the claims for the payor with the shortest time limit first.

An unprocessed claim is much easier to work with than a claim that must be appealed. Usually the claim itself is missing vital information. Evaluate the claim and the supporting documentation for missing or inaccurate information. Once you have found the problem and corrected it (or problems and corrected them), you may resubmit the corrected claim.

Duplicate claims are considered to be fraudulent double billing. Medicare considers identical claims and "tracer" claims that are automatically generated by a computer system but do not change the claim in any way to be duplicate claims. Many other payors also use this method of differentiating between duplicate claims and corrected claims. As long as at least one item on the claim form has changed, Medicare's computer system will recognize it as a corrected claim. Therefore when Medicare returns a claim as "unprocessable," you may identify and correct the errors and then simply resubmit the corrected claim.

However, a few payors require you to stamp or print the words "corrected claim" in the top or bottom margin of the claim, or both. Use a color of ink that scans well. Black scans the best. If the optical scanner does not read the information, your claim could still be mistaken for a duplicate claim. If you send electronic claims to this payor, check with the payor to see if placing the words "corrected claim" in block No. 19 on the CMS-1500 claim form is acceptable. If not, you might have to send corrected claims on paper.

APPEALS

Appeals must be filed within the time period detailed in the payor contract. Medicare requires appeals to be filed within 60 days of receipt of the MRN. Occasionally you can negotiate a new time limit for special circumstances, such as when you find a system configuration error that was repeated on every claim and the system has now been reconfigured to print the correct information. However, if the payor has no assurance that the problem is corrected and is unlikely to recur, they are unlikely to extend the time to file an appeal.

Once you determine that you must file an appeal, you should begin by calling the payor's appeals department and asking what they require for appeals. Often the payor will assign a **case number** at this time.

Preparing for an appeal is often very time-consuming. It requires a great deal of attention to detail. Many payors require completion of a payor-specific appeals form. The rendering provider usually must write a letter stating why he or she believes the claim should be paid or why the claim should be paid at a higher rate. You will probably be expected to write the letter for the physician and assemble the supporting documents. The case number must appear on every page of the appeal documents, including each piece of supporting documentation. It is wise also to include the physician's name and daytime telephone number on every page.

You should include a *copy* of the original claim and/or an *original* corrected claim, when applicable, with the letter. You should also send supporting documentation to clearly show the payor why they should take the time and go to the expense of paying employees to reconsider the payment decision. Do not skimp, but only send relevant documents. You do not want to go through the appeal process more than once!

Send a copy of the documentation from the medical record for this service only (not the entire medical record) and a copy of any other items evaluated by the physician during or in conjunction with this service (test results, problem list, medications list, etc.). You may also send copies of articles from medical journals or copies of clinical studies that support the services rendered or that influenced treatment decisions. Sometimes it helps to use a highlighter to make the most relevant sections of a long article stand out. Ask the rendering physician to help identify the best supporting documentation to send with the appeal.

The rendering physician should review every document and approve the entire appeals packet before signing the required letter. The physician's letter should also include a list of the enclosures. Usually the list of enclosures is placed at the bottom of the page directly beneath the physician's signature. Figure 13-6 is an example of a letter requesting an appeal.

The envelope should be addressed exactly as directed by the appeals department. When a payor-specific appeals form is required, this form is the first page in the packet, followed by the letter from the rendering physician. Otherwise, the letter is first. The claim form follows the letter, and the documentation from the medical record follows the claim. Other supporting documentation from the medical record is next, followed by any other patient documents. Copies of articles and clinical studies, when included, are the last items in the packet.

Send the appeal by certified mail with a return receipt requested. This gives you proof the payor

---

Lake Eola Cardiology Practice   517890 South Pioneer Drive, Orlando, FL 32897 • 634-555-4987

Letter of Appeal

January 15, 20XX

BCBS of Florida
PO Box YYYY
Jacksonville, FL

Re: Denial of payment due to lack of medical necessity

Patient: ___Margaret Zimmerman___   Case #: ___20010110MAC47___

Margaret Zimmerman was seen in my office on September 2, 20XX for an echocardiogram. This test was performed due to a significant cardiac history and significant cardiac findings. Please see the enclosed copy of my office notes dated September 1, 20XX, the lab results dated September 1, 20XX, and EKG tracing dated September 1, 20XX. All of these documents support the medical necessity of the echocardiogram for this patient. The information obtained by the echocardiogram was crucial in determining the most effective plan of care for Ms. Zimmerman.

In addition, please see the enclosed medical studies that compare patient outcomes when an echocardiogram is performed versus when an echocardiogram is not performed on patients with a clinical picture similar to Ms. Zimmerman. Clearly patient outcomes are better when the echocardiogram is performed.

I believe the echocardiogram performed on Margaret Zimmerman was medically necessary and I should receive payment for performing this vitally important procedure.

Sincerely,

Clarence Sherman MD

Clarence Sherman, M.D.
(634) 555-4987

Enclosures:
    Original claim
    Echocardiogram report dated 09/02/20XX
    Office notes dated 09/01/20XX
    Labs dated 09/01/20XX
    EKG tracing dated 09/01/20XX
    Clinical studies

FIGURE 13-6
Letter of appeal. (Courtesy Medical Compliance Management, Inc., Orlando, Fla.)

received the appeal packet and a record of the date the payor received it.

Appeals are resolved much more quickly when you follow payor procedures and make the process as simple and as pleasant as possible for everyone. If you do not hear from the payor within 2 or 3 weeks, call the payor's appeals department and politely ask if they have any further questions or if they would like to speak with the physician. Be prepared to give the payor the case number and a few details about the case so they can locate the records quickly.

POSTING PAYMENTS

The best way to track billing results so you know you are billing and receiving the correct payment for every item on every claim is to use a system that allows **line item posting** of payments. See Figure 13-7 for an example of line item posting.

With line item posting, every payment is posted to the exact line item transaction (charge) for which the payment is received. Each payment is subtracted from the remaining balance due for that exact service. You can clearly identify every remaining balance for

Date of Service	Date of Charge/ Payment	Item	Description	$ Amount	Item Balance	Total Balance
10/02/20XX	10/02/20XX	99203	New OV	+ 85.00	+ 85.00	
	10/02/20XX		Pt payment	– 10.00	+ 75.00	
	11/04/20XX		Ins 1 payment	– 45.00	+ 30.00	
	11/10/20XX		Ins 2 payment	– 20.00	+ 10.00	
	11/10/20XX		Ins write-off	– 10.00	0.00	0.00
10/09/20XX	10/09/20XX	99213	OV	+ 75.00	+ 75.00	
	10/09/20XX		Pt payment	– 10.00	+ 65.00	
	11/10/20XX		Ins 1 payment	– 40.00	+ 25.00	+ 25.00
10/17/20XX	10/17/20XX	99213	OV	+ 75.00	+ 75.00	
	10/17/20XX		Pt payment	– 10.00	+ 65.00	+ 65.00
11/07/20XX	11/07/20XX	99213	OV	+ 75.00	+ 75.00	
	11/07/20XX		Pt payment	– 10.00	+ 65.00	
	11/30/20XX		Ins 1 payment	– 30.00	+ 35.00	+ 35.00
11/14/20XX	11/14/20XX	99214	OV	+ 120.00	+ 120.00	
	11/14/20XX		Pt payment	– 10.00	+ 110.00	
	12/18/20XX		Ins 1 payment	– 60.00	+ 50.00	+ 50.00
Total Balance						+ 175.00

Jonathon Quincy—HMO with $10.00 copay is primary/Wife's HMO is secondary

+ = Charges/Amount due; – = Payments/Amount overpaid

FIGURE 13-7
Line item posting. Every payment is posted to the exact line item transaction for which the payment is received.

each service so you can always determine whether another action is required. Line item posting also makes it easier for you to determine how much of a contractual write-off there is for each service. The contractual write-off is calculated and posted after the full payment due is received.

When a patient wants to know the total remaining balance for multiple services, you can add up the remaining amounts for each service to find the total, or you can pull up the screen on your computer system that shows the total due. However, to avoid giving a patient an incorrect balance, it is wise also to use the line item screens to identify which items you expect to receive insurance payments for, and which items are clearly a patient responsibility.

The old-fashioned **ledger cards** were very adequate for posting payments when every payment was a patient responsibility, and the patient submitted the claims to the payor. Then you always knew that every charge and every balance was due from the patient.

The ledger card system works very much like a credit card statement. Charges and payments are recorded as they occur. Each new charge adds to the total to increase the balance owed. Each payment is subtracted from the total to reduce the balance owed. The balance goes up and down as new charges and new payments are recorded. See Figure 13-8 for an example of a ledger card.

Ledger cards do not work well in today's medical office environment, as the patient may only owe a small portion of the total charge, and medical plans

owe some, but not always all, of the remaining balance. When a ledger card is used to record charges and payments, trying to determine who owes what for each service is tedious, time consuming, and subject to human error. It can feel like you are trying to unscramble scrambled eggs.

Because insurance payments are tied to specific charges, but the ledger cards typically list grouped charges, it can be difficult to determine when full payment is received for a specific service. In addition, it is difficult to calculate and track the amounts owed by other payors and amounts owed by the patient. Lastly, it is difficult to calculate the contractual discount you are required to write off. In addition, when a patient has multiple charges, you cannot easily determine if all expected payments have indeed arrived.

Unless secondary payments are processed at the time the primary payment is posted, it is difficult to determine how much to bill the secondary payor. In addition, payments from secondary payors cannot easily be tied to payments from primary payors. Yet, you must determine whether there is a remaining balance for each item so you can determine whether the patient owes a balance and whether there is an **insurance write-off.**

The only way to try to track this level of information using ledger cards is to record a code number for each procedure in the "description" section for each day's charges and for each day's payments. However, this space is often too small to contain all the applicable codes.

Date	Item and description	$ Amount	Balance
10/2/XX	99203 new office visit	+ 85.00	+ 85.00
10/2/XX	Patient payment	− 10.00	+ 75.00
10/9/XX	99213 office visit	+ 75.00	+ 150.00
10/9/XX	Patient payment	− 10.00	+ 140.00
10/17/XX	99213 office visit	+ 75.00	+ 215.00
10/17/XX	Patient payment	− 10.00	+ 205.00
11/4/XX	Insurance 1 payment	− 45.00	+ 160.00
11/7/XX	99213 office visit	+ 75.00	+ 235.00
11/7/XX	Patient payment	− 10.00	+ 225.00
11/10/XX	Insurance 1 payment	− 40.00	+ 185.00
11/10/XX	Insurance 2 payment	− 20.00	+ 165.00
11/14/XX	99214 office visit	+ 120.00	+ 285.00
11/14/XX	Patient payment	− 10.00	+ 275.00
11/30/XX	Insurance 1 payment	− 30.00	+ 245.00
12/18/XX	Insurance 1 payment	− 60.00	+ 185.00

Jonathon Quincy—HMO with $10.00 copay is primary/
Wife's HMO is secondary

+ = Charges/Amount due; − = Payments/Amount overpaid

FIGURE 13-8
Ledger card. All charges and payments are posted in chronologic order.

Therefore if your current system does not allow line item posting of payments, please encourage your physician(s) to get a new system. A computerized system will increase both efficiency and accuracy. You must be able to prove that you have collected the correct payment for every service and that you have written off the correct amount.

When you post a payment, do not automatically write off the amount the EOB calls an "insurance discount" or "contractual obligation." The EOB is correct when it states that you cannot collect this amount from the patient. However, you may collect a portion or even the entire amount of the insurance discount or contractual obligation from a secondary or tertiary payor.

Once the secondary and tertiary payments exceed the patient's portion of the charge, they are applied to the insurance discount or contractual obligation for the transaction. Many collectable charges are lost when write-offs or adjustments are posted too early (before secondary and/or tertiary payors are billed) or when they are posted incorrectly, such as including collectable patient charges in an insurance write-off. Specific types of write-offs are explained in detail later in this chapter.

Clinical Application Exercise

Use Figures 13-7 and 13-8 to complete the following exercises. Answer the questions first using Figure 13-8 and then using Figure 13-7.

Date = date of service

Question	Answer for Figure 13-8	Answer for Figure 13-7
1. Have any service dates been paid in full?	_____	_____
2. Which date(s) have no insurance payment?	_____	_____
3. Which payment is less than expected?	_____	_____
4. Which date(s) received a secondary payment?	_____	_____
5. Are any dates waiting for secondary payment?	_____	_____
6. What is the insurance discount for 10/2?	_____	_____

ELECTRONIC PAYMENT POSTING

Some payors have computer systems that can automatically deposit payments in the physician's bank account and then automatically post the payments in your practice management computer system. You receive an electronic EOB for each transaction. The electronic EOB is often called an **electronic remittance voucher.**

Electronic payment posting increases the accuracy of payment entry, and it reduces the

opportunity for employee error and theft. However, an accurate payment entry does not mean the payor's payment decision is correct.

Although the automatic bank deposit saves significant time, the electronic posting of the payment does not. You still must evaluate the EOB to determine if the electronic payment was correct. If the correct payment was not received, you must still determine whether further action is required with the primary payor, and you must bill any secondary or tertiary payors. You also must determine whether the patient owes a balance. Finally, you must determine the amount of the insurance write-off, if any.

BILLING SECONDARY AND TERTIARY PAYORS

Not every patient has more than one medical plan. When a patient has additional payors, the CMS-1500 claim form filed to the primary payor has "P" printed in the top left margin under "Please do not staple in this area" and above the three small PICA boxes.

Once the primary payor's full payment is received and posted, the next step is to see if there is a secondary payor for the claim. A secondary payor is the medical plan that is second in the line of legal responsibility for paying the claim when there is more than one medical plan.

When secondary payor information is completed correctly on a claim sent to Medicare, Medicare automatically forwards the claim to Medigap payors and Medicare supplement payors that are registered with Medicare. A remark on the MRN will tell you whether Medicare forwarded the claim or whether you must send the claim yourself. Do not become complacent and assume every Medigap and supplemental claim is forwarded. Always check each transaction as you post the primary payment. You will find that occasionally a claim is not forwarded, even though claims for the same patient have been forwarded in the past.

Secondary claims are not identical to primary claims. The primary and secondary payor information is switched on the CMS-1500 claim form, so the secondary payor information is printed in the top margin and in blocks 1, 1a, 4, 6, 7, 11, 11a, 11b, 11c, and 11d. The primary payor information is printed in blocks 9, 9a, 9b, 9c, and 9d. In addition, "S" is printed in the top left margin under "Please do not staple in this area" and above the three small PICA boxes. A copy of the EOB from the primary payor must be sent with secondary claims, so secondary claims are usually submitted on paper.

Most practice management systems have an option you may select to automatically print secondary claims, and the software system makes the necessary changes. Some computer systems require you to enter specific information, such as the original date of service and the date the primary payment is posted. Check with your software manufacturer if you encounter any difficulties in printing secondary claims.

Once the primary payor's and the secondary payor's full payments are received and posted, the next step is to look for a tertiary payor for the claim. A tertiary payor is the medical plan that is third in the line of legal responsibility for paying the claim when

there are more than two medical plans. Only a few patients have three medical plans.

Tertiary claims are not identical to either primary or secondary claims. The tertiary payor information is printed on the CMS-1500 claim form in the top margin and in blocks 1, 1a, 4, 6, 7, 11, 11a, 11b, 11c, and 11d. The secondary payor information is placed in blocks 9, 9a, 9b, 9c, and 9d. In addition, "T" is printed in the top left margin under "Please do not staple in this area" and above the three small PICA boxes. A copy of the EOBs from both the primary payor and the secondary payor must accompany the claim.

Most practice management systems have an option you may select to print tertiary claims automatically, and the software system makes the necessary changes. Some computer systems require you to enter specific information, such as the original date of service and the date the secondary payment is posted. Check with your software representative if you encounter any difficulties in printing tertiary claims.

CALCULATING PATIENT BALANCE

When calculating the patient balance for a claim, you begin by determining how much of the total charge the patient is responsible for according to the primary payor's EOB or contract. Either the patient or another payor must pay this fee, but once this amount is received from a source other than the primary payor, the patient cannot usually be charged an additional amount for this claim. Figure 13-9 illustrates calculating the patient balance when there are one payor, two payors, and three payors.

Secondary and tertiary payors are not limited by the primary payor rules. Often they pay all the patient's portion and at least part of the primary payor's discount. Once the secondary payment, alone or combined with the tertiary payment, exceeds the patient's portion of the charge, the patient does not owe anything. If the patient has already made a payment for this service, refund it to the patient.

When the secondary payment, alone or combined with a tertiary payment, does not exceed the patient's portion of the charge as listed on the primary payor's EOB, subtract the secondary (and tertiary) payment from the patient's portion of the charge as listed on the primary payor's EOB, and the difference is the *"actual patient responsibility"* amount for this claim.

If the patient has already made a payment, you must determine whether the payment was more than the "actual patient responsibility" amount. If it was, refund the overage to the patient. To find the overage, subtract the "actual patient responsibility"

Mr. Busey paid a $10.00 copay on October 7, 20XX.

Primary Payor EOB (For examples 1, 2, and 3)

Name	Date Svc	Proc	Mod	Charge	Allowed	Co-ins	Ded	CO	Payment
Busey, Carl	100720XX	99214		180.00	150.00	30.00	40.00	30.00	80.00

Patient Responsibility: $70.00   CO Contractual obligation. Do not bill patient for this amount.

Secondary Payor EOB (For examples 1 and 2)

Name	Date Svc	Proc	Mod	Charge	Allowed	Primary	Patient	Payment
Busey, Carl	100720XX	99214		180.00	150.00	80.00	$10.00	60.00

Patient Responsibility: $10.00

Tertiary Payor EOB (For example 1)

Name	Date Svc	Proc	Mod	Charge	Allowed	Primary	Secondary	Payment
Busey, Carl	100720XX	99214		180.00	170.00	80.00	60.00	30.00

Patient Responsibility: $0.00

Example 1:

Calculating the patient balance when Mr. Busey has three payors

Step one: Determine Mr. Busey's responsibility for the primary payor.	$70.00
Step two: Add together any secondary and tertiary payments.	$60.00 + $30.00 = $90.00
Step three: Are the secondary and tertiary payments combined greater than $70.00?	Yes
Actual patient responsibility amount	*$0.00*
Step four: Has Mr. Busey already made a payment?	Yes, $10.00
Step five: Refund Mr. Busey the amount of his payment.	Refund $10.00

Example 2:

Calculating the patient balance when Mr. Busey has two payors

Step one: Determine Mr. Busey's responsibility for the primary payor.	$70.00
Step two: What is the amount of the secondary payment?	$60.00
Step three: Is the secondary payment greater than $70.00?	No
Step four: Subtract the secondary payment from $70.00.	$70.00 − $60.00 = $10.00
Actual patient responsibility amount	*$10.00*
Step five: Has Mr. Busey already made a payment?	Yes, $10.00
Step six: Subtract the payment from the $10.00 patient balance.	$10.00 − $10.00 = $0.00
Step seven: Mr. Busey has met his responsibility.	Do not send a bill.

Example 3:

Calculating the patient balance when Mr. Busey has one payor

Step one: Determine Mr. Busey's responsibility for the primary payor.	$70.00
Actual patient responsibility amount	*$70.00*
Step two: Has Mr. Busey already made a payment?	Yes, $10.00
Step three: Subtract the payment from the $70.00 patient balance.	$70.00 − $10.00 = $60.00
Step four: Bill Mr. Busey the remaining patient balance.	Bill $60.00

FIGURE 13-9

Calculating the patient balance when there are one payor, two payors, and three payors. Begin by determining how much of the total charge the patient is responsible for according to the primary payor's EOB or contract. Either the patient or another payor must pay this fee, but once this amount is received from a source other than the primary payor, the patient cannot usually be charged an additional amount for this claim.

amount from the patient payment. The difference is the overage.

If the patient payment did not exceed the "actual patient responsibility," subtract the patient payment from the "actual patient-responsibility" amount. The difference is the balance still owed by the patient. Send the patient a bill commonly called a "patient statement" or a "patient invoice" for this amount. Patient statements normally are sent every 2 weeks or every 4 weeks until payment is received. Some states have laws that limit the frequency of sending patient statements to no more often than every 30 days. However, every state is different. Some states have no specific laws governing collections. To find the laws applicable to your state, you may go to www.lawdog.com and search for collections laws for your state.

These rules for calculating patient payments apply to the vast majority of the medical plans you will encounter, but they do not apply to commercial indemnity plans. *The rules are different for commercial indemnity plans.*

The EOBs for indemnity plans often mirror the EOBs for other plans, but the meanings of terms are different. The allowable charge on an EOB for an indemnity plan is the usual, customary, and reasonable (UCR) charge as determined by the payor. There are no payor/physician contracts with indemnity plans, so there are no insurance discounts or contractual obligations. With indemnity plans, the patient responsibility is the entire amount remaining after payor payment(s).

At one time, the UCR charge or prevailing fee represented an average of the fees charged in the region. Today, the UCR charge or prevailing fee often represents the lowest fee the payor has on record that the physician accepted for the service.

The physician can submit a letter of protest to the payor if the UCR rate is too low, but be prepared to defend your position. By law, you cannot accept a higher allowable fee from Medicare than the lowest total fee you ever accept for the service. Anytime the UCR charge for an indemnity plan is less than Medicare's fee schedule for the service, you really should help the physician protest the fee. Even though the total payment is higher when the patient is billed correctly for the balance, payors know most medical offices follow only one set of rules when calculating the patient payment. They mistakenly bill the patient for only 20% of the allowable instead of the entire balance. This results in a lower total payment than Medicare's fee schedule and places the physician at risk in a Medicare audit. It also lowers the payment floor for future contract negotiations.

Begin by calling the payor and asking politely for the protocol to follow when protesting a fee. Usually the physician must send a letter of protest stating why the fee should be altered. See Figure 13-10 for an example of a letter of protest.

CALCULATING WRITE-OFFS

A write-off is a portion of the charge that cannot be collected or a portion of the charge that the physician has chosen not to collect. The standard charge is always recorded first for every service rendered. A write-off is the mechanism used to reduce a charge for a specific reason, usually a discount given to a specific payor or to a specific person.

While insurance plan discounts are the most common, they are not the only write-offs that occur. There are many types of write-offs. Sometimes physicians give discounts to specific patients, and occasionally physicians choose to see a patient at no charge. Even when the services are provided at no charge, the standard fee is recorded first, and then a write-off is posted to reduce the fee to zero. When the write-offs are recorded in this manner, they can be used to reduce the amount of income tax owed by the medical office.

Most patient statements mirror the way you record charges and payments. When patients cannot understand an item, they will call. Few patients understand the concept of write-offs.

Your phone will ring less often when write-off accounts clearly identify the nature of the entry. Therefore it is wise to name your write-off accounts in a manner that patients can understand and that also tells you the nature of each write-off. As most people do understand discounts, one method is to name each write-off account as a discount for a particular payor.

A write-off is posted as though it were a payment, except the amount is recorded in the adjustment column instead of the payment column. The specific write-off account, such as Medicare Discount, is named as the source of payment instead of a medical plan or a patient.

If your current computer system is not set up to allow multiple types of write-offs, ask your software supplier or technician to reconfigure the software to allow multiple write-offs.

PATIENT WRITE-OFFS

There are a variety of possible patient write-offs. The consumer credit laws require that any offer extended to one patient must also be available to every patient who asks for it. This does *not* mean you are required to offer it to *every* patient. It means you must offer it only to those patients who *ask* for it.

Lake Eola Family Practice   517860 South Pioneer Drive, Orlando, FL 32897 • 634-555-4983

Prevailing Fee Committee
BlueCross BlueShield of Florida
PO Box YYYY
Jacksonville, FL 00314

RE: Protest of Prevailing Fees

Provider #: FL012345678

Dear Committee,

I am writing to protest the prevailing fees you have assigned for services I render to BCBS plan patients. Since January 1, 20XX, I have been in the process of instituting a compliance program, and verifying that I am charging and collecting the correct amount for services I render. As a participating Medicare provider, I cannot accept a fee lower than the current year Medicare allowable fee schedule. It has been brought to my attention that accepting your prevailing fee of $50.00 for a 99214, as occurred on the attached Explanation of Benefits, would put me at risk in a Medicare audit.

My standard fees are always higher than the Medicare allowable fee schedule. The other commercial plans I bill allow an average of 90% or more of my standard fee schedule. Like BCBS, many other commercial plans pay 80% of the allowable fees, with the remainder due from the patient. My protest is with your prevailing allowable fee, not the method by which the fee is split between BCBS and the patient. Currently my practice mix is 78% commercial payors. My records show I am usually able to collect a minimum of 90% of my standard fee schedule.

Please review my standard fee schedule and the current Medicare participating provider allowable fee schedule, and let me know in writing what adjustments BCBS is willing to make to the "prevailing fees" for my services. Thank you for helping me achieve compliance.

Sincerely,

Aaron Rubin MD

Aaron Rubin, M.D.

Enclosures:
Fee Schedule for Services Rendered by Aaron Rubin, M.D., Lake Eola Family Practice
EOB from BCBS of FL

FIGURE 13-10
Letter of protest. (Courtesy Medical Compliance Management, Inc., Orlando, Fla.)

When a physician sees a patient at no charge, it is usually for one of two reasons. The first is a postoperative follow-up visit where the charges for the visit are bundled in with the charges for the procedure (the surgery). The fees for postoperative follow-up are recorded as zero because payment is received in advance as part of the payment for the surgery. There is no write-off for postoperative follow-up visits.

The second reason, called **professional courtesy,** is when the physician chooses to see a patient at no charge. When a physician gives a professional courtesy discount to a patient, you do not bill a medical plan for the service.

The responsibility for paying the "allowed" amount on a claim is usually shared between the patient and the payor. Most payors consider it fraud when a bill is submitted to the payor to collect the payor's share of the fee, but the patient is not charged the patient's share of the fee. The only exception is in cases of financial hardship, as discussed below. So remember,

to qualify as a professional courtesy discount, the entire visit must be free. The fees for the professional service are recorded in the computer with the usual charge, and the entire balance is then written off as a professional courtesy discount. Do not skip processing professional courtesy transactions just because there is no charge. Write-off accounts are used to reduce the taxable income reported to the IRS (Internal Revenue Service).

Most professional courtesy visits are given to other physicians and their immediate family members. However, professional courtesy may not be given when doing so meets the federal definition of a kickback, a type of illegal payback. Professional courtesy kickbacks are most often given in exchange for referrals. Therefore to avoid the appearance of wrongdoing, you cannot extend professional courtesy when the recipient or a family member of the recipient sends referrals to your office.

When a patient is in financial difficulty and cannot meet his or her financial responsibility, the physician may choose to give the patient a **financial hardship discount.** This means the actual patient responsibility that remains after all payors have paid is written off as a patient financial hardship discount or a patient financial hardship write-off. Financial hardship write-offs are used instead of the patient payment to meet the patient financial responsibility, and they are posted before the insurance discount is calculated and posted.

Most government and managed care programs require a written "Waiver of Payment" notice to be signed and kept on file before patient copayment, coinsurance, or deductible amounts can be written off as a hardship discount. The waivers are required because Medicare and managed care plans require the patient to pay a portion of the fee, and it is illegal to routinely waive patient copays. See Figure 13-11 for an example of a financial hardship waiver. A copy of the signed waiver is sent to each medical plan listed on the form. Medical plans track the number of waivers on file for each provider. An excessive number of waivers will cause the payor to look further. Hardship write-offs should be identified separately from professional courtesy write-offs and separately from other **patient discounts.**

Some physicians choose to give self-pay patients a discount when they pay on time. These write-offs are normally identified as a timely payment discount, a patient discount, or a patient write-off. Medicare rules specifically say it is illegal to accept more from Medicare than the least amount you are willing to accept for the service from *any other source.* Therefore patient discounts must not cause the total fee to fall below the Medicare fee schedule, or the physician could be at risk in a Medicare audit.

Every practice has a specific procedure that must be followed when a patient is given a discount. An owner usually reviews large charges before a write-off is approved. Remember, not all physicians have an ownership interest in a practice. Managers are often, but not always, given the authority to give a patient a discount. Do not ever give a patient a discount unless you have clearly been given the authority to do so.

Bad Debt Write-offs

Occasionally, you will not be able to collect a charge from a patient or from an insurance company. When this happens, the write-off does not represent a discount given freely by the physician, so it should be classified separately.

FIGURE 13-11
Waiver of payment due to financial hardship. (Courtesy Medical Compliance Management, Inc., Orlando, Fla.)

When an insurance company files for bankruptcy and does not pay remaining outstanding claims, if the payment cannot legally be collected from the patient, the loss is recorded as an insurance **bad debt write-off.** Patient bad debt should be classified separately from payor bad debt. Some state laws require a certain amount of time to pass before an account can be deemed uncollectable and written off as bad debt. You may learn the rules for your state at www.lawdog.com.

Many physicians like to list penalties in this category rather than as an insurance write-off, as a penalty is not a discount freely given by the physician. You will want to record penalties without alarming patients should the entry be recorded on a patient statement, so choose the name of this account carefully. "Insurance debt write-off" might be used to satisfy the physician while differentiating the account from the insurance discount and from true bad debt.

Insurance Write-offs

Writing off insurance discounts is the last step to occur in the claim cycle. Many physicians want to track each type of write-off, including each payor write-off. In this case, each insurance discount is named by payor or by type. Others want to lump all of them into one category called "insurance write-off." Common names for insurance write-off accounts include "[name of payor] write-off," "insurance write-off," "contractual discount," "contractual obligation," "managed care write-off," "managed care discount," "Medicare write-off," "Medicaid write-off," and many more.

Although the name of each account may vary, the process of writing off uncollectable balances does not. When all expected payments have been received, post a write-off "payment" to the adjustment column for the remaining balance to "zero out" the balance for that transaction. See Figure 13-7 for an example of how insurance write-offs are posted. In Figure 13-7, only the first transaction has completed the claim cycle and includes the insurance write-off. Once all expected payments for that transaction were received, the remaining balance was written off as an insurance write-off.

PAYMENT POLICIES

Years ago, medical offices did not need a complex financial policy. One statement posted near the check-in window and near the checkout window was sufficient: "Payment is expected at the time service is rendered."

In today's world, physicians bill many medical plans and only collect small amounts directly from patients. An official financial policy that covers numerous situations is needed to protect the physician's right to collect the money he or she has rightfully earned. See Figure 13-12 for an example of an official **financial policy statement.**

When you work in a medical office, no matter what position you fill, part of your job is to help the physician receive payment for services rendered. You are responsible for enforcing the financial policy. Just as you want to be paid for work you perform, physicians want to be paid for work they perform. You are much more likely to be paid well when you do your job well, and the physician is paid the correct amount on time for every service.

Do not offer payment terms to a patient unless you have been given the authority to do so. When you offer payment terms to a patient, you are splitting the patient's balance for a service into several equal installments and allowing the patient to make payments over time instead of paying the balance in full when it is due. Many offices have a policy that says billing managers must get approval from the owner(s) and/or doctors of the practice every time payment terms are offered.

The Fair Credit Opportunity Act says that when offering credit, you cannot discriminate based on age, race, color, national origin, gender, marital status, religious preference, income from public assistance, or a history of exercising rights under consumer credit laws. If you offer payment terms to one patient, you must consider payment terms (without discrimination) for every patient *who asks for* payment terms. Please note, however, that (1) you do not have to offer payment terms to anyone who *does not* specifically ask for them, and (2) when you do offer payment terms, they do not have to be identical from one patient to the next. Most offices have a policy that says you will run a credit check on every patient who asks for payment terms, and you will decline to offer payment terms if the credit score is below a specific rating. This is allowed as long as the same standard for the "allowed" credit score is applied to everyone.

When you deny someone credit, the Fair Credit Reporting Act says you must disclose the reason credit was denied and give the name and address of each credit reporting agency you used in reaching your decision. You do not have to disclose specifics of the individual's credit report.

In addition, the Truth-in-Lending Act, a law enforced by the Federal Trade Commission, applies to (1) anyone who charges interest or (2) anyone who agrees that payment may be split into more than four installments. Regulation Z of the Truth-in-Lending Act applies when a specific agreement is reached between the physician (or an authorized

---

Financial Policy for Lake Eola Family Practice

Basic Policy

If you do not have insurance, or if the care you receive is not a covered service for your medical plan, you must pay in full at the time of your appointment unless the billing manager has approved payment terms in advance.

Medical Plan

If you give us the proper documents, we will file your medical claims for you. If you want us to file your claims, you must give us current information about every medical plan you have, including private plans, employer plans, managed care plans, HMO, PPO, POS plans, state, federal and military programs, and any other type of medical plan you might have. Medical claim requirements vary based on the type of medical plans and the number of medical plans you have. Even if you believe a particular plan will not pay anything for this service, you still must provide us with current information about the plan or we cannot correctly file any medical claims for you.

Copayments and deductibles must be paid at the time of service. We give discounts to medical plans to avoid the additional cost of also processing and sending bills to patients.

You must allow us to make a photocopy of the front and back of each medical plan ID card and your driver's license or state ID card. You must give us your birthdate and the birthdate of the policyholder for each plan. You must give us your Social Security number and the Social Security number of the policyholder for each plan. We only use Social Security numbers for filing your medical claims and collecting payment due. We do not use Social Security numbers for any other purpose.

You must sign a statement allowing us to release your medical records to your medical plan(s), and you must sign an assignment-of-benefits statement for every medical plan allowing the plan(s) to send payment directly to Lake Eola Family Practice.

If one of your medical plans is TRICARE/CHAMPUS or CHAMPVA, you must also allow us to make a photocopy of your current military ID card.

If any of the information you supply is incorrect or if your medical plan has expired, you will be responsible for payment in full.

Noncovered Services

You are responsible for payment in full of items that are deemed noncovered services by your medical plan.

Injury

If your injury is related to an automobile accident, you must supply us with information about your automobile policy and the automobile policy of the person found to be at fault for the accident.

If your injury is work related, you must supply us with the name, address, and phone number of your employer, the name of the workers' compensation carrier, the case number, and the authorization number.

Missed Appointments

In fairness to the physician and other patients that are waiting for appointments, we require at least 24 hours' notice when canceling an appointment. You may be charged for missed appointments. Missed appointments cannot be billed to a medical plan. If you miss appointments frequently or if you do not pay for missed appointments, you may be dismissed from the practice.

I have read, understood, and agree to follow the above financial policy.

Signature of patient or legal guardian_____ Date _____

FIGURE 13-12

Financial policy statement. (Courtesy Medical Compliance Management, Inc., Orlando, Fla.)

representative) and the patient for a payment to be split into more than four installments. To meet the requirements of Regulation Z, you must use a truth-in-lending statement that details: the total balance owed, the amount of each payment, the date each payment is due, the date the final payment is due, the total finance charges (even if the amount is zero), and the interest rate listed as an annual percentage rate (APR).

There are many brands of computer accounting software that include a program that will calculate payments, total interest, and the interest annual percentage rate. The best programs allow you to print it out on an actual truth-in-lending statement form. Both the patient and the physician (or the physician's representative) should sign the "truth-in-lending" agreement, and it is placed in the patient's financial record. Each subsequent bill to the patient should then include the full balance owed and the

"minimum" payment due on the date(s) specified in the agreement. Note, however, that if the patient chooses to pay in installments without a specific agreement from the physician (or office personnel on behalf of the physician), Regulation Z does not apply.

Clinical Application Exercise

Use the information from Figure 13-13 to post payments. Mr. Schwartz has two payors. Record the payments on the worksheet in Figure 13-14. Calculate the actual patient responsibility and perform the next action. Record the insurance write-offs when all other payments due on an account have been received.

On 08/14/20XX, Edgar Schwartz paid a $10.00 co-pay at the time of his visit.
On 08/24/20XX, Edgar Schwartz paid a $10.00 co-pay at the time of his visit.
On 09/07/20XX, the payment and EOB from the primary payor, Aetna, was received:

Name	Date Svc	Proc	Mod	Charge	Allowed	Co-ins	CO	Payment
Schwartz, Edgar	081420XX	99213		120.00	96.00	10.00	24.00	86.00
Patient Responsibility: $10.00			CO Contractual obligation. Do not bill patient for this amount.					

On 09/15/20XX, Edgar Schwartz paid a $10.00 copay at the time of his visit.
On 09/17/20XX, the payment and EOB from the primary payor, Aetna, was received:

Name	Date Svc	Proc	Mod	Charge	Allowed	Co-ins	CO	Payment
Schwartz, Edgar	082420XX	99213		120.00	96.00	10.00	24.00	86.00
Patient Responsibility: $10.00			CO Contractual obligation. Do not bill patient for this amount.					

On 10/02/20XX, the payment and EOB from the secondary payor, Cigna, was received:

Name	Date Svc	Proc	Mod	Charge	Allowed	Primary	Patient	Payment
Schwartz, Edgar	081420XX	99213		120.00	100.00	86.00	$0.00	14.00
Patient Responsibility: $0.00								

On 10/07/20XX, the payment and EOB from the primary payor, Aetna, was received:

Name	Date Svc	Proc	Mod	Charge	Allowed	Co-ins	CO	Payment
Schwartz, Edgar	091520XX	99212		90.00	75.00	10.00	15.00	65.00
Patient Responsibility: $10.00			CO Contractual obligation. Do not bill patient for this amount.					

On 10/12/20XX, the payment and EOB from the secondary payor, Cigna, was received:

Name	Date Svc	Proc	Mod	Charge	Allowed	Primary	Patient	Payment
Schwartz, Edgar	082420XX	99213		120.00	100.00	86.00	$0.00	14.00
Patient Responsibility: $0.00								

On 11/05/20XX, the payment and EOB from the secondary payor, Cigna, was received:

Name	Date Svc	Proc	Mod	Charge	Allowed	Primary	Patient	Payment
Schwartz, Edgar	091520XX	99212		90.00	85.00	65.00	$0.00	20.00
Patient Responsibility: $0.00								

FIGURE 13-13

History of payments received for patient Edgar Schwartz. Record these payments on the worksheet in Figure 13-14.

CPT only © 2005. Current Procedural Terminology, 2006, Professional Edition, American Medical Association. All Rights Reserved.

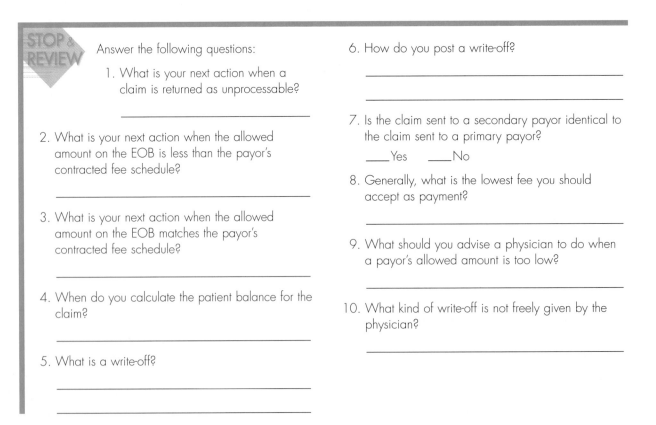

FIGURE 13-14
Posting payment worksheet.
Use this worksheet to record
the payments from
Figure 13-13.

Date of Service	Date of Charge/ Payment	Item(s)	Description	$ Amount	Item Balance	Total Balance
Balance Carried Forward						
Total Balance						

+ = Charges/Amount due; − = Payments/Amount overpaid

STOP & REVIEW

Answer the following questions:

1. What is your next action when a claim is returned as unprocessable?

_____

2. What is your next action when the allowed amount on the EOB is less than the payor's contracted fee schedule?

_____

3. What is your next action when the allowed amount on the EOB matches the payor's contracted fee schedule?

_____

4. When do you calculate the patient balance for the claim?

_____

5. What is a write-off?

_____

_____

6. How do you post a write-off?

_____

_____

7. Is the claim sent to a secondary payor identical to the claim sent to a primary payor?

____Yes   ____No

8. Generally, what is the lowest fee you should accept as payment?

_____

9. What should you advise a physician to do when a payor's allowed amount is too low?

_____

10. What kind of write-off is not freely given by the physician?

_____

Keeping Track of Financial Documentation

Just as each patient has a medical record, each patient should also have a financial record. Consumer credit laws specify that private medical information cannot be stored in a financial record. Therefore the financial record for each patient is a separate chart. It should never be stored in the patient's medical record. The financial record holds the superbills, claim copies, EOBs, and any correspondence sent and received regarding financial transactions for each patient. Ideally, the documents for each claim are clipped together. You should be able to quickly locate every available piece of financial documentation for every transaction.

Medicare remittance notices contain information for many patients in one document. The original is stored in a special file by date received. Before storing it, the entire document is photocopied and then the copy *(not the original)* is cut apart into segments for each individual patient. Make a notation somewhere on each segment where you filed the original copy of the MRN. Each segment is then ready to be filed in the patient financial records. A copy of the entire original MRN is required when filing claims to secondary or tertiary payors, and payment information about other patients is blacked out or obscured on the *copy* sent with the claim. Take care so you do not accidentally obscure information on your original MRN.

Unfortunately, not every medical practice stores financial documents in individual patient financial records. Physicians would not store medical record documentation (chart notes, lab results, etc.) in large multipatient files instead of individual patient records, yet this is exactly how many medical offices choose to store patient financial records. They usually have separate files for EOBs, superbills, and sometimes, but not always, claim copies. Some medical offices store financial records by the day, some by the week, and most by the month. Others just pitch them all in a large box. When it is full, they close the lid for storage and get another. With any of these multipatient methods, it can literally take days to match up the documents for one transaction, and often documents cannot be located even after days of searching.

PAYOR QUALITY CONTROL REQUIREMENTS

Most payor contracts require physicians to cooperate fully with payor quality assurance teams. Producing copies of documents in a timely manner is frequently another contract requirement. If a quality assurance team performs an audit and wants to see copies of EOBs from other payors for coordination of benefits, you must be able to produce the documents in a timely manner.

Quality control teams also regularly request copies of medical record documents. These also must be produced in a timely manner. If you do not respond by the assigned deadline, you often forfeit payment for the claim.

Some payor contracts allow you to bill the payor for the cost of producing copies. Read your contracts closely so you do not miss items such as this.

UPDATING FORMS AND FEE SCHEDULES

If your superbill contains diagnosis and/or procedure codes, it must be updated annually. Most payor's contracts require the physician to use current codebooks. When you bill outdated codes because the superbill lists outdated codes, you risk receiving reduced payments.

Most payors choose to impose penalties rather than deny payment for outdated codes because it is very cost effective for them to do so. If they were to deny payment, you might identify and fix the problem. Then they would have to consider full payment for each subsequent claim. However, when they merely apply a penalty and use a cleverly worded adjustment code to explain the reduced payment, many physician offices accept the reduced payment as payment-in-full for the service. If you make the same mistake repeatedly, the payor can save significant amounts of money. Of course, that also means you fail to collect significant amounts of money the physician has rightfully earned. The time allowed to make corrections is usually short, typically 60 days. After that, the money often becomes uncollectable unless you negotiate a deal with the payor.

Payor fee schedules also must be updated annually or as often as the fee schedule changes. Find out which of your commercial and managed care payors update their fee schedules twice a year. You must compare your payments to a current fee schedule, or you risk not recognizing a reduced payment. Once again, it does not take long for uncollected money to add up to a significant amount, and the time allowed to make corrections is usually short, typically 60 days. After that, the money often becomes uncollectable unless you negotiate a deal with the payor.

If you use reference charts to convey fee schedules or payor contract requirements, these also must be updated whenever a change occurs.

HOW TO USE AGING REPORTS

As you could see when you completed the exercise in posting payments, tracking just three transactions for one patient can be rather complex. You cannot rely on your memory alone to know what items require follow-up for every patient in your practice.

Aging reports are used to report the status of claims to the physician, and they are also used to identify individual transactions that require follow-up. When you use a computerized practice management system, your aging reports can be compiled to report data same data in several ways. When the same report date ranges and aging ranges are used for each type of aging report, the totals for each aging range column will match on the different reports. If they do not match, there is a problem in the way your computer system is reporting data, and you cannot rely on any of the numbers until the problem is identified and corrected.

The data can be reported by payor to identify pending insurance claims with each payor. The physician can tell at a glance which payors process claims in a timely manner. The data can be reported by payor and by patient to identify exactly which patients still have pending claims with each payor.

The data can be reported by patient to identify which patients have claims that require follow-up. The data can be reported by patient and payor to identify if the follow-up is needed with the primary payor, the secondary payor, and/or a tertiary payor.

See Figure 13-15 for examples of aging reports. Note that the totals for each date-range column match on the different reports.

If you submit claims electronically, "<30 days" should have the largest numbers, and each subsequent date range should have smaller numbers than the previous one. If you submit claims on paper, the "30-60 days" range will have the highest numbers because the payment takes longer to process. After that, each subsequent date range should have smaller numbers than the previous one. When the longer date ranges have larger numbers, it often means payor discounts have not been written off at the correct time or have been written off improperly. It also might mean that patients have not been billed for their remaining balances.

Some payor contracts will only send payment for clean claims that arrive within 60 days of the dates of service. For those payors, you want to pay close attention to the claims in the 30-to-60-day range. If you receive a denial, an unprocessed claim, or a penalized payment, you want to take action immediately. The turnaround time allowance in which you can still receive payment is now very small. Other payors allow a longer time to receive a clean claim. All unpaid claims should receive attention, but there is less urgency when the turnaround time allowance is longer.

When your follow-up reveals that a payment was not received when expected, you must take action as soon as possible. Call the payor and request the status of the claim. Always document phone calls to the payor in the patient's financial record or in the computer system if your system allows comments to be attached to specific transactions.

If the payor does not have a record of the payment, and you do not have a record to prove the payor received the claim, you will have to send another claim. To avoid the label "duplicate claim" should the payor later find the original claim, stamp or print the words "Second copy, payor denies record of original" or "tracer claim" in the top and/or bottom margin of the claim for paper claims and in block No. 19 of the CMS-1500 claim form for electronic claims. To be sure this claim is received by the payor, follow-up again soon after. Some payors view tracer claims in a bad light. Check with each payor to learn the payor-specific preferences when an original claim cannot be located. Your claims will be processed faster when you follow payor-specific preferences. The payor tracer letter in Figure 13-16 has proven to be very effective and is favored by many payors.

When you are following up on balances for patient responsibility amounts, send statements for the more recent claims, and target the older claims with polite and courteous telephone calls. Generally, the more time that has passed since the date of service, the harder it is to collect money from the patient. Only a few balances should fall in the "60-90 day" time range, and the goal is to have none fall in the ">90 day" time range. Statistics show that once a claim is more than 90 days old, there is a less than 50% chance of collecting the patient balance due. Patient tracer letters can also be sent. Figure 13-17 is an example of a patient tracer letter that has proven to be effective.

RETROSPECTIVE PAYMENT AUDITS

The Office of Inspector General, Department of Health and Human Services (OIG/HHS) released the Final Compliance Guidance for Individual and Small Group Physician Practices on September 25, 2000. The central theme of the document is lawful, honest,

Aging Report by Payor September 30, 20XX					
Payor	<30 Days	30-60 days	60-90 days	>90 days	Total
BCBS	510.00	1,240.00	208.00	30.00	1,988.00
Medicare	2,716.00	426.00	390.00	255.00	3,787.00
Total	**3,326.00**	**1,666.00**	**598.00**	**285.00**	**5775.00**

Aging Report by Payor by Patient September 30, 20XX						
Payor	Patient	<30 Days	30-60 days	60-90 days	>90 days	Total
BCBS		**510.00**	**1,240.00**	**208.00**	**30.00**	**1,988.00**
	Baker, Michael	510.00	890.00	110.00		1,510.00
	Gonzalez, Maria		350.00	98.00	30.00	478.00
Medicare		**2,716.00**	**426.00**	**390.00**	**255.00**	**3,787.00**
	Johnson, Cindy	260.00	96.00		65.00	421.00
	Lewis, Howard		150.00	390.00	150.00	690.00
	Williams, Corey	2,456.00	180.00		40.00	2,676.00
Total		**3,326.00**	**1,666.00**	**598.00**	**285.00**	**5,775.00**

Aging Report by Patient by Payor September 30, 20XX						
Patient	Payor	<30 Days	30-60 days	60-90 days	>90 days	Total
Baker, Michael		**510.00**	**890.00**	**110.00**		**1,510.00**
	BCBS	510.00	890.00	110.00		1,510.00
Gonzalez, Maria			**350.00**	**98.00**	**30.00**	**478.00**
	BCBS		350.00	98.00	30.00	478.00
Johnson, Cindy		**260.00**	**96.00**		**65.00**	**421.00**
	Medicare	260.00	96.00		65.00	421.00
Lewis, Howard			**150.00**	**390.00**	**150.00**	**690.00**
	Medicare		150.00	390.00	150.00	690.00
Williams, Corey		**2,456.00**	**180.00**		**40.00**	**2,676.00**
	Medicare	2,456.00	180.00		40.00	2,676.00
Total		**3,326.00**	**1,666.00**	**598.00**	**285.00**	**5,775.00**

Aging Report by Patient September 30, 20XX					
Patient	<30 Days	30-60 days	60-90 days	>90 days	Total
Baker, Michael	510.00	890.00	110.00		1,510.00
Gonzalez, Maria		350.00	98.00	30.00	478.00
Johnson, Cindy	260.00	96.00		65.00	421.00
Lewis, Howard		150.00	390.00	150.00	690.00
Williams, Corey	2,456.00	180.00		40.00	2,676.00
Total	**3,326.00**	**1,666.00**	**598.00**	**285.00**	**5,775.00**

FIGURE 13-15

Aging reports are used to report the status of claims to the physician, and they are also used to identify individual transactions that require follow-up.

and accurate billing, coding, and collections. The purpose is to prevent the submission of fraudulent claims. This guidance strongly recommends concurrent and/or retrospective audits as a method of monitoring accuracy in billing, coding, and collections.

Concurrent payment audits occur at the time payments are recorded. The transactions chosen for the audit are in various stages of completion. They evaluate the correctness of payments received on the day of the audit. You do this in an informal fashion when you check the payor fee schedule each time

you evaluate the payment on an EOB. Periodically, formal concurrent payment audits should be conducted to document your compliance activities.

A **retrospective payment audit** traces and evaluates the financial records for a specified number of completed transactions. The last payment and the write-offs have already been posted. You do this on an informal basis when you evaluate the entire transaction before posting write-offs. Formal retrospective payment audits should be performed periodically to document your compliance activities. When records are stored haphazardly in multi-

Dear Insurance Carrier:

Please find attached a duplicate claim which has already been submitted more than 90 days ago for consideration for payment. To date, we have received no response regarding this claim.

Should your records indicate this claim was not previously considered, we would appreciate your processing the attached claim appropriately.

In the event you have previously considered this claim, we would appreciate the disposition taken regarding the outcome of this claim by checking below:

_____ Applied to Deductible

_____ Payment to Patient

_____ Additional Info Requested from Patient

_____ Not Authorized Service and/or Provider

_____ Lapse/Cancellation of Policy for Date of Service

_____ Other (Please Explain) _____

_____

We appreciate your cooperation in resolving this outstanding claim. Should you have any questions or need additional information, please do not hesitate to contact our office at 634-555-1212.

Sincerely,   PATIENT NAME:
                                     ACCOUNT NUMBER:

FIGURE 13-16
Payor tracer letter. (Courtesy MD Consultative Services, Inc., Orlando, Fla.)

patient files, you will not be able to conduct retrospective payment audits effectively.

The following documents are needed *for each transaction* in the audit sample for a retrospective audit:

- [ ] A copy of the fee schedule and/or payor contract requirements
- [ ] A copy of each original claim form (primary, secondary, tertiary)
- [ ] A copy of the EOB for each payment received
- [ ] A copy of each patient statement
- [ ] A copy of the record for each patient payment (a printout from the management system)
- [ ] A copy of the record for each write-off (a printout from the management system)

A retrospective payment audit verifies whether correct payment was received from every source and whether correct write-offs were posted. It does not evaluate the accuracy of the superbill or the quality of medical record documentation. Clinical employees perform concurrent and/or retrospective documentation audits for those items.

You begin a retrospective payment audit by evaluating the original claim for each transaction.

- [ ] Was the claim prepared correctly? Evaluate each EOB.
- [ ] Was the correct payment received? Evaluate each patient statement.
- [ ] Were the transaction and each previous payment reported correctly?
- [ ] Were the correct patient payments received?
- [ ] Were refunds issued when overpayments were identified? Evaluate each write-off.
- [ ] Does the assigned write-off account accurately portray the entry?
- [ ] Were the write-offs posted correctly?

Dear Patient:

Please find attached a duplicate claim filed to your insurance carrier more than 90 days ago. Your insurance carrier has informed our office these services will not be considered for payment for the following reason(s):

—— Applied to Deductible

—— Payment to Patient

—— Additional Info Requested from Patient not received

—— Not Authorized Service and/or Provider

—— Lapse/Cancellation of Policy for Date of Service

—— Other (Please Explain) ————————————————————

Due to the lateness of these charges, it is now your responsibility to make immediate arrangements for payment for these services. Please indicate the account number located in box 26 on the enclosed claim form with your payment. If you feel your insurance carrier has incorrectly processed these charges, please contact them directly.

Should we not receive payrnent within 15 days for these services, collection proceedings may begin at that time.

Should you have any questions, please feel free to contact our office at 634-555-1212.

Thank you for your cooperation in resolving your account.

Sincerely yours,

FIGURE 13-17
Patient tracer letter. (Courtesy MD Consultative Services, Inc., Orlando, Fla.)

Although audit findings can be reported for each individual transaction audited, it is acceptable and it is much more common to report audit findings in a summary fashion. The entire team (often the entire staff in a small medical office) should discuss audit findings soon after the audit is completed, so shortfalls can be discussed and corrective action can be taken.

☐ Keep a log of these staff meetings.
☐ Keep the records of audit findings in a special file.

The OIG/HHS guidance states that these records must be kept the same length of time as all other medical and financial records. If the government ever audits you, you may need to prove the steps you took to meet the laws.

LEGAL ISSUES

Financial records must be kept for the same length of time as medical records: the time specified in the payor contract or the time specified in a state or federal law, whichever is longest. In most states, 7 years is the longest time period to keep medical and financial records.

You must pay special attention to the amount you may legally bill a patient. Balance billing is an outdated concept for the vast majority of the claims you file. You must meet current collections laws and you must meet payor contract requirements.

Professional courtesy write-offs may occur only when the entire service is given at no charge. You may not bill a payor for any portion of a claim when a professional courtesy discount is given. The OIG/HHS Final Compliance Guidance for Individual and Small Group Physician Practices released on 9/25/2000 clearly states that professional courtesy may not be given when doing so meets the federal definition of a kickback, and it cites the example of professional courtesy given in exchange for referrals.

Collection laws vary by state. Some states mandate how often you may call and how often you may send written correspondence. Learn the laws for your state, and follow them closely. In addition, you should always be polite and respectful when you call to collect from a patient.

In Florida, the collection laws stipulate that you may only call to collect after 9:00 AM and before 8:00 PM. You cannot call on Sunday, and you cannot call a patient at his or her place of employment unless the patient has given you permission to do so. In addition, you cannot leave a detailed message on an answering machine because someone other than the patient might hear the message. You cannot tell a spouse the nature of the call, but you can say the call is "not of a medical nature" so the patient or patient's family cannot claim you caused them undue stress and worry about the patient's medical condition. Many practices hire collections employees to make calls to patients between 6:00 PM and 8:00 PM when most people are home from work.

STOP & REVIEW

Answer the following questions:

1. Is an EOB part of the patient's medical record?_____

2. Is a superbill part of the patient's medical record?

_____

3. Where should EOBs and superbills be stored, and why?

_____

_____

4. If the largest balances on an aging report fall in the over-90-day range, what does this tell you?

_____

_____

5. If you file electronic claims, what date range on an aging report should have the largest balance?

_____

_____

6. If you file claims on paper, what date range on an aging report should have the largest balance?

_____

7. What do concurrent payment audits evaluate?

_____

8. What do retrospective payment audits evaluate?

_____

9. Is it legal to write off only patient balances for professional courtesy write-offs? Why or why not?

_____

_____

10. What is the most likely consequence if you do not respond to a payor request for additional documentation?

_____

Chapter Review

The reimbursement process follows the lifecycle of the medical claim. It begins when the patient first requests an appointment, and it ends when full payment is received and the paperwork is complete. The greatest reimbursement success occurs when employees work together as one team to oversee the claim cycle from start to finish.

While completing and submitting clean claims is very, very important, it is only the first segment of the reimbursement process. The next segment begins when a response is received from the primary payor. A document commonly called an EOB accompanies each payment and each denial of payment.

The purpose of the EOB is to explain the payor's payment decision. When you receive an EOB, read every item pertaining to each transaction, including each explanatory note. Most footnotes are error codes or claim adjustment codes, but some convey other types of information. Adjustment codes are used by payors to explain why a claim or service line item is paid differently than it was billed. In addition, Medicare often uses remark codes.

The best clues to penalties and other payment reductions are found in the explanatory notes and remarks on the EOB. However, the only way to truly know if your payment was reduced is to compare (1) the EOB to a copy of the original claim and (2) the EOB's "allowed amount" to the payor fee schedule.

An official financial policy that covers numerous situations protects the physician's right to collect the money he or she has rightfully earned. You are responsible for enforcing the financial policy.

When the allowed amount on an EOB does not match the payor fee schedule for the service, you should investigate and determine whether further action should be taken with the primary payor before considering other options. Most of the time further action is advisable, but occasionally it is not.

When a claim is returned as unprocessable, the claim can usually be corrected and rebilled. However, when the payor processes a claim and payment is either penalized or denied, the payor's decision must be evaluated to determine whether the claim may be rebilled or appealed. Begin by reading the EOB, including every footnote and every remark code.

The best way to track billing results so you know you are billing and receiving the correct payment for every claim is to use a system that allows line item posting of payments. With line item posting, every payment is posted to the exact transaction for which the payment is received. Each payment is subtracted from the remaining balance due for that specific service. You can clearly identify every remaining balance for each service, so you can always determine whether another action is required.

A write-off is a portion of the charge that cannot be collected or a portion of the charge that the physician has chosen not to collect. A write-off is posted as though it were a payment, except it is placed in the adjustment column. The specific write-off account is named as the source of payment instead of a medical plan or a patient.

Just as each patient has a medical record, each patient should also have a financial record. If a quality assurance team performs an audit and wants to see copies of EOBs from other payors for coordination of benefits, you must be able to produce the documents in a timely manner. The financial record holds the superbills, claim copies, EOBs, and any correspondence sent and received regarding financial transactions for each patient.

If your superbill contains diagnosis and/or procedure codes, it must be updated annually. Payor fee schedules also must be updated annually or as often as the fee schedule changes.

Aging reports are used to report the status of claims to the physician, and they are also used to identify individual transactions that require follow-up. If you submit claims electronically, "<30 days" should have the largest numbers, and each subsequent date range should have smaller numbers than the previous one. If you submit claims on paper, the "30-60 days" range will have the highest numbers because the payment takes longer to process. After that, each subsequent date range should have smaller numbers than the previous one. When the longer date ranges have larger numbers, it often means payor discounts have not been written off at the correct time or have been written off improperly. It also might mean that patients have not been billed for their remaining balances.

The OIG/HHS's Final Compliance Guidance for Individual and Small Group Physician Practices was released on September 25, 2000. The central theme of the document is lawful, honest, and accurate billing, coding, and collections.

Answer the following questions:

1. What is the greatest obstacle to reimbursement?

   _____

2. When does the medical claim cycle begin?

   _____

3. What happens when a preauthorization is not obtained before performing a service that requires preauthorization?

   _____

4. Who is held accountable for verifying patient eligibility and determining all possible payors?

   _____

5. What is a tertiary payor?

   _____

   _____

6. If you want to collect payment for a noncovered service, what must occur before the service is rendered?

   _____

   _____

7. Submitting a claim completes the first segment in the reimbursement process. When does the next segment begin?

   _____

8. The footnotes and symbols are used to tie together the items in the EOB with the applicable _____ that are usually located at the bottom of the page.

9. Why are error messages on EOBs often vague?

   _____

   _____

10. What are adjustment codes?

    _____

    _____

11. What tool can you create to help you decide what the next action should be when you receive an EOB from a payor?

    _____

12. What must occur before you look to see if a secondary payor may be billed?

    _____

13. Electronic posting of payments increases accuracy, but does it save time?

    _____

14. How do you know whether Medicare automatically forwarded your claim to a secondary payor?

_____

15. Are patient hardship write-offs or insurance write-offs posted first?

_____

16. Why is it a bad idea to store patient financial documents in large, multi-patient files?

_____

17. How do you know whether you may bill a payor for the cost of copying documents for the payor?

_____

18. What can happen if you do not update your superbill and a claim is filed with an outdated code?

_____

19. When the same report date and aging ranges are used for each type of aging report and the totals for each aging-range column do not match, what does this tell you?

_____

_____

20. How long should you keep patient financial records?

_____

_____

DEVELOPING CRITICAL THINKING SKILLS: ANALYZING PROBLEMS AND MAKING DECISIONS

Objectives   After completing this chapter, you should be able to:

- List at least three examples of payor contract provisions that influence scheduling, billing, or collections
- Discuss potential situations and make decisions concerning confidentiality and patient rights
- Discuss potential situations and make decisions concerning payor collections
- Discuss potential situations and make decisions concerning patient collections
- Discuss potential situations and make decisions concerning provider compliance with laws
- Discuss legal responsibilities related to each issue

Key Terms

collections agency an outside resource option to collect delinquent payments from patients.

comment period the time during which everyone may review proposed rules and requirements developed by the Secretary of Health and Human Services to meet a specific law. Anyone may submit comments and suggestions during this time.

compliance deadline the date when a "final rule" developed by the Secretary of Health and Human Services to meet a specific law becomes mandatory and is strictly enforced.

conversion number the dollar value assigned to each RVU (relative value unit) to find the allowed fee in an RBRVS (resource-based relative value system) fee schedule.

curriculum vitae an expansive résumé that documents credentials, education, work history, and specific accomplishments, such as research projects, speaking engagements, and published works.

delinquent payment or account a payment or account that is overdue.

False Claims Act a law that makes it illegal to submit a false or an inaccurate claim to the government for payment. This law covers all types of government payments, not just medical claims.

final rule the official release of new rules or standards developed by the Secretary of Health and Human

Services to meet a specific law. Once a final rule is officially released, you may begin using the rule. After an implementation period, a compliance deadline is established.

gag clause prohibits a physician from discussing with a patient the treatment options the payor does not cover, such as experimental treatments or treatments that are expensive, even when one of these treatments represents the best course of action for the patient.

proposed standard the first draft of new rules or standards developed by the Secretary of Health and Human Services to meet a specific law. After a public comment period, a final rule is developed.

Qui Tam a provision of the False Claims Act designed to allow ordinary citizens to report violations without repercussions.

relator the person who reports a violation under the False Claims Act. A whistleblower.

Stark laws laws that regulate many activities relating to consultations and referrals. They prevent physicians and other providers from profiting from the consultations and referrals they give out. They are often called the anti-kickback laws.

whistleblower a relator in a Qui Tam action; the person who reports a violation of the False Claims Act.

Introduction

In Chapters 1 through 13, you learned about medical plans, how to work together as a team to gather claim information, how to complete and file claim forms, and how to achieve reimbursement success. However, in the real world things are not always textbook perfect. Laws change and new rules are implemented nearly every year. Even when everything is done correctly, unexpected problems can and do arise.

When you know the fundamentals about how medical insurance and reimbursement function and you know what changes to look for in the future, you are better equipped to resolve medical insurance and reimbursement problems encountered in a working medical practice.

Each of the topics discussed in this chapter has been either introduced or discussed in detail in another chapter. The purpose of this chapter is to give you a sample of what can go wrong and why. Many of the topics are explained in more detail in this chapter because your knowledge level is greater now than it was when the topic was first introduced. When you finish this chapter, you will be able to analyze some of the most common problems encountered in medical practices and make appropriate decisions.

Health Insurance Portability and Accountability Act of 1996 (HIPAA)

The Health Insurance Portability and Accountability Act of 1996 (HIPAA) set many deadlines for the gradual introduction and implementation of certain requirements of the law. These HIPAA requirements influence how medical entities (physician offices, hospitals, medical plans, claim clearinghouses, etc.) conduct business.

The Secretary of the Department of Health and Human Services was given the responsibility of proposing standards, each of which has specific rules, to meet the requirements of the "Administrative Simplification" section of HIPAA. **Proposed standards** are subject to change before the **final rule** is published. When a standard is first proposed, there is a specified **comment period** during which everyone nationwide may review the standard and its rules and submit opinions and suggestions. After the comment period is closed, the opinions and suggestions are evaluated and a final rule is developed.

Once a *final rule* is published, you may begin using the standard. By the **compliance deadline,** you are *required* to use the standard. The compliance deadline also is subject to change. The period between the date the final rule is published and the date that compliance becomes mandatory is commonly called the implementation phase. You are expected to learn how to use the standard during this time. When a final rule is very complex, providers are given a longer period to learn to use the standard.

Final HIPAA standards are expected to follow the compliance schedule that appears in Table 14-1. The compliance dates are estimates, as published on the official government websites for HIPAA.

The standard for "Transactions and Code Sets" is intended to provide one set of codebooks and one set of rules that every payor and every medical provider will be required to follow. This standard was developed to ease the burden that physicians and hospitals faced of trying to meet hundreds of different sets of rules, since every payor wrote its own rules to augment or replace national rules. It also is intended to make the electronic transmission of claims easier by standardizing the claim transmission format. Currently, clearinghouses are needed to translate claims into the hundreds of electronic formats created by payors.

The "National Provider Identifier" (NPI) standard is intended to replace the collection of ID numbers given to each physician with one number per physician that is valid nationwide and that is recognized by all payors. Historically each payor issued ID numbers, and some issued different ID numbers for use with referrals or when rendering care, with a different set of ID numbers for each physician in each office location.

The "National Employer Identifier" standard is intended to replace the collection of ID numbers given to each facility, each incorporated solo physician, and each group practice with one ID number that is valid nationwide and is recognized by all payors. The employer identification number (EIN) used for tax purposes has now been named as the national employer identifier.

The "Security" standard is intended to close loopholes in laws by defining what security measures must be taken to prevent illegal access to medical information that is stored on a computer or that is

TABLE 14-1
HIPAA Standards Schedule

Standard	Proposed	Final Rule	Compliance
• Transactions and Code Sets	05/07/1998	08/17/2000	10/16/2002
small health plans			10/16/2003
• National Provider Identifier	05/17/1998	1/23/2004	5/23/2007
small health plans			5/23/2008
• National Employer Identifier	06/16/1998	5/31/2002	6/30/2004
small health plans			8/1/2005
• Security	08/12/1998	5/31/2003	4/21/2005
small health plans			4/21/2006
• Privacy	10/29/1999	2/20/2003	4/14/2003
small health plans			4/14/2004

transmitted electronically. It also defines punishment when unauthorized persons gain illegal access.

The "Privacy" standard is intended to revise the rules governing who may gain access to an individual's medical records and revise the steps that are required before access is granted. The rule makes it easier for payors to obtain records needed to make payment decisions. It also makes it easier for patients to acquire copies of their medical records and enables patients to learn who has received copies of their medical records. The privacy law adds several new record-keeping requirements for all medical entities.

Some standards are still in development. When they are officially proposed, a comment period is announced. You should begin to learn the requirements when the standard is first proposed, but you will not begin to use them until a final rule is published. Every comment submitted during the comment period is taken into consideration as the final rule is drafted. The final rule usually has modifications and is not identical to the proposed rule. All the dates are estimates and are subject to change. By the compliance date, the new standard becomes mandatory.

When you begin using a standard at the time that the final rule is first published, you can become proficient by the date of mandatory compliance. Those who wait until the standard is mandatory before they begin implementation risk penalties and sanctions as they learn the rules.

HIPAA standards that are still in development are expected to follow the schedule in Table 14-2. Sometimes it takes longer than expected to write a final rule. The final rule usually has modifications and is not identical to the proposed standard.

The "National Health Plan Identifier" standard is expected to make it easier for physicians and hospitals to identify payors and send claims to the correct payor address the first time.

The "Claims Attachments" standard is expected to provide a standardized secure method for attaching medical records, operative reports, diagnostic imaging, etc., to claims that are transmitted electronically.

As the various deadlines for implementing each phase of HIPAA draw near, you must be ready to help your practice meet the new requirements. It is essential for you to join professional organizations to keep abreast of these changes as they occur. Medical assistants, medical billers, medical coders, medical records specialists, medical office managers, medical compliance officers, and medical financial officers each have professional organizations. Each organization takes steps to keep members informed of important laws and how they apply to you personally as well as professionally. Many of these organizations are listed by name in Chapter 2.

If you have time to do the research yourself, most of this information is available on the Internet. The CMS website (http://cms.hhs.gov) and the website for the Department of Health and Human Services (http://www.hhs.gov) are good places to begin when searching for items about HIPAA and the status of proposed "Administrative Simplification" standards.

MEDICAL OFFICE CONFIDENTIALITY REQUIREMENTS

The privacy and security of patient information are closely intertwined. However, HIPAA treats privacy and security as separate issues. The final rule for the Health Information Security Act, proposed in August 1998, was released in May 2003. It redefines the way in which medical offices must handle the security of individually identifiable patient information if any information for that patient is ever placed in a computer or transmitted electronically. The proposed electronic security rules also govern hard copies of electronic documents and hard copies of other documents for every patient who has electronic documents on file. The compliance date is an estimate released by the government and may be subject to change.

TABLE 14-2
HIPAA Schedule for Standards in Development

Standard	Proposed	Final Rule	Compliance
• National Health Plan Identifier	04/2000	Unknown	Unknown
• Claims Attachments	03/2000	Unknown*	Unknown*

*No longer listed on the official government websites for HIPAA.

Since October 16, 2003, Medicare has required claims to be sent electronically. There are a few exceptions for companies that truly are unable to send electronic claims, but you must complete an application to be granted an exception and you must have a compelling reason to get approval to send paper claims.

If your medical office uses a computer or if any patient information is ever entered in a computer, including when your billing company uses a computer to send claims, security within the physician's office must prevent a patient or a visitor from seeing any *individually identifiable* patient information. Individually identifiable information is a concept borrowed from the Privacy Act and is discussed in more detail there. Many offices use a divider or a screen to prevent unauthorized people from viewing computer monitors or viewing hard copies of documents currently in use by employees.

The Security Act also requires each medical entity to take reasonable measures to prevent an unauthorized person from accessing patient information using the Internet. If your office has Internet access, you can meet this requirement by purchasing and installing a good quality computer program called a firewall. A firewall prevents unauthorized access to your system when you are online. A person skilled in using computers to steal information, commonly called a hacker, might be able to get around even the best firewall. However, having a firewall is considered a reasonable measure to meet the law because the average person online cannot gain access and the average computer hacker is not skilled enough to get around a good quality firewall.

If your practice does not own a computer and all patient documents, including billing documents, are completed *without* the use of a computer or a word processing typewriter that uses a computer chip, the proposed Health Information Security Act does not apply to your practice.

The final rule for the privacy standard, first proposed in October 1998, was released February 20, 2003. The final rule took many people by surprise because the scope was greatly expanded from the proposed rule.

Key provisions of the final rule for the privacy standard are:

☐ *Access:* People are given the right to see and copy their own medical records. Some states did not grant people this right of access, even when the patient paid the entire bill for the medical care. The only exception is for mental health. In mental health, the provider (a psychiatrist or a psychologist) may refuse to give a patient access to his or her own record if the provider determines that doing so could be detrimental to the patient.

☐ *Privacy:* The proposed rules pertained only to records stored on a computer, but the final rule pertains to all patient information, including that stored on a computer, all forms of hard-copy records, and spoken information. The inclusion of spoken information was the biggest surprise in the final rule, and spoken information is the most difficult to control. You must make a reasonable effort to avoid eavesdropping. Lower your voice and face a corner when speaking on the telephone. Do not discuss patients in public parts of your office or facility, such as elevators, hallways, and waiting rooms. Keep a partition (usually Plexiglas) between the waiting room and the receptionist.

Originally, the Privacy Act would have made patient sign-in sheets illegal, and you would not have been able to call a patient by name when you were ready for them. However, a clarification was issued 2 months after the final rule was published. The clarification clearly allows for a sign-in sheet and allows patients to be called by name.

In addition, in the final rule, business associates who require access to patient information must sign a "business associates agreement" in which they also agree to keep patient information confidential. When such an agreement is in place, the business associate can be held accountable for any breaches he or she creates.

☐ *Limits on disclosure:* In the final rule, *other than those disclosures required for treatment, payment, and normal health care operations,* health care providers and payors are required to obtain the patient's consent before disclosures of individually identifiable information occur.

This consent must be voluntary and cannot be tied to the delivery of any benefits or services. Previously, many medical practices and most payors required people to sign broad waivers of their privacy *as a condition* of receiving health care or health benefits.

Note, however, that under this standard, whoever pays for medical care may see the medical record entries related to the care paid for *without first obtaining consent from the patient*. This not only includes payors, it also includes banks and credit card companies. The only exception to this disclosure with or without consent when related to paying for medical care is psychotherapy notes. Then the patient must sign a specific consent for each individual entry that is disclosed.

In addition, patients may now ask to see a list of each disclosure of *individually identifiable* patient information from his or her records, including but not limited to who received information, what information was sent, and the date it was sent. This has greatly increased the record-keeping burden for the medical office. Please see Appendix D for more information about the provisions for disclosure.

❑ *Patient rights*: Under this rule, all businesses, not just medical businesses, must inform people of their business policies for handling *individually identifiable* information, and the person's rights regarding that information. Each business must disclose who they share information with on either a routine or occasional basis, and they must give people the option of being excluded when this information is shared. Individually identifiable information is clearly spelled out in the privacy act. It includes demographics, such as name, address, phone number, birth date, and medical record number, as well as *any* information that would cause someone to identify a specific individual. The final rule included the example of a small town where only one or two hip surgeries might be performed on a given day or even in a given week or month. If you then refer to just the procedure and the date or time of the procedure (the hip case from Thursday morning), most of the people in the town would be able to identify the exact person who had received the surgery. In that situation, it would be a violation of privacy even though the patient's name and demographics were not mentioned.

❑ *Research:* Under this rule, the patient is *not* given the right of access to his or her own medical records related to participation in a research project. Nor are they guaranteed access to the results of any research projects they participate in, even if the anticipated results did not occur and, most surprising of all, not even when a high percentage of the participants are dying. There is already controversy about this rule, so watch for changes.

❑ *Penalties:* Health care providers, payors, and clearinghouses would be subject to civil and criminal penalties (up to $25,000 per year and 10 years in jail) for violating the law. Yet, HIPAA prevents the Secretary of the Department of Health and Human Services from including a private right of action for individuals to sue for violations of the law.

❑ *Preemption:* In the final rule, federal regulations would not preempt or override stronger state laws. Instead, they would set a baseline of minimum protections to which the states could add additional provisions to better protect their citizens. A July 1999 report issued by the Health Privacy Project found that while few states have health privacy laws that protect all medical data, most states have enacted legislation to protect sensitive information, such as information pertaining to mental health, communicable diseases, and genetic testing. Please see Appendix D for more information about protected health information (PHI).

To protect patient confidentiality (both privacy and security), unauthorized people must not be given access to private medical records. Although the physical medical record is the property of the physician, the information in the record belongs to the patient. Therefore a patient must be given access to his or her medical record and may have a copy of his or her medical record, except as noted above, but the physician owns the medical record.

WHO MAY SEE PATIENT RECORDS

Rendering physicians and select employees may see a patient's medical records on a need-to-know basis. Patient consent is not required in this instance because it falls under the clause pertaining to treatment, payment, and operations (TPO).

Patients may see their own medical records except when a mental health provider denies access to specific mental health records. Parents of minor children and legal guardians may see the applicable medical records. However, spouses do not have the right to see each other's medical records or to be told individually identifiable medical information without a written consent from the patient.

Use of the patient's medical record is strictly regulated. It may not be used for any purposes other than those stated in current laws. Under the new privacy standard, when a payor pays a claim for a service, permission from the patient is not required for the payor to gain access to the medical record entry for the service. The exception to this rule is psychotherapy notes. Psychotherapy notes cannot be released to a payor without the patient's express, limited permission.

If you allow an unauthorized person access to a medical record and the information is misused, you and the person who misused the information may both be held liable for civil and criminal penalties. Under both the privacy and the security standards, the civil penalties are increased up to $25,000 per year and criminal penalties are increased to up to 10 years in prison.

PATIENT PROTECTION LAWS

The patient protection policies and procedures used in your practice must mirror current state and federal laws. You must become familiar with current laws and pending legislation so you can adapt your practice to meet the new laws as they take effect. You are not required to meet pending legislation, but you should be prepared to explain the issues to patients when they ask.

Internet search engines can help you learn about both current and pending legislation. However, it would be wise to consult the medical attorney for your practice to verify current laws before changing office policies based on an Internet search.

Many states have state-specific legislation detailing patient rights and responsibilities. To find out if additional "patient rights" legislation exists in your state, contact the insurance commissioner or the Department of Insurance. If your state has patient rights legislation, ask the insurance commissioner's office to send you a copy of the rights or see if a copy is available on the Internet. Contact information for the Department of Insurance for each state can be found in Appendix B and can be verified at Medicare's website: www.medicare.gov.

Payor Contracts

Payor contracts often play a key role in the prevention and resolution of reimbursement problems. Unfortunately, many physicians do not have their contracts professionally reviewed before they sign them, and many do not inform their employees about contract provisions. In addition, sometimes physicians do not make a photocopy of each contract before returning the signed contract to the payor. You cannot effectively meet contract requirements you do not know exist.

Problems arise when contract provisions are not followed. Additional problems arise if the physician did not seek the advice of a *medical* attorney and/or a *medical* CPA, and, as a result, unfavorable contract provisions were not identified before the contract was signed.

Most payors will not readily share specific contract provisions when you call to ask about contract requirements. They typically claim it is too difficult because they maintain multiple standard contracts as well as numerous customized contracts with literally thousands of physicians and other providers for each of their hundreds of medical plans. It is interesting that the claim adjustors employed by these same payors can readily find every contract-specific requirement when it is time to impose penalties.

It is critical for medical office employees to have access to the clauses in payor contracts that pertain to scheduling, billing, and collections. Physician substitution coverage is an example of an issue that pertains to all three: scheduling the patient when the attending physician is not available and then billing and collecting the fee when someone else provided the service. When you learn and follow payor-specific contract requirements, many reimbursement problems are prevented.

When you work as a billing manager or an office manager, you are responsible for knowing and meeting contract requirements and for sharing them with other employees on a need-to-know basis. When you work in another position in the medical office, understanding these issues will enhance your ability to meet the responsibilities of your position. In addition, this kind of knowledge can enhance opportunities for advancement.

So the key question is: How do you persuade a physician to share this critical information? When you can demonstrate that you are knowledgeable, that you understand contract confidentiality, and that you understand how and when you may use contract information, you have taken the first step toward winning the confidence of the physician.

Remember, physicians have a high level of education and special medical skills, but they seldom have time to also become experts in business. Physicians generally hire employees to handle business issues for them. Payor contracts and medical reimbursement are among the business functions in the medical office.

You can become one of the people physicians turn to for assistance when they negotiate payor contracts. Begin by learning as much as you can about payor contracts: the purpose, how to use the information, how and when contract information may be shared, and how to help physicians meet payor contract requirements. These topics are introduced in this book, and additional courses are available if you want to learn more than is offered here.

PROVIDER ENROLLMENT, CREDENTIALING, AND CONFIDENTIALITY

As a side effect of the many laws regulating payor contracts, the process of becoming an authorized provider for a medical plan has become much more complex than merely signing a contract.

Each physician must complete a long application form and attach documents to prove current licensure, educational background, clinical background, and areas of expertise. Gathering these documents and compiling the required information is more time consuming than merely updating the physician's **curriculum vitae.** A curriculum vitae is an expansive résumé that documents the physician's credentials, educational history, and work history as well as specific accomplishments, such as research projects, speaking engagements, and published works.

The payor uses this information for credentialing. Credentialing is the process of verifying credentials to establish that a person has not misrepresented accomplishments, that licensure remains current, and that the person has not been excluded from participation in federal medical plans. Even if the physician has already been credentialed by the medical plan and is merely changing practice affiliations (changing partners or opening a solo practice), credentialing can take several months. The physician is not considered an authorized provider until credentialing is complete. Often a payor-specific provider number is issued when credentialing is complete.

In the flurry of application paperwork, it is easy to forget to read the actual contract, especially if the physician has previously been a provider for the medical plan. Physicians often do not realize fees

can be negotiated, and many physicians miss the fine print that advises making a copy of the contract. The original contract is returned to the payor with the application paperwork. The payor does not routinely send the physician another copy of the entire contract; often the payor only returns a copy of the signed signature page. Staff members are then informed, "Now we accept Aetna," or whatever contract was just signed.

Antitrust laws prohibit physicians from discussing their payor contracts and fee schedules with other physicians. The intent of the legislation is to prevent large physician organizations from engaging in price fixing. Antitrust laws do not prohibit physicians from discussing contract provisions and fee schedules with employees. Payor contracts can be shared on a need-to-know basis with anyone who has a legitimate reason to see the information. This includes medical attorneys, medical CPAs, and medical business consultants, as well as practice employees. Some medical offices now require a signed confidentiality agreement from each person or company that will view any portion of any contract(s).

Physicians may overemphasize the confidentiality of payor contracts because they do not fully understand the complexities of the antitrust laws, but often it can be to avoid the problems they need to face when copies of their contracts are not in their files and they cannot argue the fee schedule and other contract provisions. If you suspect this is the situation, use diplomacy to resolve it without embarrassing or upsetting the physician. This is a common issue. Physicians are highly educated professionals. Remember to always treat them with the utmost respect.

One acceptable course of action is to ask the physician for permission to get an updated copy of each contract so you will have current fee schedules to use in the billing and collections department. With the physician's permission, you may then call provider services at each medical plan and ask for an updated copy of the contract with the current-year fee schedule attached. When it arrives, you may respectfully ask the physician for permission to review the entire contract so you can find and summarize the clauses that pertain to scheduling, billing, and collections.

The payor will probably look at the physician's claim preparation history and can make an educated guess about whether the physician or his employees are properly applying the contract. If the payor is saving a lot of money through penalties and by downcoding billed services that do not meet contract requirements, the payor is not going to be very eager to send you an updated copy of the contract.

Payors know most medical offices are not persistent. When the payor fails to respond to the first request, very few medical offices make a second request. However, the squeaky wheel almost always gets the oil. Sometimes you have to be persistent and request a contract copy from the payor more than once. Remain polite and courteous each time you talk with the payor's provider representative, but keep asking until you receive the updated contract with a current fee schedule. Then remember to call and thank the provider representative for the help you have received.

FEE SCHEDULES

Contract law is a serious matter. In February 2000, the courts ruled in favor of the payor when a hospital system wanted to exercise the right to cancel a particular payor contract without cause, as was allowed in the contract. The payor successfully argued that the hospital actually wanted to negotiate better fees before the expiration of the existing contract, and the judge agreed with the payor.

This case set a legal precedent that has become very difficult for physicians and other medical entities to overcome. To avoid facing problems such as this, ask your physician(s) to obtain the assistance of a medical CPA to negotiate realistic fees and a medical attorney to find and remove any other unfavorable contract provisions before each contract is signed or renewed.

Payor contracts discuss fees in a variety of ways. Many of them are designed to make you work to find the fee schedule, and a few are cleverly worded, which can easily mislead you about the true fee schedule.

Some payors use the resource-based relative value system (RBRVS) to calculate fees. RBRVS was introduced in Chapter 10. The payor gives a **conversion number** in the contract and tells which version of RBRVS to use when calculating the fee. The conversion number is the dollar value per relative value unit (RVU). The most common version of RBRVS is Medicare's RBRVS fee schedule, but other publishers such as McGraw-Hill and Ingenix also publish RBRVS fee schedules. These other publishers usually assign RVUs to every CPT procedure code. Medicare only assigns RVUs to the procedures that are "covered services" for Medicare.

When Medicaid uses RBRVS, they usually use Medicare's RBRVS fee schedule and assign a Medicaid conversion number (dollar value per RVU). *Only Medicaid may have a conversion number lower than Medicare's conversion number.*

Workers' compensation often has a unique RBRVS scale. When someone refers to the state's RBRVS rate, they usually mean the state's workers' compensation RBRVS fee schedule. *The "state" RBRVS usually applies only to workers' compensation claims.*

Some payors assign one conversion number (dollar value per RVU) for some services and another conversion number for other services. For example, one payor contract might assign the following conversion numbers: Medical services: 48.00, surgical services: 58.00, OB/GYN services: 54.00.

The medical office is expected to obtain a copy of the specified version of RBRVS, look up each procedure code, find the *total* number of RVUs assigned to each procedure code, and perform the mathematical calculations to determine each fee. Most RBRVS books have multiple columns. Separate columns show the breakdown between the *work* RVUs, the *overhead* (practice expense) RVUs, and the *malpractice* (risk) RVUs assigned to each procedure code both alone and with a specific modifier attached. Some RBRVS books include a column to show the assigned global periods for procedures that have global periods. Usually one of the columns gives the total number of RVUs for the procedure code or procedure code plus modifier.

The geographic practice site indicator (GPSI— pronounced "gypsy") allows for regional cost differences and expenses that are common to a given region. The RVUs and the GPSI are stable numbers within a given region. The variable is the conversion factor identified in each payor contract.

First you multiply each of the work, overhead, and malpractice RVUs by the GPSI for each factor and then add them together to get the adjusted RVUs. Then you multiply the adjusted RVUs by the conversion factor (CF) (dollar value per RVU) to find the fee for each item [adjusted RVUs: (work RVU × work GPSI) plus (overhead RVU × overhead GPSI) plus (malpractice RVU × malpractice GPSI)] × CF = $. Use a calculator and double-check each of your numbers!

For example:
The adjusted RVUs for a given procedure are 2.5.

If the conversion factor is 48.00, multiply 2.5 by 48.00 (2.5 × 48.00 = 120.00) to get a fee of $120.00.

If the conversion factor is 54.00, multiply 2.5 by 54.00 (2.5 × 54.00 = 135.00) for a fee of $135.00.

If the conversion factor is 58.00, multiply 2.5 by 58.00 (2.5 × 58.00 = 145.00) to get a fee of $145.00.

Because the law states you cannot bill Medicare a higher fee than you accept elsewhere for the same service, *you must be sure the conversion factor in each of your contracts is higher than Medicare's conversion factor.* In 2005, Medicare's conversion factor was 37.8975.

For example:

The adjusted RVUs for a given procedure are 2.5.

Medicare's conversion factor is 37.8975. Multiply 2.5 by 37.8975 (2.5 × 37.8975 = 94.74375) and round the answer to the nearest penny to get a fee of $94.74.

Note that the contract conversion factors in the previous example are higher than Medicare's conversion number, and the resulting fees are higher than Medicare's fee for a procedure assigned 2.5 total RVUs.

Medicare also publishes a fee schedule in which the RBRVS mathematical calculations have already been applied. It is listed each fall in the *Federal Register,* and it is often available on the Internet website for a state Medicare carrier. The only thing not yet applied is the GPSI. Medicare also will send a fee schedule with all the math, including the GPSI, to specific physicians upon request.

Very few other payors who use RBRVS offer that courtesy. You should take the time to do the math and create a fee schedule for each of your major payors that use RBRVS to use as a reference when you post payments.

The following illustration shows how to compare the fees for multiple conversion numbers. Each conversion number can represent a different payor, or it can represent a different specialty for the same payor. Add a column on the left for the correlating procedure code, and you also have a usable fee schedule comparison chart.

CF = conversion factor

Adjusted RVUs	CF 37.8975 Medicare	CF 48.00 Payor A	CF 54.00 Payor B	CF 58.00 Payor C
2.5	$94.74	$120.00	$135.00	$145.00
25.39	$962.22	$1,218.72	$1,371.06	$1,472.62
51.49	$1,951.34	$2,471.52	$2,780.46	$2,986.42

Other payors attach a fee schedule to the contract that specifies the "allowed" fee for each procedure code the contract authorizes the provider to render. Some of these contracts only list a few procedure codes. If your physician(s) perform more services than are included in the contract's fee schedule, ask for an expanded fee schedule that includes each possible service, or you might not receive payment when you perform the services not specifically included on the contract's fee schedule. Next, check to be sure each fee is higher than the Medicare fee for the same service.

Many payor contracts allow the *lower* of the physician's standard fee (or, as a variation, a percentage of the physician's standard fee) *or* a payor-determined fee. Details about the payor-determined fees usually are not disclosed in the contract. Payors typically claim they do not want physicians to *raise* fees to match the payor's maximum allowed fees; therefore they are justified in not revealing the payor-determined fee schedule. Many physicians honestly believe this means payments will be based on their own fee schedule. However, if you take the time to really look at what the contract says, you will see that the physician's fees are only allowed in full when they are *lower* than the payor's undisclosed fee schedule.

You must be very cautious when you find this type of language in a payor contract! More than any other contract, a payor contract with this language should be scrutinized by both a medical attorney and a medical CPA. Conceivably, it gives the payor the ability to change fees at will without committing to a written fee schedule, and the payor could set fees as low as they desire because there are no minimum fee limits. In addition, these payors are usually managed care plans that do not allow the physician to balance-bill the patient. The physician gives away a lot of legal ground for challenging fees when he or she signs this type of contract.

In addition, many payor contracts contain an obscure clause that requires the physician to continue to render services to plan patients even when the payor gives no reimbursement for the services.

Any time the payor fee schedule is lower than the Medicare fee schedule, it is very important for you to file a letter of protest. If you do not, the lower fee schedule could become your new Medicare fee schedule because you cannot charge Medicare a higher amount than you are willing to accept elsewhere for the same service. See Figure 13-10 in Chapter 13 for an example of a letter of protest.

Another method of payment that can be found in payor contracts is called capitation. Capitation was first introduced in Chapter 4. Under capitation, a physician is paid a fixed dollar amount each month for each plan member registered under the physician's care. The formulas are very complex for comparing the proposed insurance income per patient to the expected practice expenses per patient to determine whether the proposed capitation rate is appropriate. Most medical accountants enlist the aid of an actuary (a mathematician experienced in these calculations and projections) when evaluating capitation contracts. Capitation plans do not have fee schedules, and although you submit zero-balance claims, the reimbursement is received as a fixed monthly capitation payment. However, be aware that sometimes capitation payments only cover specific services and separate payment is negotiated for other services. These separately paid other services are called carve-outs.

Indemnity plans do not require payor contracts and do not publish payor fee schedules. When you do not have a payor fee schedule for one of your major payors, you can build one by tracking the allowed amounts for specific services from the EOBs you receive. Then you can compare current fees to past fees the payor paid for each service. Once again, you must remember to also compare the fees to the Medicare fee schedule and file a letter of protest anytime the payor's UCR (usual, customary, and reasonable) fee drops below the Medicare fee schedule. Remember, when a patient has an indemnity plan, you may balance-bill the patient for the entire balance of the fee not paid by the insurance plan. You are not limited to the allowed fee listed on the EOB.

CONTRACT TIME LIMITS

Most payor contracts specify numerous time limits. Some stipulate a time limit for seeing patients who request an appointment. This type of time limit is usually expressed in hours for urgent problems and days for nonurgent problems. For example, you might be required to see a patient with an urgent problem within 24 to 48 hours (today or tomorrow), and a patient with a nonurgent problem within 10 days. If this is a contract requirement, and the patient is not seen until 2 weeks (14 days) after calling for the appointment, you are in violation of the payor contract. Some payors compare the number of days between the time an authorization number is issued and the date of service on the claim to monitor this requirement. The claim payment could be penalized if the requirement is not met.

Most contracts specify a time limit from the date of service to the payor's receipt of a *clean* claim. If a clean claim is not filed within that time limit, neither the payor nor the patient is responsible for paying for the service.

Medicare allows 1 year from the end of the government fiscal year (October 1 to September 30) for the date of service. If you are seen on the last day of the fiscal year (September 30), you have 1 year to file a clean claim. If you are seen on the first day of the fiscal year (October 1), you have nearly 2 years to file a clean claim because the fiscal year doesn't end until the next September 30 and you have 1 year from the end of the fiscal year for the date of service.

Many managed care contracts have clean claim time limits that are as short as 60 days and a few are beginning to require clean claims within 30 days of the date of service. This means that even if the first claim goes out on the date of service, it is unlikely you will have more than one additional opportunity to get it right.

Most payor contracts also stipulate time limits for filing appeals regarding payment decisions. Medicare allows 60 days from the date of the Medicare remittance notice (MRN), but some others are as short as 10 days from receipt of the explanation of benefits (EOB). If you do not perform concurrent audits every day as you post payments, and you do not perform monthly retrospective payment audits, you could easily lose the opportunity to collect the correct reimbursement.

In addition, payor contracts often stipulate a time limit for producing requested documents. The time limit for documents varies widely. Some are as short as 10 days, and others are as long as 2 months. If documents are not received in the specified time, the claim is denied. It is more difficult to appeal a denial when you have failed to produce documents within the allowed window of time unless there is a valid reason for the delay, such as when a payor requests a document the payor is not authorized to receive. For example, psychotherapy notes cannot be sent to the payor unless the patient gives a specific written authorization for the release. The standard "release of records" is not enough. A release for psychotherapy notes must specify which notes (by date of service) may be released, and they must specify the exact payor the notes may be sent to.

Payor contracts also spell out how much notice the payor must give you before utilization review inspections, the length of time you must retain medical and financial records, and a payor time limit for sending payment after receipt of a clean claim.

Most payor contracts contain a clause that allows the contract to automatically renew every year if it is not canceled. Often the payor is allowed to send a letter stating that fees are changing, and if you do not respond within a specified time limit, the new fees automatically take effect.

Notice, the payor does not have to disclose the new fees, the payor is only obligated to send an announcement that the fees are changing. It is up to you to request a copy of the new fees so you may decide whether to accept them. If you do not act, the contract is renewed for another year, and the new fees take effect. The time limit might be as short as 10 days, but typically it is around 30 days.

In most practices, the physician does not open the mail. It is the responsibility of the person who opens the mail to understand the significance of a notification letter for contract renewal and/or fee change, and to make sure it gets to the physician and the billing department so they can evaluate the new fees and determine whether to accept them.

Always remember, when the physician or practice is not profitable, you cannot be given a pay raise. Notify the physician promptly when notification letters are received, and help the physician meet each time limit.

OTHER CONTRACT REQUIREMENTS

Most payor contracts require coding from current-year codebooks. Some contracts specify exact codebooks, such as "current-year ICD-9-CM, CPT-4, and HCPCS codebooks," while other contracts just say "current-year codebooks." The medical office must purchase new codebooks every year if the billing and coding employees are to meet this contract requirement.

If a contract that specifies exact codebooks does not specify the HCPCS codebook, it could mean the payor does not yet provide coverage for HCPCS codes. You should call the payor and get an answer in writing regarding this issue.

On the other hand, contracts seldom require payors to accept current-year codes on January 1, and many payors are slow to update their systems. When this occurs, your best protection is to get a written notice from the payor each year for the date they will begin to accept that year's current codes.

Although the new standards for code sets have now reached the compliance deadline and every payor is required by law to accept every CPT-4 (Level I procedures), HCPCS (Level II procedures), and ICD-9-CM (diagnosis) code when a claim arrives with any of those codes, they are not required to provide coverage for every code. In addition, they are not limited to only using those codes. Payors may still decide their own rules for what items are and are not covered services.

Some payors have specific claim form requirements, such as special words that are to be placed on the claim form, and some include payor-specific procedure codes and modifiers. Sometimes contract requirements can take precedence over national laws. If you are unsure about an issue, check with your medical attorney. When any of these contract requirements are not met, the claim could be penalized or denied, usually due to insufficient data.

Most contracts require payor-specific provider numbers. Eventually this will be replaced with the National Provider Identifier (NPI), but the earliest providers just began to sign up for an NPI in June 2005. Medicare will be the first to implement the NPI, but it will take time for other payors to adopt it and to convert their software systems to accommodate it.

Other items to look for and think about when reviewing payor contracts include:

❑ Where do you send claims?

❑ Is the payor allowed to determine the level of service? If so, is the payor required to base the decision on the official documentation guidelines and a copy of the medical record entry for the encounter?

❑ Are funds ever withheld for risk sharing? If so, when and how are they distributed? How do you know when full payment is received? Do you have the tools and the ability to meet and to track this type of plan requirement?

❑ Does a capitation contract specify how to track capitation?

❑ Does a noncapitated contract become capitated for months when a specific volume of plan patients is seen? If so, can your practice management system track the changes in reimbursement under such a plan? Are you capable of meeting and tracking this type of complex plan requirement?

❑ Is it mandatory to list other payors (i.e., primary, secondary, tertiary payors) on the claim form?

❑ Are you allowed to balance-bill patients?

❑ How many days are you given to challenge or accept changes to a contract or to a fee schedule?

❑ Independent Physician Association (IPA) contracts usually involve multiple payors. If this contract includes payors also covered by another contract, does the most recent contract specify that it replaces all previous contracts for that payor? Legal action sometimes arises from this type of contract dispute. Do you know which set of contracted billing rules to follow? Do you know which contracted fee schedule to use when posting reimbursement for patients on those plans?

❑ What hours are the physician(s) required to be available to patients, and do these requirements match the practice office hours or current methods of operation?

❑ Is substitution coverage allowed, and are there restrictions on who may provide substitution coverage? How is the claim filed when the service is provided by a substitute?

❑ What referral procedures must be followed, and what happens if they are not followed?

❑ If the payor becomes insolvent and cannot pay you, may you bill the patient?

❑ Are fees reduced if you fail to get preauthorizations?

❑ Are you required to display stickers or placards for the payor, and if so, do you have a place to display them? Can your reimbursement be reduced if they are not displayed as directed in the contract?

❑ Is the physician required to use a payor-specific formulary when prescribing medications, and if so, does the physician have a copy of the formulary? Can reimbursement be penalized if the physician does not use this formulary?

❑ Does the contract require specific levels of malpractice insurance or mandate any other insurance requirements? If so, has this requirement been met? What are the consequences if this requirement is not met?

Contracts are very complex. Important clauses are often put in the contract in a disjointed, seemingly haphazard order, similar to the manner in which they are listed above. To prevent reimbursement problems, you must have or create an easy reference so you can readily verify whether you are meeting contract requirements for each payor. See Figure 3-15 in Chapter 3 for an example of a managed care chart you can develop and use to track contract requirements for each payor. Remember to update the charts when contract requirements change.

LEGAL ISSUES

Antitrust laws prohibit physicians from discussing their contracts with other physicians. The intent of the law is to prevent large physician organizations from engaging in price fixing. These laws do not prohibit a physician from sharing contract information

with employees and other contracted professionals such as attorneys, accountants, and consultants.

In addition, many states have laws that govern payor/physician contracts:

❑ Often state laws do not allow "gag" clauses. A **gag clause** prohibits a physician from discussing with the patient any treatment option(s) the payor does not cover, such as experimental treatments or expensive treatments, even when these treatments represent the best course of action for the patient.

❑ Some state laws declare that managed care plans in that state must allow the patient to see any licensed physician in the state.

❑ In many states, it is not legal for a payor to limit fees for mental health when other medical fees are not limited. Typically, these laws only pertain to the "allowed amount" in the contract. The payor can choose how to split the fee responsibility between the payor and the patient.

For example: With standard Medicare the fee responsibility is split 80% Medicare–20% patient (80/20) for medical/surgical services and 50% Medicare–50% patient (50/50) for mental health services.

To avoid contracts with illegal clauses, it is wise to have a medical attorney review each contract before the physician signs the contract.

Answer the following questions:

1. Why do physicians sometimes not have copies of their payor contracts?

_____

_____

2. What is the payor's fee (before GPSI) for a service with 15.3 total RVUs and a conversion number of 46.89?

_____

3. Should you advise a physician to consider accepting a contract with an RBRVS conversion number of 32.99, and why or why not?

_____

4. Should you advise a physician to consider accepting a contract with an RBRVS conversion number of 68.00, and why or why not?

_____

_____

5. If a contract states in one section that the physician agrees to be available 24 hours a day, 365 days a year, and several pages later the contract states that no substitution coverage is allowed, what is the physician agreeing to when he or she signs the contract?

_____

6. The contract gives you 60 days to file a clean claim. The patient supplied an insurance card 2 years ago but recently changed from an Aetna HMO through her employer to an Aetna PPO through her husband's employer. She is an established patient, so the scheduler and the receptionist merely asked, "Are you still with Aetna?" and the patient correctly replied "Yes." The first claim submitted was returned as unprocessable with a "Patient not covered" error code. New insurance information is obtained from the patient and a corrected claim is sent to the correct Aetna medical plan, but the relationship to the insured is not revised. The claim is returned as

unprocessable with a "Patient not covered" error code. It is now more than 60 days since the date of service. What is likely to happen if you resubmit a corrected claim to the payor?

_____

7. Do antitrust laws allow physicians to share contract requirements with employees?

_____

8. Under the proposed Health Information Security Act, does the law apply to your practice if your practice is not computerized, but your billing

agency is computerized and claims are sent electronically?

_____

9. Under the proposed Privacy Standard, may patients read their medical records?

_____

10. Are you required to meet the requirements in pending legislation, and why or why not?

_____

Common Problems

There are many causes for problems you might encounter when working with medical insurance billing and collections. Some of the more common problems are discussed in this section of the chapter. Although greater detail may be provided in another chapter, do not be tempted to skip this section. New laws are discussed or new insights are presented for every topic, and some topics are presented in greater detail in this chapter to build on the knowledge you have gained throughout this course.

REFERRALS VS. CONSULTATIONS

It is very important to understand that even though many physicians believe the terms *consultation* and *referral* to be synonyms, they are not synonyms in the eyes of a payor. *For reimbursement purposes, the payor definitions of each term must be met.* The physician's confusion often arises because the exact same request form is traditionally used for both purposes, and the form is typically called a "consultation" form. Typically, there are no boxes on the form to easily designate "consultation" or "referral." Instead, the requesting physician must define the intent of the visit in writing: (1) "opinion/advice" for specific condition(s) or symptom(s), brief pertinent history (consultation) *or* (2) "advise and *treat*" specific condition(s) or symptom(s), brief pertinent history (referral).

A referral is used whenever total or partial care of the patient is transferred to another physician. "Evaluate and treat" indicates a referral. The accepting physician agrees to manage all or a specific portion of the patient's care.

A consultation is used when only an opinion or treatment advice is sought from the consulting physician. The consultant must send a written report to the requesting physician, or both physicians must document a telephone discussion.

Please read Chapter 6 for more details about the current codebook definitions and the documentation requirements for the various levels of consultations and referrals.

The Stark laws regulate many activities relating to consultations and referrals. They prevent physicians from profiting by steering consultations or referrals to a particular provider.

Stark Laws
Stark laws are designed to prevent a physician from inflating medical costs by ordering more tests or services than needed from a medical entity in which the physician has a financial interest. A financial interest can mean an ownership interest, it can mean a family member has an ownership interest, or it can mean payment or even gifts received for referrals. The physician is required to disclose his or her financial interest to patients before services are rendered. Some medical plans deny payment if they suspect Stark law violations.

The Compliance Program Guidance for Individual and Small Group Physician Practices released by the Office of Inspector General, Department of Health and Human Services (OIG/HHS) on 9/25/2000 states that routinely waiving Medicare copayments or deductibles could increase the number of Medicare patients or increase the number of visits from Medicare patients. As a result, this activity inflates medical costs. Therefore routinely waiving copayments or deductibles is also a violation of Stark laws.

The Stark laws are often called the antikickback laws. Stark I laid the initial groundwork, and Stark II further defines the financial relationships and family relationships that fall under the laws and the exemptions to the laws.

Details about the Stark laws and other health care laws are available on the Internet and from your practice attorney. For an Internet search, begin with the key words "Stark law" or "Stark laws." The metacrawler at <u>dogpile.com</u> searches multiple search engines and gives you the results from each.

VERIFYING PLAN COVERAGE

Performing or verifying patient eligibility for medical plan coverage during check-in is a critically important step in the reimbursement process. Through this process, you learn or verify where, when, how, and from whom to collect payment for services rendered. You must identify every possible payor so the correct order of payor responsibility can be determined before the first claim is sent.

Many payors have a 60-day time limit for receiving clean claims. A lot of time is wasted when the first claim is sent to the wrong payor or to the wrong billing address for the right payor. When the claim fails the first payor edit, it is rejected immediately. The claim does not go through the rest of the edits and audits. The net result is that absolutely everything else on the claim must be perfect. There can be no other errors as there is not enough turnaround time to correct another error and still receive payment for the claim.

Very few patients know and understand medical insurance law. They seldom know which medical plan must be listed first on a claim form. Many patients mistakenly think they can choose the health plan to bill first in the same manner they choose which credit card to use for the copayment, and they will feed you information in the order they choose for payor responsibility.

You must diplomatically ask the right questions to get the answers you need to make the correct decisions about payment responsibility. Figure 13-2 in Chapter 13 is a tool that asks the right questions to determine patient eligibility and the order of payor responsibility in most situations. Ideally, this is followed by verification directly with the primary payor, whether by telephone call, secure computer website, or a payor's instant verification program.

When you establish eligibility correctly before the service is rendered, numerous potential errors are prevented, and you are more likely to get a clean claim to the payor before the payor's deadline.

PAYMENT REDUCED OR DENIED

There are many potential reasons for payments to be reduced or denied. Payors consider every item on the claim to be a potential reason for a claim denial and/or penalty.

Human error can never be completely eliminated, but errors can be minimized when everyone works together. A team environment can provide an effective system of checks and balances to prevent problems before they occur. A team minimizes the potential for error as information is gathered from patients and providers and passed through the medical office on its way to the billing department, and a team verifies the quality of supporting documentation in the medical record before the billing documents even reach the billing department.

Patient Not Covered
If the eligibility process was performed correctly and a claim denial comes back with a message on the EOB that the "patient is not covered," the first item to check is the spelling of the patient's name in block No. 2 on the CMS-1500 claim form. If that is correct, look at block No. 6, "Patient's relationship to the insured." Is the correct relationship identified between the patient and the insured for the payor in the primary payor slot on the claim?

If that is correct, look at the addresses for both the patient in block No. 5 and the insured in block No. 7. Do they match payor records? If that checks out, look at the ID number in block No. 1a. Do the numbers match the numbers on the patient's ID card? A transposed number could cause the payor to not recognize the patient. Next, look at the payor's address. Does it match the address on the patient's ID card or the address in eligibility documentation?

These are the items the payor's editing system looks at to verify patient identity. If you find a problem, correct it and resubmit the claim. Then verify that your computer system now lists the information correctly so the same problem does not occur again on the next claim for this patient.

If everything matches your records and you cannot find an error, call the payor. Perhaps a step was missed in the eligibility process or perhaps the payor made a mistake.

Service or Procedure Not Covered
The first item to look at when an EOB says a service is not covered is whether the service is an official noncovered service for the medical plan or whether it is just not covered this time. Noncovered services are handled differently than a normally covered service that has been denied.

When the service is a noncovered service, look to see if a secondary payor may be billed. If not, look at the payor contract to see whether the patient may be billed. Some payors allow billing for noncovered services and others, such as Medicare, require written patient notification before the service is rendered if the patient is to be billed. See Figure 3-6 and Figure 3-7 in Chapter 3 for examples of Medicare Advance Beneficiary Notices (ABNs).

Whenever an ABN is on file, the service should be billed with a HCPCS Level II modifier (-GA) that notifies the payor that the waiver is on file. If the service is known to be a noncovered Medicare service, another modifier (-GY) also must be attached to the claim. And if you suspect a service may be denied as not meeting medical necessity requirements, yet another modifier (-GZ) must also be attached to the claim. If the patient then calls the payor, the payor will know that the patient was notified in advance and agreed to pay for the service. If you do not have an ABN signed before the service is rendered, Medicare and some other payors do not allow you to bill the patient for a noncovered service.

Pay attention to coverage issues so you can get ABNs when necessary. By doing so, you resolve the problem of nonpayment for noncovered services because you may then collect the fee from the patient.

When a service is normally covered by the payor but is not covered this time, usually medical necessity requirements were not met. You should begin by comparing the original claim to the medical record. Are the diagnoses listed correctly? Is each service linked to the single most appropriate diagnosis for that service?

Some payors allow you to link to more than one diagnosis, but many, including Medicare, do not. From the payor's point of view, if even one of the linked diagnoses is not appropriate for the billed service, the service will fail the payor's medical necessity audit.

If you cannot find the problem on your own, enlist the assistance of the physician. Figure 14-1 is an example of a form that can help you discuss this issue with the physician. If you are billing from a central billing office or a remote location, this form can be faxed to the physician. Use the completed form as supporting documentation to correct errors on the claim, when applicable, and file an appeal to have the claim reconsidered for payment. See Chapter 13 for more information about filing appeals.

Insufficient Data

An "insufficient data" error code on an EOB can apply to any field on the claim form. Sometimes it

Lake Eola Family Practice 517860 South Pioneer Drive, Orlando, FL 32897 • 634-555-4893

Provider Name ______________ Date of Service ______________

Re: Patient Name ______________ Record Number ______________

Payment was reduced or denied for ______________ service/procedure.

The billed diagnoses were: ______________

☐ Which diagnosis should this service be linked with to best support medical necessity for the charge? ______________

☐ The medical record shows the following diagnoses that were not billed on the claim: ______________

☐ Is there another diagnosis or comorbidity that supports this service? ______________

☐ The above diagnoses are correct. Please file an appeal.

Please reprocess this claim with the information listed above.

______________ Physician Signature ______________ Date

FIGURE 14-1
A request for the physician's input into an evaluation of the billed diagnoses. (Courtesy Medical Compliance Management, Inc., Orlando, Fla.)

refers to an unusual item required in the payor contract. Sometimes a required field was left blank. Sometimes incorrect or insufficient modifier(s) were used. Other times the billed service has been targeted for review and the payor is requesting additional information every time the service is billed.

Begin by reviewing the overall claim. Is anything obviously wrong? Compare each item of patient-supplied information to the claim. Is everything correct? Compare the billed service to the documentation in the medical record. Does the medical record documentation support the billed service? Could additional or different modifiers better explain the service? Do the diagnoses establish medical necessity? Does an E-code explain the cause of accidents, injuries, and/or poisonings? Is the service linked to the diagnosis code in the manner preferred by the payor?

Usually claims that have insufficient data are unprocessable. Unprocessable claims can be corrected and resubmitted. See Chapter 13 for more information about rebilling unprocessable claims.

Other Factors

There are many other factors that can influence payment.

Is the service rendered in the normal scope of practice for the specialty and experience level of the physician who performed the service? Although the American Medical Association clearly states in their CPT manual that any licensed physician may perform every service and procedure in the codebook, most payors only allow payment for services in the scope of license *and experience level* of the rendering physician. The payor's complex credentialing requirements are intended to allow the payor to direct their covered members to the best-qualified physicians for each type of service. Payors believe that medical costs will ultimately be lower with this approach because their statistics show better patient outcomes. The faster the patient recovers, the lower the overall cost of medical care.

> Most payors do not believe that a family practice physician is the best-qualified physician to perform brain surgery, so they usually will not authorize a family practice physician to perform this procedure.

Therefore authorization for a service or procedure is a different issue than authorization for a specific physician. Even participating primary care physicians must obtain authorizations for specific procedures. Often when a procedure is authorized by the payor, a separate authorization is required for the physician who will perform the service, and sometimes yet another authorization is required for the location

where the service will be performed (hospital, surgicenter). Was an authorization required to perform the service or procedure, and if so, was the authorization obtained? Was the rendering physician authorized by the payor to perform the service or procedure? Was there an authorization for the location where the service was performed?

Medical necessity plays an increasingly important role in reimbursement. Correct diagnosis coding and correct diagnosis linking are essential when meeting medical necessity requirements. Payors conduct clinical studies continuously. They know whether patient outcomes for a particular diagnosis are generally improved by specific services or procedures. The payor's goal is to get the patient well and then keep the patient well to reduce health care utilization. Payors will not pay for services that do not improve patient outcomes.

For example: If an EKG is not linked to a diagnosis that has cardiac implications, the service could be denied. Often personal or family history items are adequate to meet medical necessity requirements.

In addition, if the EKG is linked to a diagnosis with cardiac implications, but it is also linked to an irrelevant diagnosis, such as a minor abrasion on the left ankle, the payment for the service could be severely penalized.

Denials and penalties can be avoided by linking each service to the *single* most appropriate diagnosis for that service. Some payors do allow a service to be linked to more than one diagnosis; however, it is easier to consistently get it right when you try to always link to just one diagnosis. Cultivating good habits can prevent or reduce this type of denial or penalty.

Occasionally, when multiple services occur on one date, there is not enough space to list the diagnoses that are most applicable to each service. You do not have to squeeze everything onto one claim form. Complete as many claim forms as it takes to correctly report the services rendered. Burns and complex trauma often require multiple claim forms to correctly report the services rendered on one date of service.

Likewise, when there are multiple dates of service to be billed for one patient, the diagnoses might not be the same for each service. Here, too, more than one claim form might be necessary to correctly report the services.

Most payor contracts require coding to be performed from current-year codebooks. If the billed codes are outdated, truncated (missing required digits), or do not exist, the payment will be severely penalized or denied. There are a few exceptions.

Many workers' compensation plans require codes from 1995 or 1996 codebooks to avoid updating the computer systems. However, now that all medical plans are required to program their computers to accept all current medical procedure and diagnosis codes, expect workers' compensation to also begin requiring current codes.

If the documentation in the medical record does not support the billed level of service or the billed service, the payor will downcode the service and might also apply a severe penalty or might deny payment entirely.

Most medical schools do not teach physicians how to correctly code their services, and physicians seldom stay updated each year on the new billing and coding requirements. Often physicians use fast-finder guides that only list the code and an abbreviated description but do not list rules governing code usage. Physicians rarely look up synonyms to see if they have been assigned different meanings in the codebook.

Medical diagnosis synonyms are sometimes acceptable because diagnosis synonyms usually point to the same diagnosis code. However, medical procedure synonyms seldom point to the same procedure code. When synonyms are listed on a fast-finder procedure guide, the definitions almost always describe different procedures.

For example: A myringoplasty and a tympanoplasty both involve repair of the eardrum. Technically, the terms are medical synonyms. However, the codebook definitions show the myringoplasty involves repairing only the soft tissue of the eardrum, whereas the tympanoplasty involves not only soft tissue, but also bone at the points where the eardrum connects to bone. Therefore the tympanoplasty is a more complex procedure than a myringoplasty.

Physicians who only use fast-finder guides often believe that because the terms are synonyms, they can be used interchangeably. When these physicians see that a tympanoplasty has a better reimbursement rate than a myringoplasty, they often choose to bill every eardrum repair as a tympanoplasty.

Payors always use the codebook definitions to distinguish between the two terms. A payor's patterning software can easily find a pattern of billing all eardrum repairs as the more complex, and less often performed, tympanoplasty.

These physicians do not intend to commit fraud, but intent is no longer a requirement when an OIG investigation shows that this "error" is not an isolated incident.

Most payors use results of the patterning studies to give the payor justification to flag all the physician's claims for a blanket penalty. This is often more cost effective for the payor than auditing the charts for fraud and prosecuting the physician.

In addition, when the definitions of procedure synonyms differ in the complexity of the service rendered, the diagnosis code also must justify the level of complexity that is performed. Diagnosis coding and code linkage is critical when the payor makes the fine distinctions between similar, but significantly different services. Payor audits compare the service to the diagnosis to see if the level of service is justified. Consistently upcoding a service to receive increased reimbursement is classified as fraud and not abuse. Fraud is a criminal offense.

Compare the billed procedure to the codebook description of the service to see if it matches. Then check the diagnosis code to see if the diagnosis matches the level of the service rendered. This is often the time to confer with other team members, especially those with clinical expertise. You can better defend your position when the entire team agrees on an answer. The team decision should be documented in the patient's financial record for the encounter. Remember to also keep a special file to document all team decisions regarding billing problems.

Physicians sometimes choose not to participate in team meetings about billing and collections problems. When you determine that a reduced or denied payment might be related to an inappropriate procedure code chosen by the physician, you must be very diplomatic when you present the problem to the physician. Figure 14-2 shows a form to help you discuss this issue with the physician. If you are billing from a central billing office or a remote location, this form can be faxed to the physician. Use the completed form as supporting documentation to correct errors on the claim, when applicable, and to file an appeal to have the claim reconsidered for payment. This form then becomes part of the medical record for the encounter, and a copy can be placed in the financial record as well if the billing office is in a separate location from the medical office.

The medical coding concepts presented in Chapters 5, 6, and 7 of this textbook cover coding basics in more detail than many comparable textbooks. However, please remember that medical coding is a separate and distinct specialty. This book does not cover all the coding concepts. Medical coding courses that cover these coding concepts are available from many colleges, vocational schools, and trade schools.

Because compliance guidance for medical offices has now been available since September 25, 2000, recommending that accountability be included in every job description in the medical office, the

Lake Eola Family Practice   517860 South Pioneer Drive, Orlando, FL 32897 • 634-555-4893

Provider Name_____   Date of Service _____

Re: Patient Name _____   Record Number _____

Payment was reduced or denied for _____ service/procedure.

The billed diagnoses were: _____

_____

_____

☐ The codebook definition for this service is _____

_____

☐ The medical record description of the service matches _____

   defined as _____

_____

☐ The medical record shows the following diagnoses that were not billed on the claim: _____

_____

☐ Is there another diagnosis or comorbidity that supports this service? _____

_____

☐ Which code best describes the procedure actually performed?_____

☐ The service was billed correctly. Please file an appeal.

Please reprocess this claim with the information listed above.

_____   _____
Physician Signature   Date

FIGURE 14-2

A request for a physician's input into an evaluation of billed procedures. (Courtesy Medical Compliance Management, Inc., Orlando, Fla.)

federal government may now choose to hold medical billers accountable for the codes submitted on medical claims unless the responsibility for medical coding is clearly assigned to someone else, such as a physician, a certified professional coder, or a certified coding specialist. The assignment of responsibility to someone else for medical coding should be clearly documented in a job description. If the medical office you work for does not have a certified coding employee and you are asked to accept the responsibility of medical coding, you might want to consider taking a medical coding course and learning both basic and advanced coding concepts for your specialty.

The coding concepts presented in this book are intended to provide the level of coding knowledge appropriate for an entry-level billing position. Chapters 5, 6, and 7 cover the *basic* medical coding requirements in detail. Armed with this level of coding knowledge, a medical biller can actively participate in the team's system of checks and balances, preventing many problems before they occur and troubleshooting when problems do arise.

REBILLING VS. FILING AN APPEAL

Whenever payment has been denied or reduced, you must decide whether to file an appeal or rebill the encounter. If the claim was returned as unprocessable and no payment was received, rebill the claim. If payment was received, but you do not agree with the payment decision, appeal the claim. If you do not know whether to rebill or file an appeal, call the payor's provider services and ask for guidance. Chapter 13 covers rebilling and filing appeals in more detail.

Options Patients May Pursue

When the patient is a minor and when a court of law has said the adult patient is mentally incompetent and a legal guardian has been appointed, the patient may not seek medical care on his or her own except for emergency care and treatment of sexually transmitted diseases. Usually a medical plan will not pay for the care rendered unless a parent, legal guardian, or an adult who has written permission to seek care on behalf of the parent or legal guardian accompanies the minor or mentally incompetent patient. You should make a copy of the written permission for your files.

See Figure 14-3 for an example of a permission letter. If any of your patients fall in this category, give the parent or legal guardian a copy of a similar letter and ask him or her to complete it each time the patient is left in the care of someone else. Most schools have similar permission forms on file for each student, but day care centers, babysitters, medical attendants, and/or paid companions should also have permission to seek medical care while the patient is in their care.

Many times patients want to become involved in helping you collect the money due for medical services, especially if they have an indemnity plan and are financially responsible for unpaid balances. If a patient wants to become involved, make sure it is not too soon in the process. You may need to kindly ask him or her to wait until you have corrected the claim and rebilled the encounter or

filed an appeal *and* received the payor's response. However, if you have confirmed that the paperwork was prepared correctly the first time and you believe the medical plan is responsible for payment, but the payor has denied coverage, you may send a letter to the patient and enlist the patient's help. The patient can begin a protest or an objection at the same time that you file an appeal.

Advise the patient to start by calling the consumer services division of his or her medical plan. Ask the patient to keep detailed records of each phone call or written correspondence, including the date, the person contacted, and a summary of the call. Advise the patient to make a photocopy of written correspondence before mailing it, and to keep all written responses received.

Sometimes all it takes is one call from a patient or from the patient's employer with an inquiry as to why covered services are being denied for the payor to reverse a decision. Other times it takes a little more persistence.

Patients may also file an appeal of a medical plan's decision if the telephone call does not produce the desired results. The payor will require the date of service, a description of the problem, and a description of actions taken to date to attempt to correct the problem. The patient will need the

---

Permission to Seek Medical Care

_____ is caring for my child _____ in my absence.
Care Giver Name   Child Name

In the event of illness or injury _____ has my permission to
                                  Care Giver Name

seek medical care for _____ .
                       Child Name

Preferred Hospital: _____   Phone: _____
Physician: _____   Phone: _____
Health History: _____
Allergies: _____
_____

Name of Insurance Plan: _____
Insurance ID Number: _____   Insurance Group Number: _____
Name of Insured (Policyholder): _____
Insurance Mailing Address for Claims: _____
Name of Second Insurance Plan: _____
Insurance ID Number: _____   Insurance Group Number: _____
Name of Insured (Policyholder): _____
Insurance Mailing Address for Claims: _____

_____   _____   _____
Signature of Parent or Guardian   Relationship to Patient   Date

(Attach a photocopy of both sides of each insurance card and a photocopy of the driver's license or state ID for the parent or guardian.)

FIGURE 14-3
Permission to seek medical care. When the patient is a minor or is not legally responsible for making medical decisions, the patient may not seek medical care on his or her own. Usually the medical plan will not pay for medical care unless an adult who has written permission to seek care on behalf of the patient accompanies the patient. (Adapted from Brown JL: Navigating the Health Insurance Maze, unpublished manuscript, 1997.)

records he or she kept regarding previous attempts to correct the situation when describing the problem and completing the appeal paperwork.

If the services are still denied after the patient's appeal, the patient may then contact the Department of Insurance for his or her state and ask the insurance commissioner to intervene. The insurance commissioner will require paperwork similar to the patient's appeal. The insurance commissioner will need to know the date of service, a description of the problem, and a description of actions taken to date to attempt to correct the problem.

If this does not resolve the problem, the patient may contact the Better Business Bureau to report the medical plan and file a complaint that promised services have not been delivered.

The patient also has the option of either contacting an attorney to see if legal action is warranted or contacting the Department of Justice. An attorney charges fees for pursuing legal action; the Department of Justice does not charge fees unless the report is false. Remember, if a patient contacts the Department of Justice with a valid complaint, and your physician is found to be at fault, you could be out of a job. Make sure your documentation is in order before encouraging a patient to become involved in the process.

Legal Issues

Clean claims can prevent most of the problems you will encounter, and a team approach makes it easier to file a clean claim the first time around. However, payment decisions are sometimes subjective. The payor may interpret an encounter differently than you do.

There could be times when your physician must face the prospect of choosing legal action to collect the payment due from a payor. You want your physician to win, so be sure your documentation is in order and will pass an audit before legal proceedings begin.

Contract requirements might limit the legal options. Often contracts require disputes that have not been resolved by appeals to go to mediation. A medical attorney should be engaged to represent your medical practice in this action.

When there is an unresolved problem with a claim, let the patient know the steps you have taken to correct the problem. Patient statements can be used to tell the patient about your collection efforts, but also stay in telephone contact with him or her. Reassure the patient that your documentation and coding correctly portray the visit. When possible, enlist the help of the patient in resolving the problem.

When the patient also appeals a decision and does not receive satisfaction, the patient also may choose to seek legal action against either the medical plan or the physician, or both. Not every state allows patients to sue managed care plans, but patients are always allowed to sue physicians. Therefore attorneys are more likely to go after physicians than medical plans. The patient is less likely to blame the physician for the payor's inappropriate denials when he or she is partnered with you in resolving the problem.

Answer the following questions:

1. What is the primary difference between a referral and a consultation?

_____

2. The Stark laws are often called the _____ laws.

3. Why is it so important to verify plan coverage for every patient, not just new patients?

_____

4. If eligibility was performed correctly and the claim is returned with "Patient not covered" in the error code on the EOB, what do you look at to resolve the problem?

_____

5. When a claim is returned with an error code that says "Service or procedure not covered," what must you determine in order to know how to proceed?

_____

6. When a claim is returned with an error code that says "Insufficient data," where do you look to discover what data are missing?

_____

7. Do payors allow every physician to perform every procedure in the procedure codebooks?

_____

8. Once a procedure is authorized, can the patient have the physician of his or her choice perform the procedure, and why or why not?

_____

9. If a claim is penalized or denied due to lack of medical necessity, what items do you evaluate to determine whether to take further action?

10. May a patient file an appeal to a claim decision?

PATIENTS REFUSE TO PAY THEIR PORTION

Although the patient's portion of the total charge is usually small, often only a $10.00 copayment, it is sometimes difficult to collect from patients. Excuses abound for not paying copayment and deductible amounts at the time of service.

However, you never want to hear the excuse, "No one asked for the payment" or "I tried to pay, but no one would accept the payment." Always try to collect *known* copayment and deductible amounts at the time of service.

Internal Collection Methods

You will prevent many collection problems when you are diligent about enforcing the practice's financial policy. When you accept payments directly from payors, you are *required* to collect copayment, coinsurance, and deductible amounts from patients. Collecting these patient payment amounts is not an option. It is wise to make every effort to collect these funds at the time of service because when you must send patient statements for small amounts, the costs for personnel, supplies, and postage are often greater than the amount you collect.

Therefore internal collection methods always begin with collecting copayment, coinsurance, and deductible amounts at the time of service. Only patients who have more than one medical plan (and the other plan covers the payment), and patients who have prearranged payment terms in place may wait until a later date to pay these amounts. Remember, though, copayments are not collected and patient statements are not sent to designated hardship patients. When a patient has hardship papers on file, the patient responsibility amount can be written off as soon as all insurance payments are received.

Patient Statements

Ideally, patient statements are only sent when a "patient responsibility" balance remains after all insurance payments arrive.

Try not to send patient statements for transactions that still have a payor balance pending. When you do so, the phone will ring constantly as patients call to tell you to bill the insurance first. You will have

more time to complete other tasks when you do not have to answer unnecessary phone calls.

Wait until the payment from the primary payor has arrived before you bill the patient. When there is a secondary or tertiary payor, wait until all payor payments have arrived before you bill the patient.

Once you know the remaining patient balance, you also know the insurance write-off. Post the insurance write-off before printing the patient statement so the total balance due on the statement is a patient responsibility.

Many practices use an automated, cyclic approach to patient billing, and all patient statements are sent out on a regular day or days of the month. This is not an insurmountable obstacle. *Whenever an automated system is in use, you must double-check the computer system setup to verify that it automatically prints only the information you choose on the patient statements.* Each patient statement should clearly show the charge for each transaction, each payment applied to each transaction, who made each payment, the insurance discounts applied to each transaction, and the remaining balance due from the patient.

If your system does not show this information, ask the software vendor to reconfigure the system so it does. Most software systems can be configured so transactions are not printed on the patient statements unless the transaction has a payor payment (from each assigned payor) posted to the transaction. Also, ask for an override so you have the option to print a statement that includes transactions with no payor payment(s) when you need to notify a patient that a payor is too slow in paying the bill.

Remember, often 30 to 60 days have already passed since the date of service before you send the first patient statement for a claim. Statistics show that once 90 days have passed since the date of service, the likelihood of collecting from the patient is less than 50%. Therefore once you begin to send statements, send them every 2 weeks until payment is received, but give the patient 30 days to make a payment before past due notices begin to appear on the patient statements.

In some states, collection laws dictate that patient statements may only be sent once a month. You must comply with the laws of your state. You may find the laws for your state at www.lawdog.com.

Patients are given a sense of urgency, and they pay faster, when they receive statements twice a month than when they receive them once a month. In addition, when the patient can look at the statement and clearly see that all expected insurance payments were received, he or she is reassured that the payment due is correct, and is more likely to send payment.

Once three or four patient statements have been sent and no payment has been received, the physician should be notified of the account status. In most practices, the billing manager or the office manager is the person who will handle this. The physician usually decides the next course of action. Small amounts are often written off under a bad debt account due to the expense incurred when trying to collect, but large balances are not usually written off that soon. Of course, there are always a few physicians who continue collections efforts for small balances.

Past Due Accounts

When a patient's balance is past due and the patient has not arranged a payment plan, it helps to remind the patient of the amount due the day before a scheduled appointment and politely ask whether he or she plans to pay by cash, check, or credit card.

When a patient has a long history of nonpayment, in addition to reminding the patient of the amount due the day before the scheduled appointment, you may ask for the payment before the patient is seen on the day of the appointment. When the medical problem is urgent and delay is not an option, you must allow the patient to see the physician regardless of whether a payment is made on the past due account.

However, if the medical problem is not urgent, and the patient did not bring the past due payment, you may offer to wait while they go back and get it, or politely offer to reschedule the appointment for another day to give them time to get it. Remember, some payor contracts require the physician to see the patient within certain time limits. You must stay within those requirements, and you must stay within the collection laws for your state. Also, while you can try to delay service for a nonurgent problem, you cannot refuse services because of nonpayment of a past due balance unless the physician has officially withdrawn from the case and has followed the required procedures for dropping a patient. See Figure 3-14 and read that section in Chapter 3 for further details on withdrawing from a case.

When your internal collection methods fail, it might be time to consider using outside resources, such as a **collections agency.** If you have sent at least three patient statements with no response, the physician may legally choose to write off the charge. If the physician does not want to write off the charge *and* the patient has not called to make payment arrangements, the billing manager or office manager may ask the physician for approval to send the account to an outside collections agency. It is policy to get the physician's approval for every claim sent to a collections agency. An office manager should not make this decision independently unless the physician has given written authorization to do so.

Once you tell a patient that the account will be sent to collections and the patient still does not pay, you must follow through and send the account to collections, or you should write it off. It is wise to check with the practice's attorney for the laws in your state. In some states, if you threaten a patient with a collections agency, but instead continue to try to collect the account yourself, you could be leaving yourself and the practice open to a legal charge of harassment.

Outside Resources

When an aged patient balance is legally due from a patient and the physician does not want to write it off, you might be directed to send the transaction to a collections agency. The collections agency will need the patient's Social Security number and driver's license number. They require this information to find the patient and to verify that they have found the correct person. The collections agency then "owns" the account, and they will attempt to collect payment. Most collections agencies earn a percentage of the amount collected as payment for their services.

A **delinquent payment or account** is a payment or account that is overdue. When payment is not made and the patient has not contested the charge, most collections agencies choose to report the delinquent transaction to the credit bureau. Unlike medical offices, collections agencies seldom have a personal relationship with a delinquent account holder, so there are no personal reasons to delay reporting an account to the credit bureau. In fact, reporting information to the credit bureau is a vital and important part of their job. Then they continue to try to collect the money owed.

Once a delinquent transaction is reported to the credit bureau, only the agency that reported the delinquent transaction can get it removed. *If a collections agency reports a patient's delinquent account to the credit bureau, no one in your practice, including the physician, can get it removed from the patient's credit report.* Only the collections agency can get it removed.

If the delinquent transaction represents a fee that was never really owed by the patient (such as an insurance discount that was not written off) and the patient can prove it, the item can be removed from the credit report immediately. However, a collections agency is unlikely to remove a delinquent notice for any other reason.

Sometimes a patient suddenly pays a fee that has been owed for 5 years because he or she now wants to buy a house or a car and the unpaid fee shows up as a bad mark on his or her credit report. Creditors are entitled to know how difficult it was to collect the delinquent payment. The delinquent payment is reported, but the fact that the payment arrived 5 years late stays on the credit report for a full 7 years after the delinquent payment is received. The best you can do is to reassure the patient that a late payment paints a better picture on a credit report than no payment.

Legal Issues

You should always be polite when you call to collect from a patient, and you must always confirm the identity of the person you are speaking with before disclosing financial information. You may disclose information to the financially responsible parent of a child or to the legal guardian of a person who has been declared by a court of law to be mentally incompetent and therefore not legally responsible for his or her own actions.

You may not disclose financial information to the spouse of a patient or to the child of a patient. You may not disclose financial information to the domestic partner of a patient or to a close friend of a patient.

Always document every collection effort in the patient's financial record, including the date and time when there is no answer or the line is busy. Also document your efforts when you speak with someone, but the person you are required to contact is reportedly not there.

Remember, collection laws differ for each state. Learn the laws for your state and follow them closely. Some states mandate how often you may call or send written correspondence. You may not harass or threaten patients, but with proper notice, the physician can cease to provide medical care by officially withdrawing from a case.

When a patient owes a significant amount of money and cannot or will not pay, the physician has the option of choosing whether to continue to provide medical care. You cannot make this decision for the physician, and the physician cannot suddenly cease to provide medical care.

When a physician wishes to cease to provide medical care to a particular patient, regardless of the reason, formal steps must be taken and documented to terminate the physician-patient relationship. If the withdrawal from providing medical care is not handled correctly, the physician could be charged with abandonment.

A formal letter of withdrawal must be sent to the patient, and the patient must be given adequate notice to find a new physician. Unless the applicable payor contract or the laws for your state have different requirements, 30 days is usually deemed adequate notice for a patient to find a new physician. See Figure 3-14 in Chapter 3 for an example of a letter of withdrawal. The letter of withdrawal should be sent by certified mail with a return receipt requested. Both a copy of the withdrawal letter and the original signed return receipt are filed in the patient's financial record. Alternatively, you may give the letter of withdrawal to the patient in person and have the patient sign an acknowledgment that the letter was delivered.

Next, you must flag the chart and notify the schedulers and the receptionists that no appointments for this patient may be scheduled to fall after the cutoff date. However, during the 30-day interval before the cutoff date, the physician must continue to provide medical care for urgent problems.

Finally, it is important to enforce the cutoff date. When a cutoff date is not enforced, the formal process of withdrawal often must begin again.

Whether or not the physician chooses to continue rendering care, you must continue to try to collect the amount due unless the physician has chosen to write it off as a patient bad debt or as a financial hardship discount. Remember, hardship discounts come under close scrutiny by payors, so monitor the number of hardship discounts, and keep the physician updated about how many are on the books each month.

A very good resource for legal advice about collections is the practice's business attorney. Remember, though, that the attorney will send a bill for any advice given. Do not call the practice's attorney unless you have been authorized to do so.

If you have the time to do some research yourself, laws and legal opinions can be found on the Internet. The Internet Law Library was first compiled by the U.S. House of Representatives but is now maintained by an outside firm. It can be found at www.priweb.com/internetlawlibrary/511.htm. To locate laws pertaining to collections, look under the topic "bankruptcy and debt collection." Another resource is the law library at Cornell University. It can be found at www.law.cornell.edu/topics/debtor_creditor.html. Please remember that websites do change from time to time. If these sites are no longer valid, a Web search using the key terms "debt collections" or "debt collections laws" should yield good results. The website www.dogpile.com offers a metacrawler search engine that searches numerous other search engines and posts the results from each.

PHYSICIAN NONCOMPLIANCE

The changes required of physicians by the new documentation laws are not easy, and physician noncompliance with documentation requirements is a very difficult issue for a subordinate employee to cope with. Although physician noncompliance cannot be tolerated, it can be dealt with in a manner that is gentle and tactful.

Please remember that current laws require documentation in a manner that has never been standard in the medical industry. In addition, medical plans are now given free access to greatly expanded medical record documentation. This often violates a physician's deeply held beliefs regarding the confidentiality of the patient-physician relationship.

Many of the examination items that are measured by counting in the 1997 documentation guidelines are items that physicians often evaluate on every patient but only document when the findings are abnormal. This includes speech patterns, grooming habits, balance, coordination, mental alertness, condition of the skin, and much more. Now physicians *must document* these items for every patient in order to prove the work was performed. In addition, they must document every possible diagnosis, which items were ruled out, and which items are still under consideration. In other words, physicians are now required to document their thought processes as they evaluate and treat each patient.

Although it often takes seconds to evaluate these items mentally, it takes considerably longer to write it all down in the medical record, and it cannot be counted as face-to-face time unless the physician does all the writing in the presence of the patient. In addition, once you start documenting thought processes, liability increases when something is inadvertently left out.

There are many internal methods and outside resources to help physicians meet these difficult compliance requirements.

Internal Methods to Encourage Compliance

Documentation compliance cannot be achieved overnight. Do not give one short in-service and expect every required change to occur magically. Long-ingrained habits are not changed that quickly.

Do your homework first. Find a variety of documentation tools that you can present in conjunction with the documentation requirements. High-quality forms are available to gently guide the physician into fully documenting every observation. The best ones make the task seem less impossible and more achievable.

This book contains examples of many such forms, and many more are available from other suppliers. Electronic medical record software is another option to consider. However, a word of caution is needed. Some software options and some paper forms make it so easy for the physician to meet documentation requirements that physicians end up overdocumenting visits. This is acceptable as long as the level of service is given careful consideration when a code is chosen.

Remember, documentation is not the only consideration when selecting the level of service to bill. If you are going to meet medical necessity requirements, the nature of the presenting illness must be appropriate for the level of service. For example, a sore throat does not normally warrant a Level 5 service, and a heart attack normally warrants more than a Level 1 service. See Chapter 6 for more details about documentation requirements for evaluation and management (E/M) services.

When the topic is documentation compliance, physicians often respond better to suggestions from clinical support personnel, such as nurses and qualified medical assistants, than they do to suggestions from the business side of the medical practice. Get the clinical support employees involved in the team! They are in the best position to perform concurrent documentation audits on a daily basis.

Therefore the clinical support employees should learn the documentation requirements before the physicians' in-services take place. Ask the clinical support employees to screen the various documentation aids and choose the ones they think will best suit the personality and style of the physician before getting the physician involved in the process. Half the battles are won when the clinical support employees are on your side and want to help the physicians make the required transitions.

Perform a retrospective financial audit before the physicians' first in-service. Show the historical revenue collection for the practice first, then show what that revenue could have been if the documentation had met the national guidelines. Often this approach gives the physicians an acceptable reason to comply voluntarily with undesired changes.

Ask the clinical support employees to conduct the portion of the in-service that introduces the physicians to the current documentation requirements and have them offer the physicians a selection of tools to meet the new requirements. When possible, allow each physician to make the final decision about which documentation aids, software programs, and forms to use.

Ask the clinical support employees to begin concurrent monitoring of documentation as soon as the new tools or forms are in place. They can gently guide each physician until the new requirements become ingrained habits that are easily met.

At the same time, the billing and collections department may use the letters in Figures 14-1 and 14-2 to draw attention to each claim that is penalized or denied due to inadequate documentation.

In addition, when you read a payor update or newsletter that contains information the physician must know to meet current requirements, highlight the relevant parts and personally hand it to the physician to read, or ask the billing manager to do this for you. Alternatively, share the information with the entire team. Remember, your demeanor should be helpful, not critical, if you want to achieve the proper result. This approach will help the physician view you (or the billing manager) as a knowledgeable source for medical plan requirements, while also sending the message that you value his or her time enough to condense the required reading.

Outside Resources to Establish Compliance

The professional organization for your physician's specialty can be a valuable reference for updating specialty-specific documentation requirements. Encourage physicians to attend seminars and continuing education programs that focus on medical documentation, health care laws, and medical fraud and abuse (in addition to, not instead of, the seminars that are required to update and maintain their skills as physicians). This will reinforce the training provided in-house and confirm to the physician that you are a knowledgeable source for medical plan requirements.

Purchase books on these subjects and join professional organizations yourself so you remain up to date on these issues. Use the information from these resources as an authoritative reference when you must speak with a physician about a documentation issue or when you discuss a documentation issue with the entire team.

Hire outside consultants to periodically perform financial and/or documentation audits. Share the findings with the entire team.

Last Resort Options

If a physician absolutely will not change and is determined to remain noncompliant, you may need to find another job. Every time you submit a claim with false or inaccurate information, in the eyes of the law you are as guilty as the physician. Your ability to pay the penalty is not likely to be as great as the physician's ability to pay it.

The civil penalties are steep, up to $10,000 per occurrence, and the criminal penalties could include imprisonment and the forfeiture of your personal property and/or belongings purchased from your paycheck if the source of your paycheck includes money obtained from false or inaccurate claims. Furthermore, if your name is placed on the government's list of sanctioned people, medical practices that file claims to government medical programs are not allowed to hire you. Even in the most remote parts of the country, most medical practices include either Medicare or Medicaid patients.

The **False Claims Act** is a law that makes it illegal to submit a false or inaccurate claim to the government for payment. The **Qui Tam, or "whistleblower,"** provision of the False Claims Act was designed to allow ordinary people to report claim violations without repercussion. The Justice Department (DOJ) reported in February 2000 that more than half of the $3 billion recovered in civil fraud cases since 1986 under the False Claims Act's Qui Tam provisions has come from cases involving charges of health care fraud. That percentage increases every year.

The person who reports a violation of the False Claims Act is called a **relator.** Although reports can be made anonymously, relators seldom remain anonymous for long. As soon as your role as a relator is made public, you can count on receiving some form of repercussion that is not specifically prohibited by the law. Most relators are either fired or the work environment becomes so intolerable that they quit voluntarily. With the information age technology available today, your role as a relator could quickly become public knowledge across the nation. Finding a similar position in the medical industry could be challenging.

In addition, although the Qui Tam law states that whistleblowers may receive a share of the revenue obtained through penalties or saved by stopping the alleged violations, there are many loopholes in this law. In reality, only about 30% of those who report wrongdoings to the OIG/HHS or the DOJ ever see any money from whistleblowing. Those who do receive money often must wait 5 years or more as the alleged violations are investigated, tried in court, and then appealed to each level of the legal system.

Your entire family will feel the effects if you decide to take a Qui Tam action and report a noncompliant physician. Do you have their support?

Be very sure that the wrongdoing you report is valid and verifiable. Store your proof of the wrongdoing and a record of your actions to correct the problem in a secure place away from work. Are you strong enough to withstand the challenges to your competency and the doubts that will be cast about your objectivity, your abilities, and the accuracy of violations you report?

Even if you choose to quit and do not file an official report, still keep records about the noncompliant physician's violations and your efforts to correct the problem. If a government audit later reveals the problem, you will want to be able to prove what you knew, when you knew it, and what actions you took to try to correct it.

Remember, patients can also become whistleblowers. Some payors ask patients to regularly review their bills and promptly report each questionable item. Even though patients often don't understand their bills and sometimes are too sick to remember each service or item on the bill, a few payors offer patients incentives to report suspected wrongdoing. As a result, a few patients are overzealous and some even manufacture complaints. Yet, this fact remains: a patient complaint has the same potential as any other complaint to spark an audit because the payor has an obligation to try to learn the truth.

Answer the following questions:

1. Unless the patient has a secondary payor, when should you collect copayments, coinsurance, and deductible amounts?

_____

2. When may the physician choose to legally write off a copayment amount?

_____

3. When more than 90 days have passed since the date of service, what is the likelihood of collecting from the patient?

_____

4. If a collections agency reports a delinquent bill to the credit bureau, can the physician get it removed?

_____

5. What laws should you know before you call a patient to collect money owed the physician?

_____

6. Is it realistic to expect a physician to change documentation habits and come into compliance after one short in-service about documentation?

_____

7. What employee(s) are in the best position to perform documentation audits?

_____

8. If a physician absolutely will not change his or her documentation patterns to come into compliance with federal laws, what should you do and why?

_____

9. What is another name for a Qui Tam action?

_____

10. What is a person who reports a violation of the False Claims Act called?

_____

Chapter Review

You must become familiar with current and pending laws so you can adapt your practice to meet the provisions of new laws as they take effect.

The Health Information Security Act and the Privacy Act are redefining the way in which medical offices handle security and privacy. A high standard of security must be met when medical records are stored or transmitted electronically. Use of the patient's medical record information is strictly regulated. Unauthorized people must not be given access to private medical records. Yet, payors no longer are required to obtain permission from the patient to access most medical records for claims they pay. The patient protection policies and procedures used in your practice must mirror current state and federal laws.

Payor contracts are very complex. Antitrust laws prohibit physicians from discussing their payor contracts with other physicians, but antitrust laws do not prohibit physicians from discussing contract provisions with employees. Payor contracts can be shared on a need-to-know basis with anyone who has a legitimate reason to see the information.

Payor contracts discuss fees in a variety of ways. Many of them are designed to make you work to find the fees, and some seem to follow your practice fee schedule, but actually do not unless your fees are less than the payor's undisclosed fee schedule.

Most payor contracts specify numerous time limits. Most payor contracts require coding from current-year codebooks. Payor contracts also can cover many other items. To avoid contracts with illegal clauses, it is wise to have a medical attorney review each contract before the physician signs the contract.

Stark laws are designed to prevent a physician from inflating medical costs by ordering more tests or services than needed from a medical entity in which the physician has a financial interest. The Stark laws are often called the antikickback laws.

Performing or verifying patient eligibility for medical plan coverage during check-in is a critically important step in the reimbursement process. You must learn where, when, how, and from whom to collect payment for services rendered. There are many potential reasons for payments to be reduced or denied. Payors consider every item on the claim to be a potential reason for a claim denial and/or penalty. Many other factors can influence payment. Clean claims can prevent most of the problems you will encounter, and a team approach makes it easier to file a clean claim the first time around.

There are many causes for problems you will encounter when working with medical insurance. Procedure synonyms often cause problems. For reimbursement purposes, "consultation" and "referral" are not synonyms.

Many times patients want to become involved in helping you collect the money due for medical services, especially if they have an indemnity plan and are financially responsible for unpaid balances. You can advise patients, but be sure your paperwork is in order first because it probably will be required when the payor evaluates the patient's request.

Although the patient's portion of the payment is usually small, often only a $10.00 copayment, sometimes it is difficult to collect even this small amount. Collection laws differ for each state, but they must be followed.

When you accept payments directly from payors, you are required to collect copayment amounts from patients. Internal collection methods begin with collecting copayments, coinsurance, and deductible amounts at the time of service unless specific circumstances exist.

Patient statements are only sent when a balance remains after all insurance payments arrive. Once you know the remaining patient balance, you also know the insurance write-off. Post the insurance write-off before printing the patient statement so the total balance due on the statement is a patient responsibility amount.

A collections agency will need the patient's Social Security number and driver's license number to effectively find the patient and request payment. When payment is not made and the patient has not contested the charge, most collections agencies report delinquent transactions to the credit bureau. Once a delinquent transaction is reported to the credit bureau, only the agency that reported the delinquent transaction can get it removed.

Provider noncompliance cannot be tolerated, but it can be dealt with in a tactful and gentle manner. There are many internal methods and outside resources to help physicians meet difficult compliance requirements.

If a physician absolutely will not change and is determined to remain noncompliant, find other work. Every time you submit a claim with false or inaccurate information, in the eyes of the law you are as guilty as the physician.

Answer the following questions:

1. What is a curriculum vitae?

   _____

   _____

2. When a fee schedule does not list all the codes your practice bills, what should you do?

   _____

   _____

3. Indemnity plans do not require payor-physician contracts. Should you expect full payment using your practice fee schedule? Why or why not?

   _____

4. What does "RBRVS" stand for?

   _____

5. Can you send an appeal any time you want to? Why or why not?

   _____

6. Is the payor ever allowed to determine the level of service, and if so, why?

   _____

   _____

7. Where do you learn how to bill capitation services for a specific payor?

   _____

8. How do you know whether you may balance-bill a patient?

   _____

9. What tool helps you remember contract requirements?

   _____

10. May a patient's spouse see the patient's medical record without a written consent from the patient? Why or why not?

    _____

11. What is Medicare's time limit for filing a clean claim?

   _____

12. Working together as a team minimizes human error.
    ____True   ____False

13. When an EOB says "patient not covered," it always means that eligibility was not performed.
    ____True   ____False

14. When an EOB says "patient or procedure not covered," it always means this is a noncovered service.
    ____True   ____False

15. When a vital piece of information is missing on the claim, what error code is most often used on the EOB?

   _____

16. Physicians always code services correctly.
    ____True   ____False

17. It is best to collect patient payment on the day of the appointment.
    ____True   ____False

18. The physician can remove a history of delinquent payments reported by a collections agency from the patient's credit report.
    ____True   ____False

19. Continuing education is one option for helping a noncompliant physician come into compliance.
    ____True   ____False

20. If you become a relator in a Qui Tam action, you will definitely collect a lot of money.
    ____True   ____False

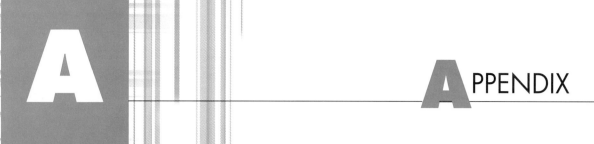

APPENDIX

1997 Examination Tables*

TABLE A-1A
General Multi-System Examination

Organ System/Body Area	Elements of General Multi-System Examination
Constitutional	❏ Measurement of any three of the following seven vital signs: (1) sitting or standing blood pressure, (2) supine blood pressure, (3) pulse rate and regularity, (4) respiration, (5) temperature, (6) height, (7) weight (may be measured and recorded by ancillary staff) ❏ General appearance of patient (e.g., development, nutrition, body habitus, deformities, attention to grooming)
Eyes	❏ Inspection of conjunctiva and lids ❏ Examination of pupils and irises (e.g., reaction to light and accommodation, size, and symmetry) ❏ Ophthalmoscopic examination of optic discs (e.g., size, C/D ratio, appearance) and posterior segments (e.g., vessel changes, exudates, hemorrhages)
Ears, Nose, Mouth, and Throat	❏ External inspection of ears and nose (e.g., overall appearance, scars, lesions, masses) ❏ Otoscopic examination of external auditory canals and tympanic membranes ❏ Assessment of hearing (e.g., whispered voice, finger rub, tuning fork) ❏ Inspection of nasal mucosa, septum, turbinates ❏ Inspection of lips, teeth, and gums ❏ Examination of oropharynx: oral mucosa, salivary glands, hard and soft palates, tongue, tonsils, and posterior pharynx
Neck	❏ Examination of neck (e.g., masses, overall appearance, symmetry, tracheal position, crepitus) ❏ Examination of thyroid (e.g., enlargement, tenderness, mass)
Respiratory	❏ Assessment of respiratory effort (e.g., intercostal retractions, use of accessory muscles, diaphragmatic movement) ❏ Percussion of chest (e.g., dullness, flatness, hyperresonance) ❏ Auscultation of lungs (e.g., breath sounds, adventitious sounds, rubs)

Cardiovascular	❏ Palpitation of heart (e.g., location, size, thrills)
	❏ Auscultation of heart with notation of abnormal sounds and murmurs
	❏ Examination of:
	   ❏ Carotid arteries (e.g., pulse amplitude, bruits)
	   ❏ Abdominal aorta (e.g., size, bruits)
	   ❏ Femoral arteries (e.g., pulse amplitude, bruits)
	   ❏ Pedal pulses (e.g., pulse amplitude)
	   ❏ Extremities for edema and/or varicosity *Continued.*

*Source: Department of Health and Human Services, Centers for Medicare and Medicaid Services.

TABLE A-1A
General Multi-System Examination—cont'd

Organ System/Body Area	Elements of General Multi-System Examination
Chest (Breasts)	❑ Inspection of breasts (e.g., symmetry, nipple discharge) ❑ Palpation of breasts and axillae (e.g., masses, lumps, tenderness)
Gastrointestinal (Abdomen)	❑ Examination of abdomen with notation of presence of masses or tenderness ❑ Examination of liver and spleen ❑ Examination for presence or absence of hernia ❑ Examination, when indicated, of anus, perineum and rectum, including sphincter tone, presence of hemorrhoids, rectal masses ❑ Obtain stool sample for occult blood test when indicated

Genitourinary	MALE:
	❑ External examination of the scrotal contents (e.g., hydrocele, spermatocele, tenderness of cord, testicular mass)
	❑ Examination of the penis
	❑ Digital rectal examination of prostate gland (e.g., size, symmetry, nodularity, tenderness)
	FEMALE:
	❑ Pelvic examination (with or without specimen collection for smears and cultures), including:
	  ❑ Examination of external genitalia (e.g., general appearance, hair distribution, lesions) and vagina (e.g., general appearance, estrogen effect, discharge, lesions, pelvic support, cystocele, rectocele)
	  ❑ Examination of urethra (e.g., masses, tenderness, scarring)
	  ❑ Examination of bladder (e.g., fullness, masses, tenderness)
	  ❑ Cervix (e.g., general appearance, lesions, discharge)
	  ❑ Uterus (e.g., size, contour, position, mobility, tenderness, consistency, descent or support)
	  ❑ Adnexa/parametria (e.g., masses, tenderness, organomegaly, nodularity)

Lymphatic	❑ Palpation of lymph nodes in two or more areas:
	  ❑ Neck
	  ❑ Axillae
	  ❑ Groin
	  ❑ Other

Musculoskeletal	❑ Examination of gait and station
	❑ Inspection and/or palpatation of digits and nails (e.g., clubbing, cyanosis, inflammatory conditions, petechiae, ischemia, infection, nodes)
	❑ Examination of joints, bones and muscles of one or more of the following six areas: (1) head and neck; (2) spine, ribs and pelvis; (3) right upper extremity; (4) left upper extremity; (5) right lower extremity; and (6) left lower extremity. The examination of a given area includes:
	  ❑ Inspection and/or palpatation with notation of presence of any misalignment, asymmetry, crepitation, defects, tenderness, masses, effusions
	  ❑ Assessment of range of motion, with notation of any pain, crepitation, or contracture
	  ❑ Assessment of stability with notation of any dislocation (luxation), subluxation, or laxity
	  ❑ Assessment of muscle strength and tone (e.g., flaccid, cogwheel, spastic) with notation of any atrophy or abnormal movements

Skin	❑ Inspection of skin and subcutaneous tissue (e.g., rashes, lesions, ulcers) ❑ Palpation of skin and subcutaneous tissue (e.g., induration, subcutaneous nodules, tightening)
Neurological	❑ Test cranial nerves with notation of any deficits ❑ Examination of deep tendon reflexes with notation of pathologic reflexes (e.g., Babinski) ❑ Examination of sensation (e.g., touch, pin, vibration, proprioception)

Psychiatric	❑ Description of patient's judgment and insight
	❑ Brief assessment of mental status, including:
	  ❑ Orientation to time, place, and person
	  ❑ Recent and remote memory
	  ❑ Mood and affect (e.g., depression, anxiety, agitation)

TABLE A-1B
Content and Documentation Requirements—General Multi-System Examination

Level of Exam	Perform and Document
Problem Focused	One to five elements identified by a bullet
Expanded Problem-Focused	At least six elements identified by a bullet
Detailed	At least two elements identified by a bullet from each of six areas/systems Or At least 12 elements identified by a bullet in two or more areas/systems
Comprehensive	Perform all elements identified by a bullet in at least nine organ systems or body areas And Document at least two elements identified by a bullet from each of nine areas/systems

TABLE A-2A
Cardiovascular Examination

Organ System/Body Area	Elements of Cardiovascular Examination
Constitutional	❑ Measurement of any three of the following seven vital signs: (1) sitting or standing blood pressure; (2) supine blood pressure; (3) pulse rate and regularity; (4) respiration; (5) temperature; (6) height; and (7) weight (may be measured by ancillary staff) ❑ General appearance of patient (e.g., development, nutrition, body habitus, deformities, attention to grooming)
Head and Face	
Eyes Ears, Nose, Mouth, and Throat	❑ Inspection of conjunctiva and lids (e.g., xanthelasma) ❑ Inspection of teeth, gums, and palate ❑ Inspection of oral mucosa with notation of presence of pallor or cyanosis
Neck	❑ Examination of jugular veins (e.g., distention; a, v, or cannon a waves) ❑ Examination of thyroid (e.g., enlargement, tenderness, mass)
Respiratory	❑ Assessment of respiratory effort (e.g., intercostal retractions, use of accessory muscles, diaphragmatic movement) ❑ Auscultation of lungs (e.g., breath sounds, adventitious sounds, rubs)

Cardiovascular	❑ Palpation of heart (e.g., location, size, and forcefulness of the point of maximal impact; thrills; lifts; palpable S3 or S4)
	❑ Auscultation of heart including sounds, abnormal sounds and murmurs
	❑ Measurement of blood pressure in two or more extremities when indicated (e.g., aortic dissection, coarctation)
	❑ Examination of:
	   ❑ Carotid arteries (e.g., waveform, pulse amplitude, bruits, apical-carotid delay)
	   ❑ Abdominal aorta (e.g., size, bruits)
	   ❑ Femoral arteries (e.g., pulse amplitude, bruits)
	   ❑ Pedal pulses (e.g., pulse amplitude)
	   ❑ Extremities for peripheral edema and/or varicosities

Chest (Breast)	
Gastrointestinal (Abdomen)	❑ Examination of abdomen with notation of presence of masses or tenderness ❑ Examination of liver and spleen ❑ Obtain stool sample for occult blood from patients who are being considered for thrombolytic or anticoagulant therapy
Genitourinary (Abdomen)	
Lymphatic	
Musculoskeletal	❑ Examination of the back with notation of kyphosis or scoliosis ❑ Examination of gait with notation of ability to undergo exercise testing and/or to participate in exercise programs ❑ Assessment of muscle strength and tone (e.g., flaccid, cogwheel, spastic) with notation of any atrophy and abnormal movements
Extremities	❑ Inspection and palpation of digits and nails (e.g., clubbing, cyanosis, inflammation, petechiae, ischemia, infections, Osler's nodes)
Skin	❑ Inspection and/or palpation of skin and subcutaneous tissue (e.g., stasis dermatitis, ulcers, scars, xanthomas)

Neurological/Psychiatric	❑ Brief assessment of mental status, including:
	   ❑ Orientation to time, place, and person
	   ❑ Mood and affect (e.g., depression, anxiety, agitation)

TABLE A-2B
Content and Documentation Requirements—Cardiovascular Examination

Level of Exam	Perform and Document
Problem Focused	One to five elements identified by a bullet
Expanded Problem–Focused	At least six elements identified by a bullet
Detailed	At least 12 elements identified by a bullet
Comprehensive	Perform all elements identified by a bullet; document every element in each shaded box and at least one element in each unshaded box

TABLE A-3A
Ear, Nose, and Throat Examination

System/Body Area	Elements of Ear, Nose, and Throat Examination
Constitutional	❏ Measurement of any three of the following seven vital signs: (1) sitting or standing blood pressure; (2) supine blood pressure; (3) pulse rate and regularity; (4) respiration; (5) temperature; (6) height; and (7) weight (may be measured and recorded by ancillary staff) ❏ General appearance of patient (e.g., development, nutrition, body habitus, deformities, attention to grooming) ❏ Assessment of ability to communicate (e.g., use of sign language or any other communication aids) and quality of voice
Head and Face	❏ Inspection of head and face (e.g., overall appearance, scars, lesions, and masses) ❏ Palpation and/or percussion of face with notation of presence or absence of sinus tenderness ❏ Examination of salivary glands ❏ Assessment of facial strength
Eyes	❏ Test ocular motility, including primary gaze alignment
Ears, Nose, Mouth, and Throat	❏ Otoscopic examination of external auditory canals and tympanic membranes, including pneumootoscopy with notation of mobility of membranes ❏ Assessment of hearing with tuning forks and clinical speech reception thresholds (e.g., whispered voice, finger rub) ❏ External inspection of ears and nose (e.g., overall appearance, scars, lesions, and masses) ❏ Inspection of nasal mucosa, septum, and turbinates ❏ Inspection of lips, teeth, and gums ❏ Examination of oropharynx: oral mucosa, hard and soft palates, tongue, tonsils, and posterior pharynx (e.g., asymmetry, lesions, hydration of mucosal surfaces) ❏ Inspection of pharyngeal walls and pyriform sinuses (e.g., pooling of saliva, asymmetry, lesions) ❏ Examination by mirror of larynx, including the condition of the epiglottis, false vocal cords, true vocal cords, and mobility of larynx (use of mirror not required in children) ❏ Examination by mirror of nasopharynx including appearance of the mucosa, adenoids, posterior choanae, and eustachian tubes (use of mirrors not required in children)
Neck	❏ Examination of neck (e.g., masses, overall appearance, symmetry, tracheal position, crepitus) ❏ Examination of thyroid (e.g., enlargement, tenderness, mass)
Respiratory	❏ Inspection of chest, including symmetry, expansion and/or assessment of respiratory effort (e.g., intercostal retractions, use of accessory muscles, diaphragmatic movement) ❏ Auscultation of lungs (e.g., breath sounds, adventitious sounds, rubs)
Cardiovascular	❏ Auscultation of heart with notation of abnormal sounds and murmurs ❏ Examination of peripheral vascular system by observation (e.g., swelling, varicosities) and palpation (e.g., pulses, temperature, edema, tenderness)

TABLE A-3A
Ear, Nose, and Throat Examination—cont'd

System/Body Area	Elements of Ear, Nose, and Throat Examination
Chest (Breasts)	
Gastrointestinal (Abdomen)	
Genitourinary	
Lymphatic	❑ Palpation of lymph nodes in neck, axillae, groin, or other location
Musculoskeletal	
Extremities	
Skin	

Neurological/Psychiatric	❑ Test cranial nerves with notation of any deficits
	❑ Brief assessment of mental status including:
	   ❑ Orientation to time, place, and person
	   ❑ Mood and affect (e.g., depression, anxiety, agitation)

TABLE A-3B
Content and Documentation Requirements—Ear, Nose, and Throat Examination

Level of Exam	Perform and Document
Problem Focused	One to five elements identified by a bullet
Expanded Problem-Focused	At least six elements identified by a bullet
Detailed	At least 12 elements identified by a bullet
Comprehensive	Perform all elements identified by a bullet; document every element in each shaded box and at least one element in each unshaded box

TABLE A-4A
Eye Examination

System/Body Area	Elements of Eye Examination
Constitutional	
Head and Face	

Eyes	❑ Test visual acuity (does not include determination of refractive error)
	❑ Gross visual field testing by confrontation
	❑ Test ocular motility, including primary gaze alignment
	❑ Inspection of bulbar and palpebral conjunctivae
	❑ Examination of ocular adnexae, including lids (e.g., ptosis or lagophthalmos), lacrimal glands, lacrimal drainage, orbits, and preauricular lymph nodes
	❑ Examination of pupils and irises, including shape, direct and consensual reaction (afferent pupil), size (e.g., anisocoria), and morphology
	❑ Slit lamp examination of the corneas including epithelium, stroma, endothelium, and tear film
	❑ Slit lamp examination of the anterior chambers, including depth, cells, and flare
	❑ Slit lamp examination of the lenses, including clarity, anterior and posterior capsule, cortex, and nucleus
	❑ Measurement of intraocular pressures (except in children and patients with trauma or infectious disease)
	❑ Ophthalmoscopic examination through dilated pupils (unless contraindicated) of:
	   ❑ Optic discs, including size, C/D ratio, appearance (e.g., atrophy, cupping, tumor elevation), and nerve fiber layer
	   ❑ Posterior segments, including retina and vessels (e.g., exudates and hemorrhages)

Continued.

TABLE A-4A
Eye Examination—cont'd

System/Body Area	Elements of Eye Examination
Ears, Nose, Mouth and Throat	
Neck	
Respiratory	
Cardiovascular	
Chest (Breasts)	
Gastrointestinal (Abdomen)	
Genitourinary	
Lymphatic	
Musculoskeletal	
Extremities	
Skin	

Neurological/Psychiatric	❑ Brief assessment of mental status including:
	   ❑ Orientation to time, place, and person
	   ❑ Mood and affect (e.g., depression, anxiety, agitation)

TABLE A-4B
Content and Documentation Requirements—Eye Examination

Level of Exam	Perform and Document
Problem Focused	One to five elements identified by a bullet
Expanded Problem-Focused	At least six elements identified by a bullet
Detailed	At least nine elements identified by a bullet
Comprehensive	Perform all elements identified by a bullet; document every element in each shaded box and at least one element in each unshaded box

TABLE A-5A
Genitourinary Examination

System/Body Area	Elements of Genitourinary Examination
Constitutional	❑ Measurement of any three of the following seven vital signs: (1) sitting or standing blood pressure; (2) supine blood pressure; (3) pulse rate and regularity; (4) respiration; (5) temperature; (6) height; and (7) weight (may be measured by ancillary staff) ❑ General appearance of patient (e.g., development, nutrition, body habitus, deformities, attention to grooming)
Head and Face	
Eyes	
Ears, Nose, Mouth, and Throat	
Neck	❑ Examination of the neck (e.g., masses, overall appearance, symmetry, tracheal position, crepitus) ❑ Examination of thyroid (e.g., enlargement, tenderness, mass)
Respiratory	❑ Assessment of respiratory effort (e.g., intercostal retractions, use of accessory muscles, diaphragmatic movement) ❑ Auscultation of lungs (e.g., breath sounds, adventitious sounds, rubs)
Cardiovascular	❑ Auscultation of heart with notation of abnormal sounds and murmurs ❑ Examination of peripheral vascular system by observation (e.g., swelling, varicosities) and palpation (e.g., pulses, temperature, edema, tenderness)
Chest (Breasts)	❑ (See Genitourinary [Female].)
Gastrointestinal (Abdomen)	❑ Examination of abdomen with notation of presence of masses or tenderness ❑ Examination for presence or absence of hernia ❑ Examination of liver and spleen ❑ Obtain stool sample for occult blood test when indicated

TABLE A-5A
Genitourinary Examination—cont'd

System/Body Area	Elements of Genitourinary Examination

Genitourinary	**MALE:**
	❑ Inspection of anus and perineum
	❑ Examination (with or without specimen collection for smears and cultures) of genitalia, including:
	  ❑ Scrotum (e.g., lesions, cysts, rashes)
	  ❑ Epididymis (e.g., size, symmetry, masses)
	  ❑ Testes (e.g., size, symmetry, masses)
	  ❑ Urethral meatus (e.g., size, location, lesions, drainage)
	  ❑ Penis (e.g., lesions, presence or absence of foreskin, foreskin retractability, plaque, masses, scarring, deformities)
	❑ Digital rectal examination, including:
	  ❑ Prostate gland (e.g., size, symmetry, nodularity, tenderness)
	  ❑ Seminal vesicles (e.g., symmetry, tenderness, masses, enlargement)
	  ❑ Sphincter tone, presence of hemorrhoids, rectal masses

Genitourinary	**FEMALE:**
	Includes at least seven of the following 11 elements identified by bullets:
	❑ Inspection and palpation of breasts (e.g., masses or lumps, tenderness, symmetry, nipple discharge)
	❑ Digital rectal examination including sphincter tone, presence of hemorrhoids, rectal masses
	❑ Pelvic examination (with or without specimen collection for smears or cultures), including:
	  ❑ External genitalia (e.g., general appearance, hair distribution, lesions)
	  ❑ Urethral meatus (e.g., size, location, lesions, prolapse)
	  ❑ Urethra (e.g., masses, tenderness, scarring)
	  ❑ Bladder (e.g., fullness, masses, tenderness)
	  ❑ Vagina (e.g., general appearance, estrogen effect, discharge, lesions, pelvic support, cystocele, rectocele)
	  ❑ Cervix (e.g., general appearance, lesions, discharge)
	  ❑ Uterus (e.g., size, contour, position, mobility, tenderness, consistency, descent, or support)
	  ❑ Adnexa/parametria (e.g., masses, tenderness, organomegaly, nodularity)
	  ❑ Anus and perineum

Lymphatic	❑ Palpation of lymph nodes in neck, axillae, groin, or other location
Musculoskeletal	
Extremities	
Skin	❑ Inspection and/or palpation of skin and subcutaneous tissue (e.g., rashes, lesions, ulcers)

Neurological/Psychiatric	❑ Brief assessment of mental status, including:
	  ❑ Orientation to time, place, and person
	  ❑ Mood and affect (e.g., depression, anxiety, agitation)

TABLE A-5B
Content and Documentation Requirements—Genitourinary Examination

Level of Exam	Perform and Document
Problem Focused	One to five elements identified by a bullet
Expanded Problem-Focused	At least six elements identified by a bullet
Detailed	At least 12 elements identified by a bullet
Comprehensive	Perform all elements identified by a bullet; document every element in each shaded box and at least one element in each unshaded box

TABLE A-6A
Hematologic/Lymphatic/Immunologic Examination

System/Body Area	Elements of Hematologic/Lymphatic/Immunologic Examination
Constitutional	☐ Measurement of any three of the following seven vital signs: (1) sitting or standing blood pressure; (2) supine blood pressure; (3) pulse rate and regularity; (4) respiration; (5) temperature; (6) height; and (7) weight (may be measured by ancillary staff) ☐ General appearance of patient (e.g., development, nutrition, body habitus, deformities, attention to grooming)
Head and Face	☐ Palpation and/or percussion of face with notation of presence or absence of sinus tenderness
Eyes	☐ Inspection of conjunctivae and lids
Ears, Nose, Mouth and Throat	☐ Otoscopic examination of external auditory channels and tympanic membranes ☐ Inspection of nasal mucosa, septum, and turbinates ☐ Inspection of teeth and gums ☐ Examination of oropharynx (e.g., oral mucosa, hard and soft palates, tongue, tonsils, posterior pharynx)
Neck	☐ Examination of the neck (e.g., masses, overall appearance, symmetry, tracheal position, crepitus) ☐ Examination of thyroid (e.g., enlargement, tenderness, mass)
Respiratory	☐ Assessment of respiratory effort (e.g., intercostal retractions, use of accessory muscles, diaphragmatic movement) ☐ Auscultation of lungs (e.g., breath sounds, adventitious sounds, rubs)
Cardiovascular	☐ Auscultation of heart with notation of abnormal sounds and murmurs ☐ Examination of peripheral vascular system by observation (e.g., swelling, varicosities) and palpation (e.g., pulses, temperature, edema, tenderness)
Chest (Breasts)	
Gastrointestinal (Abdomen)	☐ Examination of abdomen with notation of presence of masses or tenderness ☐ Examination of liver and spleen
Genitourinary	
Lymphatic	☐ Palpation of lymph nodes in neck, axillae, groin, or other location
Musculoskeletal	
Extremities	☐ Inspection and palpation of digits and nails (e.g., clubbing, cyanosis, inflammation, petechiae, ischemia, infections, nodes)
Skin	☐ Inspection and/or palpation of skin and subcutaneous tissue (e.g., rashes, lesions, ulcers, ecchymoses, bruises)

Neurological/Psychiatric	☐ Brief assessment of mental status, including:
	  ☐ Orientation to time, place, and person
	  ☐ Mood and affect (e.g., depression, anxiety, agitation)

TABLE A-6B
Content and Documentation Requirements—Hematologic/Lymphatic/Immunologic Examination

Level of Exam	Perform and Document
Problem Focused	One to five elements identified by a bullet
Expanded Problem-Focused	At least six elements identified by a bullet
Detailed	At least 12 elements identified by a bullet
Comprehensive	Perform all elements identified by a bullet; document every element in each shaded box and at least one element in each unshaded box

TABLE A-7A
Musculoskeletal Examination

System/Body Area	Elements of Musculoskeletal Examination
Constitutional	❑ Measurement of any three of the following seven vital signs: (1) sitting or standing blood pressure; (2) supine blood pressure; (3) pulse rate and regularity; (4) respiration; (5) temperature; (6) height; and (7) weight (may be measured by ancillary staff) ❑ General appearance of patient (e.g., development, nutrition, body habitus, deformities, attention to grooming)
Head and Face	
Eyes	
Ears, Nose, Mouth, and Throat	
Neck	
Respiratory	
Cardiovascular	❑ Examination of peripheral vascular system by observation (e.g., swelling, varicosities) and palpation (e.g., pulses, temperature, edema, tenderness)
Chest (Breasts)	
Gastrointestinal (Abdomen)	
Genitourinary	
Lymphatic	❑ Palpation of lymph nodes in neck, axillae, groin, or other location

Musculoskeletal	❑ Examination of gait and station
	❑ Examination of joint(s), bone(s), and muscle(s)/tendon(s) of four of the following six areas: (1) head and neck, (2) spine, ribs and pelvis, (3) right upper extremity, (4) left upper extremity, (5) right lower extremity, and (6) left lower extremity. The examination of a given area includes:
	  ❑ Inspection, percussion, and palpation with notation of any misalignment, asymmetry, crepitation, defects, tenderness, masses, or effusions
	  ❑ Assessment of range of motion with notation of any pain (e.g., straight leg raising), crepitation, or contracture
	  ❑ Assessment of stability with notation of any dislocation (luxation), subluxation, or laxity
	  ❑ Assessment of muscle strength and tone (e.g., flaccid, cogwheel, spastic) with notation of any atrophy or abnormal movements
	NOTE: For the comprehensive level of examination, all four of the elements identified by a bullet must be performed and documented for each of the four anatomic areas. For the three lower levels of examination, each element is counted separately for each body area. For example, assessing range of motion in two extremities constitutes two elements.

Extremities	(See Musculoskeletal and Skin.)
Skin	❑ Inspection and/or palpation of the skin and subcutaneous tissue (e.g., scars, rashes, lesions, café-au-lait spots, ulcers) in four of the following six areas: (1) head and neck, (2) trunk, (3) right upper extremity, (4) left upper extremity, (5) right lower extremity, and (6) left lower extremity. NOTE: For the comprehensive level, the examination of all four anatomical areas must be documented and performed. For the three lower levels of examination, each body area is counted separately. For example, inspection of the skin and subcutaneous tissue in two extremities counts as two elements.

Neurological/Psychiatric	❑ Test coordination (e.g., finger/nose, heel/knee/shin, rapid alternating movements in the upper and lower extremities, evaluation of fine motor coordination in young children)
	❑ Examination of deep tendon reflexes and/or nerve stretch test with notation of pathologic reflexes (e.g., Babinski)
	❑ Examination of sensation (e.g., by touch, pin, vibration, proprioception)
	❑ Brief assessment of mental status, including:
	  ❑ Orientation to time, place, and person
	  ❑ Mood and affect (e.g., depression, anxiety, agitation)

TABLE A-7B
Content and Documentation Requirements—Musculoskeletal Examination

Level of Exam	Perform and Document
Problem Focused	One to five elements identified by a bullet
Expanded Problem-Focused	At least six elements identified by a bullet
Detailed	At least 12 elements identified by a bullet
Comprehensive	Perform all elements identified by a bullet; document every element in each shaded box and at least one element in each unshaded box

TABLE A-8A
Neurologic Examination

System/Body Area	Elements of Neurologic Examination
Constitutional	☐ Measurement of any three of the following seven vital signs: (1) sitting or standing blood pressure; (2) supine blood pressure; (3) pulse rate and regularity; (4) respiration; (5) temperature; (6) height; and (7) weight (may be measured by ancillary staff) ☐ General appearance of patient (e.g., development, nutrition, body habitus, deformities, attention to grooming)
Head and Face	
Eyes	☐ Ophthalmoscopic examination of optic discs (e.g., size, C/D ratio, appearance) and posterior segments (e.g., vessel changes, exudates, hemorrhages)
Ears, Nose, Mouth, and Throat	
Neck	
Respiratory	
Cardiovascular	☐ Examination of carotid arteries (e.g., pulse amplitude, bruits) ☐ Auscultation of heart with notation of abnormal sounds and murmurs ☐ Examination of peripheral vascular system by observation (e.g., swelling, varicosities) and palpation (e.g., pulses, temperature, edema, tenderness)
Chest (Breasts)	
Gastrointestinal (Abdomen)	
Genitourinary	
Lymphatic	

Musculoskeletal	☐ Examination of gait and station
	☐ Assessment of motor function, including:
	  ☐ Muscle strength in upper and lower extremities
	  ☐ Muscle tone in upper and lower extremities (flaccid, cog wheel, spastic) with notation of any atrophy or abnormal movements (e.g., fasciculation, tardive dyskinesia)

Extremities	(See Musculoskeletal.)
Skin	

Neurological	☐ Evaluation of higher integrative functions, including:
	  ☐ Orientation to time, person, and place
	  ☐ Recent and remote memory
	  ☐ Attention span and concentration
	  ☐ Language (e.g., naming objects, repeating phrases, spontaneous speech)
	  ☐ Fund of knowledge (e.g., awareness of current events, past history, vocabulary)
	☐ Test the following cranial nerves:
	  ☐ 2nd cranial nerve (e.g., visual acuity, visual fields, fundi)
	  ☐ 3rd, 4th, and 6th cranial nerves (e.g., pupils, eye movement)
	  ☐ 5th cranial nerve (e.g., facial sensation, corneal reflexes)
	  ☐ 7th cranial nerve (e.g., facial symmetry, strength)
	  ☐ 8th cranial nerve (e.g., hearing with tuning fork, whispered voice and/or finger rub)
	  ☐ 9th cranial nerve (e.g., spontaneous or reflex palate movements)
	  ☐ 11th cranial nerve (e.g., shoulder shrug strength)
	  ☐ 12th cranial nerve (e.g., tongue protrusion)

Neurological	☐ Examination of sensation (e.g., by touch, pin, vibration, proprioception) ☐ Examination of deep tendon reflexes in upper and lower extremities with notation of pathologic reflexes (e.g., Babinski) ☐ Test coordination (e.g., finger/nose, heel/knee/shin, rapid alternating movements in the upper and lower extremities, evaluation of fine motor coordination in young children)
Psychiatric	

TABLE A-8B
Content and Documentation Requirements—Neurologic Examination

Level of Exam	Perform and Document
Problem Focused	One to five elements identified by a bullet
Expanded Problem-Focused	At least six elements identified by a bullet
Detailed	At least 12 elements identified by a bullet
Comprehensive	Perform all elements identified by a bullet; document every element in each shaded box and at least one element in each unshaded box

TABLE A-9A
Psychiatric Examination

System/Body Area	Elements of Psychiatric Examination
Constitutional	☐ Measurement of any three of the following seven vital signs: (1) sitting or standing blood pressure; (2) supine blood pressure; (3) pulse rate and regularity; (4) respiration; (5) temperature; (6) height; and (7) weight (may be measured by ancillary staff) ☐ General appearance of patient (e.g., development, nutrition, body habitus, deformities, attention to grooming)
Head and Face	
Eyes	
Ears, Nose, Mouth, and Throat	
Neck	
Respiratory	
Cardiovascular	
Chest (Breasts)	
Gastrointestinal (Abdomen)	
Genitourinary	
Lymphatic	
Musculoskeletal	☐ Assessment of muscle strength (e.g., flaccid, cogwheel, spastic) with notation of any atrophy and abnormal movements ☐ Examination of gait and station
Extremities	
Skin	
Neurological	

Psychiatric	☐ Description of speech, including: rate, volume, articulation, coherence, and spontaneity with notation of abnormalities (e.g., perseveration, paucity of language)
	☐ Description of thought processes, including rate of thoughts; content of thoughts (e.g., logical vs. illogical, tangential); abstract reasoning; and computation
	☐ Description of associations (e.g., loose, tangential, circumstantial, intact)
	☐ Description of abnormal or psychotic thoughts, including hallucinations, delusions, preoccupation with violence, homicidal or suicidal ideation, and obsessions
	☐ Description of the patient's judgment (e.g., concerning everyday activities and social situations) and insights (e.g., concerning psychiatric condition)
	☐ Complete mental status examination, including:
	  ☐ Orientation to time, place and person
	  ☐ Recent and remote memory
	  ☐ Attention span and concentration
	  ☐ Language (e.g., naming objects, repeating phrases)
	  ☐ Fund of knowledge (e.g., awareness of current events, past history, vocabulary)
	  ☐ Mood and affect (e.g., depression, anxiety, agitation, hypomania, lability)

TABLE A-9B
Content and Documentation Requirements—Psychiatric Examination

Level of Exam	Perform and Document
Problem Focused	One to five elements identified by a bullet
Expanded Problem-Focused	At least six elements identified by a bullet
Detailed	At least nine elements identified by a bullet
Comprehensive	Perform all elements identified by a bullet; document every element in each shaded box and at least one element in each unshaded box

TABLE A-10A
Respiratory Examination

System/Body Area	Elements of Respiratory Examination
Constitutional	❑ Measurement of any three of the following seven vital signs: (1) sitting or standing blood pressure; (2) supine blood pressure; (3) pulse rate and regularity; (4) respiration; (5) temperature; (6) height; and (7) weight (may be measured by ancillary staff) ❑ General appearance of patient (e.g., development, nutrition, body habitus, deformities, attention to grooming)
Head and Face	
Eyes	
Ears, Nose, Mouth, and Throat	❑ Inspection of nasal mucosa, septum, and turbinates ❑ Inspection of teeth and gums ❑ Examination of oropharynx (e.g., oral mucosa, hard and soft palates, tongue, tonsils, and posterior pharynx)
Neck	❑ Examination of neck (e.g., masses, overall appearance, symmetry, tracheal position, crepitus) ❑ Examination of thyroid (e.g., enlargement, tenderness, mass) ❑ Examination of jugular veins (e.g., distention; a, v, or cannon a waves)
Respiratory	❑ Inspection of chest with notation of symmetry and expansion ❑ Assessment of respiratory effort (e.g., intercostal retractions, use of accessory muscles, diaphragmatic movement) ❑ Percussion of chest (e.g., dullness, flatness, hyperresonance) ❑ Palpation of chest (e.g., tactile fremitus) ❑ Auscultation of lungs (e.g., breath sounds, adventitious sounds, rubs)
Cardiovascular	❑ Auscultation of heart, including sounds, abnormal sounds, and murmurs ❑ Examination of peripheral vascular system by observation (e.g., swelling, varicosities) and palpation (e.g., pulses, temperature, edema, tenderness)
Chest (Breasts)	
Gastrointestinal (Abdomen)	❑ Examination of abdomen with notation of presence of masses or tenderness ❑ Examination of liver and spleen
Genitourinary	
Lymphatic	❑ Palpation of lymph nodes in neck, axillae, groin, or other location
Musculoskeletal	❑ Assessment of muscle strength and tone (e.g., flaccid, cogwheel, spastic) with notation of any atrophy or abnormal movements ❑ Examination of gait and station
Extremities	❑ Inspection and palpation of digits and nails (e.g., clubbing, cyanosis, inflammation, petechiae, ischemia, infections, nodes)
Skin	❑ Inspection and/or palpation of skin and subcutaneous tissue (e.g., rashes, lesions, ulcers)

Neurological/Psychiatric	❑ Brief assessment of mental status, including:
	   ❑ Orientation to time, place, and person
	   ❑ Mood and affect (e.g., depression, anxiety, agitation)

TABLE A-10B
Content and Documentation Requirements—Respiratory Examination

Level of Exam	Perform and Document
Problem Focused	One to five elements identified by a bullet
Expanded Problem-Focused	At least six elements identified by a bullet
Detailed	At least 12 elements identified by a bullet
Comprehensive	Perform all elements identified by a bullet; document every element in each shaded box and at least one element in each unshaded box

TABLE A-11A
Skin Examination

System/Body Area	Elements of Skin Examination
Constitutional	☐ Measurement of any three of the following seven vital signs: (1) sitting or standing blood pressure; (2) supine blood pressure; (3) pulse rate and regularity; (4) respiration; (5) temperature; (6) height; and (7) weight (may be measured by ancillary staff) ☐ General appearance of patient (e.g., development, nutrition, body habitus, deformities, attention to grooming)
Head and Face	
Eyes	☐ Inspection of conjunctivae and lids
Ears, Nose, Mouth, and Throat	☐ Inspection of lips, teeth, and gums ☐ Examination of oropharynx (e.g., oral mucosa, hard and soft palates, tongue, tonsils, posterior pharynx)
Neck	☐ Examination of thyroid (e.g., enlargement, tenderness, mass)
Respiratory	
Cardiovascular	☐ Examination of peripheral vascular system by observation (e.g., swelling, varicosities) and palpation (e.g., pulses, temperature, edema, tenderness)
Chest (Breasts)	
Gastrointestinal (Abdomen)	☐ Examination of liver and spleen
Genitourinary	☐ Examination of anus for condyloma and other lesions
Lymphatic	☐ Palpation of lymph nodes in neck, axillae, groin, or other location
Musculoskeletal	
Extremities	☐ Inspection and palpation of digits and nails (e.g., clubbing, cyanosis, inflammation, petechiae, ischemia, infections, nodes)

Skin	☐ Palpation of scalp and inspection of hair of scalp, eyebrows, face, chest, pubic area (when indicated), and extremities
	☐ Inspection and/or palpation of skin and subcutaneous tissue (e.g., rashes, lesions, ulcers, susceptibility to and presence of photo damage) in 8 of the following 10 areas:
	  ☐ Head, including the face and neck
	  ☐ Chest, including breasts and axillae
	  ☐ Abdomen
	  ☐ Genitalia, groin, buttocks
	  ☐ Back
	  ☐ Right upper extremity
	  ☐ Left upper extremity
	  ☐ Right lower extremity
	  ☐ Left lower extremity
	NOTE: For the comprehensive level, the examination of at least eight anatomic areas must be performed and documented. For the three lower levels of examination, each body area is counted separately. For example, inspection and/or palpation of the skin and subcutaneous tissue of the right upper extremity and left upper extremity constitutes two elements.
	☐ Inspection of eccrine and apocrine glands of skin and subcutaneous tissue with identification and location of any hyperhidrosis, chromhidrosis, or bromhidrosis

Neurological/Psychiatric	☐ Brief assessment of mental status, including:
	  ☐ Orientation to time, place, and person
	  ☐ Mood and affect (e.g., depression, anxiety, agitation)

TABLE A-11B
Content and Documentation Requirements—Skin Examination

Level of Exam	Perform and Document
Problem Focused	One to five elements identified by a bullet
Expanded Problem-Focused	At least six elements identified by a bullet
Detailed	At least 12 elements identified by a bullet
Comprehensive	Perform all elements identified by a bullet; document every element in each shaded box and at least one element in each unshaded box

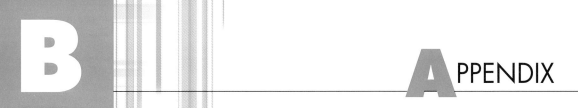

APPENDIX B

Directory of State Contacts

All states:	American Cancer Society	800-227-2345	www.cancer.org
	Medicare	800-633-4227	www.medicare.gov
	Medicare COB	800-999-1118	http://cms.hhs.gov/medicare/cob
	OIG/DHHS	800-447-8477	www.hhs.gov
	Black Lung	800-638-7072	http://www.dol.gov/esa/regs/compliance/owcp/
	National Cancer Institute	800-422-6237	www.cancer.gov
	Railroad Medicare Carrier:		
	Palmetto Government	800-833-4455	www.palmettogba.com
	Benefits Administrators		
	Social Security	800-772-1213	www.socialsecurity.gov
	Department of Veterans Affairs	800-827-1000	www.va.gov

State	Type	Agency	Telephone	Toll Free	Website
Alabama	DMERC	Palmetto Government Benefits Administrators (GBA)	—	800-583-2236	—
	ESRD	Network 8, Inc.	601-936-9260	877-936-9260	—
	Health Department	Alabama Department of Public Health	334-206-5300	—	www.adph.org
	Insurance Department	Insurance Department of Alabama	334-269-3550	800-433-3966	www.aldoi.gov/
	CMS Carrier	BCBS of Alabama	—	800-292-8855	—
	CMS FI	BCBS of Alabama	—	800-292-8855	www.almedicare.com
	Medicaid	Alabama Medicaid Agency	334-242-5000	800-362-1504	www.medicaid.state.al.us/

Continued.

State	Type	Agency	Telephone	Toll Free	Website
	QIO (PRO)	Alabama Quality Assurance Foundation	205-977-4205	800-760-3540	www.aqaf.com
	SHIP	Alabama Department of Senior Services	334-242-5743	800-243-5463	www.adss.state.al.us/
	SCHIP	State Children's Health Insurance—ALL Kids	334-206-5568	888-373-5437	www.adph.org/allkids/
Alaska	DMERC	CIGNA (Connecticut General Life Insurance Company of North America)	—	800-899-7095	http://cignamedicare.com
	ESRD	Northwest Renal Network—Network 16	206-923-0714	800-262-1514	—
	Health Department	Alaska Department of Health and Social Services	907-465-3030	—	www.state.ak.us
	Insurance Department	Insurance Division of Alaska	907-269-7900	800-467-8725	www.dced.state.ak.us/insurance
	CMS Carrier	Noridian Mutual Insurance Co.	—	800-444-4606	—
	CMS FI	Premera Blue Cross	—	877-602-7896	—
	Medicaid	Alaska Department of Health and Social Services	907-465-3355	800-780-9972	www.hss.state.ak.us/
	QIO (PRO)	QualisHealth	—	800-445-6941	www.qualishealth.org
	SHIP	Alaska Medicare Information	907-269-3654	800-478-6065	www.state.ak.us/local/akpages/ADMIN/dss/
	SCHIP	State Child Health Insurance—Denali KidCare	907-269-6529	888-318-8890	www.hss.state.ak.us/dhcs/denalikidcare/
American Samoa	DMERC	CIGNA (Connecticut General Life Insurance Company of North America)	—	800-899-7095	http://cignamedicare.com
	ESRD	TransPacific Renal Network—No. 17	415-472-8590	800-232-3773	www.network17.org
	Health Department	Hawaii Department of Health	808-586-4400	—	www.hawaii.gov/health
	Insurance Department	Office of the Governor of American Samoa	684-633-4116	—	—
	CMS Carrier	Noridian Mutual Insurance Company	—	800-444-4606	—
	CMS FI	United Government Services	866-264-4990	—	—
	Medicaid	Department of Human Services of Hawaii	808-524-3370	800-316-8005	www.med-quest.us/
	QIO (PRO)	Mountain-Pacific Quality Health Foundation	808-545-2550	800-524-6550	www.mpqhf.org
	SHIP	PLUS	808-586-7299	888-875-9229	www.hawaii.gov/eoa/index.html
	SCHIP	American Samoa Child Health Insurance Program	684-633-4590	—	—
Arizona	DMERC	CIGNA (Connecticut General Life Insurance Company of North America)	—	800-899-7095	http://cignamedicare.com

State	Type	Agency	Telephone	Toll Free	Website
	ESRD	Intermountain ESRD Network—Network 15	303-831-8818	800-783-8818	—
	Health Department	Arizona Department of Health Services	602-417-4000	—	www.hs.state.az.us/division.htm
	Insurance Department	Arizona Department of Insurance	602-912-8444	800-325-2548	www.id.state.az.us/
	CMS Carrier	Noridian Mutual Insurance Co.	—	800-444-4606	—
	CMS FI	BCBS of Arizona	—	877-602-7909	—
	Medicaid	Health Care Cost Containment of Arizona	602-417-7000	800-962-6690	www.ahcccs.state.az.us
	QIO (PRO)	Health Services Advisory Group, Inc.	602-264-6382	800-359-9909	www.hsag.com
	SHIP	Arizona State Health Insurance Assistance Program	602-542-6595	800-432-4040	www.de.state.az.us/aaa/programs/ship/
	SCHIP	State Child Health Insurance—Arizona KidsCare	602-417-5437	877-764-5437	www.kidscare.state.az.us/
Arkansas	DMERC	Palmetto Government Benefits Administrators (GBA)	—	800-583-2236	—
	ESRD	End Stage Renal Disease Network 13	405-942-6000	800-472-8664	www.network13.org
	Health Department	Arkansas Department of Health	501-661-2000	800-482-5400	www.healthyarkansas.com/health.html
	Insurance Department	Department of Insurance of Arkansas	501-371-2782	800-224-6330	www.state.ar.us/insurance/
	CMS Carrier	BCBS of Arkansas	—	800-482-5525	—
	CMS FI	BCBS of Arkansas	—	877-356-2368	—
	Medicaid	Department of Human Services of Arkansas	501-682-8292	800-482-5431	www.medicaid.state.ar.us/
	QIO (PRO)	Arkansas Foundation for Medical Care	479-649-8501	800-272-5528	www.afmc.org
	SHIP	State Health Insurance Assistance Program of Arkansas	501-371-2782	800-224-6330	www.accessarkansas.org/insurance/
	SCHIP	State Child Health Insurance—ARKids First	501-682-8269	800-482-5431	www.arkidsfirst.com/
California	DMERC	CIGNA (Connecticut General Life Insurance Company of North America)	—	800-899-7095	http://cignamedicare.com
	ESRD—South	Southern California Renal Disease Council—Network 18	323-962-2020	800-637-4767	www.esrdnetwork18.org
	ESRD—Pacific	TransPacific Renal Network—No. 17	415-472-8590	800-232-3773	www.network17.org
	Health Department	California Department of Health Services	916-445-4171	—	www.dhs.cahwnet.gov/home/contactinfo
	Insurance Department	Department of Consumer Insurance of California	213-897-8921	800-927-4357	www.insruance.ca.gov/index.html
	CMS Carrier	National Heritage Insurance Company	—	800-952-8627	www.medicarenhic.com
	CMS FI	United Government Services	877-647-6528	866-804-0684	—

Continued.

State	Type	Agency	Telephone	Toll Free	Website
	Medicaid	California Department of Health Services	916-636-1980	800-541-5555	www.medi-cal.ca.gov
	QIO (PRO)	Lumetra	415-677-2000	800-841-1602	www.cmri-ca.org
	SHIP	Health Insurance Counsel and Advocacy Program of California	—	800-434-0222	www.aging.ca.gov
	SCHIP	State Child Health Insurance—Healthy Families	—	800-880-5305	www.healthyfamilies. ca.gov/
Colorado	DMERC	Palmetto Government Benefits Administrators (GBA)	—	800-583-2236	www.palmettogba.com
	ESRD	Intermountain ESRD Network 15	303-831-8818	800-783-8818	—
	Health Department	Colorado Department of Public Health and Environment	303-692-2035	—	www.cdphe.state.co. us/cdphehom.asp
	Insurance Department	Department of Insurance of Colorado	303-894-7499	800-930-3745	www.dora.state.co. us/insurance/
	CMS Carrier	Noridian Mutual Insurance Company	800-444-4606	800-332-6681	www.noridian medicare.com
	CMS FI	TrailBlazer Health Enterprises, LLC	—	800-442-2620	www.the-medicare. com
	Medicaid	Department Health Care Policy and Financing of Colorado	303-866-2993	800-221-3943	www.chcpf.state.co.us
	QIO (PRO)	Colorado Foundation for Medial Care	303-695-3300	800-727-7086	www.cfmc.org
	SHIP	Colorado State Health Insurance Assistance Program	303-899-5151	888-696-7213	www.colorado medicare.com
	SCHIP	Colorado Child Health Plus	303-692-2960	800-359-1991	www.cchp.org
Connecticut	DMERC	HealthNow DMERC	—	800-842-2052	http://umd.nycpic. com
	ESRD	ESRD Network of New England—Network 1	203-387-9332	866-286-3773	—
	Health Department	Connecticut Department of Public Health	860-509-8000	—	www.dph.state.ct.us
	Insurance Department	Department of Insurance of Connecticut	860-297-3800	800-203-3447	www.state.ct.us/cid/
	CMS Carrier	First Coast Service Options, Inc.	—	800-982-6819	—
	CMS FI	Empire Medical Services	—	800-442-8430	—
	Medicaid	Department of Social Services of Connecticut	860-424-4908	800-842-1508	www.dss.state.ct.us
	QIO (PRO)	Qualidigm	860-632-2008	800-553-7590	www.qualidigm.org
	SHIP	CHOICES	860-424-5245	800-994-9422	www.ctelerlyservices. state.ct.us/
	SCHIP	State Child Health Insurance—HUSKY Plan	—	877-284-8759	www.huskyhealth. com/
Delaware	DMERC	HealthNow DMERC	—	800-842-2052	http://umd.nycpic. com
	ESRD	ESRD Network 4, Inc.	412-325-2250	800-548-9205	—
	Health Department	Delaware Health and Social Services	302-255-9040	—	www.state.de.us/dhss

State	Type	Agency	Telephone	Toll Free	Website
	Insurance Department	Insurance Department of Delaware—Consumer Services Division	302-739-6775	800-282-8611	www.state.de.us/inscom
	CMS Carrier	TrailBlazer Health Enterprises, LLC	—	800-444-4606	www.mytrailblazer.com
	CMS FI	Empire Medical Services	—	800-442-8430	—
	Medicaid	Delaware Health and Social Services	302-255-9660	800-372-2022	www.state.de.us/dhss/
	QIO (PRO)	Quality Insights of Delaware	302-478-3600	866-475-9669	www.qualityinsights.org
	SHIP	ELDERinfo	302-739-6266	800-336-9500	www.state.de.us/inscom/elindex.htm
	SCHIP	Delaware Healthy Children Program	302-255-9774	800-996-9969	www.state.de.us/dhss/healthychildren.html
District of Columbia	DMERC	Adminastar Federal, Inc.	—	800-270-2313	—
	ESRD	Mid-Atlantic Renal Coalition Network 5	804-794-3757	866-651-6272	—
	Health Department	District of Columbia Department of Health	202-442-5988	—	http://dchealth.dc.gov/index.asp
	Insurance Department	Department of Insurance and Security Regulations of Washington, DC	202-727-8000	—	http://disr.washingtondc.gov/information/rights/insurance
	CMS Carrier	TrailBlazer Health Enterprises, LLC	—	800-444-4606	www.mytrailblazer.com
	CMS FI	Care First of Maryland, Inc. (d.b.a. BCBS MD)	410-252-5310	800-655-1636	—
	Medicaid	District of Columbia Department of Health	202-526-6266	888-557-1116	http://dchealth.dc.gov/about/
	QIO (PRO)	Delmarva Foundation for Medical Care, Inc.	410-822-0697	800-645-0011	www.dfmc.og
	SHIP	Washington, DC, Health Insurance Counseling Project	202-739-0668	—	http://dcoa.dc.gov/dcoa/site/default.asp
	SCHIP	State Child Health Insurance—DC Healthy Families	—	888-557-1116	www.dchealth.dc.gov/services/
Florida	DMERC	Palmetto Government Benefits Administrators (GBA)	—	800-583-2236	www.palmettogba.com
	ESRD	Florida Medical Quality Assurance, Inc.—Network 7	813-383-1530	800-826-3773	—
	Health Department	Florida Department of Health	580-245-4494	—	www.doh.state.fl.us
	Insurance Department	Department of Insurance of Florida	850-413-3100	800-342-2762	www.fldfs.com
	CMS Carrier	First Coast Service Options, Inc.	—	800-333-7586	—
	CMS FI	First Coast Service Options, Inc.	—	800-333-7586	—
	Medicaid	Agency for Health Care Administration of Florida	850-488-3560	888-419-3456	www.fdhc.state.fl.us/Medicaid/

Continued.

State	Type	Agency	Telephone	Toll Free	Website
	QIO (PRO)	Florida Medical Quality Assurance	813-354-9111	800-844-0795	www.fmqai.com
	SHIP	SHINE (Serving Health Insurance Needs of Elders)	850-414-2060	800-963-5337	http://elderaffairs. state.fl.us/doea/ english/shrine.html
	SCHIP	Florida KidCare	—	888-540-5437	www.floridakidcare. org
Georgia	DMERC	Palmetto Government Benefits Administrators (GBA)	—	800-583-2236	www.palmettogba.com
	ESRD	Southeastern Kidney Council—Network 6	919-855-0882	800-524-7139	—
	Health Department	Georgia Department of Community Health	404-656-4507	—	www.dch.state.ga.us
	Insurance Department	Department of Insurance of Georgia	404-656-2070	800-656-2298	www.gainsurance.org
	CMS Carrier	Cahaba Government Benefits Administrators (GBA)	—	800-727-0827	—
	CMS FI	BCBS of Georgia	—	800-322-3380	—
	Medicaid	Georgia Department of Community Health	770-570-3300	866-322-4260	www.communityhealth. state.ga.us//
	QIO (PRO)	Georgia Medical Care Foundation	404-982-7575	800-979-7217	www.gmcf.org
	SHIP	GeorgiaCares	404-657-5334	800-669-8387	www.state.ga.us/ departments/dhr/
	SCHIP	PeachCare for Kids	—	877-427-3224	www.peachcare.org/ dehome.asp
Guam	DMERC	CIGNA (Connecticut General Life Insurance Company of North America)	—	800-899-7095	http://cignamedicare. com
	ESRD	TransPacific Renal Network—No. 17	415-472-8590	800-232-3773	www.network17.org
	Health Department	Hawaiian Department of Health	808-586-4400	—	www.hawaii.gov/ health
	Insurance Department	Department of Revenue and Taxation of Guam	671-475-1817	—	—
	CMS Carrier	Noridian Mutual Insurance Company	—	800-444-4606	—
	CMS FI	United Government Services	—	866-264-4990	—
	QIO (PRO)	Mountain-Pacific Quality Health Foundation	808-545-2550	800-524-6550	www.mpqhf.org
	SHIP	PLUS	808-586-7299	888-875-9229	www.hawaii.gov/ eoa/
	SCHIP	Guam Department of Health Care Financing	617-735-7282	—	—
Hawaii	DMERC	CIGNA (Connecticut General Life Insurance Company of North America)	—	800-447-8477	http://cignamedicare. com
	ESRD	TransPacific Renal Network—No. 17	415-472-8590	800-232-3773	www.network17.org
	Health Department	Hawaiian Department of Health	808-586-4400	—	www.hawaii.gov/ health

State	Type	Agency	Telephone	Toll Free	Website
	Insurance Department	Insurance Division of Hawaii, Department of Commerce and Consumer Affairs	808-586-2790	800-974-4000	www.state.hi.us/dcca/ins/
	CMS Carrier	Noridian Mutual Insurance Company	—	800-444-4606	—
	CMS FI	United Government Services	—	866-264-4990	—
	Medicaid	Department of Human Services of Hawaii	808-524-3370	800-316-8005	www.med-quest.us/
	QIO (PRO)	Mountain-Pacific Quality Health Foundation	808-545-2550	800-524-6550	www.mpqhf.org.
	SHIP	PLUS	808-586-7299	888-875-9229	www.hawaii.gov/eoa/index.html
	SCHIP	Department of Human Services of Hawaii	—	—	www.med-quest.us/
Idaho	DMERC	CIGNA (Connecticut General Life Insurance Company of North America)	—	800-899-7095	http://cignamedicare.com
	ESRD	Northwest Renal Network—No. 16	206-923-0714	800-262-1514	—
	Health Department	Idaho Department of Health and Welfare	208-334-5500	—	www.state.id.us/dhw
	Insurance Department	Department of Insurance of Idaho	208-334-4250	800-721-3272	www.doi.state.id.us/
	CMS Carrier	CIGNA (Connecticut General Life Insurance Company of North America)	—	800-627-2782	—
	CMS FI	Medicare Northwest	—	866-804-0681	http://medicare.regence.com
	Medicaid	Idaho Department of Health and Welfare	208-334-5747	877-200-5441	www.state.id.us/dhw/medicaid/
	QIO (PRO)	QualisHealth	—	800-445-6941	www.qualishealth.org
	SHIP	Senior Health Insurance Benefits Advisors of Idaho	—	800-247-4422	www.doi.state.id.us/shba/shibahealth.aspx
	SCHIP	Idaho Children's Health Insurance Program	—	800-926-2588	www.idahocareline.org
Illinois	DMERC	Adminastar Federal, Inc.	—	800-270-2313	—
	ESRD	The Renal Network—Network 9/10	317-257-8265	800-456-6919	—
	Health Department	Illinois Public Health Department	217-782-4977	—	www.idph.state.il/us/
	Insurance Department	Department of Insurance of Illinois	312-814-2427	86-445-5364	www.ins.state.il.us/
	CMS Carrier	Wisconsin Physician Services	—	800-642-6930	—
	CMS FI	Adminastar Federal, Inc.	—	877-602-2430	—
	Medicaid	Department of Public Aid of Illinois	217-782-2570	800-226-0768	www.dpaillinois.com
	QIO (PRO)	Illinois Foundation for Medical Care	515-223-2900	800-383-2856	www.ifmc.org
	SHIP	Senior Health Insurance Program of Illinois	217-785-9021	800-548-9034	www.ins.state.il.us/

Continued.

State	Type	Agency	Telephone	Toll Free	Website
	SCHIP	Illinois KidCare	—	866-468-7543	www.kidcareillinois.com/
Indiana	DMERC	Adminastar Federal, Inc.	—	800-270-2313	—
	ESRD	The Renal Network—Network 9/10	317-257-8265	800-456-6919	—
	Health Department	Indiana State Department of Health	317-233-1325	—	www.in.gov/isdh
	Insurance Department	Insurance Department of Indiana—Consumer Services Division	317-232-2385	800-622-4461	www.in.gov/idoi
	CMS Carrier	Adminastar Federal, Inc.	—	800-622-4792	—
	CMS FI	Adminastar Federal, Inc.	—	877-602-2430	—
	Medicaid	Family and Social Services Administration of Indiana	317-233-4455	—	www.in.gov/fssa/healthcare/
	QIO (PRO)	Health Care Excel, Inc.	812-234-1499	800-288-1499	www.hce.org
	SHIP	Indiana Senior Health Insurance Information Program	317-232-5299	800-452-4800	www.in.gov/indoi/shiip
	SCHIP	Hoosier Healthwise	—	800-889-9949	www.state.in.us/fssa/hoosier_healthwise/
Iowa	DMERC	CIGNA (Connecticut General Life Insurance Company of North America)	—	800-899-7095	http://cignamedicare.com
	ESRD	ESRD Network 12	816-880-9990	800-444-9965	http://network12.org
	Health Department	Iowa Department of Public Health	515-281-7689	—	www.idph.state.ia.us
	Insurance Department	Insurance Division of Iowa	515-281-6867	800-35-4664	http://www/shiip.state.is.us/
	CMS Carrier	Noridian Mutual Insurance Company	—	800-532-1285	www.noridianmedicare.com
	CMS FI	Cahaba Government Benefits Administrators (GBA)	—	877-910-8139	—
	Medicaid	Department of Human Services of Iowa	515-327-5121	800-338-8366	www.dhs.state.ia/us
	QIO (PRO)	Iowa Foundation for Medical Care	515-233-2900	800-752-7014	www.ifmc.org
	SHIP	Senior Heath Insurance Information Program of Iowa	515-281-5705	800-351-4664	www.shiip.state.ia.us/
	SCHIP	hawk-i	—	800-257-8563	www.hawk-i.org/
Kansas	DMERC	CIGNA (Connecticut General Life Insurance Company of North America)	—	800-899-7095	http://cignamedicare.com
	ESRD	ESRD Network 12	816-880-9990	800-444-9965	http://network12.org
	Health Department	Kansas Department on Aging	785-296-1500	—	www.kdhe.state.ks.us/
	Insurance Department	Insurance Department of Kansas	785-296-3071	800-432-244	www.ksinsurance.org/
	CMS Carrier	BCBS of Kansas	—	800-432-3531	—
	CMS FI	BCBS of Kansas	—	800-445-7170	—
	Medicaid	Kansas Department of Social and Rehabilitation Services	785-274-4200	800-792-4884	www.srskansas.org/hcp/

State	Type	Agency	Telephone	Toll Free	Website
	QIO (PRO)	Kansas Foundation for Medical Care	785-273-2552	800-432-0407	www.kfmc.org
	SHIP	Senior Health Insurance Counseling for Kansas	316-337-7386	800-860-5260	www.agingkansas.org/shick
	SCHIP	HealthWave Program	—	800-792-4884	www.kansashealthwave.org
Kentucky	DMERC	Palmetto Government Benefits Administrators (GBA)	—	800-583-2236	—
	ESRD	The Renal Network— Network 9/10	317-257-8265	800-456-6919	—
	Health Department	Kentucky Cabinet for Health Services	502-564-6930	—	www.chs.ky.gov/
	Insurance Department	Kentucky Office of Insurance	502-564-3630	800-595-6053	www.doi.state.ky.us/
	CMS Carrier	Adminastar Federal, Inc.	—	800-583-2236	—
	CMS FI	Adminastar Federal, Inc.	—	877-602-2430	—
	Medicaid	Kentucky Cabinet for Health and Family Services	502-564-2687	800-635-2570	http://chs.ky.gov/dms/
	QIO (PRO)	Health Care Excel, Inc.	502-339-7442	800-288-1499	www.hce.org
	SHIP	Kentucky State Health Insurance Assistance Program	502-564-6930	877-293-7447	http://chs.state.ky/us/aging
	SCHIP	Kentucky Children Health Insurance Program	—	877-524-4718	http://chs.ky.gov/kchip/
Louisiana	DMERC	Palmetto Government Benefits Administrators (GBA)	—	800-583-2236	—
	ESRD	End Stage Renal Disease Network 13	405-942-6000	800-472-8664	www.network13.org
	Health Department	Louisiana Department of Health and Hospital	225-342-9500	—	www.dhh.state.la.us
	Insurance Department	Department of Insurance of Louisiana	225-342-5900	800-259-5300	www.ldi.state.la.us/
	CMS Carrier	BCBS of Arkansas	—	800-462-9666	www.lamedicare.com
	CMS FI	Trispan Health Services	—	800-932-7644	www.trispan.com
	Medicaid	Louisiana Department of Health and Hospital	225-342-5774	888-342-6207	www.dhh.state.la.us
	QIO (PRO)	Louisiana Health Care Review	225-926-6353	800-433-4958	www.lhrc.org
	SHIP	Louisiana Senior Health Insurance Information Program	225-342-5301	800-259-5301	www.ldi.state.la.gov/
	SCHIP	LaChip	—	800-252-2447	www.dhh.state.la.us/MEDICAID/LaCHIP/
Maine	DMERC	HealthNow DMERC	—	800-842-2052	http://umd.nycpic.com
	ESRD	End Stage Renal Disease Network of New England— Network 1	203-387-9332	866-286-3773	—
	Health Department	Maine Department of Human Services	207-287-2736	—	www.state.me.us/dhs
	Insurance Department	Bureau of Insurance of Maine	207-624-8475	800-300-5000	www.maineinsurancereg.org

Continued.

State	Type	Agency	Telephone	Toll Free	Website
	CMS Carrier	National Heritage Insurance Company	—	800-492-0919	—
	CMS FI	Associated Hospital Services	—	888-896-4997	—
	Medicaid	Maine Department of Human Services	207-287-3094	800-321-5557	www.state.me.us/bms
	QIO (PRO)	Northeast Health Care Quality Foundation	603-749-1641	800-772-0151	www.medicarequality.org
	SHIP	Maine State Health Insurance Assistance Program	207-623-1797	800-750-5353	www.maine.gov/dhs/beas/hiap/
	SCHIP	Maine Care	—	877-543-7669	www.maine.gov/dhs/bfi/cubcare/
Maryland	DMERC	Adminastar Federal, Inc.	—	800-270-2313	—
	ESRD	Mid-Atlantic Renal Coalition—Network 5	804-794-3757	866-651-6272	—
	Health Department	Maryland Department of Health and Mental Hygiene	410-767-6860	877-463-3464	www.dhmh.state.md.us
	Insurance Department	Insurance Administration of Maryland	410-468-2000	800-492-6116	www.mdinsurance.state.md.us/
	CMS Carrier	TrailBlazer Health Enterprises, LLC	—	800-444-4606	www.mytrailblazer.com
	CMS FI	Care First of Maryland (d.b.a. BCBS of MD)	410-252-5310	800-655-1636	—
	Medicaid	Department of Human Resources of Maryland	410-767-5800	800-492-5231	www.dhr.state.md.us/fia/medicaid.htm
	QIO (PRO)	Delmarva Foundation for Medical Care, Inc.	410-822-0697	800-492-5811	www.dfmc.org
	SHIP	Maryland Senior Health Insurance Assistance Program	410-767-1100	800-243-3425	www.mdoa.state.md.us/Services/ship.html
	SCHIP	Maryland Children's Health Insurance Program	—	800-456-8900	www.dhmh.state.md.us/mma/mchp/
Massachusetts	DMERC	HealthNow DMERC	—	800-842-2052	http://umd.nycpic.com
	ESRD	End Stage Renal Disease Network of New England—Network 1	203-387-9332	866-286-3773	—
	Health Department	Massachusetts Department of Public Health	617-624-6000	800-850-6968	www.state.ma.us/dph
	Insurance Department	Commonwealth of Massachusetts	617-521-7794	—	www.state.ma.us/consumer/
	CMS Carrier	National Heritage Insurance Company	781-741-3330	800-882-1228	—
	CMS FI	Associated Hospital Services	—	888-896-4997	—
	Medicaid	Office of Health and Human Services of Massachusetts	617-628-4141	800-325-5231	www.state.ma.us/dma
	QIO (PRO)	MassPRO	781-890-0011	800-252-5533	www.masspro.org
	SHIP	Serving Health Information Needs of Elders	—	800-243-4636	www.800ageinfo.com

State	Type	Agency	Telephone	Toll Free	Website
	SCHIP	Massachusetts Children's Health Insurance Program	—	800-841-2900	www.state.ma.us/dma
Michigan	DMERC	Adminastar Federal, Inc.	—	800-270-2313	—
	ESRD	Renal Disease Network 11—Upper Midwest	651-644-9877	800-973-3773	www.esrdnet11.org
	Health Department	Michigan Department Community Health	517-373-3500	—	www.michigan.gov/mdch
	Insurance Department	Financial and Insurance Services of Michigan	517-373-0220	877-999-6442	www.cis.state.mmi.us/ofis/
	CMS Carrier	Wisconsin Physician Services	—	800-482-4045	—
	CMS FI	BCBS Wisconsin (d.b.a. United Government Services)	—	866-804-0666	—
	Medicaid	Michigan Department Community Health	517-335-5500	800-642-3195	www.michigan.gov/mdch
	QIO (PRO)	Michigan Peer Review Organization	248-465-7300	800-365-5899	www.mpro.org
	SHIP	Michigan Medicare/Medicaid Assistance Program	517-886-0899	800-803-7174	www.mymmap.org
	SCHIP	MIChild	—	888-988-6300	www.michigan.gov/mdch/
Minnesota	DMERC	Adminastar Federal, Inc.	—	800-270-2313	—
	ESRD	Renal Disease Network 11—Upper Midwest	651-644-9877	800-973-3773	www.esrdnet11.org
	Health Department	Minnesota Department of Health	651-215-5800	—	www.health.state.mn.us
	Insurance Department	Department of Commerce of Minnesota	651-296-4026	800-657-3602	www.commerce.state.mn.us/
	CMS Carrier	Wisconsin Physician Services	—	800-352-2762	—
	CMS FI	Noridian Mutual Insurance Company	—	800-330-5935	—
	Medicaid	Department of Human Services of Minnesota	651-297-3933	—	www.dhs.state.mn.us/
	QIO (PRO)	Stratis Health	952-854-3306	800-444-3423	www.stratishealth.org
	SHIP	Minnesota SHIP/Senior LinkAge Line	651-296-2770	800-333-2433	www.mnaging.org/
	SCHIP	MinnesotaCare	651-297-3862	800-657-3672	www.dhs.state.mn.us/HealthCare/
Mississippi	DMERC	Palmetto Government Benefits Administrators (GBA)	—	800-583-2236	—
	ESRD	Network 8, Inc.	601-936-9260	877-936-9260	—
	Health Department	Mississippi State Department of Health	601-576-7400	—	www.msdh.state.ms.us/
	Insurance Department	Department of Insurance of Mississippi	601-359-356	800-562-2957	www.doi.state.ms.us/
	CMS Carrier	Cahaba Government Benefits Administrators (GBA)	—	800-682-5417	—
	CMS FI	Trispan Health Services	—	800-932-7644	www.trispan.com

Continued.

State	Type	Agency	Telephone	Toll Free	Website
	Medicaid	Office of the Governor of Mississippi	601-359-6050	800-421-2408	www.dom.state.ms.us/
	QIO (PRO)	Information and Quality Healthcare	601-957-175	800-844-0600	www.iqh.org
	SHIP	Mississippi Insurance Counsel and Assistance Program	601-359-4929	800-948-3090	www.mdhs.state.ms.us/
	SCHIP	Mississippi Health Benefits Program	—	877-543-7669	www.dom.state.ms.us/CHIP/chip.html
Missouri	DMERC	CIGNA (Connecticut General Life Insurance Company of North America)	—	800-899-7095	http://cignamedicare.com
	ESRD	End Stage Renal Disease Network 12	816-880-9990	800-444-9965	http://network12.org
	Health Department	Missouri Department of Health and Senior Services	207-287-2826	—	www.dhss.state.mo.us/
	Insurance Department	Insurance Department of Missouri—Consumer Services Division	573-751-2640	800-726-7390	www.insurance.mo.gov
	CMS Carrier	BCBS of Kansas	—	800-892-5900	—
	CMS FI	Mutual of Omaha Insurance Companies	—	877-647-6528	www.mutualmedicare.com
	Medicaid	Department of Social Services of Missouri	573-751-4815	800-392-2161	www.dss.state.mo.us/dms/pages/
	QIO (PRO)	Missouri Patient Care Review Foundation	573-893-7900	800-347-1016	www.mpcrf.org
	SHIP	CLAIM Program of Missouri	573-893-7900	800-390-3330	www.missouriclaim.org
	SCHIP	MC+ for Kids	—	888-275-5908	www.dss.state.mo.us/mcplus
Montana	DMERC	CIGNA (Connecticut General Life Insurance Company of North America)	—	800-899-7095	http://cignamedicare.com
	ESRD	Northwest Renal Network—Network 18	206-923-0714	800-262-1514	—
	Health Department	Montana Department of Public Health and Human Services	406-444-5622	406-444-1970	www.dphhs.state.mt.us
	Insurance Department	Insurance Department of Montana —Consumer Services Division	406-444-2040	800-332-6148	http://sao.state.mt.us
	CMS Carrier	BCBS of Montana	406-444-8350	800-332-6146	—
	CMS FI	BCBS of Montana	406-791-4086	866-737-8928, ext. 4086	—
	Medicaid	Montana Department of Health and Human Services	406-444-5900	800-362-8312	www.dphhs.state.mt.us/
	QIO (PRO)	Mountain-Pacific Quality Health Foundation	406-443-4020	800-497-8032	www.mpqhf.org
	SHIP	Senior and Long Term Care Division of Montana	406-444-4077	800-551-3191	www.dphhs.state.mt.us/sltc/
	SCHIP	Montana Children's Health Insurance Plan	406-444-6971	877-543-7669	www.dphhs.mt.gov

State	Type	Agency	Telephone	Toll Free	Website
Nebraska	DMERC	CIGNA (Connecticut General Life Insurance Company of North America)	—	800-899-7095	http://cignamedicare.com
	ESRD	End Stage Renal Disease Network 12	816-880-9990	800-444-9965	http://network12.org
	Health Department	Nebraska Health and Human Services System	402-471-3121	—	www.hhs.state.ne.us
	Insurance Department	Nebraska Department of Insurance—Consumer Services Division	402-471-2201	800-234-7119	www.nol.org/home/NDOI
	CMS Carrier	BCBS of Kansas	—	800-633-1113	—
	CMS FI	BCBS of Nebraska	—	877-602-7775	—
	Medicaid	Nebraska Health and Human Services System	402-471-3121	800-430-3244	www.hhs.state.ne.us
	QIO (PRO)	Cimro of Nebraska	402-476-1399	800-247-3004	www.comronebraska.org
	SHIP	Nebraska State Health Insurance Information Program	402-471-2201	800-234-7119	www.nol.org/home/NDOI/
	SCHIP	Nebraska Kids Connection	—	800-632-5437	www.hhs.state.ne.us/med/kidsconx.htm
Nevada	DMERC	CIGNA (Connecticut General Life Insurance Company of North America)	—	800-899-7095	—
	ESRD	Intermountain End Stage Renal Disease Network—Network 15	303-831-8818	800-783-8818	—
	Health Department	Nevada Department Human Resources, Aging Division	775-687-4210	—	http://hr.state.nv.us
	Insurance Department	Insurance Division of Nevada—Department of Business and Industry	775-687-4270	800-992-0900	http://doi.state.nv.us/
	CMS Carrier	Noridian Mutual Insurance Company	—	800-444-4606	—
	CMS FI	Mutual of Omaha Insurance Companies	—	877-647-6528	www.mutualmedicare.com
	Medicaid	Nevada Department Human Resources, Aging Division	702-486-5000	—	http://dhcfp.state.nv.us/
	QIO (PRO)	Healthinsight	702-385-9933	800-748-6773	www.healthinsight.org
	SHIP	State Health Insurance Advisory Program of Nevada	702-486-3478	800-307-4444	www.nvaging.net/ship/ship_main.htm
	SCHIP	Nevada Check Up	775-684-3777	—	www.nevadacheckup.state.nv.us/
New Hampshire	DMERC	HealthNow DMERC	—	800-842-2052	http://umd.nycpic.com
	ESRD	End Stage Renal Disease Network of New England—Network 1	203-387-9332	866-286-3773	—
	Health Department	New Hampshire Department of Health and Human Services	603-271-4238	—	www.dhhs.state.nh.us/DHHS/DHHS_SITE/

Continued.

State	Type	Agency	Telephone	Toll Free	Website
	Insurance Department	Insurance Department of New Hampshire—Consumer Services Division	603-271-2261	800-852-3416	www.state.nh.us/insurance/
	CMS Carrier	National Heritage Insurance Company	—	800-447-1142	www.medicarenhic.com/
	CMS FI	Anthem Health Plans—New Hampshire—Vermont	603-695-7000	800-522-8323	—
	Medicaid	New Hampshire Department of Health and Human Services	603-271-5254	800-852-3345	www.dhhs.state.nh.us
	QIO (PRO)	Northeast Health Care Quality Foundation	603-749-1641	800-772-0151	www.medicarequality.org
	SHIP	Health Insurance Counseling, Education, and Assistance Services	603-225-9000	800-852-3388	www.nhhelpline.org/hiceas/hiceas/
	SCHIP	Healthy Kids	—	877-464-2447	www.nhhealthykids.com/
New Jersey	DMERC	HealthNow DMERC	—	800-842-2052	http://umd.nycpic.com
	ESRD	Trans-Atlantic Renal Council—Network 3	609-490-0310	888-877-8400	—
	Health Department	New Jersey Department of Health and Senior Services	609-292-7837	—	www.state.nj.us/health/index.shtml
	Insurance Department	Insurance Department of New Jersey—Consumer Services Division	609-292-5316	800-446-7467	www.state.nj.us/dobi/index.html
	CMS Carrier	Empire Medical Services	—	800-462-9306	—
	CMS FI	BCBS of Tennessee (d.b.a. Riverbend Government Benefits)	—	866-641-2007	—
	Medicaid	Department of Health and Human Services of New Jersey	609-588-2600	800-356-1561	www.state.nj.us/humanservices/
	QIO (PRO)	Peer Review Organization of New Jersey, Inc.	732-238-5570	800-624-4557	www.pronj.org
	SHIP	New Jersey Department of Health and Senior Services	609-943-3433	800-792-8820	www.state.nj.us/health/senior/ship.htm
	SCHIP	New Jersey Family Care	—	800-701-0710	www.njfamilycare.org
New Mexico	DMERC	Palmetto Government Benefits Administrators (GBA)	—	800-583-2236	—
	ESRD	Intermountain End Stage Renal Disease Network—Network 15	303-831-8818	800-783-8818	—
	Health Department	New Mexico Department of Health	505-827-2613	—	www.health.state.nm.us
	Insurance Department	Department of Insurance of New Mexico	505-827-4601	800-947-4722	www.nmprc.health.state.nm.us
	CMS Carrier	BCBS of Arkansas	—	800-423-2925	—
	CMS FI	TrailBlazer Health Enterprises, LLC	—	800-442-2620	www.the-medicare.com

State	Type	Agency	Telephone	Toll Free	Website
	Medicaid	Department of Human Services of New Mexico	505-827-3100	888-997-2583	www.state.nm.us/hsd/mad/Index.html
	QIO (PRO)	New Mexico Medical Review Association	505-998-9898	800-279-6824	www.nmmra.org
	SHIP	New Mexico Aging and Long Term Care Department	505-476-4828	800-432-2080	www.nmaging.state.nm.us/
	SCHIP	New Mexikids/SCHIP	—	888-997-2583	www.state.nm..us/hsd/mad/OtherDocs/
New York	DMERC	HealthNow DMERC	—	800-842-2052	http://umd.nypic.com
	ESRD	End Stage Renal DiseaseNetwork of New York—Network 2	212-289-4524	800-238-3773	—
	Health Department	New York State Department of Health	518-486-9057	—	www.health.state.ny.us/
	Insurance Department	Insurance Department of New York	212-480-6400	800-342-3736	www.ins.state.ny.us/
	CMS Carrier	Empire Medical Services	—	800-442-8430	—
	CMS FI	Empire Medical Services	—	800-442-8430	—
	Medicaid	New York State Department of Health	518-747-8887	800-541-2831	www.health.state.ny.us/nysdoh/medicaid/
	QIO (PRO)	Island Peer Review Organization	516-326-7767	800-331-7767	www.ipro.com
	SHIP	Health Insurance Information, Counseling, and Assistance Program	212-869-3850	800-333-4114	www.hiicap.state.ny.us/
	SCHIP	New York Child Health Plus	—	800-698-4543	www.health.state.ny.us/nysdoh/chplus/
North Carolina	DMERC	Palmetto Government Benefits Administrators (GBA)	—	800-583-2236	—
	ESRD	Southeastern Kidney Council—Network 6	919-855-0882	800-524-7139	—
	Health Department	North Carolina Department of Health and Human Services	919-733-4534	—	www.dhh.state.nc.us
	Insurance Department	Department of Insurance of North Carolina	919-733-0111	800-443-9354	www.ncshiipc.com
	CMS Carrier	CIGNA (Connecticut General Life Insurance Company of North America)	—	800-672-3071	—
	CMS FI	Palmetto Government Benefits Administrators (GBA)	—	800-685-1512	—
	Medicaid	North Carolina Department of Health and Human Services	919-857-4011	800-662-7030	www.dhhs.state.nc.us/dma/
	QIO (PRO)	Medical Review of North Carolina	919-380-9860	800-722-0468	www.mrnc.org
	SHIP	North Carolina Senior Health Insurance Information Program	919-733-0111	800-443-9354	www.ncshiip.com/
	SCHIP	North Carolina Health Choice for Children	919-857-4262	800-367-2229	www.dhhs.state.nc.us/dma/cpcont.htm

Continued.

State	Type	Agency	Telephone	Toll Free	Website
North Dakota	DMERC	CIGNA (Connecticut General Life Insurance Company of North America)	—	800-899-7095	http://cignamedicare.com
	ESRD	Renal Disease Network 11—Upper Midwest	651-644-9877	800-973-3773	www.esrdnet11.org
	Health Department	North Dakota Department of Health	701-328-2372	—	www.health.state.nd.us
	Insurance Department	North Dakota Insurance Department	701-328-2440	800-247-0560	www.state.nd.us/ndins/
	CMS Carrier	Noridian Mutual Insurance Company	—	800-247-2267	—
	CMS FI	Noridian Mutual Insurance Company	701-277-2363	800-247-2267	—
	Medicaid	Department of Human Services of North Dakota	701-328-2332	800-755-2604	http://lnotes.state.nd/us
	QIO (PRO)	North Dakota Health Care Review, Inc.	701-852-4231	800-472-2902	www.ndhcri.org
	SHIP	North Dakota Insurance Department	701-328-2440	800-247-0560	www.state.nd.us/ndins/
	SCHIP	Healthy Steps	—	800-755-2604	www.state.nd.us/childrenshealth
Northern Mariana Islands	DMERC	CIGNA (Connecticut General Life Insurance Company of North America)	—	800-899-7095	http://cignamedicare.com
	ESRD	TransPacific Renal Network—No. 17	415-472-8590	800-232-3773	www.network17.org
	Health Department	Hawaii Department of Health	808-586-4400	—	www.hawaii.gov/health
	Insurance Department	Economic Development/Bank and Insurance Northern Mariana Islands	670-664-3017	—	www.commerce.gov.mp
	CMS Carrier	Noridian Mutual Insurance Company	—	800-444-4606	—
	CMS FI	United Government Services	—	866-264-4990	—
	Medicaid	Department of Human Services of Hawaii	808-524-3370	800-316-8005	www.med-quest.us/
	QIO (PRO)	Mountain-Pacific Quality Health Foundation	808-545-2550	800-524-6550	www.mpqhf.org
	SHIP	PLUS	808-586-7299	888-875-9229	www.haaii.gov/eoa/index.html
Ohio	DMERC	Adminastar Federal, Inc.	—	800-270-2313	—
	ESRD	The Renal Network—Network 9/10	317-257-8265	800-456-6919	—
	Health Department	Ohio Department of Health	614-466-3543	—	www.odh.state.oh.us
	Insurance Department	Consumer Services Division of Ohio	614-644-2658	800-686-1526	www.ohioinsurance.gov/
	CMS Carrier	Palmetto Government Benefits Administrators (GBA)	—	800-282-0530	www.palmettogba.com
	CMS FI	Adminastar Federal, Inc.	—	877-602-2430	—

State	Type	Agency	Telephone	Toll Free	Website
	Medicaid	Ohio Department of Job and Family Services—Health Plans	614-728-3288	800-324-8680	www.state.oh.us/odjfs/
	QIO (PRO)	Ohio KePRO, Inc.	216-477-9604	800-589-7337	www.ohiokeproinc.com
	SHIP	Senior Health Insurance Info Program of Ohio	614-644-3458	800-686-1578	www.ohioinsurnace.gov/
	SCHIP	Healthy Start	—	800-324-8680	www.state.oh.us/odjufs/ohp/bcps/schip/
Oklahoma	DMERC	Palmetto Government Benefits Administrators (GBA)	—	800-583-2236	—
	ESRD	End Stage Renal Disease Network 13	405-942-6000	800-472-8664	www.network13.org
	Health Department	Oklahoma State Department of Health	405-271-5600	—	www.health.state.ok.us
	Insurance Department	Insurance Department of Oklahoma—Consumer Services Division	405-521-2828	800-522-0071	www.od.state.ok.us/
	CMS Carrier	BCBS of Arkansas	—	800-522-9079	—
	CMS FI	Chisholm Administrative Services	—	877-910-8153	www.bcbsok.com
	Medicaid	Health Care Authority of Oklahoma	405-522-7300	800-522-0114	www.ohca.state.ok.us/
	QIO (PRO)	OK Foundation for Medical Quality, Inc.	405-840-2891	800-522-3414	www.ofmq.com
	SHIP	Oklahoma Senior Health Insurance Counseling Program	504-521-6628	800-763-2828	www.oid.state.ok.us/consumer/shicp.html
	SCHIP	SoonerCare	—	800-987-7767	www.okdhs.org/medapp/
Oregon	DMERC	CIGNA (Connecticut General Life Insurance Company of North America)	—	800-899-7095	http://cignamedicare.com
	ESRD	Northwest Renal Network—Network 16	206-923-0714	800-262-1514	—
	Health Department	Oregon Department of Human Services	503-947-5107	—	www.dhs.state.or.us/
	Insurance Department	Insurance Division of Oregon—Consumer and Business Division	503-947-7263	800-727-4134	www.oregonshiba.org
	CMS Carrier	Noridian Mutual Insurance Company	—	800-444-4606	—
	CMS FI	Medicare Northwest	—	866-804-0681	—
	Medicaid	Oregon Department of Human Services	503-845-5772	800-527-5772	www.dhs.state.or.us/
	QIO (PRO)	Oregon Medical Professional Review Organization	503-279-0100	800-344-4354	www.ompro.org
	SHIP	Oregon Senior Health Insurance Benefits Assistance	503-947-7984	800-722-4134	www.oregonshiba.org
	SCHIP	Oregon Health Plan	503-945-5772	800-527-5772	www.dhs.state.or.us/healthplan/

Continued.

State	Type	Agency	Telephone	Toll Free	Website
Pennsylvania	DMERC	HealthNow DMERC	—	800-842-2052	http://umd.nypic.com
	ESRD	End Stage Renal Disease Network 4, Inc.	412-325-2250	800-548-9205	—
	Health Department	Pennsylvania Department of Health	—	877-724-3258	www.dsf.health.state.pa.us/health/site/
	Insurance Department	Insurance Department of Pennsylvania	717-787-2317	877-881-6388	www.insurance.state.pa.us
	CMS Carrier	HGS Administrators of Pennsylvania	800-382-1274	800-633-4227	—
	CMS FI	Veritus Medical Services	—	800-633-4227	—
	Medicaid	Department of Public Welfare of Pennsylvania	717-787-1870	800-692-7462	www.dpw.state.pa.us/omap/dpwomap.asp
	QIO (PRO)	Quality Insights of Pennsylvania	304-346-9864	877-346-6180	www.qipa.org
	SHIP	APRISE	724-925-4213	800-783-7067	www.state.pa.us/
	SCHIP	Pennsylvania Children's Health Insurance Program	—	800-986-5437	www.insurance.state.pa.us/html/chip.html
Puerto Rico	DMERC	Palmetto Government Benefits Administrators (GBA)	—	800-583-2236	—
	ESRD	Trans-Atlantic Renal Council—Network 3	609-490-0310	888-877-8400	—
	Insurance Department	Commissioner of Insurance of Puerto Rico	787-722-8686	888-722-8686	—
	CMS Carrier	Triple S, Inc.	—	800-981-7015	www.triples.1-medi1org
	CMS FI	Cooperative De Seguros De Vida (COSVI)	787-758-9720	866-863-8598	—
	Medicaid	Medicaid Office of Puerto Rico and Virgin Isles	787-765-1230	—	—
	QIO (PRO)	QIPRO, Inc.	787-641-1240	800-981-5062	www.qipro.org
	SHIP	Puerto Rico State Health Insurance Assistance Program	787-721-4300	877-725-4300	—
	CHIP	Children's Health Insurance Program	—	877-543-7669	—
Rhode Island	DMERC	HealthNow DMERC	—	800-842-2052	www.umd.nypic.com
	ESRD	End Stage Renal Disease Network of New England—Network 1	203-387-9332	866-286-3773	—
	Health Department	Rhode Island Department of Health	401-222-2231	—	www.healthri.org
	Insurance Department	Department of Business Regulation of Rhode Island—Insurance Division	401-222-2223	—	www.dbr.state.ri.us/
	CMS Carrier	Arkansas BCBS	401-459-1000	800-662-5170	—
	CMS FI	Arkansas BCBS	401-459-1000	800-662-5170	—
	Medicaid	Department of Human Services of Rhode Island	401-462-5300	—	www.dhs.state.ri.us/

State	Type	Agency	Telephone	Toll Free	Website
	QIO (PRO)	Rhode Island Quality Partners, Inc.	401-528-3200	800-662-5028	www.riqualitypartners.org
	SHIP	Rhode Island Senior Health Insurance Program	401-462-3000	—	www.dbr.state.ri.us/
	SCHIP	Rite Care	401-462-1300	—	www.dhs.state.ri.us/dhs/famchild/shcare.
South Carolina	DMERC	Palmetto Government Benefits Administrators (GBA)	—	800-583-2236	—
	ESRD	Southeastern Kidney Council—Network 6	919-855-0882	800-524-7139	—
	Health Department	South Carolina Department of Health and Human Services	803-898-2500	—	www.dhhs.state.sc.us/default.htm
	Insurance Department	Department of Insurance of South Carolina	803-737-6160	800-768-3467	www.doi.state.sc.us/
	CMS Carrier	Palmetto Government Benefits Administrators (GBA)	—	800-583-2236	—
	CMS FI	Palmetto Government Benefits Administrators (GBA)	—	800-583-2236	—
	Medicaid	South Carolina Department Health and Human Services	803-898-2500	888-549-0820	www.dhhs.state.sc.us
	QIO (PRO)	Carolina Medical Review	803-731-8225	800-922-3089	www.mrnc.org
	SHIP	Bureau of Senior Services of South Carolina	803-898-2850	800-868-9095	www.caresouth-carolina.com/vantage
	SCHIP	Partners for Healthy Children	—	888-549-0820	www.dhhs.state.sc.us/InsideDHHS/
South Dakota	DMERC	CIGNA (Connecticut General Life Insurance Company of North America)	—	800-899-7095	http://cignamedicare.com
	ESRD	Renal Disease Network 11—Upper Midwest	651-644-9877	800-973-3773	www.esrdnet11.org
	Health Department	South Dakota Department of Health	605-773-3495	800-452-7691	www.state.sd.us/doh/
	Insurance Department	Insurance Department of South Dakota—Consumer Services Division	605-773-3563	—	www.state.sd.us/drr2/reg/insurance
	CMS Carrier	Noridian Mutual Insurance Company	—	800-437-4762	—
	CMS FI	Cahaba Government Benefits Administrators (GBA)	—	877-910-8139	—
	Medicaid	Department of Social Services of South Dakota	605-773-3495	800-452-7691	www.state.sd.us/scial/MedElig
	QIO (PRO)	South Dakota Foundation for Medical Care, Inc.	605-336-3505	800-658-2285	www.sdfmc.org
	SHIP	Adult Services and Aging of South Dakota	605-773-3656	800-536-8197	www.state.sd.us/social/ASA/SHINE

Continued.

State	Type	Agency	Telephone	Toll Free	Website
	SCHIP	South Dakota Children's Health Insurance Program	—	800-305-3064	www.state.sd.us/ social/medical/CHIP/
Tennessee	DMERC	Palmetto Government Benefits Administrators (GBA)	—	800-583-2236	—
	ESRD	Network 8, Inc.	601-936-9260	877-936-9260	—
	Health Department	Tennessee Department of Health	615-741-3111	—	www.state.tn.us/health
	Insurance Department	Tennessee Department of Insurance—Commerce and Insurance	615-741-4955	800-525-2816	www.state.tn.us/ commerce/
	CMS Carrier	CIGNA (Connecticut General Life Insurance Company of North America)	—	800-342-8900	—
	CMS FI	BCBS of Tennessee (d.b.a. Riverbend GBA)	—	866-641-2007	—
	Medicaid	Department of Health	615-741-0192	800-669-1851	www.state.tn.us/ health/
	QIO (PRO)	Q Source	901-682-0381	800-528-2655	www.qsource.org
	SHIP	Tennessee Commission on Aging and Disability	615-741-2056	877-801-0044	www.state.tn.us/ commerce/
	SCHIP	TennCare	—	800-669-1851	www.state.tn.us/ tenncare/
Texas	DMERC	Palmetto Government Benefits Administrators (GBA)	—	800-583-2236	—
	ESRD	End Stage Renal Disease Network of Texas—Network 14	972-503-3215	877-886-4435	—
	Health Department	Texas Department of Health	512-458-7111	888-963-7111	www.thd.state.tx.us
	Insurance Department	Insurance Department of Texas	512-463-6515	800-252-3439	www.tdi.state.tx.us
	CMS Carrier	TrailBlazer Health Enterprises, LLC	—	800-442-2620	www.trailblazerhealth. com
	CMS FI	TrailBlazer Health Enterprises, LLC	—	800-442-2620	www.the-medicare. com
	Medicaid	Health and Human Services Commission of Texas	512-424-6500	888-834-7406	www.hhsc.state.tx.us
	QIO (PRO)	Texas Medical Foundation	512-329-6610	800-725-8315	www.tmf.org
	SHIP	Department on Aging of Texas (SHIP)	512-438-3200	800-252-9240	www.tdoa.state.tx.us
	SCHIP	TexCare Partnership	—	—	www.texcarepartner ship.com
Utah	DMERC	CIGNA (Connecticut General Life Insurance Company of North America)	—	800-899-7095	http://cignamedicare. com
	ESRD	Intermountain End Stage Renal Disease Network—Network 15	303-831-8818	800-783-8818	—
	Health Department	Utah Department of Health	801-538-6101	—	www.health.utah.gov

State	Type	Agency	Telephone	Toll Free	Website
	Insurance Department	Office of Consumer Health Assistance of Utah	801-538-3077	866-350-6242	www.insurance.utah.gov
	CMS Carrier	Regence BCBS of Utah	—	800-426-3477	http://utmedicare regents.com
	CMS FI	Regence BCBS of Utah	—	866-804-0681	—
	Medicaid	Utah Department of Health	801-538-6155	800-662-9651	http://health.utah.gov/medicaid/
	QIO (PRO)	HealthInsight	702-385-9933	800-274-2290	www.healthinisght.org
	SHIP	Aging and Adult Services of Utah	801-538-3910	800-541-7735	www.hsdaas.utah.gov/
	SCHIP	Utah Children's Health Insurance Program	—	800-543-7669	www.utahchip.org
Vermont	DMERC	HealthNow DMERC	—	800-842-2052	http://nypic.com
	ESRD	End Stage Renal Disease Network of New England— Network 1	203-387-9332	866-286-3773	—
	Health Department	Vermont Department of Health	802-863-7200	800-464-4343	www.healthy vermonters.info
	Insurance Department	Banking, Insurance, Securities, and Health Care Administration of Vermont	802-828-2900	800-631-7788	www.bishca.state.vt.us/
	CMS Carrier	National Heritage Insurance Company	—	800-447-1142	www.medicarenhic.com/
	CMS FI	Anthem Health Plans of New Hampshire-Vermont	603-695-7000	800-522-8323	—
	Medicaid	Agency of Human Services of Vermont	802-241-2800	800-250-8427	www.dpath.state.vt.us/
	QIO (PRO)	Northeast Health Care Quality Foundation	603-749-1641	800-772-0151	www.medicarequality.org
	SHIP	Area Agency on Aging of Vermont	802-751-0428	800-642-5119	www.medicarehelpvt.net/
	SCHIP	Dr. Dynasaur	—	800-250-8427	www.path.state.vt.us/Programs_Pages/Healthcare/drdynasaur.htm
Virgin Islands	DMERC	Palmetto Government Benefits Administrators (GBA)	—	800-583-2236	—
	ESRD	Trans-Atlantic Renal Council—Network 3	609-490-0310	888-877-8400	—
		Insurance Department Division of Banking and Insurance of Virgin Islands	340-773-6449	—	www.ltg.gov.di
	CMS Carrier	Triple S, Inc.	340-776-8311, ext. 1005	800-981-7015	www.triples.1-medi1org
	CMS FI	Cooperative De Seguros De Vida (COSVI)	787-758-9720	866-863-8598	—
	Medicaid	Medicaid Office Puerto Rico and Virgin Islands	787-765-1230	—	—
	QIO (PRO)	Virgin Islands Medical Institute	340-712-2444	—	www.networkvi.com/vimi_files

Continued.

State	Type	Agency	Telephone	Toll Free	Website
	SHIP	State Health Insurance Assistance Program of Virgin Islands	340-776-8311, ext. 1005	—	—
	SCHIP	Virgin Islands Bureau of Health Insurance and Medical Assistance	—	—	—
Virginia	DMERC	Adminastar Federal, Inc.	—	800-270-2313	—
	ESRD	Mid-Atlantic Renal Coalition—Network 5	804-794-3757	866-651-6272	—
	Health Department	Virginia Department of Health	804-864-7001	—	www.vdh.state.va.us
	Insurance Department	Insurance Department of Virginia	804-371-9691	800-552-7945	www.state.va.us/scc
	CMS Carrier	TrailBlazer Health Enterprises, LLC	—	800-444-4606	www.mytrailblazer.com
	CMS FI	United Government Services	—	877-768-5471	—
	Medicaid	Department of Social Services of Virginia	804-726-4231	—	www.dss.state.va.us/benefit/medicaid
	QIO (PRO)	Virginia Health Quality Center	804-289-5320	800-545-3814	www.vhqc.com
	SHIP	Virginia Insurance Counseling and Assistance Program	804-662-9333	800-552-3402	www.aging.state.va.us/
	SCHIP	Family Access to Medical Security Insurance Plan	—	866-873-2647	www.famis.org/
Washington	DMERC	CIGNA (Connecticut General Life Insurance Company of North America)	—	800-899-7095	http://cignamedicare.com
	ESRD	Northwest Renal Network—Network 16	206-923-0714	800-2662-1514	—
	Health Department	Washington State Department of Health	—	800-525-0127	www.doh.wa.gov/
	Insurance Department	Statewide Health Insurance Benefits Advisors of Washington	206-389-2747	800-397-4422	www.insurance.wa.gov/
	CMS Carrier	Noridian Mutual Insurance Company	—	800-444-4606	—
	CMS FI	Premera Blue Cross	—	877-602-7896	—
	Medicaid	Washington State Department of Social and Health Services	800-562-6188	800-562-3022	http://fortress.wa.gov/dshs/maa/
	QIO (PRO)	QualisHealth	—	800-445-6941	www.qualishealth.org
	SHIP	Statewide Health Insurance Benefits Advisors of Washington	—	800-397-4422	www.insurance.wa.gov/
	SCHIP	Washington Children's Health Insurance Program	—	877-543-7669	http://fortress/wa.gov/dshs/maa/CHIP/Index.html
West Virginia	DMERC	Adminastar Federal, Inc.	—	800-270-2313	—
	ESRD	Mid-Atlantic Renal Coalition—Network 5	804-794-3757	866-651-6272	—
	Health Department	West Virginia Department of Health and Human Services	304-558-0684	—	www.wv.gov/ www.wvdhhr.org

State	Type	Agency	Telephone	Toll Free	Website
	Insurance Department	West Virginia Insurance Commissioner	304-558-3386	888-879-9842	—
	CMS Carrier	Palmetto Government Benefits Administrators (GBA)	—	800-848-0106	—
	CMS FI	United Government Services	—	877-768-8571	—
	Medicaid	West Virginia Department of Health and Human Services	304-558-1700	—	www.wvdhhr.org/bms/
	QIO (PRO)	West Virginia Medical Institute, Inc.	304-346-9864	800-642-8686, ext. 2266	www.wvmi.org
	SHIP	Bureau of Senior Services of West Virginia	304-558-3317	877-987-4463	www.state.wv.us/seniorservices
	SCHIP	West Virginia Children's Health Insurance Program	304-558-2732	877-982-2447	www.wvchip.org/
Wisconsin	DMERC	Adminastar Federal, Inc.	—	800-270-2313	—
	ESRD	Renal Disease Network 11—Upper Midwest	651-644-9877	800-973-3773	www.esrdnet11.org
	Health Department	Wisconsin Department of Health and Family Services	608-266-1865	—	www.dhfs.state.wi.us
	Insurance Department	Office of Commissioner of Insurance of Wisconsin	608-266-3585	800-236-8517	www.oci.wi.gov
	CMS Carrier	Wisconsin Physician Services	—	877-567-7176	—
	CMS FI	BCBS of Wisconsin (d.b.a. United Government Services)	—	800-531-9695	—
	Medicaid	Wisconsin Department of Health and Family Services	608-221-5720	800-362-3002	www.dhfs.stat.wi.us/medicaid/index.htm
	QIO (PRO)	MetaStar, Inc.	608-274-1940	800-362-2320	www.metastar.com
	SHIP	State Health Insurance Assistance Program of Wisconsin	—	800-242-1060	www.dhfs.state.wi.us/aging/index.htm
	SCHIP	Badger Care	—	800-362-3002	www.dhfs.state.wi.us/badgercare/index.htm
Wyoming	DMERC	CIGNA (Connecticut General Life Insurance Company of North America)	—	800-899-7095	http://cignamedicare.com
	ESRD	Intermountain End Stage Renal Disease Network—Network 15	303-831-8818	800-783-8818	—
	Health Department	Wyoming Department of Health	307-777-7531	—	http://wdh.state.wy.us/main/index.asp
	Insurance Department	Insurance Department of Wyoming	307-777-7401	800-438-5768	http://insurance.state.wy.us/
	CMS Carrier	Noridian Mutual Insurance Company	—	800-442-2371	—
	CMS FI	BCBS of Wyoming	—	888-557-2301	—
	Medicaid	Wyoming Department of Health	307-777-7531	888-996-8678	http://wdhfs.state.wy.us/

Continued.

State	Type	Agency	Telephone	Toll Free	Website
	QIO (PRO)	Mountain-Pacific Quality Health Foundation	406-443-4020	800-497-8232	www.mpqhf.org
	SHIP	State Health Insurance Information Program of Wyoming	307-856-6880	800-856-4398	www.wyomingseniors.com/
	SCHIP	Wyoming Kid Care	—	888-996-8786	http://kidcare.state.wy.us/index.htm

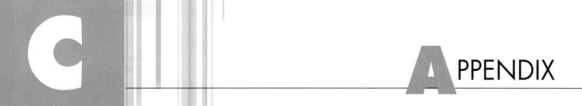

Lake Eola Family Practice Associates

Lake Eola Associates Practice Information and Fee Schedule
Practice Information

Practice Tax ID No.	Group Medicare NPI	Group BCBS PIN No.	All Others: Group ID No.
59-xx234567	78XX901234	B78901X	89012A

Medical Staff Information

Provider	Medicare NPI	BCBS Provider Number	All Other: Use SSN Provider Number
Eric Anderson, MD	123XX45678	BC1234A	123xx6789
Todd Wilson, MD	234XX56789	BC2345A	234xx7890
Aaron Rubin, MD	345XX67890	BC3456A	345xx8901
Javier Gomez, MD	456XX78901	BC4567A	456xx9012
Bruce James, PA	567XX89012	BC5678A	567xx0123
Cassandra Lewis, ARNP	678XX90123	BC6789A	678xx1234

Fee Schedule

Code	Description	Office	Medicare	Aetna	BCBS	Medicaid
99201	New visit, level 1	48.00	39.21	45.00	43.00	29.00
99202	New visit, level 2	72.00	61.47	68.00	65.00	46.00
99203	New visit, level 3	100.00	86.64	96.00	92.00	75.00
99204	New visit, level 4	150.00	125.06	130.00	135.00	100.00
99205	New visit, level 5	200.00	155.50	160.00	175.00	120.00
99211	Established visit, level 1	40.00	19.40	32.00	28.00	15.00
99212	Established visit, level 2	8.00	33.97	45.00	40.00	29.00
99213	Established visit, level 3	75.00	45.72	68.00	60.00	40.00
99214	Established visit, level 4	140.00	70.71	110.00	125.00	58.00
99215	Established visit, level 5	190.00	105.81	160.00	175.00	89.00
93000	12-lead EKG; interpretation/report	65.00	28.01	55.00	48.00	24.00
90703	Tetanus toxoid, IM	5.00	(Excluded)	5.00	4.70	3.00
90788	Antibiotic injection, IM	10.00	4.65	5.00	4.70	3.00
J0540	Procaine penicillin G to 1,200,000 units	8.00	(Excluded)	4.50	6.00	3.00
J0570	Penicillin G to 1,200,000 units	8.00	(Excluded)	4.50	6.00	3.00
90782	Injection, subcutaneous or IM	10.00	4.30	5.00	4.70	3.75
J3420	Vitamin B12 to 1000 µg	5.00	(Excluded)	3.00	4.50	2.50
J2175	Demerol 100 mg	5.00	(Excluded)	5.00	3.80	2.50
A6448	Compression bandage	10.00	(Bundled)	7.00	6.50	5.00
A4570	Splints	25.00	(Excluded)	15.00	22.00	10.00

Case Study 1: Carolyn Jones

Lake Eola Family Practice   517860 South Pioneer Drive, Orlando, FL 32897 • 634-555-4893

Patient Registration Form

Have you been seen in this office in the past 3 years? ✔ Yes ___ No   **Do you have a living will?** _No_

Today's Date _5/28/2005_   Home Phone _634-555-7654_   Work Phone _None_

Patient Name (Last name, First name, Middle initial) _Jones, Carolyn_

Street Address _8976543 S. Pioneer Dr._   City _Orlando_   State _FL_   Zip _32897_

Date of Birth _3/28/1976_   Age _29_   Gender: _X_ Female ___ Male   Social Security # _670-XX-1234_

Marital Status: _X_ Married ___ Single ___ Widowed ___ Divorced ___ Other   Driver's License # _B654-XX-1099_

Is the patient a student? ___ Full Time ___ Part Time _X_ No   Is the patient employed? ___ Full Time ___ Part Time _X_ No

Patient's Employer Name & Address _N/A_

School Name & Address _N/A_

Emergency Contact Person _Carl Jones_   Relationship _Husband_   Phone _634-555-7654_

Referring Physician Name & Phone Number _None_

Insurance Plan and Responsible Party Information

Insurance Company Name _Blue Cross Blue Shield_   Address _PO Box YYYY_

City _Jacksonville_   State _FL_   Zip _39782_   Phone _1-800-555-1212_

Policy # _____   Group # _87654C_   ID # _HBDCC0127B_

Policy Holder's Name _Carl Jones_   Address _8976543 S. Pioneer_

City _Orlando_   State _FL_   Zip _32897_   Phone _634-555-7654_

Policy Holder's Date of Birth _7/10/1972_   Social Security # _901-XX-4567_   Driver License # _B659-XX-8899_

Gender: _X_ Male ___ Female   Relationship to patient: ___ Self _X_ Spouse ___ Parent ___ Guardian ___ Other

Policy Holder's Employer's Name _Martin Marietta Corp_   Address _517992 S. Pioneer Dr._

City _Orlando_   State _FL_   Zip _32897_   Phone _634-555-1290_

Secondary Insurance Company Name _None_   Address _____

City _____   State _____   Zip _____   Phone _____

Secondary Policy # _____   Group # _____   ID # _____

Secondary Policy Holder's Name _____   Phone _____   Address _____

City _____   State _____   Zip _____   Relationship to patient: ___ Self ___ Spouse ___ other

Secondary Policy Holder's Date of Birth _____   Social Security # _____   Driver License # _____

Authorizations

It is customary to pay for all services on the date rendered unless other arrangements were made before your appointment. The patient and the guarantor are responsible for all deductibles and copays at the time of the visit and any other fees in accordance with insurance contracts. The patient and guarantor are responsible for all elective or noncovered services and any services that are not considered medically necessary.

Financially responsible person if patient is student or unemployed _Carl Jones_   Phone _634-555-7654_

I authorize the release of any medical information necessary to process this claim and I request that payment of medical benefits be made directly to Lake Eola Family Practice. I hereby acknowledge that I am fully responsible for payment as listed above.

Signed _Carolyn Jones_   Date _5/28/2005_   Time _2:15 PM_

Template © 1998 Medical Compliance Management, Inc.

FIGURE C-1, A

Lake Eola Family Practice   517860 South Pioneer Drive, Orlando, FL 32897 • 634-555-4893

Problem List – Medication List

Patient Name _Carolyn Jones_ DOB _3/28/1976_

Allergies & allergic response _NKA_

Referring Physician & ID # _None_

	Problem (e.g., acute or chronic diagnosis, injury,↑ BP)	Date Identified	Date Resolved
1	Candidiasis vaginitis – mod.	5/28/2005	
2			
3			
4			
5			
6			
7			
8			
9			
10			
11			
12			
13			
14			
15			

	All Medications (with dosage & instructions) (include prescription and over-the-counter medications)	Start Date	Discontinue Date
1	OrthoNovum	5/28/2005	
2	Nystatin Vaginal Suppositories	5/28/2005	6/11/2005
3			
4			
5			
6			
7			
8			
9			
10			

Template © 1998 Medical Compliance Management, Inc.

FIGURE C-1, B

Name _Jones, Carolyn_   Date _05_/_28_/_2005_

HPI Chief Complaint:

White vaginal discharge & vaginal
itching x 1 week

Renew BCP

Current Meds.:

OrthoNovum

Past/Family History

① Father has emphysema
② Spouse smokes cigarettes

THIS SECTION TO BE COMPLETED BY PATIENT.

Personal/Social History

Are you... ☐ single   ☒ married
    ☐ live in partner   ☐ divorced

Do you have children? ☒ Yes   ☐ No
Ages of child(ren) _2, 3_
No. of pregnancies _2_ Miscarriages _0_
Occupation _Mother_

	Yes	No
a. Are your immunizations up to date?	☒	☐

Date of last tetanus shot: _May 1994_

b. Concerns about your breasts, menstruation, pain or bleeding with intercourse, vaginal itching or discharge?	☒	☐

c. Approximate date of last pelvic exam. _Nov 04_
d. Approximate date of last pap test _Nov 04_

e. Are you sexually active now?	☒	☐

   ☐ same sex   ☒ opposite sex
   ☒ single partner   ☐ multiple partners

Have you had more than 4 lifetime partners?	☐	☒

f. Birth control method _OrthoNovum_

		Yes	No
g.	Do you have concerns about sexual orientation, sexually transmitted diseases, exposure to AIDS or other sexual concerns?	☐	☒
h.	Do you feel safe/comfortable in your home, with your family, and/or your partner relationship?	☒	☐
i.	Do you smoke or use tobacco products now?	☒	☐
j.	Do you use recreational drugs?	☐	☒
k.	Do you drink alcohol?	☒	☐

   ☒ daily   ☐ weekly   ☐ rarely
   # of drinks _2-3_
If yes, do you drink: ☒ beer, ☐ wine, ☐ liquor

Review of Systems

Are you concerned about?
(circle concerns)

		Yes	No
1.	Recent changes in health status	☐	☒
2.	Eye problems: vision, pain, tearing	☐	☒
3.	Ears, nose, mouth, throat problems	☐	☒
4.	Heart problems: chest pain, blood pressure	☐	☒
5.	Lung problems: coughing, wheezing, infections	☐	☒

		Yes	No
6.	Abdominal pain, stomach, bowel problems	☐	☒
7.	Kidney or bladder problems	☐	☒
8.	Muscle, bone, joint or back problems	☐	☒
9.	Skin, hair or nail problems	☐	☒
10.	Neurologic problems: headaches, dizziness, numbness	☐	☒
11.	Nervousness, anxiety, depression, suicidal thoughts	☐	☒
12.	Excessive thirst and urine output, recent weight changes	☐	☒
13.	Anemia, bruising, blood clots, swollen glands	☐	☒
14.	Food allergies, hayfever, eczema, asthma, decreased immunity	☐	☒
	Do you have any other concerns?	☐	☒

_____
_____
_____
_____

Carolyn Jones   _5/28/05_
Patient's Signature   Date

Provider Comments:

b. vag. discharge/itching x 1 week
f. OrthoNovum BCP x 2 yrs
i. smokes 2 pks/day

Todd Wilson MD   _5/28/05_
Provider's Signature   Date

☒ PFSH and ROS have been reviewed.   ☐ Unresolved problems from previous visit have been addressed.

Anticipatory Guidance

☐ Nutrition
☐ Exercise
☐ Calcium
☐ Multi vit. with folate

☐ Dental care
☐ Cardiovascular risks
☐ Sun exposure
☒ Smoking cessation
☒ Alcohol/drugs
☐ Sexual issues

☒ STD prevention
☐ Self exam. breasts, skin, oral cavity
☐ School/Work
☐ Family
☐ Recreation/ Hobbies
☐ Safety/Injury/Gun Safety

☐ Auto seat belts
☐ Smoke detectors
☐ Domestic violence
☐ Stress
☐ Educational handouts

©1995 Piermed, Inc. Rev. 6/98 (800) 998-1908   500-02

Female 19-39

FIGURE C-1, C

Name _Jones, Carolyn_____ DOB _03_/_28_/_1976_ Age __29__ Chart No. | JONCOO6 |

Assessment

9a   Monilial vulvo-vaginitis

Plan

Nystatin Vag. Supp.
qd x 2 wks.
Renew BCP x 6 mos.

_Todd Wilson MD_____   ___prn_____
Provider's Signature   Return Visit

FOLD HERE   FOLD HERE

Physical Exam

Ht. _5' 6"_ Wt. _120#_ Temp. _98.4°_ Resp. __18__

B.P. sit. or stand. _110_ / _76_   Supine ___ /____

Pulse rate and regularity _72, regular_____

Circle abnormal and pertinent normal findings
Describe abnormalities above.
☑ Normal   ☒ Abnormal

1. Constitutional
a. ☑ gen. appear., development, body shape,
      nutrition, deformities, grooming

2. Eyes
a. ☑ conjunctiva, lids
b. ☑ pupils, irises
c. ☐ fundi (optic discs, vessels, exudate, hemorr.)

3. Ears, Nose, Throat & Mouth
a. ☑ appearance of ears, appearance of nose
b. ☑ auditory canals, tympanic membranes
c. ☐ hearing (whis. voice, finger rub, tun. fork)
d. ☑ nasal mucosa, sputum, turbinates
e. ☐ lips, teeth, gums
f. ☐ oropharynx (mucosa, saliv. glands, hard &
      soft palates, tongue, tonsils, post. pharynx)

4. Neck
a. ☑ appearance, masses, symmetry, tracheal
      position, crepitus
b. ☑ thyroid (enlargement, tenderness, mass)

5. Respiratory
a. ☑ respiratory effort (intercostal retractions)
      use of accessory muscles, diaphragm move.
b. ☐ percussion (dullness, flatness, hyper-reson.)
c. ☐ palpation (tactile fremitus)
d. ☑ auscultation (breath sounds, rhonchi, wheezes,
      rales, rubs)

6. Cardiovascular
a. ☐ palpation (location of p.m.i., size, thrill)
b. ☑ auscultation (abnormal sounds, murmurs)
c. ☑ carotid arteries (pulse amplitude, bruits)
d. ☐ abdominal aorta (size, bruits)
e. ☐ femoral arteries (pulse amplitude, bruits)
f. ☑ pedal pulses (pulse amplitude)
g. ☑ extremities (edema, varicosities)

7. Chest (Breasts)
a. ☐ inspection (size, symmetry, nipple discharge)
b. ☐ palpation of breasts & axillae (masses,
      lumps, tenderness)

8. Gastrointestinal (Abdomen)
a. ☑ examination for masses, tenderness
b. ☑ examination of liver, spleen
c. ☐ examination for presence or absence of hernia
d. ☑ examination of (when indicated) anus, perineum,
      rectum: (sphincter tone, hemorrhoids, masses)
e. ☐ stool for occult blood when indicated

9. Genitourinary
Pelvic Exam (with or without specimen collection
for smears or cultures), including:
a. ☒ Ext. Genitalia (eg. gen. app., hair distrib.,
      lesions) and vagina (eg. gen. app., esrogen eff.,
      lesions, pelvic support, cystocele, rectocele)
b. ☑ Urethra (eg. masses, tender., scarring)
c. ☑ Bladder (eg. fullness, masses, tender.)
d. ☑ Cervix (eg. gen. app., lesions, disch.)
e. ☑ Uterus (eg. size, contour, position, mobility,
      tender., consistency, descent or support)
f. ☑ Adnexia / Parametria (eg. masses, tender.,
      organomegaly, nodularity)

10. Lymphatic
a. ☑ palpation of lymph nodes in 2 or more areas:
      (Circle: neck, axillae, groin, other)

11. Musculoskeletal
a. ☑ examination of gait and station
b. ☑ inspection and/or palpation of digits & nails
      (clubbing, cyanosis, inflammatory conditions,
      petechiae, ischemia, infections, nodes)
c. ☐ assessment of range of motion (pain,
      crepitation, contracture)
d. ☐ Examination of joint, bone, & muscle of 1 or
      more of the following 6 areas (circle)
      • head/neck   • rt. upper extremities
      • spine, ribs, & pelvis • lt. upper extremities
      • rt. lower extremities • lt. lower extremities
e. ☐ inspect, and/or palpation (misalign, asymmetry,
      crepitation, defects, tender., masses, effusion)
f. ☐ assessment of stability: dislocation (luxation),
      subluxation or laxity
g. ☑ muscle strength & tone (flaccid, cogwheel,
      spastic), atrophy or abnormal movement

12. Skin
a. ☑ inspection of skin & sub-Q tissue (rashes,
      lesion, ulcers)
b. ☐ palpation of skin & sub-Q tissue (induration,
      sub-Q nodules, tightening)

13. Neurology
a. ☐ test cranial nerves: notation of deficits
b. ☐ examination of DTR's with notation of
      pathological reflexes (eg. Babinski)
c. ☐ examination of sensation (touch, pain,
      vibration, proprioception)

14. Psychiatric
a. ☐ description of patient's judgment & insight
      Brief assessment of mental status:
b. ☑ orientation to time, place, & person
c. ☑ recent & remote memory
d. ☑ mood & affect (depression, anxiety, agitation)
e. ☐ other _____

Procedures and Immunizations

☐ Hearing   ☐ Glucose   ☐ Cholesterol
☐ Vision   ☐ PT   ☐ HDL/LDL
☐ CBC   ☐ TSH   ☐ CXR
            ☐ Urine   ☐ EKG

☐ PAP Test
☐ Chlamydia screen (high risk or pregnancy)
☐ Rubella Screen (or vaccination history)

Are immunizations current?
☒ Yes ☐ No

☐ dT
☐ Hep B
☐ Influenza

Drug Allergies:

NKA

© 1995 Piermed, Inc. Rev

| Female 19-39 | Date / Time 5/28/2005 3 PM | Summary Monilial Vaginitis | ☐ Referral 500-06 |

FIGURE C-1, D

Lake Eola Family Practice

517860 South Pioneer Drive, Orlando, FL 32897 • 634-555-4893

Superbill   #456298

Weight _120_ BP _110/76_ TPR _98.4°-72-18_

Account Number JONC006	Doctor Todd Wilson MD	Date of Service 05/28/2005

Patient Name Jones, Carolyn	Date of Birth 03/28/1976	LMP May 15, 2000

Insurance BCBS of FL	Responsible Party Carl Jones	Phone Number 634-555-7654

Address PO Box YYYY	Referring Physician and ID # None

City Jacksonville	State FL	Zip 39782

New Patient

```
__ 99201 H[PF]   E[PF]   MDM[S]   10 min
__ 99202 H[EPF]  E[EPF]  MDM[S]   20 min
__ 99203 H[D]    E[D]    MDM[LC]  30 min
__ 99204 H[C]    E[C]    MDM[MC]  45 min
__ 99205 H[C]    E[C]    MDM[HC]  60 min
```

✓ Established Patient

```
__ 99211 H[N/A]  E[N/A]  MDM[N/A] 5 min
__ 99212 H[PF]   E[PF]   MDM[S]   10 min
X  99213 H[EPF]  E[EPF]  MDM[LC]  15 min
__ 99214 H[D]    E[D]    MDM[MC]  25 min
__ 99215 H[C]    E[C]    MDM[HC]  40 min
```

Reason For Visit

__ Authorization _____
   Expiration Date _____
__ Annual exam, complex due to (history, condition): _____
_____
__ Annual exam, simple
__ Follow-up, condition _____
__ Follow-up, post procedure, no condition or complication _____
   Procedure/date _____
__ Follow-up, post procedure, with condition or complication _____
   Procedure/date _____
X_ New Problem _Vag itching/discharge_
__ Post-op, no condition or complication Surgery/date _____
__ Post-op, with conditions or complication
_____
   Surgery/date _____
__ Pre-op _____
__ Procedure _____
__ Second surgical opinion _____
__ Other (Accident, Decision for surgery) ___
_____

Procedures

⇒ Place to be done: _____
⇒ Date to be done: _____
__ Authorization _____
   Expiration date _____
__ Biopsy, type/site _____
_____
__ Cautery, type/site _____
_____
__ Destruction of lesion(s), extensive, site: ___
_____
__ Destruction of lesion(s), simple, site: ___
_____
__ Emergency surgery (list above), reason: ___
_____
__ Excision, type/site _____
_____
__ I & D abscess, type/site: _____
_____
__ Insertion/Removal of IUD, type _____
__ Major surgery, type/site _____
_____
__ Minor surgery, type/site _____
_____
__ Sonogram _____
__ Other _____
_____

Miscellaneous

__ Immunization _____
__ Injection _____
__ Supplies
__ Surgical tray

_X_ Patient Teaching (Preventive medicine)
_No_   Handouts – STD,
Charge   Smoking – ETOH
__ Other _____
_____
_____

Outside Lab

__ Beta HCG, Serum
__ Biopsy/Pathology
__ Biopsy, Mult./Pathology
__ CBC
__ Cholesterol
__ Culture, throat
__ Cultures (source) _____
__ Glucose, __1hr glucose, __3hr glucose
__ Estrogen
__ Herpes simplex, AB
__ Mononucleosis
__ Pap Smear
__ PT__PTT
__ Sed rate
__ SMAC
__ Urinalysis, w/micro
__ HIV
__ Other _____
_____
_____
_____

Diagnosis Codes

1. _112.1_
2. _____
3. _____
4. _____

Appointment in _prn_ Weeks
Procedure in _____ Weeks
Sent Labs to _____
Call in _prn_ Mos./Weeks

Previous Balance $ _0_
Co-Pay $ _10.00_
Paid Today (Cash)/Check $ _10.00_
(Yes)-No All Diagnosis, Procedures, & VS above are documented in Record
Doctor's Signature _Todd Wilson MD_

New Charges $ _75.00_
New Balance $ _65.00_
Check Number _____

Template © 1998 Medical Compliance Management, Inc.,
CPT only © American Medical Association. All Rights Reserved.

FIGURE C-1, E

Case Study 2: Enrique Sanchez

Lake Eola Family Practice   517860 South Pioneer Drive, Orlando, FL 32897 • 634-555-4893

Patient Registration Form

Have you been seen in this office in the past 3 years? ✔ Yes ___ No   Do you have a living will? _No_

Today's Date _2/15/2005_ ___ Home Phone _634-555-1998_ ___ Work Phone _634-555-1650_

Patient Name (Last name, First name, Middle initial) _Sanchez, Enrique_

Street Address _4592176 Spur Lane_ ___ City _Orlando_ ___ State _FL_ ___ Zip _32897_

Date of Birth _4/29/1967_ ___ Age _38_ ___ Gender: ___ Female _X_ Male ___ Social Security # _234-XX-7890_

Marital Status: ___ Married _X_ Single ___ Widowed ___ Divorced ___ Other ___ Driver's License # _B692-XX-1699_

Is the patient a student? ___ Full Time ___ Part Time _X_ No Is the patient employed? _X_ Full Time ___ Part Time ___ No

Patient's Employer Name & Address _Harcourt Brace, 1579 Ocean Port, Orlando_

School Name & Address _N/A_

Emergency Contact Person _Miriam Sanchez_ ___ Relationship _Mother_ ___ Phone _555-1212_ ~~Puerto Rico~~

Referring Physician Name & Phone Number _None_

Insurance Plan and Responsible Party Information

Insurance Company Name _Aetna_ ___ Address _PO Box WW_

City _Tampa_ ___ State _FL_ ___ Zip _32897_ ___ Phone _800-555-1212_

Policy # _____ Group # _HB6792_ ___ ID # _HB634XX816501_

Policy Holder's Name _Sanchez, Enrique_ ___ Address _4592176 Spur Lane_

City _Orlando_ ___ State _FL_ ___ Zip _32897_ ___ Phone _634-555-1998_

Policy Holder's Date of Birth _4/29/1967_ ___ Social Security # _234-XX-7890_ ___ Driver License # _B692-XX-1699_

Gender: _X_ Male ___ Female ___ Relationship to patient: _X_ Self ___ Spouse ___ Parent ___ Guardian ___ Other

Policy Holder's Employer's Name _Harcourt Brace_ ___ Address _1579 Ocean Port_

City _Orlando_ ___ State _FL_ ___ Zip _32897_ ___ Phone _634-555-1650_

Secondary Insurance Company Name _None_ ___ Address _____

City _____ State _____ Zip _____ Phone _____

Secondary Policy # _____ Group # _____ ID # _____

Secondary Policy Holder's Name _____ Phone _____ Address _____

City _____ State _____ Zip _____ Relationship to patient: ___ Self ___ Spouse ___ other

Secondary Policy Holder's Date of Birth _____ Social Security # _____ Driver License # _____

Authorizations

It is customary to pay for all services on the date rendered unless other arrangements were made before your appointment. The patient and the guarantor are responsible for all deductibles and copays at the time of the visit and any other fees in accordance with insurance contracts. The patient and guarantor are responsible for all elective or noncovered services and any services that are not considered medically necessary.

Financially responsible person if patient is student or unemployed _____ Phone _____

I authorize the release of any medical information necessary to process this claim and I request that payment of medical benefits be made directly to Lake Eola Family Practice. I hereby acknowledge that I am fully responsible for payment as listed above.

Signed _Enrique Sanchez_ ___ Date _2/15/2005_ ___ Time _10:00 AM_

Template © 1998 Medical Compliance Management, Inc.

FIGURE C-2, A

Lake Eola Family Practice   517860 South Pioneer Drive, Orlando, FL 32897 • 634-555-4893

Problem List – Medication List

Patient Name ___Sanchez, Enrique_____ DOB _04/29/1967_

Allergies & allergic response ___Penicillin – hives, itching_____

Referring Physician & ID # ___None_____

	Problem (e.g., acute or chronic diagnosis, injury,↑ BP)	**Date Identified**	**Date Resolved**
1	Gastric ulcer	10/1/1996	12/5/1996
2	Epigastric pain	2/15/2005	
3			
4			
5			
6			
7			
8			
9			
10			
11			
12			
13			
14			
15			

	All Medications (with dosage & instructions) (include prescription and over-the-counter medications)	**Start Date**	**Discontinue Date**
1	Tagamet 800 mg ÷ PO BID	10/1/1996	12/5/1996
2	Mylanta ÷ TBSP PO q 6 h prn	12/5/1996	
3	Tums chew ÷ PO qid prn	12/5/1996	
4			
5			
6			
7			
8			
9			
10			

Template © 1998 Medical Compliance Management, Inc.

FIGURE C-2, B

Name _Sanchez, Enrique_____ Date _02_/_15_/_2005_

HPI Chief Complaint:

C/O Abd pain – upper abd – x 2 mos.
   Pain ↑ after meals & during night
No Nausa, No Vomiting
No Diarrhea, Occ. constipation
↑ Stress at work→deadlines, travel

Current Meds.:

OTC Mylanta T̄ TBSP prn
OTC Tums T̄ prn

Past/Family History

Hx gastric ulcer 4 years ago
   Treated c̄ Tagamet 800 mg BID x 2 mos.
   No recurrence.
No Tobacco. 1-2 beer/wine q d
Father died at age 35 from GI bleed with gastric
   ulcer (Puerto Rico)
Mother alive & well in Puerto Rico
1 Brother c̄ Hx gastric ulcers.

THIS SECTION TO BE COMPLETED BY PATIENT.

Personal/Social History

Are you... ☒ single ☐ married
☐ live in partner ☐ divorced ☐ widow

Do you have children? ☐ Yes ☒ No
Ages of child(ren) _____

Occupation _Editor – Textbooks_

                             Yes No
a. Are your immunizations up to date? ☒ ☐
   Date of last tetanus shot: _1995_

b. Do you have any pain or blood
   on urination? ☐ ☒

c. Do you have lesions, sores or
   drainage from penis? ☐ ☒

d. Do you have any lumps, swelling,
   tenderness or pain in groin, scrotum,
   or testicles? ☐ ☒

e. Are you sexually active now? ☐ ☐
   ☐ same sex ☒ opposite sex
   ☒ single partner ☐ multiple partners

   Have you had more than 4
   lifetime partners? ☒ ☐

f. Do you use condoms? ☒ ☐

g. Do you have concerns about sexual
   orientation, sexually transmitted
   diseases, or exporsure to HIV or
   other sexual concerns? ☐ ☒

h. Do you feel safe/comfortable in
   your home, with your family, and/or
   your partner relationship? ☒ ☐

i. Do you smoke or use tobacco
   products now? ☐ ☒

j. Do you use recreational drugs? ☐ ☒

k. Do you drink alcohol? ☒ ☐
   ☒ daily ☐ weekly ☐ rarely
   # of drinks _1-2_
   If yes, do you drink: ☒ beer, ☒ wine, ☐ liquor

Review of Systems
Are you concerned about?
(circle concerns) Yes No
1. Recent changes in health status ☒ ☐
2. Eye problems: vision, pain, tearing ☐ ☒
3. Ears, nose, mouth, throat problems ☐ ☒
4. Heart problems: chest pain, blood pressure ☐ ☒
5. Lung problems: coughing, wheezing,
   infections ☐ ☒

                          Yes No
6. (Abdominal pain, stomach, bowel problems ☒ ☐
7. Kidney or bladder problems ☐ ☒
8. Muscle, bone, joint or back problems ☐ ☒
9. Skin, hair or nail problems ☐ ☒
10. Neurologic problems: headaches,
    dizziness, numbness ☐ ☒
11. (Nervousness, anxiety, depression,
    suicidal thoughts ☒ ☐
12. Excessive thirst and urine output,
    recent weight changes ☐ ☒
13. Anemia, bruising, blood clots,
    swollen glands ☐ ☒
14. Food allergies, hayfever, eczema,
    asthma, decreased immunity ☐ ☒

Do you have any other concerns? ☐ ☒

_____
_____
_____
_____

Enrique Sanchez   _2/15/05_
Patient's Signature   Date

Provider Comments: 6. Epigastric Pain off & on x 2 mos, ↑severity last 24 hours
Pain↑p̄ meals & during night. Pain awakens him from a sound sleep
11. Nervous because father died from GI bleed.

Javier Gomez   _2/15/05_

☒ PFSH and ROS have been reviewed.   ☐ Unresolved problems from previous visit have been addressed.   Provider's Signuture   Date

Anticipatory Guidance

☐ Nutrition
☐ Exercise
☐ Dental care
☐ Cardiovascular risks

☐ Sun exposure
☐ Smoking cessation
☒ Alcohol/drugs
☐ Sexual issues
☐ STD prevention
☐ Self exam: testes, skin, oral cavity

☐ School/Work
☐ Family
☐ Recreation/Hobbies
☐ Safety/ Injury/Gun Safety
☐ Auto seat belts
☐ Smoke detectors

☐ Domestic violence
☒ Stress
☒ Educational handouts

500-01

Male19-39

FIGURE C-2, C

Name __Sanchez, Enrique__   DOB __04/29/1967__ Age __38__ Chart No. | SANE056 |

Assessment

8a. Epigastric abd. Pain

   R/O recurrent peptic ulcer
   R/O duodenal ulcer
   R/O reflux syndrome
   R/O angina

8e. hemocult stool negative

14d. Very anxious. Is nearing age of father when
   father died from GI bleed.
   Doesn't know if father had PUD

Plan

1. Stat CBC – draw at hospital
   & call results.
2. Schedule EGD ASAP at Lake
   Eola Hospital
3. Cont. OTC meds for now

Javier Gomez MD   _Tomorrow_
Provider's Signature   Return Visit

FOLD HERE   FOLD HERE

Physical Exam

Ht. _5' 7"_ Wt. _180_ Temp. _97.6_ Resp. _22_

B.P. sit. or stand. _124_ / _70_   Supine ___ / ___

Pulse rate and regularity _110, regular –_
                              Thready
Circle abnormal and pertinent normal findings
Describe abnormalities above.

☑ Normal   ☒ Abnormal

1. Constitutional
a. ☑ gen. appear., development, body shape,
   nutrition, deformities, grooming

2. Eyes
a. ☑ conjunctiva, lids
b. ☑ pupils, irises
c. ☐ fundi (optic discs, vessels, exudate, hemorr.)

3. Ears, Nose, Throat & Mouth
a. ☑ appearance of ears, appearance of nose
b. ☑ auditory canals, tympanic membranes
c. ☐ hearing (whis. voice, finger rub, tun. fork)
d. ☑ nasal mucosa, sputum, turbinates
e. ☑ lips, teeth, gums
f. ☑ oropharynx (mucosa, saliv. glands, hard &
   soft palates, tongue, tonsils, post. pharynx)

4. Neck
a. ☑ appearance, masses, symmetry, tracheal
   position, crepitus
b. ☑ thyroid (enlargement, tenderness, mass)

5. Respiratory
a. ☑ respiratory effort (intercostal retractions)
   use of accessory muscles, diaphragm move.
b. ☑ percussion (dullness, flatness, hyper-reson.)
c. ☐ palpation (tactile fremitus)
d. ☑ auscultation (breath sounds, rhonchi, wheezes,
   rales, rubs)

6. Cardiovascular
a. ☑ palpation (location of p.m.i., size, thrill)
b. ☑ auscultation (abnormal sounds, murmurs)
c. ☑ carotid arteries (pulse amplitude, bruits)
d. ☑ abdominal aorta (size, bruits)
e. ☑ femoral arteries (pulse amplitude, bruits)
f. ☑ pedal pulses (pulse amplitude)
g. ☑ extremities (edema, varicosities)

7. Chest (Breasts)
a. ☐ inspection (size, symmetry, nipple discharge)
b. ☐ palpation of breasts & axillae (masses,
   lumps, tenderness)

8. Gastrointestinal (Abdomen)
a. ☒ examination for masses, (tenderness)
b. ☑ examination of liver, spleen
c. ☑ examination for presence or absence of hernia
d. ☑ examination of (when indicated) anus, perineum,
   rectum: (sphincter tone, hemorrhoids, masses)
e. ☑ stool for occult blood when indicated

9. Genitourinary
a. ☑ scrotum (hydrocele, spermatocele,
   tenderness of cord, testicular mass)
b. ☑ examination of penis
c. ☑ digital exam of prostate (size, symmetry,
   nodularity, tenderness)

10. Lymphatic
a. ☑ palpation of lymph nodes in 2 or more areas:
   (Circle: (neck) axillae, (groin), other)

11. Musculoskeletal
a. ☑ examination of gait and station
b. ☑ inspection and/or palpation of digits & nails
   (clubbing, cyanosis, inflammatory conditions,
   petechiae, ischemia, infections, nodes)
c. ☑ assessment of range of motion (pain,
   crepitation, contracture)

d. ☑ Examination of joint, bone, & muscle of 1 or
   more of the following 6 areas (circle)
   ⦿ head/neck   • rt. upper extremities
   ⦿ spine, ribs, & pelvis • lt. upper extremities
   • rt. lower extremities   • lt. lower extremities
e. ☐ inspect, and/or palpation (misalign, asymmetry,
   crepitation, defects, tender., masses, effusion)
f. ☐ assessment of stability: dislocation (luxation),
   subluxation or laxity
g. ☐ muscle strength & tone (flaccid, cog wheel,
   spastic), atrophy or abnormal movement

12. Skin
a. ☑ inspection of skin & sub-Q tissue (rashes,
   lesion, ulcers)
b. ☐ palpation of skin & sub-Q tissue (induration,
   sub-Q nodules, tightening)

13. Neurology
a. ☐ test cranial nerves: notation of deficits
b. ☑ examination of DTR's with notation of
   pathological reflexes (eg. Babinski)
c. ☐ examination of sensation (touch, pain,
   vibration, proprioception)

14. Psychiatric
a. ☐ description of patient's judgment & insight
   Brief assessment of mental status:
b. ☑ orientation to time, place, & person
c. ☑ recent & remote memory
d. ☒ mood & affect (depression, (anxiety,) agitation)
e. ☐ other

Procedures and Immunizations

Are immunizations current?
☒ Yes ☐ No

☐ Hearing   ☐ Glucose   ☐ Cholesterol   ☐ CXR
☐ Vision   ☐ PT   ☐ HDL/LDL   ☐ EKG
☒ CBC   ☐ Urine   ☐ TSH

☐ dT   ☐ Hep B   ☐ Influenza

Drug Allergies:

PCN

**Male
19-39**

Date / Time
2/15/2005 11:00 AM

Summary
Epigastric pains, R/O PUD

☐ Referral

500-06

© 1995 Piermed, Inc. Rev

FIGURE C-2, D

Lake Eola Family Practice

517860 South Pioneer Drive, Orlando, FL 32897 • 634-555-4893

Superbill   #456298

Weight _180_   BP _124/70_   TPR _97.6°-110-22_

Account Number SANE056	Doctor Javier Gomez MD	Date of Service 2/15/2005
Patient Name Sanchez, Enrique	Date of Birth 04/29/1967	LMP N/A
Insurance AETNA	Responsible Party SELF	Phone Number 634-555-1998
Address PO Box WW	Referring Physician and ID # None	
City Tampa	State FL	Zip 32897	

New Patient

- __ 99201 H[PF] E[PF] MDM[S] 10 min
- __ 99202 H[EPF] E[EPF] MDM[S] 20 min
- __ 99203 H[D] E[D] MDM[LC] 30 min
- __ 99204 H[C] E[C] MDM[MC] 45 min
- __ 99205 H[C] E[C] MDM[HC] 60 min

✓ Established Patient

- __ 99211 H[N/A] E[N/A] MDM[N/A] 5 min
- __ 99212 H[PF] E[PF] MDM[S] 10 min
- __ 99213 H[EPF] E[EPF] MDM[LC] 15 min
- __ 99214 H[D] E[D] MDM[MC] 25 min
- X 99215 H[C] E[C] MDM[HC] 40 min

Reason For Visit

- __ Authorization _____
  Expiration Date _____
- __ Annual exam, complex due to (history, condition): _____
- __ Annual exam, simple
- __ Follow-up, condition _____
- __ Follow-up, post procedure, no condition or complication _____
  Procedure/date _____
- __ Follow-up, post procedure, with condition or complication _____
  Procedure/date _____
- X New Problem _Abd Pain-Epigastric_
- __ Post-op, no condition or complication
  Surgery/date _____
- __ Post-op, with conditions or complication
  _____
  Surgery/date _____
- __ Pre-op _____
- __ Procedure _____
- __ Second surgical opinion _____
- X Other (Accident, (Decision for surgery) __
  EGD

Procedures

- ⇒ Place to be done: _Lake Eola Hospital_
- ⇒ Date to be done: _ASAP_
- X Authorization _Get Auth._
  Expiration date _____
- __ Biopsy, type/site _____
- __ Cautery, type/site _____
- __ Destruction of lesion(s), extensive, site: __
  _____
- __ Destruction of lesion(s), simple, site: _____
  _____
- __ Emergency surgery (list above), reason: __
  _____
- __ Excision, type/site _____
  _____
- __ I & D abscess, type/site: _____
  _____
- __ Insertion/Removal of IUD, type _____
- __ Major surgery, type/site _____
  _____
- __ Minor surgery, type/site _____
  _____
- __ Sonogram _____
- X Other _EGD – Schedule_

Miscellaneous

- __ Immunization _____
- __ Injection _____
- __ Supplies
- __ Surgical tray

✓ Patient Teaching (Preventive medicine)

No   Stress   ⟩ Handouts
Charge ETOH

- __ Other _____
  _____
  _____
  _____

Outside Lab

- __ Beta HCG, Serum
- __ Biopsy/Pathology
- __ Biopsy, Mult./Pathology
- X CBC _–Draw @ Hospital._
- __ Cholesterol
- __ Culture, throat
- __ Cultures (source) _____
- __ Glucose, __1hr glucose, __3hr glucose
- __ Estrogen
- __ Herpes simplex, AB
- __ Mononucleosis
- __ Pap Smear
- __ PT __PTT
- __ Sed rate
- __ SMAC
- __ Urinalysis, w/micro
- __ HIV
- __ Other
  Make CBC Stat – Send Now.
  _____
  _____

Diagnosis Codes

1. _789.06_
2. _300.00_
3. _V12.71_
4. _____

Appointment in _____ Weeks
Procedure in _ASAP_ Weeks
Sent Labs to_____
Call in _Tomorrow_ Mos./Weeks

Previous Balance $ _0_
Co-Pay $ _10.00_
Paid Today (Cash)/Check $ _10.00_
(Yes)/No All Diagnosis, Procedures, & VS above are documented in Record
Doctor's Signature _Javier Gomez MD_

New Charges $ _190.00_
New Balance $ _180.00_
Check Number _____

Template © 1998 Medical Compliance Management, Inc.,
CPT only © American Medical Association. All Rights Reserved.

FIGURE C-2, E

Case Study 3: Miriam Gonzalez

Lake Eola Family Practice   517860 South Pioneer Drive, Orlando, FL 32897 • 634-555-4893

Patient Registration Form

Have you been seen in this office in the past 3 years? ___ Yes ✔ No   **Do you have a living will?** Yes

Today's Date _6/2/2005_ Home Phone _634-555-1200_ Work Phone _634-555-1555_

Patient Name (Last name, First name, Middle initial) _Gonzalez, Miriam_

Street Address _597652 Spur Lane_ City _Orlando_ State _FL_ Zip _32897_

Date of Birth _2/14/1949_ Age _56_ Gender: _X_ Female ___ Male Social Security # _345-XX-8999_

Marital Status: _X_ Married ___ Single ___ Widowed ___ Divorced ___ Other Driver's License # _B621-XX-1099_

Is the patient a student? ___ Full Time _X_ Part Time ___ No Is the patient employed? _X_ Full Time ___ Part Time ___ No

Patient's Employer Name & Address _Western Time-Shares, 1245 Spur Lane_

School Name & Address _UCF – Alafaya Trail – Orlando_

Emergency Contact Person _Jorges Gonzalez_ Relationship _Husband_ Phone _634-555-1200_

Referring Physician Name & Phone Number _None_

Insurance Plan and Responsible Party Information

Insurance Company Name _BC BS of FL_ Address _PO Box YYYY_

City _Jacksonville_ State _FL_ Zip _39782_ Phone _800-555-1212_

Policy # _BC345XX8999_ Group # _WTS 012_ ID # _____

Policy Holder's Name _Miriam Gonzalez_ Address _Same_

City _____ State _____ Zip _____ Phone _____

Policy Holder's Date of Birth _2/14/1949_ Social Security # _345-XX-8999_ Driver License # _B621-XX-1099_

Gender: ___ Male _X_ Female Relationship to patient: _X_ Self ___ Spouse ___ Parent ___ Guardian ___ Other

Policy Holder's Employer's Name _Western Time Shares_ Address _1245 Spur Lane_

City _Orlando_ State _FL_ Zip _32897_ Phone _634-555-1555_

Secondary Insurance Company Name _BC BS of FL_ Address _PO Box YYYY_

City _Jacksonville_ State _FL_ Zip _32897_ Phone _800-555-1212_

Secondary Policy # _MM567XX0001_ Group # _MM1976_ ID # _____

Secondary Policy Holder's Name _Jorges Gonzalez_ Phone _Same_ Address _Same_

City _____ State _____ Zip _____ Relationship to patient: ___ Self _X_ Spouse ___ other

Secondary Policy Holder's Date of Birth _6/21/1942_ Social Security # _567-XX-0001_ Driver License # _B682-XX-1099_

Employed by Martin Marietta Corp.

Authorizations

It is customary to pay for all services on the date rendered unless other arrangements were made before your appointment. The patient and the guarantor are responsible for all deductibles and copays at the time of the visit and any other fees in accordance with insurance contracts. The patient and guarantor are responsible for all elective or noncovered services and any services that are not considered medically necessary.

Financially responsible person if patient is student or unemployed _Jorges Gonzalez_ Phone _634-555-1200_

I authorize the release of any medical information necessary to process this claim and I request that payment of medical benefits be made directly to Lake Eola Family Practice. I hereby acknowledge that I am fully responsible for payment as listed above.

Signed _Miriam Gonzalez_ Date _6/2/2005_ Time _11:30 AM_

Template © 1998 Medical Compliance Management, Inc.

FIGURE C-3, A

Lake Eola Family Practice   517860 South Pioneer Drive, Orlando, FL 32897 • 634-555-4893

Problem List – Medication List

Patient Name _Gonzalez, Miriam_ DOB _02/14/1949_

Allergies & allergic response _Hay fever   No Medication Allergies_

Referring Physician & ID # _None_

	Problem (e.g., acute or chronic diagnosis, injury,↑ BP)	**Date Identified**	**Date Resolved**
1	Allergic rhinitis	06/02/2005	
2	Allergic bronchitis	06/02/2005	
3	Allergic serous otitis media	06/02/2005	
4			
5			
6			
7			
8			
9			
10			
11			
12			
13			
14			
15			

	All Medications (with dosage & instructions) (include prescription and over-the-counter medications)	**Start Date**	**Discontinue Date**
1	OTC Tylenol cold & allergy q 12 h prn		06/02/2005
2	Amoxicillin 500mg PO BID x 10 days	06/02/2005	
3	Hycodan 5 ml q 6 h prn	06/02/2005	
4	Tylenol ES ÷ PO q 4-6 h prn (OTC)	06/02/2005	
5			
6			
7			
8			
9			
10			

Template © 1998 Medical Compliance Management, Inc.

FIGURE C-3, B

Name _Gonzalez, Miriam_   Date _06_/_02_/_2005_

HPI Chief Complaint:

Cough due to seasonal allergies x 2 wks –
not improving c̄ OTC meds
Cough is now productive c̄ yellow to green
sputum. Denies Fever.
Bad taste in mouth has↓appetite _
lost 5 lbs in past 2 wks.

Current Meds.:

OTC Tylenol cold & allergy q 12h prn
Taken x 2 wks

Past/Family History

Hx seasonal allergies x 20 years usually
controlled c̄ OTC meds
Parents/Siblings all alive & well c̄ no major
health problems

Note: Moved here from New York City
2 months ago. Signed release for records to
be transferred here.

THIS SECTION TO BE COMPLETED BY PATIENT.

Personal/Social History

Are you... ☐ single ☒ married
☐ live in partner ☐ divorced ☐ widow

Do you have children? ☒ Yes ☐ No
Ages of child(ren) _16, 19, 24, 28_
No. of pregnancies _6_ Miscarriages _2_
Occupation _Time-share Sales_

	Yes	No
a. Do you have concerns about your breasts? (circle): changes in size or shape, changes in skin color, lumps, tenderness, ulcerations, discharge or blood from nipple, inverted nipple	☐	☒
b. Concerns about menstruation, (irregular bleeding patterns, hot flashes,) pain or bleeding with intercourse, itching, burning or discharge?	☒	☐
c. Do you take hormones (estrogen)?	☐	☒
d. Concerns about lesions, lumps or swelling on your vulva or vagina?	☐	☒
e. Do you have urine leakage?	☒	☐

Only c̄ coughing

f. Approximate date of last pelvic exam. _2/2000_
g. Approximate date of last pap test _2/2000_
h Approximate date of last mammogram _3/2000_

	Yes	No
i. Are you sexually active now?	☒	☐
☐ same sex ☒ opposite sex		
☒ single partner ☐ multiple partners		
j. Do you have other sexual concerns?	☐	☒
k. Do you feel safe/comfortable in your home, with your family, and/or your partner relationship?	☒	☐
l. Do you smoke or use tobacco products now?	☐	☒
m. Do you use recreational drugs?	☐	☒
n. Do you drink alcohol?	☒	☐
☐ daily ☐ weekly ☒ rarely		
# of drinks _1-2_		
If yes, do you drink: ☐ beer, ☒ wine, ☐ liquor		

Review of Systems

Are you concerned about?
(circle concerns)

	Yes	No
1. Recent changes in health status	☒	☐
2. Eye problems: vision, pain, tearing	☐	☒

	Yes	No
3. Ears, nose, mouth, throat problems	☐	☒
4. Heart problems: chest pain, blood pressure	☐	☒
5. Lung problems: (coughing,) wheezing, infections _x 2 weeks_	☒	☐
6. Abdominal pain, stomach, bowel problems	☐	☒
7. Kidney or bladder problems	☐	☒
8. Muscle, bone, joint or back problems	☐	☒
9. Skin, hair or nail problems	☐	☒
10. Neurologic problems: headaches, dizziness, numbness	☐	☒
11. Nervousness, anxiety, depression, suicidal thoughts	☐	☒
12. Excessive thirst and urine output, (recent weight changes) _lost 5 lb_	☒	☐
13. Anemia, bruising, blood clots, swollen glands	☐	☒
14. Food allergies, (hayfever,) eczema, asthma, decreased immunity	☒	☐
Do you have any other concerns?	☐	☒

Miriam Gonzalez   _6/2/05_
Patient's Signature   Date

Provider Comments: Moved to Orlando 2 months ago. Sent for records.

b. menopausal symptoms x 1 year – unchanged. e. leaks urine c̄ coughing only. Will give Keagal instructions.
5, 14 – Cough x 2 wks due to hayfever. Concerned that cough not improved & now productive.

Javier Gomez   _2/6/05_

☒ PFSH and ROS have been reviewed.   ☐ Unresolved problems from previous visit have been addressed.   Provider's Signature   Date

Anticipatory Guidance

☐ Nutrition
☐ Calcium
☐ Exercise
☐ Dental care

☐ Sun exposure
☐ Smoking cessation
☐ Alcohol/drugs
☐ Cardiovascular risks
☐ Aspirin prophylaxis
☒ Osteoporosis risks
☐ Estrogen

☐ Self exam. breasts, skin, oral cavity
☐ Sexual issues
☐ STD prevention
☒ Menopause , Keagal
☐ Menopause bleeding
☐ Work
☐ Family

☐ Safety/ Injury/Gun Safety
☐ Auto seat belts
☐ Smoke detectors
☐ Domestic violence
☐ Stress
☐ Recreation/Hobbies
☒ Educational handouts

500-04

FIGURE C-3, C

Name _Gonzalez, Miriam_____ DOB _02/_14_/1949_ Age _56_ Chart No. | GONM022 |

Assessment

3b. Tympanic membranes pink & slightly bulging
3d. Nasal mucosa congested c̄ clear drainage
3f. Pharynz reddened. Sputum yellow to green
5b. Chest percussion dull
5d. Bilat. rales & rhonchi lower lobes. No rubs. No wheezes.
10a. Post cervical lymph nodes palpable

Dx Acute bronchitis – bilat. 2° hay-fever
      Otitis media – Bilat. – serous allergic
      Allergic Rhinitis, acute pharyingitis
      R/O Pneumonia

Plan

1. CXR – Lake Eola Hospital
2. CBC   ⎫ Smith Klein
3. Sputum culture   ⎬ Beechum
                              ⎭ Labs.

Rx
Amoxicillin 500 mg PO BID
   Begin p̄ cultures
Hycodan 5 ml q 6 h prn
Tylenol ESTq 4-6 h prn (OTC)

_Javier Gomez_____   _2/6/2005_
Provider's Signature   Return Visit

FOLD HERE ▼   FOLD HERE ▼

Physical Exam

Ht. _5' 3"_ Wt. _95#_ Temp. _100.4°_ Resp. _24_

B.P. sit. or stand. _100_ / _72_ Supine ___ / ___

Pulse rate and regularity _102, regular_
                                    Thready
Circle abnormal and pertinent normal findings
Describe abnormalities above.
☑ Normal   ☒ Abnormal

1. Constitutional
a. ☑ gen. appear., development, body shape,
        nutrition, deformities, grooming

2. Eyes
a. ☑ conjunctiva, lids
b. ☑ pupils, irises
c. ☐ fundi (optic discs, vessels, exudate, hemorr.)

3. Ears, Nose, Throat & Mouth
a. ☑ appearance of ears, appearance of nose
b. ☒ auditory canals, tympanic membranes
c. ☐ hearing (whis. voice, finger rub, tun. fork)
d. ☑ nasal mucosa, sputum, turbinates
e. ☑ lips, teeth, gums
f. ☒ oropharynx (mucosa, saliv. glands, hard &
        soft palates, tongue, tonsils, post. pharynx)

4. Neck
a. ☑ appearance, masses, symmetry, tracheal
        position, crepitus
b. ☑ thyroid (enlargement, tenderness, mass)

5. Respiratory
a. ☑ respiratory effort (intercostal retractions)
        use of accessory muscles, diaphragm move.
b. ☒ percussion (dullness), flatness, hyper-reson.)
c. ☑ palpation (tactile fremitus)
d. ☒ auscultation (breath sounds, (rhonchi), wheezes,
        (rales), rubs)

6. Cardiovascular
a. ☑ palpation (location of p.m.i., size, thrill)
b. ☑ auscultation (abnormal sounds, murmurs)
c. ☑ carotid arteries (pulse amplitude, bruits)
d. ☐ abdominal aorta (size, bruits)
e. ☐ femoral arteries (pulse amplitude, bruits)
f. ☑ pedal pulses (pulse amplitude)
g. ☑ extremities (edema, varicosities)

7. Chest (Breasts)
a. ☐ inspection (size, symmetry, nipple discharge)
b. ☐ palpation of breasts & axillae (masses,
        lumps, tenderness)

8. Gastrointestinal (Abdomen)
a. ☑ examination for masses, tenderness
b. ☑ examination of liver, spleen
c. ☑ examination for presence or absence of hernia
d. ☐ examination of (when indicated) anus, perineum,
        rectum: (sphincter tone, hemorrhoids, masses)
e. ☐ stool for occult blood when indicated

9. Genitourinary
Pelvic Exam (with or without specimen collection
for smears or cultures), including:
a. ☐ Ext. Genitalia (eg. gen. app., hair distrib.,
        lesions) and vagina (eg. gen. app., estrogen eff.,
        lesions, pelvic support, cystocele, rectocele)
b. ☐ Urethra (eg. masses, tender., scarring)
c. ☐ Bladder (eg. fullness, masses, tender.)
d. ☐ Cervix (eg. gen. app., lesions, disch.)
e. ☐ Uterus (eg. size, contour, position, mobility,
        tender., consistency, descent or support)
f. ☐ Adnexia / Parametria (eg. masses, tender.,
        organomegally, nodularity)

10. Lymphatic
a. ☒ palpation of lymph nodes in 2 or more areas:
        (Circle: (neck) (axillae) groin, other)

11. Musculoskeletal
a. ☑ examination of gait and station
b. ☑ inspection and/or palpation of digits & nails
        (clubbing, cyanosis, inflammatory conditions,
        petechiae, ischemia, infections, nodes)
c. ☑ assessment of range of motion (pain,
        crepitation, contracture)
d. ☑ Examination of joint, bone, & muscle of 1 or
        more of the following 6 areas (circle)
        ⊙ head/neck   • rt. upper extremities
        ⊙ spine, ribs, & pelvis • lt. upper extremities
        • rt. lower extremities • lt. lower extremities
e. ☐ inspect, and/or palpation (misalign, asymmetry,
        crepitation, defects, tender., masses, effusion)
f. ☐ assessment of stability: dislocation (luxation),
        subluxation or laxity
g. ☐ muscle strength & tone (flaccid, cogwheel,
        spastic), atrophy or abnormal movement

12. Skin
a. ☑ inspection of skin & sub-Q tissue (rashes,
        lesion, ulcers)
b. ☑ palpation of skin & sub-Q tissue (induration,
        sub-Q nodules, tightening)

13. Neurology
a. ☐ test cranial nerves: notation of deficits
b. ☑ examination of DTR's with notation of
        pathological reflexes (eg. Babinski)
c. ☐ examination of sensation (touch, pain,
        vibration, proprioception)

14. Psychiatric
a. ☐ description of patient's judgment & insight
        Brief assessment of mental status:
b. ☑ orientation to time, place, & person
c. ☑ recent & remote memory
d. ☐ mood & affect (depression, anxiety, agitation)
e. ☐ other _____

Procedures and Immunizations

☐ Hearing   ☐ PT   ☐ Triglyceride   ☐ Stool Guaiac   Are immunizations current?
☐ Vision   ☐ TSH   ☒ CXR   ☐ Sigmoidoscopy   ☐ Yes ☐ No
☒ CBC   ☐ Urine   ☐ EKG   ☐ dT
☐ Glucose   ☐ Cholesterol ☐ PAP Test   ☒ Culture, sputum ☐ Hep B
             ☐ HDL/LDL   ☐ Mammogram   ☐ Influenza

Drug Allergies:

NKA

© 1995 Piermed, Inc. Rev

Female
40-59

Date / Time   Summary   Allergic Rhinitis
6/02/2005 PM   Allergic Bronchitis
                              Allergic Serous Otitis Media

☐ Referral

500-06

FIGURE C-3, D

Lake Eola Family Practice

517860 South Pioneer Drive, Orlando, FL 32897 • 634-555-4893

Superbill   #456298

Weight _95#_   BP _100/72_   TPR _100.4°-102-24_

Account Number GONM022	Doctor Javier Gomez MD	Date of Service 06/02/2005
Patient Name Gonzalez, Miriam	Date of Birth 02/14/1949	LMP 05/10/2000
Insurance BCBS FL/BCBS FL	Responsible Party Miriam Gonzalez	Phone Number 634-555-1200
Address PO Box YYYY	Referring Physician and ID # None	
City Jacksonville	State FL	Zip 39782	

✓ New Patient

- __ 99201 H[PF]   E[PF]   MDM[S]   10 min
- __ 99202 H[EPF] E[EPF] MDM[S]   20 min
- __ 99203 H[D]   E[D]   MDM[LC] 30 min
- _X_ 99204 H[C]   E[C]   MDM[MC] 45 min
- __ 99205 H[C]   E[C]   MDM[HC] 60 min

Established Patient

- __ 99211 H[N/A] E[N/A] MDM[N/A] 5 min
- __ 99212 H[PF]   E[PF]   MDM[S]   10 min
- __ 99213 H[EPF] E[EPF] MDM[LC] 15 min
- __ 99214 H[D]   E[D]   MDM[MC] 25 min
- __ 99215 H[C]   E[C]   MDM[HC] 40 min

Reason For Visit

- __ Authorization _____
    Expiration Date _____
- __ Annual exam, complex due to (history, condition): _____
- __ Annual exam, simple
- __ Follow-up, condition _____
- __ Follow-up, post procedure, no condition or complication _____
    Procedure/date _____
- __ Follow-up, post procedure, with condition or complication _____
    Procedure/date _____
- _X_ New Problem _Cough X 2 wks_
- __ Post-op, no condition or complication
    Surgery/date _____
- __ Post-op, with conditions or complication _____
    Surgery/date _____
- __ Pre-op _____
- __ Procedure _____
- __ Second surgical opinion _____
- __ Other (Accident, Decision for surgery) __
    _____

Procedures

- ⇒ Place to be done: _____
- ⇒ Date to be done: _____
- __ Authorization _____
    Expiration date _____
- __ Biopsy, type/site _____
- __ Cautery, type/site _____
- __ Destruction of lesion(s), extensive, site: __
- __ Destruction of lesion(s), simple, site: _____
- __ Emergency surgery (list above), reason: __
- __ Excision, type/site _____
- __ I & D abscess, type/site: _____
- __ Insertion/Removal of IUD, type _____
- __ Major surgery, type/site _____
- __ Minor surgery, type/site _____
- __ Sonogram _____
- __ Other _____

Miscellaneous

- __ Immunization _____
- __ Injection _____
- __ Supplies
- __ Surgical tray

X Patient Teaching (Preventive medicine)
Brochures only – No Charge

X Other   _CXR* Schedule at Lake Eola_
Hospital
*Get Authorization
Reason: Rales/Rhonchi

Outside Lab

- __ Beta HCG, Serum
- __ Biopsy/Pathology
- __ Biopsy, Mult./Pathology
- _X_ CBC **
- __ Cholesterol
- __ Culture, throat
- _X_ Cultures (source) _Sputum **_
- __ Glucose, __ 1hr glucose, __ 3hr glucose
- __ Estrogen
- __ Herpes simplex, AB
- __ Mononucleosis
- __ Pap Smear
- __ PT __ PTT
- __ Sed rate
- __ SMAC
- __ Urinalysis, w/micro
- __ HIV
- __ Other _____
    ** Labs to be done at SKB due
    to insurance requirements

Diagnosis Codes

1. _466.0_
2. _381.04_
3. _462_
4. _477.9_

Appointment in _10 days_ ~~Weeks~~

Procedure in _____ Weeks

Sent Labs to _____

Call in _____ Mos./Weeks

Previous Balance $ _Ø_

Co-Pay $ _10.00_

Paid Today Cash/(Check) $ _10.00_

(Yes)-No All Diagnosis, Procedures, & VS above are documented in Record

Doctor's Signature _Javier Gomez MD_

New Charges $ _150.00_

New Balance $ _140.00_

Check Number _0140_

Template © 1998 Medical Compliance Management, Inc.,
CPT only © American Medical Association. All Rights Reserved.

FIGURE C-3, E

Case Study 4: John Williams

Lake Eola Family Practice   517860 South Pioneer Drive, Orlando, FL 32897 • 634-555-4893

Patient Registration Form

Have you been seen in this office in the past 3 years? ___Yes _✓_ No   **Do you have a living will?** _No_

Today's Date ___9/6/2005___   Home Phone ___634-555-9111___   Work Phone _____

Patient Name (Last name, First name, Middle initial) ___Williams, John___

Street Address ___5971294 Rodeo Circle___ City ___Orlando___ State _FL_ Zip _32897_

Date of Birth _6/12/1955_ Age _49_ Gender: ___Female _X_ Male   Social Security # _Confidential_

Marital Status: _X_ Married ___Single ___Widowed ___Divorced ___Other   Driver's License # _B629-XX-5799_

Is the patient a student? ___Full Time ___Part Time _X_ No Is the patient employed? _X_ Full Time ___Part Time ___No

Patient's Employer Name & Address ___Williams Car Dealership___

~~School Name~~ & Address ___18754 Spur Lane, Orlando___

Emergency Contact Person _Janice Williams_   Relationship _Wife_   Phone _Same_

Referring Physician Name & Phone Number ___N/A___

Insurance Plan and Responsible Party Information

Insurance Company Name _Aetna HMO_   Address _PO Box WW_

City ___Tampa___ State _FL_ Zip _32897_ Phone _800-555-1212_

Policy # _____ Group # _WCD2700_ ID # _ACFJ667992_

Policy Holder's Name _John Williams_   Address _Same_

City _____ State _____ Zip _____ Phone _____

Policy Holder's Date of Birth _____ Social Security # _____ Driver License # _____

Gender: _X_ Male ___Female   Relationship to patient: _X_ Self ___Spouse ___Parent ___Guardian ___Other

Policy Holder's Employer's Name ___Same___   Address _____

City _____ State _____ Zip _____ Phone _____

Secondary Insurance Company Name ___None___   Address _____

City _____ State _____ Zip _____ Phone _____

Secondary Policy # _____ Group # _____ ID # _____

Secondary Policy Holder's Name _____ Phone _____ Address _____

City _____ State _____ Zip _____ Relationship to patient: ___Self ___Spouse ___other

Secondary Policy Holder's Date of Birth _____ Social Security # _____ Driver License # _____

Authorizations

It is customary to pay for all services on the date rendered unless other arrangements were made before your appointment. The patient and the guarantor are responsible for all deductibles and copays at the time of the visit and any other fees in accordance with insurance contracts. The patient and guarantor are responsible for all elective or noncovered services and any services that are not considered medically necessary.

Financially responsible person if patient is student or unemployed _____ Phone _____

I authorize the release of any medical information necessary to process this claim and I request that payment of medical benefits be made directly to Lake Eola Family Practice. I hereby acknowledge that I am fully responsible for payment as listed above.

Signed ___John Williams___   Date _6 Sept 2005_ Time _4 PM_

Template © 1998 Medical Compliance Management, Inc.

FIGURE C-4, A

Lake Eola Family Practice   517860 South Pioneer Drive, Orlando, FL 32897 • 634-555-4893

Problem List – Medication List

Patient Name ___Williams, John___   DOB ___06/12/1955___

Allergies & allergic response ___Adhesive tape – blisters   No drug Allergies___

Referring Physician & ID # ___None___

	Problem (e.g., acute or chronic diagnosis, injury, ↑ BP)	**Date Identified**	**Date Resolved**
1	Bleeding rectal hemorrhoids	09/06/2005	
2			
3			
4			
5			
6			
7			
8			
9			
10			
11			
12			
13			
14			
15			

	All Medications (with dosage & instructions) (include prescription and over-the-counter medications)	**Start Date**	**Discontinue Date**
1			
2			
3			
4			
5			
6			
7			
8			
9			
10			

Template © 1998 Medical Compliance Management, Inc.

FIGURE C-4, B

Name Williams, John   Date 09/06/2005

HPI Chief Complaint:

Bleeding hemorrhoids
   Hx hemorrhoids x 2 years
   Slight bleeding off & on x 1 month, no↑
Recent weight gain,↑fatigue, Trouble sleeping.

Current Meds.:

None

Past/Family History

Parents both alive & well
No significant Family Hx

THIS SECTION TO BE COMPLETED BY PATIENT.

Personal/Social History

Are you... ☐ single ☒ married
☐ live in partner ☐ divorced ☐ widow

Do you have children? ☒ Yes ☐ No
Ages of child(ren) 20, 23

Occupation Business Owner
            Car Dealership

	Yes	No
a. Have you had (circle) any recent health concerns: changes in the way you feel, weight loss or gain, increased tiredness or weakness, problems with sleep, changes in your overall happiness?	☒	☐
b. Do you have any pain or blood on urination?	☐	☒
c. Do you have lesions, sores or drainage from penis?	☐	☒
d. Do you have any lumps, swelling, tenderness or pain in groin, scrotum, or testicles?	☐	☒
e. Do you have any difficulty getting or sustaining an erection?	☐	☒
f. Are you sexually active now?	☒	☐

☐ same sex ☒ opposite sex
☒ single partner ☐ multiple partners

	Yes	No
Have you had more than 4 lifetime partners?	☒	☐
g. Do you use condoms?	☐	☒
h. Do you have concerns about sexual orientation, sexually transmitted diseases, or exposure to HIV or other sexual concerns?	☐	☒
i. Do you feel safe/comfortable in your home, with your family, and/or your partner relationship?	☒	☐
j. Do you smoke or use tobacco products now?	☒	☐
k. Do you use recreational drugs?	☐	☒
l. Do you drink alcohol?	☒	☐

☐ daily ☒ weekly ☐ rarely
# of drinks 2-3

If yes, do you drink: ☒ beer, ☒ wine, ☒ liquor

Review of Systems
Are you concerned about?
(circle concerns)

	Yes	No
1. Recent changes in health status	☒	☐
2. Eye problems: vision, pain, tearing	☐	☒

	Yes	No
3. Ears, nose, mouth, throat problems	☐	☒
4. Heart problems: chest pain, blood pressure	☐	☒
5. Lung problems: coughing, wheezing, infections	☐	☒
6. Abdominal pain, stomach, bowel problems	☒	☐
7. Kidney or bladder problems	☐	☒
8. Muscle, bone, joint or back problems	☐	☒
9. Skin, hair or nail problems	☐	☒
10. Neurologic problems: headaches, dizziness, numbness	☐	☒
11. Nervousness, anxiety, depression, suicidal thoughts	☐	☒
12. Excessive thirst and urine output, recent weight changes	☐	☒
13. Anemia, bruising, blood clots, swollen glands	☐	☒
14. Food allergies, hayfever, eczema, asthma, decreased immunity	☐	☒
Do you have any other concerns?	☐	☒

John Williams   9/6/05
Patient's Signuture   Date

Provider Comments: a. Weight gain of 10 lbs in last month, Trouble sleeping due to
rectal pain with BM is causing↑fatigue.
J. Smokes 1/2 pk/day

Eric Anderson MD   9/6/05
Provider's Signature   Date

☒ PFSH and ROS have been reviewed. ☐ Unresolved problems from previous visit have been addressed.

Anticipatory Guidance

☐ Nutrition
☐ Exercise
☐ Dental care
☐ Sun exposure

☒ Smoking cessation
☒ Alcohol/drugs
☐ Cardiovascular risks
☐ Aspirin prophylaxis
☐ Sexual issues
☐ Self exam: testes, skin, oral cavity

☐ STD prevention
☐ Work
☐ Family
☐ Recreation/Hobbies
☐ Safety/ Injury/Gun Safety
☐ Auto seat belts

☐ Smoke detectors
☐ Domestic violence
☐ Stress
☒ Educational handouts

©1995 Piermed, Inc. Rev. 6/98 (800) 998-1908

500-03

Male 40-59

FIGURE C-4, C

Name __Williams, John__   DOB _06_/_12_/_1955_ Age _49_ Chart No. [WILJOO9]

Assessment

8d.

2 small hemorrhoids noted just inside rectum on
anterior wall. Each measures 2cm x 3cm, and both
are bleeding slightly. Sigmoidoscopy did not reveal
any further problems. Bleeding stopped with cautery.

No other significant problems

Plan

① Procto foam p̄ each BM x 2 weeks.
② Surfak ī PO BID
③ CBC today and repeat in 2 weeks

Eric Anderson MD   _2 wks_
Provider's Signature   Return Visit

FOLD HERE   FOLD HERE

Physical Exam

Ht. _6' 2"_ Wt. _240#_ Temp. _98.2_ Resp. _18_

B.P. sit. or stand. _140_ / _84_ Supine ___ / ___

Pulse rate and regularity _86, regular_

Circle abnormal and pertinent normal findings
Describe abnormalities above.

☑ Normal   ☒ Abnormal

1. Constitutional
a. ☑ gen. appear., development, body shape,
        nutrition, deformities, grooming

2. Eyes
a. ☑ conjunctiva, lids
b. ☑ pupils, irises
c. ☐ fundi (optic discs, vessels, exudate, hemorr.)

3. Ears, Nose, Throat & Mouth
a. ☑ appearance of ears, appearance of nose
b. ☑ auditory canals, tympanic membranes
c. ☐ hearing (whis. voice, finger rub, tun. fork)
d. ☑ nasal mucosa, sputum, turbinates
e. ☐ lips, teeth, gums
f. ☑ oropharynx (mucosa, saliv. glands, hard &
        soft palates, tongue, tonsils, post. pharynx)

4. Neck
a. ☑ appearance, masses, symmetry, tracheal
        position, crepitus
b. ☑ thyroid (enlargement, tenderness, mass)

5. Respiratory
a. ☑ respiratory effort (intercostal retractions)
        use of accessory muscles, diaphragm move.
b. ☐ percussion (dullness, flatness, hyper-reson.)
c. ☐ palpation (tactile fremitus)
d. ☑ auscultation (breath sounds, rhonchi, wheezes,
        rales, rubs)

6. Cardiovascular
a. ☐ palpation (location of p.m.i., size, thrill)
b. ☑ auscultation (abnormal sounds, murmurs)
c. ☐ carotid arteries (pulse amplitude, bruits)
d. ☐ abdominal aorta (size, bruits)
e. ☑ femoral arteries (pulse amplitude, bruits)
f. ☑ pedal pulses (pulse amplitude)
g. ☑ extremities (edema, varicosities)

7. Chest (Breasts)
a. ☐ inspection (size, symmetry, nipple discharge)
b. ☐ palpation of breasts & axillae (masses,
        lumps, tenderness)

8. Gastrointestinal (Abdomen)
a. ☑ examination for masses, tenderness
b. ☑ examination of liver, spleen
c. ☑ examination for presence or absence of hernia
d. ☒ examination of (when indicated) anus, perineum,
        rectum: (sphincter tone, (hemorrhoids), masses)
e. ☒ stool for occult blood when indicated

9. Genitourinary
a. ☑ scrotum (hydrocele, spermatocele,
        tenderness of cord, testicular mass)
b ☑ examination of penis
c. ☑ digital exam of prostate (size, symmetry,
        nodularity, tenderness)

10. Lymphatic
a. ☑ palpation of lymph nodes in 2 or more areas:
        (Circle: (neck,) axillae, (groin,) other)

11. Musculoskeletal
a. ☑ examination of gait and station
b. ☑ inspection and/or palpation of digits & nails
        (clubbing, cyanosis, inflammatory conditions,
        petechiae, ischemia, infections, nodes)
c. ☐ assessment of range of motion (pain,
        crepitation, contracture)

d. ☐ Examination of joint, bone, & muscle of 1 or
        more of the following 6 areas (circle)
        • head/neck   • rt. upper extremities
        • spine, ribs, & pelvis • lt. upper extremities
        • rt. lower estremities • lt. lower extremities
e. ☐ inspect, and/or palpation (misalign, asymmetry,
        crepitation, defects, tender., masses, effusion)
f. ☐ assessment of stability: dislocation (luxation),
        subluxation or laxity
g. ☑ muscle strength & tone (flaccid, cogwheel,
        spastic), atrophy or abnormal movement

12. Skin
a. ☑ inspection of skin & sub-Q tissue (rashes,
        lesion, ulcers)
b. ☐ palpation of skin & sub-Q tissue (induration,
        sub-Q nodules, tightening)

13. Neurology
a. ☐ test cranial nerves: notation of deficits
b. ☑ examination of DTR's with notation of
        pathological reflexes (eg. Babinski)
c. ☐ examination of sensation (touch, pain,
        vibration, proprioception)

14. Psychiatric
a. ☐ description of patient's judgment & insight
        Brief assessment of mental status:
b. ☑ orientation to time, place, & person
c. ☑ recent & remote memory
d. ☐ mood & affect (depression, anxiety, agitation)
e. ☐ other

Procedures and Immunizations

☐ Hearing   ☐ Glucose   ☐ Cholesterol   ☐ TSH
☐ Vision   ☐ PT   ☐ HDL/LDL   ☐ CXR
☒ CBC   ☐ Urine   ☐ Triglyceride ☐ EKG

☐ Stool Guaiac
☒ Sigmoidoscopy

Are immunizations current?
☐ Yes ☐ No

☐ dT ☐ Hep B
☐ Influenza

Drug Allergies:

NKA

© 1995 Piermed, Inc. Rev

Male
40-59

Date / Time
09/06/2005 5:00 PM

Summary
Bleeding Hemorrhoids

☐ Referral

500-06

FIGURE C-4, D

Lake Eola Family Practice   517860 South Pioneer Drive, Orlando, FL 32897 • 634-555-4893

Superbill   #456298   Weight _240_ BP _140/84_ TPR _98.2°-86-18_

Account Number WILJ009	Doctor Eric Anderson MD		Date of Service 09/06/2005
Patient Name Williams, John		Date of Birth 06/12/1955	LMP N/A
Insurance AETNA HMO	Responsible Party SELF		Phone Number 634-555-9111
Address PO Box WW		Referring Physician and ID # None	
City Tampa	State FL	Zip 32897	

✓ New Patient

___ 99201 H[PF]   E[PF]   MDM[S]   10 min
_X_ 99202 H[EPF]   E[EPF]   MDM[S]   20 min
_X_ 99203 H[D]   E[D]   MDM[LC]   30 min
___ 99204 H[C]   E[C]   MDM[MC]   45 min
___ 99205 H[C]   E[C]   MDM[HC]   60 min

Established Patient

___ 99211 H[N/A]   E[N/A]   MDM[N/A]   5 min
___ 99212 H[PF]   E[PF]   MDM[S]   10 min
___ 99213 H[EPF]   E[EPF]   MDM[LC]   15 min
___ 99214 H[D]   E[D]   MDM[MC]   25 min
___ 99215 H[C]   E[C]   MDM[HC]   40 min

Reason For Visit

___ Authorization _____
     Expiration Date _____
___ Annual exam, complex due to (history, condition):
     _____
___ Annual exam, simple
___ Follow-up, condition _____
___ Follow-up, post procedure, no condition or complication _____
     Procedure/date _____
___ Follow-up, post procedure, with condition or complication _____
     Procedure/date _____
_X_ New Problem _Bleeding hemorrhoids_
___ Post-op, no condition or complication
     Surgery/date _____
___ Post-op, with conditions or complication
     Surgery/date _____
$22000 ___ Pre-op _____
_X_ Procedure _Sigmoidoscopy_
___ Second surgical opinion _____
___ Other (Accident, Decision for surgery) ___

Procedures

⇒ Place to be done: _Office_
⇒ Date to be done: _Now_
_X_ Authorization _A69728_
     Expiration date _12/06/2000_
___ Biopsy, type/site _____

___ Cautery, type/site _____

___ Destruction of lesion(s), extensive, site: ___
     _____
___ Destruction of lesion(s), simple, site: _____

___ Emergency surgery (list above), reason: ___

___ Excision, type/site _____

___ I & D abscess, type/site: _____

___ Insertion/Removal of IUD, type _____
___ Major surgery, type/site _____
     _45334_
_X_ Minor surgery, type/site _Sigmoidoscopy_
     w/cautery bleeding hemorrhoids
___ Sonogram _____
___ Other _____

Miscellaneous

___ Immunization _____
___ Injection _____
___ Supplies
___ Surgical tray

___ Patient Teaching (Preventive medicine)
     _____
     _____
___ Other
     _____
     _____
     _____
     _____

Outside Lab

___ Beta HCG, Serum
___ Biopsy/Pathology
___ Biopsy, Mult./Pathology
_X_ CBC _–Today– SKB Labs_
___ Cholesterol
___ Culture, throat
___ Cultures (source) _____
___ Glucose, ___1hr glucose, ___3hr glucose
___ Estrogen
___ Herpes simplex, AB
___ Mononucleosis
___ Pap Smear
___ PT___PTT
___ Sed rate
___ SMAC
___ Urinalysis, w/micro
___ HIV
_X_ Other _Repeat CBC in 2 wks @ SKB_
     Labs (HMO Lab)
     _____
     _____

Diagnosis Codes

1. _455.2_
2. _____
3. _____
4. _____

Appointment in __2__ Weeks
Procedure in _____ Weeks
~~Sent~~ Labs to _Send Patient to SKB Labs_
Call in _____ Mos./Weeks

Previous Balance $ ___0___
Co-Pay $ _10.00_
Paid Today Cash/(Check) $ _10.00_
Yes-No All Diagnosis, Procedures, & VS above are documented in Record
Doctor's Signature ___ _Eric Anderson MD_

New Charges $ _380.00_
New Balance $ _370.00_
Check Number __5976__

Template © 1998 Medical Compliance Management, Inc.,
CPT only © American Medical Association. All Rights Reserved.

FIGURE C-4, E

Case Study 5: Joselyn Brown

Lake Eola Family Practice   517860 South Pioneer Drive, Orlando, FL 32897 • 634-555-4893

Patient Registration Form

Have you been seen in this office in the past 3 years? ✔ Yes ___ No   **Do you have a living will?** Yes

Today's Date ___02/15/2005___ Home Phone ___634-555-1500___ Work Phone ___N/A___

Patient Name (Last name, First name, Middle initial) ___Brown, Joselyn___

Street Address ___1259556 Spur Ln___ City ___Orlando___ State ___FL___ Zip ___32897___

Date of Birth ___10/27/1927___ Age __77__ Gender: _X_ Female ___ Male   Social Security # ___789-XX-5678___

Marital Status: ___Married ___Single _X_Widowed ___Divorced ___Other   Driver's License # ___None___

Is the patient a student? ___Full Time ___Part Time _X_No   Is the patient employed? ___Full Time ___Part Time _X_No

Patient's Employer Name & Address ___N/A___

School Name & Address ___N/A___

Emergency Contact Person ___Sarah Andrews___ Relationship ___Daughter___ Phone ___634-555-1500___

Referring Physician Name & Phone Number ___Dr. George Slater   634-555-2525___

Insurance Plan and Responsible Party Information

Insurance Company Name ___Medicare___ Address ___PO Box ZZZZ___

City ___Jacksonville___ State ___FL___ Zip ___39782___ Phone ___800-555-1212___

Policy # _____ Group # _____ ID # ___789XX5678D___

Policy Holder's Name ___Joselyn Brown___ Address ___Same___

City _____ State ___ Zip ___ Phone _____

Policy Holder's Date of Birth ___10/27/1927___ Social Security # ___789-XX-5678___ Driver License # ___None___

Gender: ___Male ___Female   Relationship to patient: _X_Self ___Spouse ___Parent ___Guardian ___Other

Policy Holder's Employer's Name ___None___ Address _____

City _____ State ___ Zip ___ Phone _____

Secondary Insurance Company Name ___Medicaid___ Address ___PO Box XXX___

City ___Tallahassee___ State ___FL___ Zip ___32897___ Phone ___800-555-1212___

Secondary Policy # _____ Group # _____ ID # ___789XX5678D___

Secondary Policy Holder's Name ___Joselyn Brown___ Phone ___Same___ Address ___Same___

City _____ State ___ Zip ___ Relationship to patient: _X_Self ___Spouse ___ other

Secondary Policy Holder's Date of Birth ___10/27/1927___ Social Security # ___789-XX-5678___ Driver License # ___None___

Authorizations

It is customary to pay for all services on the date rendered unless other arrangements were made before your appointment. The patient and the guarantor are responsible for all deductibles and copays at the time of the visit and any other fees in accordance with insurance contracts. The patient and guarantor are responsible for all elective or noncovered services and any services that are not considered medically necessary.

Financially responsible person if patient is student or unemployed ___Joselyn Brown___ Phone ___634-555-1500___

I authorize the release of any medical information necessary to process this claim and I request that payment of medical benefits be made directly to Lake Eola Family Practice. I hereby acknowledge that I am fully responsible for payment as listed above.

Signed ___Sarah Andrews for Joselyn Brown___ Date ___2/15/2005___ Time ___10:15 AM___

Template © 1998 Medical Compliance Management, Inc.

FIGURE C-5, A

Lake Eola Family Practice   517860 South Pioneer Drive, Orlando, FL 32897 • 634-555-4893

Problem List – Medication List

Patient Name ___Brown, Joselyn___   DOB ___10/27/1927___

Allergies & allergic response ___None___

Referring Physician & ID # ___George Slater MD A90026___

	Problem (e.g., acute or chronic diagnosis, injury,↑ BP)	**Date Identified**	**Date Resolved**
1	Malignant hypertension	10/18/1987	
2	Malignant hypertensive encephalopathy	02/15/2005	
3			
4			
5			
6			
7			
8			
9			
10			
11			
12			
13			
14			
15			

	All Medications (with dosage & instructions) (include prescription and over-the-counter medications)	**Start Date**	**Discontinue Date**
1	Catapres 0.1 mg PO qd	10/18/1987	
2	Lasix 5 mg PO BID	5/15/1996	
3	K-Dur 10 mEq PO QD	5/15/1996	
4			
5			
6			
7			
8			
9			
10			

Template © 1998 Medical Compliance Management, Inc.

FIGURE C-5, B

Name Brown, Joselyn   Date 02/15/2005

HPI Chief Complaint:

1. Frontal headaches constant x 1 week, not relieved c̄ Tylenol
2. Dizziness off & on
3. Blurry vision & eye pain today
4. Has not taken Rx in 1 week

Current Meds.:

1. Catapus 0.1 mg PO QD
2. Lasix 5 mg PO BID
3. K-Dur 10 m Eq PO QD

Past/Family History

1. Mother Hx HTN, Died age 52–CVA
2. 2 sisters Hx HTN, Died ages 62, 68–CVA
3. Father died age 36–Gunshot wound
4. All six children Hx HTN–Living
5. Widowed 15 years ago.
6. Lives c̄ daughter Sarah Andrews. Sarah has Power of Attorney for medical decisions.
7. Personal Hx Malignant HTN x 15 years

THIS SECTION TO BE COMPLETED BY PATIENT.

Personal/Social History

Are you... ☐ single ☐ married
☐ live in partner ☐ divorced ☒ widow

Do you have children? ☒ Yes ☐ No
Ages of child(ren) 38, 40, 41, 45, 52, 54
No. of pregnancies 9 Miscarriages 3
Occupation None
If retired, how do you spend your time?
Helping daughter

	Yes	No
a. Do you have concerns about your breasts? (circle): changes in size or shape, changes in skin color, lumps, tenderness, ulcerations, discharge or blood from nipple, inverted nipple	☐	☒
b. Do you have menstrual bleeding?	☐	☒
If so, ☐ rarely ☐ monthly ☐ more than monthly		
c. Do you take hormones (estrogen)?	☐	☒
d. Concerns about lesions, lumps or swelling on your vulva or vagina?	☐	☒
e. Do you have vaginal dryness, itching or pain?	☐	☒
f. Do you have urine leakage?	☐	☒

g. Approximate date of last pelvic exam. Jun 2003
h. Approximate date of last pap test Jun 2003
i. Approximate date of last mammogram Jun 2003

	Yes	No
j. Are you sexually active now?	☐	☒
k. Do you have other sexual concerns?	☐	☒
l. Do you feel safe/comfortable in your home, with your family, and/or your partner relationship?	☒	☐
m. Do you smoke or use tobacco products now?	☐	☒
n. Do you use recreational drugs?	☐	☒
o. Do you drink alcohol?	☒	☐

☒ daily ☐ weekly ☐ rarely
# of drinks 1-2
If yes, do you drink: ☒ beer, ☐ wine, ☐ liquor

Review of Systems
Are you concerned about?
(circle concerns)

	Yes	No
1. Recent changes in health status	☒	☐
2. Eye problems: vision, pain, tearing	☒	☐
3. Ears, nose, mouth, throat problems	☐	☒
4. Heart problems: chest pain, blood pressure	☒	☐

	Yes	No
5. Lung problems: coughing, wheezing, infections	☐	☒
6. Abdominal pain, stomach, bowel problems	☐	☒
7. Kidney or bladder problems	☐	☒
8. Muscle, bone, joint or back problems	☐	☒
9. Skin, hair or nail problems	☐	☒
10. Neurologic problems: headaches, dizziness, numbness	☒	☐
11. Nervousness, anxiety, depression, suicidal thoughts	☒	☐
12. Excessive thirst and urine output, recent weight changes	☐	☒
13. Anemia, bruising, blood clots, swollen glands	☐	☒
14. Food allergies, hayfever, eczema, asthma, decreased immunity	☐	☒
Do you have any other concerns?	☐	☒

Sarah Andrews
for Joselyn Brown   2/15/05
Patient's Signature   Date

Provider Comments: 2. Vision Blurry today c̄ pain in eyes.
10. Frontal headache x 1 week–no relief from Tylenol. Has refused to take RX for past week.
11. States is afraid of dying.

Aaron Rubin MD   2/15/05
☐ PFSH and ROS have been reviewed.   ☐ Unresolved problems from previous visit have been addressed.   Provider's Signature   Date

Anticipatory Guidance

☐ Nutrition
☐ Calcium/Multi-vitamin
☐ Exercise/Recreation/Hobbies
☐ Dental care
☐ Sun exposure

☐ Smoking cessation
☐ Alcohol/drugs
☐ Cardiovascular risks
☐ Aspirin prophylaxis
☐ Osteoporosis risks/Estrogen
☐ Self exam. breasts, skin, oral cavity
☐ Sexual issues

☐ STD prevention
☐ Menopause
☐ Work/Retirement
☐ Family
☐ Safety/ Injury/Gun Safety
☐ Auto seat belts
☐ Smoke detectors

☐ Domestic violence
☐ Hot water <120°
☐ Fall prevention
☐ CPR for family members
☐ Stress
☐ Living Will
☐ Medical Power of Attorney

500-06

Female 60+

FIGURE C-5, C

Name _Brown, Joselyn_ DOB _10_/_27_/_1927_ Age _77_ Chart No. | BROJ008 |

Assessment

(2c) Eyes bulging c̄ evidence of retinal bleeding

(6c) Corotid bruit on Ⓡ

(6g) +4 pitting edema bilat ankles/feet

(11a) Lists to left & Ⓛ foot drags

(11e.,g.) Muscles on Ⓛ flaccid c̄ noticeable drooping of facial muscles on Ⓛ (non-dominant)

(13.a.-c.) ↓ reflexes, sensation on Ⓛ

(14.b.-d) anxious & confused. Knows name, but not time or place

Dx: Hypertensive Encephalopathy

Plan

(1) Admit to Lake Eola Hospital to stabilize

(2) Patient has Living Will— No CPR — Daughter — Sarah Andrews — has power of attorney for medical decisions.

Aaron Rubin MD   _2/15/05_

Provider's Signature   Return Visit

FOLD HERE   FOLD HERE

Physical Exam

Ht. _5' 4"_ Wt. _110#_ Temp. _97.6°_ Resp. _20_

B.P. sit. or stand. _240_/_120_ Supine _220_/_110_

Pulse rate and regularity _110, regular_
                          Bounding

Circle abnormal and pertinent normal findings
Describe abnormalities above.

☑ Normal   ☒ Abnormal

1. Constitutional
a. ☑ gen. appear., development, body shape, nutrition, deformities, grooming

2. Eyes
a. ☑ conjunctiva, lids
b. ☑ pupils, irises
c. ☒ fundi (optic discs, vessels, exudate, (hemorr.))

3. Ears, Nose, Throat & Mouth
a. ☑ appearance of ears, appearance of nose
b. ☑ auditory canals, tympanic membranes
c. ☐ hearing (whis. voice, finger rub, tun. fork)
d. ☑ nasal mucosa, sputum, turbinates
e. ☐ lips, teeth, gums
f. ☑ oropharnyx (mucosa, saliv. glands, hard & soft palates, tongue, tonsils, post. pharynx)

4. Neck
a. ☑ appearance, masses, symmetry, tracheal position, crepitus
b. ☑ thyroid (enlargement, tenderness, mass)

5. Respiratory
a. ☑ respiratory effort (intercostal retractions) use of accessory muscles, diaphragm move.
b. ☐ percussion (dullness, flatness, hyper-reson.)
c. ☐ palpation (tactile fremitus)
d. ☑ auscultation (breath sounds, rhonchi, wheezes, rales, rubs)

6. Cardiovascular
a. ☑ palpation (location of p.m.i., size, thrill)
b. ☑ auscultation (abnormal sounds, murmurs)
c. ☒ carotid arteries (pulse amplitude, (bruits)) Ⓡ
d. ☑ abdominal aorta (size, bruits)
e. ☑ femoral arteries (pulse amplitude, bruits)
f. ☑ pedal pulses (pulse amplitude)
g. ☒ extremities (edema, varicosities) +4 pitting

7. Chest (Breasts)
a. ☑ inspection (size, symmetry, nipple discharge)
b. ☑ palpation of breasts & axillae (masses, lumps, tenderness)

8. Gastrointestinal (Abdomen)
a. ☑ examination for masses, tenderness
b. ☑ examination of liver, spleen
c. ☐ examination for presence or absence of hernia
d. ☐ examination of (when indicated) anus, perineum, rectum: (sphincter tone, hemorrhoids, masses)
e. ☐ stool for occult blood when indicated

9. Genitourinary
Pelvic Exam (with or without specimen collection for smears or cultures), including:
a. ☐ Ext. Genitalia (eg. gen. app., hair distrib., lesions) and vagina (eg. gen. app., estogen eff., lesions, pelvic support, cystocele, rectocele)
b. ☐ Urethra (eg. masses, tender., scarring)
c. ☐ Bladder (eg. fullness, masses, tender.)
d. ☐ Cervix (eg. gen. app., lesions, disch.)
e. ☐ Uterus (eg. size, contour, position, mobility, tender., consistency, descent or support)
f. ☐ Adnexia / Parametria (eg. masses, tender., organomegally, nodularity)

10. Lymphatic
a. ☑ palpation of lymph nodes in 2 or more areas: (Circle: (neck), (axillae), groin, other)

11. Musculoskeletal
a. ☑ examination of gait and station
b. ☑ inspection and/or palpation of digits & nails (clubbing, cyanosis, inflammatory conditions, petechiae, ischemia, infections, nodes)
c. ☑ assessment of range of motion (pain, crepitation, contracture)
d. ☑ Examination of joint, bone, & muscle of 1 or more of the following 6 areas (circle)
   • head/neck   • rt. upper extremities
   • spine, ribs, & pelvis   • lt. upper extremities
   • rt. lower extremities   • lt. lower extremities
e. ☒ inspect, and/or palpation (misalign, (asymmetry), crepitation, defects, tender., masses, effusion)
f. ☐ assessment of stability: dislocation (luxation), subluxation or laxity
g. ☒ muscle strength & tone ((flaccid), cogwheel, spastic), atrophy or abnormal movement

12. Skin
a. ☑ inspection of skin & sub-Q tissue (rashes, lesion, ulcers)
b. ☐ palpation of skin & sub-Q tissue (induration, sub-Q nodules, tightening)

13. Neurology
a. ☒ test cranial nerves: notation of deficits
b. ☒ examination of DTR's with notation of pathological reflexes (eg. Babinski)
c. ☒ examination of sensation (touch, pain, vibration, proprioception)

14. Psychiatric
a. ☐ description of patient's judgment & insight
   Brief assessment of mental status:
b. ☒ orientation to time, place, & person
c. ☒ recent & remote memory
d. ☐ mood & affect (depression, anxiety, agitation)
e. ☐ other _____

Procedures and Immunizations

☐ Hearing	☐ PT	☐ Triglyceride	☐ Stool Guaiac
☐ Vision	☐ TSH	☐ CXR	☐ Sigmoidoscopy
☐ CBC	☐ Urine	☐ EKG	
☐ Glucose	☐ Cholesterol	☐ PAP Test	
	☐ HDL/LDL	☐ Mammogram	

Are immunizations current?
☐Yes ☐No
☐ dT
☐ Hep B
☐ Influenza
☐ Pnuemonia

Drug Allergies:

NKA

Female 60+

Date / Time
02/15/2005 11 AM

Summary
Hypertensive Encephalopathy

☐ Referral

500-06

FIGURE C-5, D

Lake Eola Family Practice

517860 South Pioneer Drive, Orlando, FL 32897 • 634-555-4893

Superbill   #456298

Weight _110#_ BP _240/120_ TPR _97.6°-110-20_

Account Number	Doctor	Date of Service
BROJ008	Aaron Rubin MD	02/15/2005

Patient Name	Date of Birth	LMP
Brown, Joselyn	10/27/1927	N/A

Insurance	Responsible Party	Phone Number
Medicare/Medicaid	Joselyn Brown	None

Address	Referring Physician and ID #
PO Box ZZZZ	A90026 George Slater MD

City	State	Zip
Jacksonville	FL	39782

New Patient

__ 99201	H[PF]	E[PF] MDM[S]	10 min
__ 99202	H[EPF]	E[EPF] MDM[S]	20 min
__ 99203	H[D]	E[D] MDM[LC]	30 min
__ 99204	H[C]	E[C] MDM[MC]	45 min
__ 99205	H[C]	E[C] MDM[HC]	60 min

Established Patient

__ 99211	H[N/A]	E[N/A] MDM[N/A]	5 min
__ 99212	H[PF]	E[PF] MDM[S]	10 min
__ 99213	H[EPF]	E[EPF] MDM[LC]	15 min
__ 99214	H[D]	E[D] MDM[MC]	25 min
X 99215	H[C]	E[C] MDM[HC]	40 min

Reason For Visit

__ Authorization _____

   Expiration Date _____

__ Annual exam, complex due to (history, condition):

_____

__ Annual exam, simple

X Follow-up, condition _HTN_

__ Follow-up, post procedure, no condition or complication _____

   Procedure/date _____

__ Follow-up, post procedure, with condition or complication _____

   Procedure/date _____

X New Problem _Blurred Vision/HA_

__ Post-op, no condition or complication
   Surgery/date _____

__ Post-op, with conditions or complication

   Surgery/date _____

__ Pre-op _____

__ Procedure _____

__ Second surgical opinion _____

__ Other (Accident, Decision for surgery) __

_____

Procedures

⇒ Place to be done: _____

⇒ Date to be done: _____

__ Authorization _____

   Expiration date _____

__ Biopsy, type/site _____

__ Cautery, type/site _____

__ Destruction of lesion(s), extensive, site: __

_____

__ Destruction of lesion(s), simple, site: ___

_____

__ Emergency surgery (list above), reason: __

_____

__ Excision, type/site _____

_____

__ I & D abscess, type/site: _____

_____

__ Insertion/Removal of IUD, type _____

__ Major surgery, type/site _____

_____

__ Minor surgery, type/site _____

_____

__ Sonogram _____

__ Other _____

_____

Miscellaneous

__ Immunization _____

__ Injection _____

__ Supplies

__ Surgical tray

__ Patient Teaching (Preventive medicine)

_____

X Other _Admit to hospital_
   ASAP. Dx: Hypertensive
   Encephlopathy, R/O CVA

_____

Outside Lab

__ Beta HCG, Serum
__ Biopsy/Pathology
__ Biopsy, Mult./Pathology
__ CBC
__ Cholesterol
__ Culture, throat
__ Cultures (source) _____
__ Glucose, __1hr glucose, __3hr glucose
__ Estrogen
__ Herpes simplex, AB
__ Mononucleosis
__ Pap Smear
__ PT__PTT
__ Sed rate
__ SMAC
__ Urinalysis, w/micro
__ HIV
__ Other _____

_____

_____

_____

Diagnosis Codes

1. _437.2_ _____

2. _V17.1_ _____

3. _V17.4_ _____

4. _____

Appointment in _____/___ Weeks

Procedure in _____ Weeks

Sent Labs to_____

Call in _____ Mos./Weeks

Previous Balance $ ___0___

Co-Pay $ ___0___

Paid Today Cash/Check $ ___0___

Yes-No All Diagnosis, Procedures, & VS above are documented in Record

Doctor's Signature _Aaron Rubin MD_

New Charges $ _190.00_

New Balance $ _190.00_

Check Number _____

Template © 1998 Medical Compliance Management, Inc.,
CPT only © American Medical Association. All Rights Reserved.

FIGURE C-5, E

Case Study 6: David Anderson

Lake Eola Family Practice

517860 South Pioneer Drive, Orlando, FL 32897 • 634-555-4893

Patient Registration Form

Have you been seen in this office in the past 3 years? ✔ Yes ___ No   Do you have a living will? Yes

Today's Date _3 Mar 2005_ Home Phone _634-555-5186_ Work Phone _634-555-4560_

Patient Name (Last name, First name, Middle initial) _Anderson, David_

Street Address _5967 Rodeo Circle_ City _Orlando_ State _FL_ Zip _32897_

Date of Birth _8 Feb 1931_ Age _74_ Gender: ___ Female _X_ Male Social Security # _465-XX-3210_

Marital Status: ___ Married ___ Single ___ Widowed _X_ Divorced ___ Other Driver's License # _B658-XX-5699_

Is the patient a student? ___ Full Time ___ Part Time _X_ No Is the patient employed? ___ Full Time _X_ Part Time ___ No

Patient's Employer Name & Address _Winn Dixie Super Market, 2757 Spur Rd_

School Name & Address _N/A_

Emergency Contact Person _William Anderson_ Relationship _Son_ Phone _555-789-5200_

Referring Physician Name & Phone Number _None_

Insurance Plan and Responsible Party Information

Insurance Company Name _Medicare_ Address _PO Box ZZZZ_

City _Jacksonville_ State _FL_ Zip _39782_ Phone _800-555-1212_

Policy # _____ Group # _____ ID # _465XX3210A_

Policy Holder's Name _David A. Anderson_ Address _5967 Rodeo Circle_

City _Orlando_ State _FL_ Zip _32897_ Phone _634-555-5186_

Policy Holder's Date of Birth _8 Feb 1931_ Social Security # _465-XX-3210_ Driver License # _B658-XX-5699_

Gender: _X_ Male ___ Female Relationship to patient: _X_ Self ___ Spouse ___ Parent ___ Guardian ___ Other

Policy Holder's Employer's Name _Winn Dixie Super MKT_ Address _2757 Spur Rd_

City _Orlando_ State _FL_ Zip _32897_ Phone _634-555-4560_

Secondary Insurance Company Name _BC BS of FL_ Address _PO Box YYYY_

City _Jacksonville_ State _FL_ Zip _39782_ Phone _800-555-1212_

Secondary Policy # _____ Group # _WD6472_ ID # _465XX3210A_

Secondary Policy Holder's Name _David A. Anderson_ Phone _634-555-5186_ Address _5967 Rodeo Circle_

City _Orlando_ State _FL_ Zip _32897_ Relationship to patient: _X_ Self ___ Spouse ___ other

Secondary Policy Holder's Date of Birth _8 Feb 1931_ Social Security # _465-XX-3210_ Driver License # _B658-XX-5699_

Policy Through Employer – Winn Dixie Supermarket

Authorizations

It is customary to pay for all services on the date rendered unless other arrangements were made before your appointment. The patient and the guarantor are responsible for all deductibles and copays at the time of the visit and any other fees in accordance with insurance contracts. The patient and guarantor are responsible for all elective or noncovered services and any services that are not considered medically necessary.

Financially responsible person if patient is student or unemployed _____ Phone _____

I authorize the release of any medical information necessary to process this claim and I request that payment of medical benefits be made directly to Lake Eola Family Practice. I hereby acknowledge that I am fully responsible for payment as listed above.

Signed _David A. Anderson_ Date _3 Mar 2005_ Time _9:15 AM_

Template © 1998 Medical Compliance Management, Inc.

FIGURE C-6, A

Lake Eola Family Practice   517860 South Pioneer Drive, Orlando, FL 32897 • 634-555-4893

Problem List – Medication List

Patient Name ___Anderson, David_____ DOB _02/08/1931_

Allergies & allergic response ___Sulpha drugs – anaphylaxis_____

Referring Physician & ID # ___None_____

	Problem (e.g., acute or chronic diagnosis, injury,↑ BP)	**Date Identified**	**Date Resolved**
1	Enlarged prostate	9/1/2004	
2	Blood in urine	3/3/2005	
3			
4			
5			
6			
7			
8			
9			
10			
11			
12			
13			
14			
15			

	All Medications (with dosage & instructions) (include prescription and over-the-counter medications)	**Start Date**	**Discontinue Date**
1			
2			
3			
4			
5			
6			
7			
8			
9			
10			

Template © 1998 Medical Compliance Management, Inc.

FIGURE C-6, B

Name Anderson, David   Date 03/03/2005

HPI Chief Complaint:

Blood in urine since yesterday
   Hx prostate hypertrophy. Was advised
to have surgery 6 months ago,
   but has been putting it off.
Doesn't feel empties bladder completely
x 1 week.

Current Meds.:

None

Past/Family History

Father died at 62 from prostate cancer.
Mother died at age 45 from a heart attack.

THIS SECTION TO BE COMPLETED BY PATIENT.

Personal/Social History

Are you...   ☐ single   ☐ married
☐ live in partner   ☒ divorced   ☐ widow

Do you have children?   ☒ Yes   ☐ No
Ages of child(ren) _38, 40, 42_

Occupation/Retired _Bookkeeper_
(Retired Accountant)

	Yes	No
a. Do you have any problems with (circle) memory, recent changes in hearing or vision,↑ injuries, problems with sleep, in your overall happiness?	☒	☐
b. Do you have any difficulty starting a urine stream, dribbling, pain or blood on urination or awake up at night to urinate If so, number of times _3-4_	☒	☐
c. Do you have lesions, sores or drainage from penis?	☐	☒
d. Do you have any lumps, swelling, tenderness or pain in groin, scrotum, or testicles?	☐	☒
e. Do you have any difficulty getting or sustaining an erection?	☐	☒

	Yes	No
f. Are you sexually active now?	☒	☐
g. Do you use condoms?	☒	☐
h. Do you have other sexual concerns?	☐	☒
i. Have you needed help with (circle) shopping, chores, walking, climbing stairs, going to the bathroom, bathing, dressing, taking medication?	☐	☒
j. Do you feel safe/comfortable in your home, with your family, and/or your partner relationship?	☒	☐
k. Do you smoke or use tobacco products now?	☐	☒
l. Do you use recreational drugs?	☐	☒
m. Do you drink alcohol?	☐	☒

☐ daily   ☐ weekly   ☒ rarely

# of drinks _____

If yes, do you drink: ☐ beer, ☐ wine, ☒ liquor

Review of Systems
Are you concerned about?
(circle concerns)

	Yes	No
1. Recent changes in health status	☒	☐
2. Eye problems: vision, pain, tearing	☐	☒

	Yes	No
3. Ears, nose, mouth, throat problems	☐	☒
4. Heart problems: chest pain, blood pressure	☐	☒
5. Lung problems: coughing, wheezing, infections	☐	☒
6. Abdominal pain, stomach, bowel problems	☐	☒
7. Kidney or bladder problems	☒	☐
8. Muscle, bone, joint or back problems	☐	☒
9. Skin, hair or nail problems	☐	☒
10. Neurologic problems: headaches, dizziness, numbness	☐	☒
11. Nervousness, anxiety, depression, suicidal thoughts	☐	☒
12. Excessive thirst and urine output, recent weight changes	☐	☒
13. Anemia, bruising, blood clots, swollen glands	☐	☒
14. Food allergies, hayfever, eczema, asthma, decreased immunity	☐	☒
Do you have any other concerns?	☐	☒

David Anderson   3/3/05
Patient's Signature   Date

Provider Comments:

a. Problems c̄ sleep related to frequent urination @ night – 3-4 x/night
b. Blood in urine since yesterday

Bruce James PA   3/3/05

☒ PFSH and ROS have been reviewed.   ☒ Unresolved problems from previous visit have been addressed. | Provider's Signature   Date

Anticipatory Guidance

☐ Nutrition	☐ Smoking cessation	☐ Work/Retirement	☐ Fall prevention
☐ Multi-vitamins	☐ Alcohol/drugs	☐ Family	☐ CPR for family members
☐ Exercise	☐ Cardiovascular risks	☐ Recreation/Hobbies	☐ Domestic violence
☐ Dental care	☐ Aspirin prophylaxis	☐ Safety/ Injury/Gun Safety	☐ Stress
☐ Sun exposure	☐ Self exam. testes, skin, oral cavity	☐ Auto seat belts	☐ Living Will
	☐ Sexual issues	☐ Smoke detectors	☐ Medical Power of Attorney
	☐ STD prevention	☐ Hot water <120°	☐ Educational handouts

©1995 Piermed, Inc. Rev. 6/98 (800) 998-1908

500-05

Male 60+

FIGURE C-6, C

Name _Anderson, David_   DOB _02_ / _08_ / _1931_   Age _74_   Chart No. | ANDD057 |

Assessment

(9c) ↑ Hypertrophy of prostate gland
Urine pink – tinged.

Dx: Enlarged prostate
Blood in urine
R/O Prostate malignancy
R/O Prostatitis

Plan

(1) Consultation with
Urologist today
(2) Return prn

Bruce James PA   _PRN_
Provider's Signature   Return Visit

FOLD HERE   FOLD HERE

Physical Exam

Ht. _5' 7"_ Wt. _189_ Temp. _98.6°_ Resp. _20_

B.P. sit. or stand. _130_ / _84_   Supine ___ / ___

Pulse rate and regularity _86, regular_

Circle abnormal and pertinent normal findings
Describe abnormalities above.

☑ Normal   ☒ Abnormal

1. Constitutional
a. ☑ gen. appear., development, body shape,
nutrition, deformities, grooming

2. Eyes
a. ☑ conjunctiva, lids
b. ☑ pupils, irises
c. ☐ fundi (optic discs, vessels, exudate, hemorr.)

3. Ears, Nose, Throat & Mouth
a. ☑ appearance of ears, appearance of nose
b. ☑ auditory canals, tympanic membranes
c. ☐ hearing (whis. voice, finger rub, tun. fork)
d. ☑ nasal mucosa, sputum, turbinates
e. ☑ lips, teeth, gums
f. ☑ oropharnyx (mucosa, saliv. glands, hard &
soft palates, tongue, tonsils, post. pharynx)

4. Neck
a. ☐ appearance, masses, symmetry, tracheal
position, crepitus
b. ☐ thyroid (enlargement, tenderness, mass)

5. Respiratory
a. ☑ respiratory effort (intercostal retractions)
use of accessory muscles, diaphragm move.
b. ☐ percussion (dullness, flatness, hyper-reson.)
c. ☐ palpation (tactile fremitus)
d. ☑ auscultation (breath sounds, rhonchi, wheezes,
rales, rubs)

6. Cardiovascular
a. ☐ palpation (location of p.m.i., size, thrill)
b. ☑ auscultation (abnormal sounds, murmurs)
c. ☐ carotid arteries (pulse amplitude, bruits)
d. ☐ abdominal aorta (size, bruits)
e. ☐ femoral arteries (pulse amplitude, bruits)
f. ☐ pedal pulses (pulse amplitude)
g. ☑ extremities (edema, varicosities)

7. Chest (Breasts)
a. ☐ inspection (size, symmetry, nipple discharge)
b. ☐ palpation of breasts & axillae (masses,
lumps, tenderness)

8. Gastrointestinal (Abdomen)
a. ☑ examination for masses, tenderness
b. ☑ examination of liver, spleen
c. ☑ examination for presence or absence of hernia
d. ☑ examination of (when indicated) anus, perineum,
rectum: (sphincter tone, hemorrhoids, masses)
e. ☐ stool for occult blood when indicated

9. Genitourinary
a. ☑ scrotum (hydrocele, spermatocele,
tenderness of cord, testicular mass)
b ☑ examination of penis
c. ☒ digital exam of prostate (size, symmetry,
nodularity, tenderness)

10. Lymphatic
a. ☑ palpation of lymph nodes in 2 or more areas:
(Circle: neck, axillae, groin, other)

11. Musculoskeletal
a. ☑ examination of gait and station
b. ☑ inspection and/or palpation of digits & nails
(clubbing, cyanosis, inflammatory conditions,
petechiae, ischemia, infections, nodes)
c. ☐ assessment of range of motion (pain,
crepitation, contracture)

d. ☐ Examination of joint, bone, & muscle of 1 or
more of the following 6 areas (circle)
• head/neck   • rt. upper extremities
• spine, ribs, & pelvis   • lt. upper extremities
• rt. lower estremities   • lt. lower extremities
e. ☐ inspect, and/or palpation (misalign, asymmetry,
crepitation, defects, tender., masses, effusion)
f. ☐ assessment of stability: dislocation (luxation),
subluxation or laxity
g. ☑ muscle strength & tone (flaccid, cogwheel,
spastic), atrophy or abnormal movement

12. Skin
a. ☑ inspection of skin & sub-Q tissue (rashes,
lesion, ulcers)
b. ☐ palpation of skin & sub-Q tissue (induration,
sub-Q nodules, tightening)

13. Neurology
a. ☑ test cranial nerves: notation of deficits
b. ☐ examination of DTR's with notation of
pathological reflexes (eg. Babinski)
c. ☐ examination of sensation (touch, pain,
vibration, proprioception)

14. Psychiatric
a. ☐ description of patient's judgment & insight
Brief assessment of mental status:
b. ☑ orientation to time, place, & person
c. ☑ recent & remote memory
d. ☐ mood & affect (depression, anxiety, agitation)
e. ☐ other

Procedures and Immunizations

☐ Hearing   ☐ Glucose   ☐ Cholesterol   ☐ TSH
☐ Vision   ☐ PT   ☐ HDL/LDL   ☐ CXR
☐ CBC   ☐ Urine   ☐ Triglyceride ☐ EKG

☐ Stool Guaiac
☐ Sigmoidoscopy

Are immunizations current?
☐ Yes ☐ No

☐ dT ☐ Hep B
☐ Influenza

Drug Allergies:

Sulpha drugs

© 1995 Plermed, Inc. Rev

**Male
60+**

Date / Time
10:00 AM 3/3/2005

Summary
Blood in Urine; Prostate Hypertrophy

☐ Referral

500-06

FOLD HERE

FIGURE C-6, D

Lake Eola Family Practice

517860 South Pioneer Drive, Orlando, FL 32897 • 634-555-4893

Superbill   #456298

Weight _____ BP _____ TPR _____

Account Number ANDD057	Doctor Bruce James PA	Date of Service 03/03/2005
Patient Name Anderson, David A.	Date of Birth 02/08/1931	LMP N/A
Insurance BCBS FL/Medicare	Responsible Party David Anderson	Phone Number 634-555-5186
Address PO Box YYYY	Referring Physician and ID # None	
City Jacksonville	State FL	Zip 39782	

New Patient

___99201 H[PF]   E[PF]   MDM[S]   10 min
___99202 H[EPF] E[EPF] MDM[S]   20 min
___99203 H[D]   E[D]   MDM[LC] 30 min
___99204 H[C]   E[C]   MDM[MC] 45 min
___99205 H[C]   E[C]   MDM[HC] 60 min

✓ Established Patient

___99211 H[N/A] E[N/A] MDM[N/A] 5 min
___99212 H[PF]   E[PF]   MDM[S]   10 min
X_99213 H[EPF] E[EPF] MDM[LC] 15 min
___99214 H[D]   E[D]   MDM[MC] 25 min
___99215 H[C]   E[C]   MDM[HC] 40 min

Reason For Visit

___Authorization _____
      Expiration Date _____
___Annual exam, complex due to (history,
      condition): _____
      _____
___Annual exam, simple
X_Follow-up, condition _Prostate_
___Follow-up, post procedure, no condition or
      complication _____
      Procedure/date _____
___Follow-up, post procedure, with condition or
      complication _____
      Procedure/date _____
X_New Problem _Blood in urine_
___Post-op, no condition or complication
      Surgery/date _____
___Post-op, with conditions or complication
      _____
      Surgery/date _____
___Pre-op _____
___Procedure _____
___Second surgical opinion _____
___Other (Accident, Decision for surgery) ___
      _____

Procedures

⇒ Place to be done: _____
⇒ Date to be done: _____
___ Authorization _____
      Expiration date _____
___ Biopsy, type/site _____

___ Cautery, type/site _____
      _____
___ Destruction of lesion(s), extensive, site: ___
      _____
___ Destruction of lesion(s), simple, site: _____

___ Emergency surgery (list above), reason: ___
      _____
___ Excision, type/site _____
      _____
___ I & D abscess, type/site: _____

___ Insertion/Removal of IUD, type _____
___ Major surgery, type/site _____

___ Minor surgery, type/site _____

___ Sonogram _____
___ Other _____

Miscellaneous

___ Immunization _____
___ Injection _____
___ Supplies
___ Surgical tray

Patient Teaching (Preventive medicine)

___ _____
X Other   _Stat consult c̄ Dr. Peters,_
Urology _____
_____

Outside Lab

___ Beta HCG, Serum
___ Biopsy/Pathology
___ Biopsy, Mult./Pathology
___ CBC
___ Cholesterol
___ Culture, throat
___ Cultures (source) _____
___ Glucose, ___1hr glucose, ___3hr glucose
___ Estrogen
___ Herpes simplex, AB
___ Mononucleosis
___ Pap Smear
___ PT ___PTT
___ Sed rate
___ SMAC
___ Urinalysis, w/micro
___ HIV
___ Other _____
_____
_____
_____

Diagnosis Codes

1. _599.7_ _____
2. _600.00_ _____
3. _____
4. _____

Appointment in __prn__ Weeks
Procedure in _____ Weeks
Sent Labs to_____
Call in _____ Mos./Weeks

Previous Balance $ ___0___
Co-Pay $ ___2 Payors___
Paid Today Cash/Check $ ___0___
(Yes)-No All Diagnosis, Procedures, & VS above are documented in Record
Doctor's Signature ___Bruce James PA___

New Charges $ ___75.00___
New Balance $ ___75.00___
Check Number _____

FIGURE C-6, E

Case Study 7: Deborah Feinstein

Lake Eola Family Practice   517860 South Pioneer Drive, Orlando, FL 32897 • 634-555-4893

Patient Registration Form

Have you been seen in this office in the past 3 years? ___Yes ✓ No   **Do you have a living will?** No

Today's Date _12/23/2005_   Home Phone _634-555-9852_   Cell/Work Phone _634-555-9537_

Patient Name (Last name, First name, Middle initial) _Feinstein, Deborah_

Street Address _1527659 Spur Estates Circle_ City _Orlando_   State _FL_   Zip _32897_

Date of Birth _4/8/1966_ Age _39_ Gender: _X_ Female ___Male Social Security # _567-XX-8901_

Marital Status: _X_ Married ___Single ___Widowed ___Divorced ___Other Driver's License # _B567-XX-8901_

Is the patient a student? ___Full Time ___Part Time _X_ No Is the patient employed? _X_ Full Time ___Part Time ___No

Patient's Employer Name & Address _Walt Disney World, Lake Buena Vista, Florida_

School Name & Address _None_

Emergency Contact Person _Lawrence Feinstein_   Relationship _Husband_ Cell Phone _634-555-9538_

Referring Physician Name & Phone Number _Lawrence Feinstein, M.D. 634-555-9538_

Insurance Plan and Responsible Party Information

Insurance Company Name _BC BS of Florida_   Address _PO Box YYYY_

City _Jacksonville_   State _FL_   Zip _39782_   Phone _800-555-1212_

Policy # _____ Group # _WDW16794A_ ID # _567XX8901-A_

Policy Holder's Name _Deborah Feinstein_   Address _Same_

City _____ State _____ Zip _____ Phone _____

Policy Holder's Date of Birth _____ Social Security # _____ Driver License # _____

Gender: ___Male _X_ Female Relationship to patient: _X_ Self ___Spouse ___Parent ___Guardian ___Other

Policy Holder's Employer's Name _Walt Disney World_   Address _Lake Buena Vista_

City _Orlando_   State _FL_ Zip _32897_   Phone _800-W-Disney_

Secondary Insurance Company Name _None_   Address _____

City _____ State _____ Zip _____ Phone _____

Secondary Policy # _____ Group # _____ ID # _____

Secondary Policy Holder's Name _____ Phone _____ Address _____

City _____ State _____ Zip _____ Relationship to patient: ___Self ___Spouse ___other

Secondary Policy Holder's Date of Birth _____ Social Security # _____ Driver License # _____

Authorizations

It is customary to pay for all services on the date rendered unless other arrangements were made before your appointment. The patient and the guarantor are responsible for all deductibles and copays at the time of the visit and any other fees in accordance with insurance contracts. The patient and guarantor are responsible for all elective or noncovered services and any services that are not considered medically necessary.

Financially responsible person if patient is student or unemployed _____ Phone _____

I authorize the release of any medical information necessary to process this claim and I request that payment of medical benefits be made directly to Lake Eola Family Practice. I hereby acknowledge that I am fully responsible for payment as listed above.

Signed _Deborah Feinstein_   Date _12/23/2005_ Time _8:00 AM_

Template © 1998 Medical Compliance Management, Inc.

FIGURE C-7, A

Lake Eola Family Practice   517860 South Pioneer Drive, Orlando, FL 32897 • 634-555-4893

Problem List – Medication List

Patient Name _Feinstein, Deborah_ DOB _04/08/1966_

Allergies & allergic response _None_

Referring Physician & ID # _Lawrence Feinstein MD   A62189   (spouse)_

	Problem (e.g., acute or chronic diagnosis, injury,↑ BP)	**Date Identified**	**Date Resolved**
1	Chronic LLQ Abd Pain	12/23/2005	
2	Risky behavior	12/23/2005	
3			
4			
5			
6			
7			
8			
9			
10			
11			
12			
13			
14			
15			

	All Medications (with dosage & instructions) (include prescription and over-the-counter medications)	**Start Date**	**Discontinue Date**
1	Lo dose Premarin (Rx from GYN)	1981	
2			
3			
4			
5			
6			
7			
8			
9			
10			

Template © 1998 Medical Compliance Management, Inc.

FIGURE C-7, B

Name _Feinstein, Deborah_   Date _12_ / _23_ / _2005_

HPI Chief Complaint:

1. Chronic abd pain x 19 years $\bar{c}$ ↑ in past year
2. Hx multiple surgeries for abd. adhesions and other problems
3. Has seen 6 MD's this year for same problem.

Current Meds.:

4. Low dose Premarin

Past/Family History

1. TAH – ruptured tubal pregnancy – 1981
2. RSO and adhesions 1984
3. LSO and adhesions 1992
4. Appy and adhesions 1996
5. Marijuana use mixed $\bar{c}$ ETOH past 3 years to deal $\bar{c}$ pain
6. Marital problems since 1992 –
7. Multiple sexual partners – both sexes.
8. Parents and siblings all alive and well.
9. Husband is Plastic Surgeon

THIS SECTION TO BE COMPLETED BY PATIENT.

Personal/Social History

Are you... ☐ single ☒ married
☐ live in partner ☐ divorced

Do you have children? ☐ Yes ☒ No
Ages of child(ren) _____
No. of pregnancies _1_ Miscarriages _1_
Occupation _Costume Designer_

	Yes	No
a. Are your immunizations up to date?	☒	☐

Date of last tetanus shot: _1996_

b. Concerns about your breasts, menstruation, pain or bleeding with intercourse, vaginal itching or discharge? ☐ Yes ☒ No
c. Approximate date of last pelvic exam. _5/2005_
d. Approximate date of last pap test _5/2005_

e. Are you sexually active now? ☒ Yes ☐ No
☒ same sex ☐ opposite sex
☐ single partner ☒ multiple partners

Have you had more than 4 lifetime partners? ☒ Yes ☐ No

f. Birth control method _Hysterectomy_

g. Do you have concerns about sexual orientation, sexually transmitted diseases, exposure to AIDS or other sexual concerns? ☒ Yes ☐ No
h. Do you feel safe/comfortable in your home, with your family, and/or your partner relationship? ☒ Yes ☐ No
i. Do you smoke or use tobacco products now? ☐ Yes ☒ No
j. Do you use recreational drugs? ☒ Yes ☐ No
k. Do you drink alcohol? ☒ Yes ☐ No
☒ daily ☐ weekly ☐ rarely
# of drinks _3-4_
If yes, do you drink: ☐ beer, ☒ wine, ☒ liquor

Review of Systems
Are you concerned about?
(circle concerns)

	Yes	No
1. Recent changes in health status	☐	☒
2. Eye problems: vision, pain, tearing	☐	☒
3. Ears, nose, mouth, throat problems	☐	☒
4. Heart problems: chest pain, blood pressure	☐	☒
5. Lung problems: coughing, wheezing, infections	☐	☒

	Yes	No
6. Abdominal pain, stomach, bowel problems	☒	☐
7. Kidney or bladder problems	☐	☒
8. Muscle, bone, joint or back problems	☐	☒
9. Skin, hair or nail problems	☐	☒
10. Neurologic problems: headaches, dizziness, numbness	☐	☒
11. Nervousness, anxiety, depression, suicidal thoughts	☒	☐
12. Excessive thirst and urine output, recent weight changes	☐	☒
13. Anemia, bruising, blood clots, swollen glands	☐	☒
14. Food allergies, hayfever, eczema, asthma, decreased immunity	☐	☒
Do you have any other concerns?	☒	☐

Please do not reveal Drug
use or sexual activity to my
spouse

Deborah Feinstein   _12/23/2005_
Patient's Signature   Date

Provider Comments:
Wants prescription pain meds. Has seen multiple MDs in last few months for same complaint, but denies Rx for Pain med. States copes by using ETOH & marijuana.

Eric Anderson MD   _12/23/2005_

☒ PFSH and ROS have been reviewed.   ☐ Unresolved problems from previous visit have been addressed.   Provider's Signature   Date

Anticipatory Guidance

☐ Nutrition
☐ Exercise
☐ Calcium
☐ Multi vit. with folate

☐ Dental care
☐ Cardiovascular risks
☐ Sun exposure
☐ Smoking cessation
☒ Alcohol/drugs
☒ Sexual issues

☒ STD prevention
☒ Self exam. breasts, skin, oral cavity
☐ School/Work
☐ Family
☐ Recreation/ Hobbies
☐ Safety/Injury/Gun Safety

☐ Auto seat belts
☐ Smoke detectors
☐ Domestic violence
☐ Stress
☒ Educational handouts

©1995 Piermed, Inc. Rev. 6/98 (800) 998-1908

Female 19-39

500-02

FIGURE C-7, C

Name _Feinstein, Deborah_   DOB _04_/_08_/_1966_ Age _39_ Chart No. | FEIN006 |

Assessment

8.   Abd flat c̄ numerous scars. +BS x 4
     Tenderness LLQ. Pt reports BM qd- Brown, formed.

14. Very anxious and tense. Reported behavior shows a
     lack of judgment. Demonstrates a lack of insight into
     risky behavior

Dx: LLQ Abd Pain—chronic
     Risky sexual behavior & damaging lifestyle.
     R/O abuse Rx & Recreational Drugs
     R/O ETOH abuse

Plan

① Drug screen
② HIV test
③ VDRL
④ Refer to pain clinic
⑤ Refer to Psychologist

Eric Anderson MD   _4 wks_
Provider's Signature   Return Visit

FOLD HERE   FOLD HERE

Physical Exam

Ht. _5' 7"_ Wt. _114#_ Temp. _97.8°_ Resp. _18_

B.P. sit. or stand. _112_ / _72_   Supine ___ / ___

Pulse rate and regularity _72, regular_

Circle abnormal and pertinent normal findings
Describe abnormalities above.

☑ Normal   ☒ Abnormal

1. Constitutional
a. ☑ gen. appear., development, body shape,
     nutrition, deformities, grooming _Immaculate_

2. Eyes
a. ☑ conjunctiva, lids
b. ☒ pupils, irises _Dilated_
c. ☑ fundi (optic discs, vessels, exudate, hemorr.)

3. Ears, Nose, Throat & Mouth
a. ☑ appearance of ears, appearance of nose
b. ☑ auditory canals, tympanic membranes
c. ☑ hearing (whis. voice, finger rub, tun. fork)
d. ☑ nasal mucosa, sputum, turbinates
e. ☑ lips, teeth, gums
f. ☐ oropharnyx (mucosa, saliv. glands, hard &
     soft palates, tongue, tonsils, post. pharynx)

4. Neck
a. ☑ appearance, masses, symmetry, tracheal
     position, crepitus
b. ☐ thyroid (enlargement, tenderness, mass)

5. Respiratory
a. ☑ respiratory effort (intercostal retractions)
     use of accessory muscles, diaphragm move.
b. ☐ percussion (dullness, flatness, hyper-reson.)
c. ☐ palpation (tactile fremitus)
d. ☑ auscultation (breath sounds, rhonchi, wheezes,
     rales, rubs)

6. Cardiovascular
a. ☐ palpation (location of p.m.i., size, thrill)
b. ☑ auscultation (abnormal sounds, murmurs)
c. ☑ carotid arteries (pulse amplitude, bruits)
d. ☑ abdominal aorta (size, bruits)
e. ☑ femoral arteries (pulse amplitude, bruits)
f. ☐ pedal pulses (pulse amplitude)
g. ☑ extremities (edema, varicosities)

7. Chest (Breasts)
a. ☑ inspection (size, symmetry, nipple discharge)
b. ☑ palpation of breasts & axillae (masses,
     lumps, tenderness) _Breast Implants present_

8. Gastrointestinal (Abdomen)
a. ☒ examination for masses, (tenderness) _LLQ_
b. ☑ examination of liver, spleen
c. ☑ examination for presence or absence of hernia
d. ☑ examination of (when indicated) anus, perineum,
     rectum: (sphincter tone, hemorrhoids, masses)
e. ☐ stool for occult blood when indicated

9. Genitourinary
Pelvic Exam (with or without specimen collection
for smears or cultures), including:
a. ☑ Ext. Genitalia (eg. gen. app., hair distrib.,
     lesions) and vagina (eg. gen. app., esrogen eff.,
     lesions, pelvic support, cystocele, rectocele)
b. ☑ Urethra (eg. masses, tender., scarring)
c. ☑ Bladder (eg. fullness, masses, tender.)
d. ☑ Cervix (eg. gen. app., lesions, disch.)
e. ☒ Uterus (eg. size, contour, position, mobility,
     tender., consistency, descent or support) _Absent_
f. ☒ Adnexia / Parametria (eg. masses, tender.,
     organomegaly, nodularity)

10. Lymphatic
a. ☑ palpation of lymph nodes in 2 or more areas:
     (Circle: (neck), (axillae), (groin), other)

11. Musculoskeletal
a. ☑ examination of gait and station
b. ☑ inspection and/or palpation of digits & nails
     (clubbing, cyanosis, inflammatory conditions,
     petechiae, ischemia, infections, nodes)
c. ☑ assessment of range of motion (pain,
     crepitation, contracture)
d. ☑ Examination of joint, bone, & muscle of 1 or
     more of the following 6 areas (circle)
     ⊙head/neck   ⊙rt. upper extremities
     ⊙spine, ribs, & pelvis ⊙lt. upper extremities
     ⊙rt. lower estremities ⊙lt. lower extremities
e. ☐ inspect, and/or palpation (misalign, asymmetry,
     crepitation, defects, tender., masses, effusion)
f. ☑ assessment of stability: dislocation (luxation),
     subluxation or laxity
g. ☑ muscle strength & tone (flaccid, cogwheel,
     spastic), atrophy or abnormal movement

12. Skin
a. ☑ inspection of skin & sub-Q tissue (rashes,
     lesion, ulcers)
b. ☐ palpation of skin & sub-Q tissue (induration,
     sub-Q nodules, tightening)

13. Neurology
a. ☑ test cranial nerves: notation of deficits
b. ☑ examination of DTR's with notation of
     pathological reflexes (eg. Babinski)
c. ☐ examination of sensation (touch, pain,
     vibration, proprioception)

14. Psychiatric
a. ☒ description of patient's judgment & insight
     Brief assessment of mental status:
b. ☑ orientation to time, place, & person
c. ☑ recent & remote memory
d. ☒ mood & affect (depression, (anxiety), agitation)
e. ☐ other ___

Procedures and Immunizations

Are immunizations current? ☐Yes ☐No

☐ Hearing   ☐ Glucose   ☐ Cholesterol   ☐ PAP Test   ☐ dT
☐ Vision   ☐ PT   ☐ HDL/LDL   ☐ Chlamydia screen ☐ Hep B
☐ CBC   ☐ TSH   ☐ CXR   (high risk or pregnancy) ☐ Influenza
            ☐ Urine   ☐ EKG   ☐ Rubella Screen
                                          (or vaccination history)

Drug Allergies:

NKA

| Female 19-39 | Date / Time 12/23/2005 8:30 AM | Summary | Chronic LLQ Abd Pain | ☐ Referral |

500-06

© 1995 Pfiermed, Inc. Rev

FIGURE C-7, D

Lake Eola Family Practice   517860 South Pioneer Drive, Orlando, FL 32897 • 634-555-4893

Superbill   #456298

Weight _114#_   BP _112/72_   TPR _98.4° –72-18_

Account Number	Doctor	Date of Service
FEID006	Eric Anderson MD	12/23/2005

Patient Name	Date of Birth	LMP
Feinstein, Deborah	04/08/1966	N/A

Insurance	Responsible Party	Phone Number
BCBS of FL	Self	634-555-9852

Address	Referring Physician and ID #
PO Box YYYY	(Husband) Lawrence Feinstein MD

City	State	Zip	
Jacksonville	FL	39782	A62189

✓ New Patient

- __ 99201 H[PF] E[PF] MDM[S] 10 min
- __ 99202 H[EPF] E[EPF] MDM[S] 20 min
- __ 99203 H[D] E[D] MDM[LC] 30 min
- __ 99204 H[C] E[C] MDM[MC] 45 min
- _X_ 99205 H[C] E[C] MDM[HC] 60 min

Established Patient

- __ 99211 H[N/A] E[N/A] MDM[N/A] 5 min
- __ 99212 H[PF] E[PF] MDM[S] 10 min
- __ 99213 H[EPF] E[EPF] MDM[LC] 15 min
- __ 99214 H[D] E[D] MDM[MC] 25 min
- __ 99215 H[C] E[C] MDM[HC] 40 min

Reason For Visit

- __ Authorization _____
  Expiration Date _____
- __ Annual exam, complex due to (history, condition): _____
- __ Annual exam, simple
- __ Follow-up, condition _____
- __ Follow-up, post procedure, no condition or complication _____
  Procedure/date _____
- __ Follow-up, post procedure, with condition or complication _____
  Procedure/date _____
- __ New Problem _____
- __ Post-op, no condition or complication
  Surgery/date _____
- __ Post-op, with conditions or complication
  Surgery/date _____
- __ Pre-op _____
- __ Procedure _____
- __ Second surgical opinion _____
- _X_ Other (Accident, Decision for surgery) ___
  Repeat Eval–Chronic LLQ pain

Procedures

- ⇒ Place to be done: _____
- ⇒ Date to be done: _____
- __ Authorization _____
  Expiration date _____
- __ Biopsy, type/site _____
- __ Cautery, type/site _____
- __ Destruction of lesion(s), extensive, site: ___
- __ Destruction of lesion(s), simple, site: ___
- __ Emergency surgery (list above), reason: ___
- __ Excision, type/site _____
- __ I & D abscess, type/site: _____
- __ Insertion/Removal of IUD, type _____
- __ Major surgery, type/site _____
- __ Minor surgery, type/site _____
- __ Sonogram _____
- __ Other _____

Miscellaneous

- __ Immunization _____
- __ Injection _____
- __ Supplies
- __ Surgical tray

- __ Patient Teaching (Preventive medicine)
  _____
- _X_ Other _Refer to Psychologist_
- _X_ _Refer to Pain Clinic_
  _____

Outside Lab

- __ Beta HCG, Serum
- __ Biopsy/Pathology
- __ Biopsy, Mult./Pathology
- __ CBC
- __ Cholesterol
- __ Culture, throat
- __ Cultures (source) _____
- __ Glucose, __1hr glucose, __3hr glucose
- __ Estrogen
- __ Herpes simplex, AB
- __ Mononucleosis
- __ Pap Smear
- __ PT __PTT
- __ Sed rate
- __ SMAC
- __ Urinalysis, w/micro
- _X_ HIV _86703 $15.00_
- _X_ Other _____
  VDRL 86592 $15.00
  Drug Screen
  _80100 $15.00_

Diagnosis Codes

1. _789.04_
2. _V69.2_
3. _V69.8_
4. _____

Appointment in _4_ Weeks

Procedure in _____ Weeks

Sent Labs to_____

Call in _____ Mos./Weeks

Previous Balance $ ___0___

20% Co-Pay $ ___49.00___

Paid Today Cash/Check $ ___49.00___

New Charges $ ___245.00___

New Balance $ ___196.00___

Check Number _____

Yes-No All Diagnosis, Procedures, & VS above are documented in Record

Doctor's Signature ___Eric Anderson MD___

FIGURE C-7, E

Case Study 8: Samuel Clark

Lake Eola Family Practice   517860 South Pioneer Drive, Orlando, FL 32897 • 634-555-4893

Patient Registration Form

Have you been seen in this office in the past 3 years? ✔ Yes ___ No   **Do you have a living will?** No

Today's Date _4/22/2005_   Home Phone _634-555-1500_   Work Phone _____

Patient Name (Last name, First name, Middle initial) _Clark, Samuel_

Street Address _2967514 Spur Ln_   City _Orlando_   State _FL_   Zip _32897_

Date of Birth _2/5/1995_   Age _10_   Gender: ___ Female _X_ Male   Social Security # _____

Marital Status: ___ Married _X_ Single ___ Widowed ___ Divorced ___ Other   Driver's License # _____

Is the patient a student? _X_ Full Time ___ Part Time ___ No   Is the patient employed? ___ Full Time ___ Part Time _X_ No

Patient's Employer Name & Address _None_

School Name & Address _Rodeo Elementary_

Emergency Contact Person _Ginger Clark_   Relationship _Mother_ Phone _634-555-1500_

Referring Physician Name & Phone Number _None_

Insurance Plan and Responsible Party Information

Insurance Company Name _BC BS_   Address _PO Box YYYY_

City _Jacksonville_   State _FL_   Zip _39782_   Phone _800-555-1212_

Policy # _____   Group # _MD890_   ID # _598XX5432C1_

Policy Holder's Name _Daniel Clark_   Address _2967514 Spur_

City _Orlando_   State _FL_   Zip _39782_   Phone _634-555-1500_

Policy Holder's Date of Birth _12/5/1965_   Social Security # _598-XX-5432_   Driver License # _B752-XX-1999_

Gender: ___ Male ___ Female   Relationship to patient: ___ Self ___ Spouse _X_ Parent ___ Guardian ___ Other

Policy Holder's Employer's Name _McDonald's_   Address _5980 Spur_

City _Orlando_   State _FL_   Zip _39782_   Phone _____

Secondary Insurance Company Name _Aetna_   Address _PO Box WWW_

City _Tampa_   State _FL_   Zip _32897_   Phone _800-555-1212_

Secondary Policy # _____   Group # _LEH5743_   ID # _ACHC59738_

Secondary Policy Holder's Name _Ginger Clark_   Phone _634-555-1500_ Address _2967514 Spur_

City _Orlando_   State _FL_ Zip _32897_   Relationship to patient: ___ Self ___ Spouse _X_ Parent/Other

Secondary Policy Holder's Date of Birth _6/15/1967_ Social Security # _598-XX-7632_ Driver License # _B752-XX-1889_
Works for Lake Eola Hospital

Authorizations

It is customary to pay for all services on the date rendered unless other arrangements were made before your appointment. The patient and the guarantor are responsible for all deductibles and copays at the time of the visit and any other fees in accordance with insurance contracts. The patient and guarantor are responsible for all elective or noncovered services and any services that are not considered medically necessary.

Financially responsible person if patient is student or unemployed _Daniel Clark_   Phone _634-555-1500_

I authorize the release of any medical information necessary to process this claim and I request that payment of medical benefits be made directly to Lake Eola Family Practice. I hereby acknowledge that I am fully responsible for payment as listed above.

Signed _Ginger Clark_   Date _1/22/05_   Time _10:00 AM_

Template © 1998 Medical Compliance Management, Inc.

FIGURE C-8, A

Lake Eola Family Practice   517860 South Pioneer Drive, Orlando, FL 32897 • 634-555-4893

Problem List – Medication List

Patient Name ___Clark, Samuel_____ DOB __02/05/1995__

Allergies & allergic response ___None_____

Referring Physician & ID # ___None_____

	Problem (e.g., acute or chronic diagnosis, injury,↑ BP)	**Date Identified**	**Date Resolved**
1	Fx Ⓛ radius (Greenstick)	04/22/2005	
2	Deep abrasion 2cm x 4cm Ⓡ upper arm	04/22/2005	
3			
4			
5			
6			
7			
8			
9			
10			
11			
12			
13			
14			
15			

	All Medications (with dosage & instructions) (include prescription and over-the-counter medications)	**Start Date**	**Discontinue Date**
1	OTC Triple antibiotic ung. Ⓡ arm qd	04/22/2005	
2			
3			
4			
5			
6			
7			
8			
9			
10			

Template © 1998 Medical Compliance Management, Inc.

FIGURE C-8, B

Name _Clark, Samuel_ **DOB** _02_/_05_/_1995_ **Chart #** _CLAS031_ **Seen With:** ☒ Mth. ☐ Fth. ☐ Other_____

Physical Exam ☑ NL ☒ Abn. (Circle Abn.)

Temp _98.2°_ P _88_ R _20_ BP_110/70_ Peak Fl _____

Constitutional... ☐	looks ill 1+, 2+, 3+ Hydration ☐ _____
Fontanel .... ☐	
Eyes .... ☑	red, drainage (clear, pur.), Fundi ☐_____
Ears: .Rtm....... ☑	red, dull, thick, ↓mobility, retract., bulging fluid (ser, pur), perf. scarred, tube (in, out)
Ltm ...... ☑	red, dull, thick, ↓mobility, retract., bulging fluid (ser, pur), perf. scarred, tube (in, out)
Ext. Canal .... ☑	cerumen, swollen, tender, pur. drainage
Nose .... ☑	drainage (watery, mucoid, pur.), Sinuses ☐
Mouth/Throat .... ☑	ulcers, drainage (mucoid, pur.) inj. _____
Tonsils	enlarged 1+, 2+, 3+, 4+, exudate, petechiae
Lymphatic .... ☑	_____
Neck .... ☑	_____
Cardiovascular ☑	_____
Respiratory ..... ☑	rhonchi, wheezes, rales, ↓br. sounds, retract.
R _Cl_ L _Cl_	resp. distress 0, 1+, 2+, 3+ _____

		CPT
Gastrointestinal ☑	_____	**PF**
Genitourinary.... ☑	_____	**EPF**
Musculoskeletal ☒	_Greenstick Fx (L) radius_	**D**
Skin .... ☒	_Deep Abrasion 4cm x 2cm_	**C**
Neurological ..... ☑	_(R) upper arm_	

History   ☒ Positive ☑ Negative   ☐ Follow-up visit

Chief complaint/duration: _Fell at school during PE._
Abrasions (R) arm, Severe Pain (L) arm

restless ☐	fussy ☐	awake at night ☐	↓ appetite ☐

Fever .... ☐	Earache .... ☐	Back pain .... ☐	Vomiting .... ☐
Congestion ...... ☐	Sw. glands ...... ☐	Mus/Jnt pain .... ☒	Diarrhea .... ☐
Cough .... ☐	Red Eyes ...... ☐	Abd. pain .... ☐	Urinary sx .... ☐
Sore Throat ..... ☐	Headache .... ☐	Constipation .... ☐	Skin rash .... ☐

Scraped (R) arm on rusty fence as fell over fence,
landing on (L) arm while catching a flyball during PE.
No loss of consciousness.

		Over ☐	CPT
Systems reviewed.......... ☒	Family/Social Hx reviewed .... ☐		**PF**
Past Hx reviewed........... ☒	Immunizations current? Yes ☐ No ☒		**EPF**
			D
Current Meds: _none_			**C**
Drug Allergies? Yes ☐ No ☒			

Treatment   ① X-ray (L) Forearm
② Applied fiberglass cast (L) arm
③ Irrigated abrasion (R) upper arm

Provider's Sig. ➤ _Todd Wilson MD_   Over ☒

CPT
SF
LC
MC
HC

☐ Report back in 24 hrs. ☐ Call in 48 hrs., prn ☒ Re-examine _48 Hrs_

Sick	Date / Time 10:30 AM 04/22/2005	Age 10 yr	Weight 75#	Height 50"	Diagnosis: _Fx (L) Radius, Abrasion (R) arm_	☐ After Hrs. ☐ Referral

©1991 Piermed, Inc. Rev 5/99

FIGURE C-8, C

Review of Systems   ☒ Positive ☑ Negative   (all positive findings must be described)

1. Constitutional Symptoms .... ☑	6. Gastrointestinal .... ☑	11. Psychiatric .... ☑
2. Eyes .... ☑	7. Genitourinary .... ☑	12. Endocrine .... ☑
3. Ears, Nose, Mouth, Throat.............. ☑	8. Musculoskeletal .... ☒	13. Hematologic/Lymphatic .... ☑
4. Cardiovascular .... ☑	9. Integumentary (skin and/or breast).. ☒	14. Allergic/Immunologic .... ☑
5. Respiratory .... ☑	10. Neurologic .... ☑	

Treatment con't.

④ Applied triple antibiotic ung. to Abrasion (R) upper arm and wrapped c̄ elastic bandage

Instructions:

① Keep ice on (L) arm over cast

② Change bandage daily (R) upper arm

③ Return in 48 hours for recheck

④ Tetanus Toxoid .5 ml IM now

Todd Wilson MD

Pediaforms® (292-27)   Piermed, Inc. • (800) 998-1908

FIGURE C-8, D

Lake Eola Family Practice

517860 South Pioneer Drive, Orlando, FL 32897 • 634-555-4893

Superbill   #456298

Weight _75#_   BP _110/70_   TPR _98.2°–88-20_

Account Number _CLAS031_	Doctor _Todd Wilson MD_	Date of Service _04/22/2005_
Patient Name _Clark, Samuel_	Date of Birth _02/15/1995_	LMP _N/A_
Insurance _Aetna/BCBS FL_	Responsible Party _Daniel Clark_	Phone Number _634-555-1500_
Address _PO Box WWW_	Referring Physician and ID # _None_	
City _Tampa_	State _FL_ Zip _32897_	

New Patient

___99201 H[PF]   E[PF]   MDM[S]   10 min
___99202 H[EPF] E[EPF] MDM[S]   20 min
___99203 H[D]   E[D]   MDM[LC] 30 min
___99204 H[C]   E[C]   MDM[MC] 45 min
___99205 H[C]   E[C]   MDM[HC] 60 min

✓ Established Patient

___99211 H[N/A] E[N/A] MDM[N/A] 5 min
___99212 H[PF]   E[PF]   MDM[S]   10 min
___99213 H[EPF] E[EPF] MDM[LC] 15 min
_X_99214 H[D]   E[D]   MDM[MC] 25 min
___99215 H[C]   E[C]   MDM[HC] 40 min

Reason For Visit

___Authorization _____
     Expiration Date _____
___Annual exam, complex due to (history, condition):
_____
___Annual exam, simple
___Follow-up, condition _____
___Follow-up, post procedure, no condition or complication _____
     Procedure/date _____
___Follow-up, post procedure, with condition or complication _____
     Procedure/date _____
_X_New Problem _Injury both arms_
___Post-op, no condition or complication
     Surgery/date _____
___Post-op, with conditions or complication

     Surgery/date _____
___Pre-op _____ 29065
_X_Procedure (L) long arm cast
___Second surgical opinion _____ $125.00
___Other (Accident, Decision for surgery) ___

Procedures

⟹ Place to be done: _____
⟹ Date to be done: _____
___Authorization _____
     Expiration date _____
___Biopsy, type/site _____
_____
___Cautery, type/site _____
_____
___Destruction of lesion(s), extensive, site: ___
_____
___Destruction of lesion(s), simple, site: _____
_____
___Emergency surgery (list above), reason: ___
_____
___Excision, type/site _____
_____
___I & D abscess, type/site: _____
_____
___Insertion/Removal of IUD, type _____
___Major surgery, type/site _____
_____
___Minor surgery, type/site _____
_____
___Sonogram _____
_X_Other _Closed Tx Fx (L) radius_
     $250.00   25500

Miscellaneous

_X_Immunization _Tetanus Toxoid .5ml_
___Injection _____ $5.00
_X_Supplies _Elastic Bandage roll_
___Surgical tray _____ $10.00

Patient Teaching (Preventive medicine)
_X_ Xray (L) Forearm–2 views
     $35.00   73090
_X_ Other _irrigate and dress wounds_
     (R) upper arm
_____
_____
_____

Outside Lab

___Beta HCG, Serum
___Biopsy/Pathology
___Biopsy, Mult./Pathology
___CBC
___Cholesterol
___Culture, throat
___Cultures (source) _____
___Glucose, ___1hr glucose, ___3hr glucose
___Estrogen
___Herpes simplex, AB
___Mononucleosis
___Pap Smear
___PT___PTT
___Sed rate
___SMAC
___Urinalysis, w/micro
___HIV
___Other _____
_____
_____
_____

Diagnosis Codes

1. _813.81_
2. _912.0_
3. _E849.4_
4. _E888,1_

Appointment in _48 hours_ Weeks	Previous Balance $ ___0___ New Charges $ _565.00_
Procedure in _____ Weeks	Co-Pay $ ___(2 Payors)___ New Balance $ _565.00_
Sent Labs to_____	Paid Today Cash/Check $ _____ Check Number _____
Call in _____ Mos./Weeks	Yes-No All Diagnosis, Procedures, & VS above are documented in Record

Template © 1998 Medical Compliance Management, Inc.,
CPT only © American Medical Association. All Rights Reserved.

Doctor's Signature ___Todd Wilson MD___

FIGURE C-8, E

Case Study 9: Nancy Robbins

Lake Eola Family Practice

517860 South Pioneer Drive, Orlando, FL 32897 • 634-555-4893

Patient Registration Form

Have you been seen in this office in the past 3 years? ✔ Yes ___ No   Do you have a living will? No

Today's Date _8/21/2005_   Home Phone _634-555-1970_   Work Phone (Mother's) _634-555-2462_

Patient Name (Last name, First name, Middle initial) _Robbins, Nancy_

Street Address _2965988 Rodeo Circle_   City _Orlando_   State _FL_   Zip _32897_

Date of Birth _12/18/1997_   Age _7_   Gender: _X_ Female ___ Male   Social Security # _678-XX-8765_

Marital Status: ___ Married _X_ Single ___ Widowed ___ Divorced ___ Other   Driver's License # _None_

Is the patient a student? _X_ Full Time ___ Part Time ___ No   Is the patient employed? ___ Full Time ___ Part Time _X_ No

Patient's Employer Name & Address _None_

School Name & Address _Rodeo Elementary_

Emergency Contact Person _Katie Robbins_   Relationship _Mother_   Phone _634-555-1970_

Referring Physician Name & Phone Number _None_

Insurance Plan and Responsible Party Information

Insurance Company Name _Medicaid_   Address _PO Box XXX_

City _Tallahassee_   State _FL_   Zip _32897_   Phone _800-555-1212_

Policy # _____   Group # _____   ID # _345XX89123_

Policy Holder's Name _Nancy Robbins_   Address _2965988 Rodeo Circle_

City _Orlando_   State _FL_   Zip _32897_   Phone _634-555-1970_

Policy Holder's Date of Birth _12/18/1992_   Social Security # _678-XX-8765_   Driver License # _None_

Gender: ___ Male _X_ Female   Relationship to patient: _X_ Self ___ Spouse ___ Parent ___ Guardian ___ Other

Policy Holder's Employer's Name _None_   Address _____

City _____   State _____   Zip _____   Phone _____

Secondary Insurance Company Name _None_   Address _____

City _____   State _____   Zip _____   Phone _____

Secondary Policy # _____   Group # _____   ID # _____

Secondary Policy Holder's Name _____   Phone _____   Address _____

City _____   State _____   Zip _____   Relationship to patient: ___ Self ___ Spouse ___ other

Secondary Policy Holder's Date of Birth _____   Social Security # _____   Driver License # _____

Authorizations

It is customary to pay for all services on the date rendered unless other arrangements were made before your appointment. The patient and the guarantor are responsible for all deductibles and copays at the time of the visit and any other fees in accordance with insurance contracts. The patient and guarantor are responsible for all elective or noncovered services and any services that are not considered medically necessary.

Financially responsible person if patient is student or unemployed _Katie Robbins_   Phone _634-555-1970_

I authorize the release of any medical information necessary to process this claim and I request that payment of medical benefits be made directly to Lake Eola Family Practice. I hereby acknowledge that I am fully responsible for payment as listed above.

Signed _Katie Robbins (Mother)_   Date _8/21/2005_   Time _3:00 PM_

Template © 1998 Medical Compliance Management, Inc.

FIGURE C-9, A

Lake Eola Family Practice   517860 South Pioneer Drive, Orlando, FL 32897 • 634-555-4893

Problem List – Medication List

Patient Name ___Robbins, Nancy_____ DOB _12/18/1997___

Allergies & allergic response __None Known_____

Referring Physician & ID # __None_____

	Problem (e.g., acute or chronic diagnosis, injury,↑ BP)	**Date Identified**	**Date Resolved**
1	℞ Serous otitis media	4/5/2002	4/15/2002
2	℞ Serous otitis media	6/28/2004	7/12/2004
3	Bilat Serous otitis media	08/21/2005	
4			
5			
6			
7			
8			
9			
10			
11			
12			
13			
14			
15			

	All Medications (with dosage & instructions) (include prescription and over-the-counter medications)	**Start Date**	**Discontinue Date**
1	Amoxil 5ml PO TID	4/5/2002	4/15/2002
2	Amoxil 5ml PO TID	6/28/2004	6/08/2004
3	Amoxil 5ml PO TID	08/21/2005	
4	Children's Tylenol PO q 6° prn fever	08/21/2005	
5			
6			
7			
8			
9			
10			

Template © 1998 Medical Compliance Management, Inc.

FIGURE C-9, B

Name _Robbins, Nancy_ DOB _12_/_18_/_1997_ Chart # _ROBN016_ Seen With: ☒ Mth. ☐ Fth. ☐ Other_____	

Physical Exam   ☑NL ☒ Abn. (Circle Abn.)

Temp _101.6°_ P _110_ R _20_ BP _100/60_ Peak Fl _____

Constitutional... ☒ looks ill 1+, ②+ 3+ Hydration ☐ _____

Fontanel .... ☐

Eyes .... ☑ red, drainage (clear, pur.), Fundi ☐_____

Ears: .Rtm....... ☒ (red,) dull, thick, ↓mobility, retract. (bulging)
  fluid (ser,) pur), perf. scarred, tube (in, out)

Ltm ...... ☒ (red,) dull, thick, ↓mobility, retract. (bulging)
  fluid (ser,)pur), perf. scarred, tube (in, out)

Ext. Canal .... ☑ cerumen, swollen, tender, pur. drainage

Nose .... ☒ drainage (watery) mucoid, pur.), Sinuses ☑

Mouth/Throat .... ☑ ulcers, drainage (mucoid, pur.) inj. _____

Tonsils .... enlarged ①+, 2+, 3+, 4+, exudate, petechiae

Lymphatic .... ☑ _____

Neck .... ☑ _____

Cardiovascular ☑ _____

Respiratory ...... ☑ rhonchi, wheezes, rales, ↓br. sounds, retract.

R___ L___ resp. distress 0, 1+, 2+, 3+ _____

Gastrointestinal ☑ _____

Genitourinary .... ☑ _____

Musculoskeletal ☑ _____

Skin .... ☑ _____

Neurological .... ☑

CPT / PF / EPF / D / C

History   ☒ Positive ☑ Negative ☐ Follow-up visit

Chief complaint/duration: _C/O Earache since this AM,_
Fever 101° since noon. Tylenol @ noon

restless ☐	fussy ☐	awake at night ☐	↓ appetite ☐

Fever .... ☒	Earache .... ☒	Back pain .... ☐	Vomiting .... ☐
Congestion ...... ☐	Sw. glands...... ☐	Mus/Jnt pain .... ☐	Diarrhea .... ☐
Cough .... ☐	Red Eyes .... ☐	Abd. pain .... ☐	Urinary sx .... ☐
Sore Throat ..... ☐	Headache .... ☐	Constipation .... ☐	Skin rash .... ☐

Acute serous otitis media, Bilat

Over ☐

Systems reviewed.......... ☒   Family/Social Hx reviewed .... ☐

Past Hx reviewed............ ☒   Immunizations current? Yes☒ No ☐

Current Meds: _none_

Drug Allergies? Yes☐ No ☒

CPT / PF / EPF / D / C

Treatment _Amoxil 5 ml TID x 10 days_
Tylenol + chewable q 6° prn fever

Provider's Sig. ➤ _Cassandra Lewis ARNP_   Over ☐

CPT / SF / LC / MC / HC

☐ Report back in 24 hrs.   ☐ Call in 48 hrs., prn   ☒ Re-examine _14 days_

Sick	Date / Time 4:00 PM 08/21/2005	Age 7	Weight 45#	Height 42"	Diagnosis: _Bilat Serous Otitis Media_	☐ After Hrs. ☐ Referral

©1991 Piermed, Inc. Rev 5/99

FIGURE C-9, C

Review of Systems   ☐ Positive ☐ Negative   (all positive findings must be described)

1. Constitutional Symptoms .... ☐
2. Eyes .... ☐
3. Ears, Nose, Mouth, Throat............ ☐
4. Cardiovascular .... ☐
5. Respiratory .... ☐
6. Gastrointestinal .... ☐
7. Genitourinary .... ☐
8. Musculoskeletal .... ☐
9. Integumentary (skin and/or breast).. ☐
10. Neurologic .... ☐
11. Psychiatric .... ☐
12. Endocrine .... ☐
13. Hematologic/Lymphatic .... ☐
14. Allergic/Immunologic .... ☐

Pediaforms® (292-27)

Piermed, Inc. • (800) 998-1908

FIGURE C-9, D

Lake Eola Family Practice

517860 South Pioneer Drive, Orlando, FL 32897 • 634-555-4893

Superbill   #456298

Weight __45#__ BP _110/60_ TPR _101.6°–110-20_

Account Number ROBN016	Doctor Cassandra Lewis ARNP		Date of Service 08/21/2005
Patient Name Robbins, Nancy		Date of Birth 12/18/1997	LMP N/A
Insurance Medicaid	Responsible Party (Mother) Katie Robbins		Phone Number 634-555-1970
Address PO Box XXX		Referring Physician and ID # None	
City Tallahassee	State FL	Zip 32897	

New Patient

__99201	H[PF]	E[PF]	MDM[S]	10 min
__99202	H[EPF]	E[EPF]	MDM[S]	20 min
__99203	H[D]	E[D]	MDM[LC]	30 min
__99204	H[C]	E[C]	MDM[MC]	45 min
__99205	H[C]	E[C]	MDM[HC]	60 min

✓ Established Patient

__99211	H[N/A]	E[N/A]	MDM[N/A]	5 min
X 99212	H[PF]	E[PF]	MDM[S]	10 min
__99213	H[EPF]	E[EPF]	MDM[LC]	15 min
__99214	H[D]	E[D]	MDM[MC]	25 min
__99215	H[C]	E[C]	MDM[HC]	40 min

Reason For Visit

__Authorization _____
  Expiration Date _____
__Annual exam, complex due to (history, condition): _____

__Annual exam, simple
__Follow-up, condition _____
__Follow-up, post procedure, no condition or complication _____
  Procedure/date _____
__Follow-up, post procedure, with condition or complication _____
  Procedure/date _____
X New Problem _Earache_

__Post-op, no condition or complication
  Surgery/date _____
__Post-op, with conditions or complication
_____
  Surgery/date _____
__Pre-op _____
__Procedure _____
__Second surgical opinion _____
__Other (Accident, Decision for surgery) ___
_____

Procedures

⇒ Place to be done: _____
⇒ Date to be done: _____
__ Authorization _____
  Expiration date _____
__ Biopsy, type/site _____

__ Cautery, type/site _____

__ Destruction of lesion(s), extensive, site: __

__ Destruction of lesion(s), simple, site: ___

__ Emergency surgery (list above), reason: __

__ Excision, type/site _____

__ I & D abscess, type/site: _____

__ Insertion/Removal of IUD, type _____
__ Major surgery, type/site _____

__ Minor surgery, type/site _____

__ Sonogram _____
__ Other _____

Miscellaneous

__ Immunization _____
__ Injection _____
__ Supplies
__ Surgical tray

__ Patient Teaching (Preventive medicine)
_____
_____
__ Other _____
_____
_____
_____
_____

Outside Lab

__ Beta HCG, Serum
__ Biopsy/Pathology
__ Biopsy, Mult./Pathology
__ CBC
__ Cholesterol
__ Culture, throat
__ Cultures (source) _____
__ Glucose, __1hr glucose, __ 3hr glucose
__ Estrogen
__ Herpes simplex, AB
__ Mononucleosis
__ Pap Smear
__ PT __PTT
__ Sed rate
__ SMAC
__ Urinalysis, w/micro
__ HIV
__ Other _____
_____
_____
_____

Diagnosis Codes

1. _381.01_
2. _____
3. _____
4. _____

Appointment in __2__ Weeks
Procedure in _____ Weeks
Sent Labs to_____
Call in _____ Mos./Weeks

Previous Balance $ ___0___
Co-Pay $ ___0___
Paid Today Cash/Check $ _____

New Charges $ _48.00_
New Balance $ _48.00_
Check Number _____

Yes-No All Diagnosis, Procedures, & VS above are documented in Record
Doctor's Signature ___Cassandra Lewis ARNP___

FIGURE C-9, E

Case Study 10: Rajid Jayaguro

Lake Eola Family Practice   517860 South Pioneer Drive, Orlando, FL 32897 • 634-555-4893

Patient Registration Form

Have you been seen in this office in the past 3 years? ___Yes ✔ No   **Do you have a living will?** ✔___

Today's Date __6/10/2005__   Home Phone __634-555-2790__   Work Phone _____

Patient Name (Last name, First name, Middle initial) __Jayaguro, Rajid__

Street Address __4575432 Spur Ln__   City __Orlando__   State __FL__   Zip __32897__

Date of Birth __3/17/1922__   Age __83__   Gender: ___Female _X_ Male   Social Security # __543-XX-0123__

Marital Status: ___Married ___Single _X_ Widowed ___Divorced ___Other   Driver's License # __B521-XX-87654__

Is the patient a student? ___Full Time ___Part Time _X_ No   Is the patient employed? ___Full Time ___Part Time _X_ No

Patient's Employer Name & Address __None__

School Name & Address __None__

Emergency Contact Person __Pareen Jayaguro__   Relationship __Daughter-in-law__ Phone __634-555-2790__

Referring Physician Name & Phone Number __None__

Insurance Plan and Responsible Party Information

Insurance Company Name __Medicare__   Address __PO Box ZZZZ__

City __Jacksonville__   State __FL__   Zip __39782__   Phone __800-555-1212__

Policy # _____   Group # _____   ID # __543XX-0123F1__

Policy Holder's Name __Rajid Jayaguro__   Address __Same__

City _____   State _____   Zip _____   Phone _____

Policy Holder's Date of Birth _____   Social Security # _____   Driver License # _____

Gender: _X_ Male ___Female   Relationship to patient: _X_ Self ___Spouse ___Parent ___Guardian ___Other

Policy Holder's Employer's Name __None__   Address _____

City _____   State _____   Zip _____   Phone _____

Secondary Insurance Company Name __BC BS Medigap D__   Address __PO Box YYYY__

City __Jacksonville__   State __FL__   Zip __39782__   Phone __800-555-1212__

Secondary Policy # _____   Group # _____   ID # __543XX0123F1__

Secondary Policy Holder's Name __Rajid Jayaguro__   Phone __Same__   Address _____

City _____   State _____   Zip _____   Relationship to patient: ___Self ___Spouse ___other

Secondary Policy Holder's Date of Birth _____   Social Security # _____   Driver License # _____

Authorizations

It is customary to pay for all services on the date rendered unless other arrangements were made before your appointment. The patient and the guarantor are responsible for all deductibles and copays at the time of the visit and any other fees in accordance with insurance contracts. The patient and guarantor are responsible for all elective or noncovered services and any services that are not considered medically necessary.

Financially responsible person if patient is student or unemployed __Rajid Jayaguro__   Phone __634-555-2790__

I authorize the release of any medical information necessary to process this claim and I request that payment of medical benefits be made directly to Lake Eola Family Practice. I hereby acknowledge that I am fully responsible for payment as listed above.

Signed __Rajid Jayaguro__   Date __6/10/2005__   Time __11:00 AM__

Template © 1998 Medical Compliance Management, Inc.

FIGURE C-10, A

Lake Eola Family Practice   517860 South Pioneer Drive, Orlando, FL 32897 • 634-555-4893

Problem List – Medication List

Patient Name ___Jayaguro, Rajid_____ DOB __03/17/1922___

Allergies & allergic response ___Codeine – hives, itching_____

Referring Physician & ID # ___None_____

	Problem (e.g., acute or chronic diagnosis, injury,↑ BP)	**Date Identified**	**Date Resolved**
1	Chronic Pyelonephritis	June 2004	
2	Sprain Ⓛ wrist	6/10/2005	
3			
4			
5			
6			
7			
8			
9			
10			
11			
12			
13			
14			
15			

	All Medications (with dosage & instructions) (include prescription and over-the-counter medications)	**Start Date**	**Discontinue Date**
1	Bactrim DS ÷ PO qd	June 2004	
2	Darvocet N ÷ PO q 4h prn pain	6/10/2005	
3			
4			
5			
6			
7			
8			
9			
10			

Template © 1998 Medical Compliance Management, Inc.

FIGURE C-10, B

Name **Jayaguro, Rajid**   Date _06_/_10_/_2005_

HPI Chief Complaint:

(1.) Tripped over family dog 2 hours ago
at home and injured (L) wrist.

(2) Reports pain in wrist when moving (L)
hand and wrist

(3.) Denies any other injuries

Current Meds.:

(1.) Bactrim DS ⊤ PO QD

Past/Family History

(1.) Personal Hx Chronic Pyelonephritis

(2) Moved to Orlando last month to live with
son's family since son now travels
on business.

(3) Parents live in India
Father age 99 – alive and well
Mother age 98 – alive and well

THIS SECTION TO BE COMPLETED BY PATIENT.

Personal/Social History

Are you... ☐ single ☐ married
☐ live in partner ☐ divorced ☒ widow

Do you have children? ☒ Yes ☐ No
Ages of child(ren) _45_
Occupation/Retired _Mathematics Professor_

	Yes	No
a. Do you have any problems with (circle) memory, recent changes in hearing or vision,↑ injuries, problems with sleep, in your overall happiness?	☐	☒
b. Do you have any difficulty starting a urine stream, dribbling, pain or blood on urination or awake up at night to urinate If so, number of times _____	☐	☒
c. Do you have lesions, sores or drainage from penis?	☐	☒
d. Do you have any lumps, swelling, tenderness or pain in groin, scrotum, or testicles?	☐	☒
e. Do you have any difficulty getting or sustaining an erection?	☒	☐

	Yes	No
f. Are you sexually active now?	☐	☒
g. Do you use condoms?	☐	☒
h. Do you have other sexual concerns?	☐	☒
i. Have you needed help with (circle) shopping, chores, walking, climbing stairs, going to the bathroom, bathing, dressing, taking medication?	☐	☒
j. Do you feel safe/comfortable in your home, with your family, and/or your partner relationship?	☒	☐
k. Do you smoke or use tobacco products now?	☐	☒
l. Do you use recreational drugs?	☐	☒
m. Do you drink alcohol?	☐	☒

☐ daily   ☐ weekly   ☐ rarely
# of drinks _____
If yes, do you drink: ☐ beer, ☐ wine, ☐ liquor

Review of Systems
Are you concerned about?
(circle concerns)

	Yes	No
1. Recent changes in health status	☐	☒
2. Eye problems: vision, pain, tearing	☐	☒

	Yes	No
3. Ears, nose, mouth, throat problems	☐	☒
4. Heart problems: chest pain, blood pressure	☐	☒
5. Lung problems: coughing, wheezing, infections	☐	☒
6. Abdominal pain, stomach, bowel problems	☐	☐
7. Kidney or bladder problems	☒	☐
8. Muscle, bone, joint or back problems	☒	☐
9. Skin, hair or nail problems	☐	☒
10. Neurologic problems: headaches, dizziness, numbness	☐	☒
11. Nervousness, anxiety, depression, suicidal thoughts	☐	☒
12. Excessive thirst and urine output, recent weight changes	☐	☒
13. Anemia, bruising, blood clots, swollen glands	☐	☒
14. Food allergies, hayfever, eczema, asthma, decreased immunity	☐	☒
Do you have any other concerns?	☐	☒

7. Chronic Pyelonephritis
8. Injured (L) wrist

Rajid Jayaguro   _6/10/05_
Patient's Signuture   Date

Provider Comments:

7. Chronic pyelonephritis controlled c̄ Bactrim DS ⊤ PO QD

Aaron Rubin MD   _6/10/05_

☒ PFSH and ROS have been reviewed.   ☐ Unresolved problems from previous visit have been addressed. | Provider's Signature   Date

Anticipatory Guidance

☐ Nutrition
☐ Multi-vitamins
☐ Exercise
☐ Dental care
☐ Sun exposure

☐ Smoking cessation
☐ Alcohol/drugs
☐ Cardiovascular risks
☐ Aspirin prophylaxis
☐ Self exam. testes, skin, oral cavity
☐ Sexual issues
☐ STD prevention

☐ Work/Retirement
☐ Family
☐ Recreation/Hobbies
☐ Safety/ Injury/Gun Safety
☐ Auto seat belts
☐ Smoke detectors
☐ Hot water <120°

☐ Fall prevention
☐ CPR for family members
☐ Domestic violence
☐ Stress
☐ Living Will
☐ Medical Power of Attorney
☐ Educational handouts

©1995 Piermed, Inc. Rev. 6/98 (800) 998-1908

500-05

Male 60+

FIGURE C-10, C

Name **Jayaguro, Rajid**   DOB _03_/_17_/_1922_   Age _83_   Chart No. **JAYR001**

Assessment

(11c.)   Pain with movement (L) wrist/hand
(11d)   x-ray of (L) wrist is WNL
(11g.)   ↓strength (L) upper extremity 2° pain

Dx: ① Sprained (L) wrist
     ② Chronic Pyelonephritis

Plan

①   Soft Splint (L) wrist
②   Apply ice to (L) wrist x 24 hrs
③   Rx Darvocet N⁺̄ q4h prn
④   CBC, UA c̄ culture
⑤   Continue Bactrim

Aaron Rubin MD   **2 wks**
Provider's Signature   Return Visit

FOLD HERE   FOLD HERE

Physical Exam

Ht. _5' 3"_ Wt. _128#_ Temp. _98.6°_ Resp. _16_

B.P. sit. or stand. _110_ / _68_   Supine ___ / ___

Pulse rate and regularity _62, regular_
                      Strong

Circle abnormal and pertinent normal findings
Describe abnormalities above.
     ☑ Normal   ☐ Abnormal

1. Constitutional
a. ☑ gen. appear., development, body shape, nutrition, deformities, grooming

2. Eyes
a. ☑ conjunctiva, lids
b. ☑ pupils, irises
c. ☑ fundi (optic discs, vessels, exudate, hemorr.)

3. Ears, Nose, Throat & Mouth
a. ☑ appearance of ears, appearance of nose
b. ☑ auditory canals, tympanic membranes
c. ☐ hearing (whis. voice, finger rub, tun. fork)
d. ☑ nasal mucosa, sputum, turbinates
e. ☐ lips, teeth, gums
f. ☑ oropharynx (mucosa, saliv. glands, hard & soft palates, tongue, tonsils, post. pharynx)

4. Neck
a. ☑ appearance, masses, symmetry, tracheal position, crepitus
b. ☑ thyroid (enlargement, tenderness, mass)

5. Respiratory
a. ☑ respiratory effort (intercostal retractions) use of accessory muscles, diaphragm move.
b. ☐ percussion (dullness, flatness, hyper-reson.)
c. ☐ palpation (tactile fremitus)
d. ☑ auscultation (breath sounds, rhonchi, wheezes, rales, rubs)

6. Cardiovascular
a. ☐ palpation (location of p.m.i., size, thrill)
b. ☑ auscultation (abnormal sounds, murmurs)
c. ☑ carotid arteries (pulse amplitude, bruits)
d. ☐ abdominal aorta (size, bruits)
e. ☐ femoral arteries (pulse amplitude, bruits)
f. ☑ pedal pulses (pulse amplitude)
g. ☑ extremities (edema, varicosities)

7. Chest (Breasts)
a. ☑ inspection (size, symmetry, nipple discharge)
b. ☑ palpation of breasts & axillae (masses, lumps, tenderness)

8. Gastrointestinal (Abdomen)
a. ☑ examination for masses, tenderness
b. ☑ examination of liver, spleen
c. ☑ examination for presence or absence of hernia
d. ☑ examination of (when indicated) anus, perineum, rectum: (sphincter tone, hemorrhoids, masses)
e. ☐ stool for occult blood when indicated

9. Genitourinary
a. ☑ scrotum (hydrocele, spermatocele, tenderness of cord, testicular mass)
b. ☑ examination of penis
c. ☑ digital exam of prostate (size, symmetry, nodularity, tenderness)

10. Lymphatic
a. ☑ palpation of lymph nodes in 2 or more areas: (Circle: (neck,) axillae, (groin,) other)

11. Musculoskeletal
a. ☑ examination of gait and station
b. ☑ inspection and/or palpation of digits & nails (clubbing, cyanosis, inflammatory conditions, petechiae, ischemia, infections, nodes)
c. ☒ assessment of range of motion ((pain,) crepitation, contracture)

Procedures and Immunizations

☐ Hearing   ☐ Glucose   ☐ Cholesterol   ☐ TSH
☐ Vision   ☐ PT   ☐ HDL/LDL   ☐ CXR
☒ CBC   ☒ Urine   ☐ Triglyceride   ☐ EKG

☐ Stool Guaiac
☐ Sigmoidoscopy

Are immunizations current?
☐ Yes ☐ No

☐ dT ☐ Hep B
☐ Influenza

d. ☒ Examination of joint, bone, & muscle of 1 or more of the following 6 areas (circle)
    •head/neck   ●rt. upper extremities
    •spine, ribs, & pelvis   ●lt. upper extremities
    ●rt. lower extremities   ●lt. lower extremities
e. ☑ inspect, and/or palpation (misalign, asymmetry, crepitation, defects, tender., masses, effusion)
f. ☑ assessment of stability: dislocation (luxation), subluxation or laxity
g. ☒ muscle strength & tone (flaccid, cogwheel, spastic), atrophy or abnormal movement

12. Skin
a. ☑ inspection of skin & sub-Q tissue (rashes, lesion, ulcers)
b. ☑ palpation of skin & sub-Q tissue (induration, sub-Q nodules, tightening)

13. Neurology
a. ☐ test cranial nerves: notation of deficits
b. ☑ examination of DTR's with notation of pathological reflexes (eg. Babinski)
c. ☑ examination of sensation (touch, pain, vibration, proprioception)

14. Psychiatric
a. ☐ description of patient's judgment & insight
    Brief assessment of mental status:
b. ☑ orientation to time, place, & person
c. ☑ recent & remote memory
d. ☑ mood & affect (depression, anxiety, agitation)
e. ☐ other

Drug Allergies:

Codeine

☐ 1995 Piermed, Inc. Rev

Male 60+

Date / Time   11:30 AM 06/10/2005

Summary   *Sprain (L) wrist; Chronic Pyelonephritis*

☐ Referral

500-06

FIGURE C-10, D

Lake Eola Family Practice 517860 South Pioneer Drive, Orlando, FL 32897 • 634-555-4893

Superbill #456298

Weight _128#_ BP _110/68_ TPR _98.6°—62-16_

Account Number _JAYR001_	Doctor _Aaron Rubin MD_	Date of Service _06/10/2005_
Patient Name _Jayaguro, Rajid_	Date of Birth _03/17/1922_	LMP _N/A_
Insurance _Medicare/Medigap_	Responsible Party _Rajid Jayaguro_	Phone Number _634-555-2790_
Address _PO Box ZZZZ_	Referring Physician and ID # _None_	
City _Jacksonville_	State _FL_	Zip _39782_	

✓ New Patient

___ 99201 H[PF] E[PF] MDM[S] 10 min
___ 99202 H[EPF] E[EPF] MDM[S] 20 min
___ 99203 H[D] E[D] MDM[LC] 30 min
_X_ 99204 H[C] E[C] MDM[MC] 45 min
___ 99205 H[C] E[C] MDM[HC] 60 min

Established Patient

___ 99211 H[N/A] E[N/A] MDM[N/A] 5 min
___ 99212 H[PF] E[PF] MDM[S] 10 min
___ 99213 H[EPF] E[EPF] MDM[LC] 15 min
___ 99214 H[D] E[D] MDM[MC] 25 min
___ 99215 H[C] E[C] MDM[HC] 40 min

Reason For Visit

___ Authorization _____
    Expiration Date _____
___ Annual exam, complex due to (history, condition): _____
___ Annual exam, simple
___ Follow-up, condition _____
___ Follow-up, post procedure, no condition or complication
    Procedure/date _____
___ Follow-up, post procedure, with condition or complication _____
    Procedure/date _____
_X_ New Problem _(L) wrist injury_
___ Post-op, no condition or complication Surgery/date _____
___ Post-op, with conditions or complication
    Surgery/date _____
___ Pre-op _____
___ Procedure _____
___ Second surgical opinion _____
___ Other (Accident, Decision for surgery) ___
    _____

Procedures

⇒ Place to be done: _____
⇒ Date to be done: _____
___ Authorization _____
    Expiration date _____
___ Biopsy, type/site _____
_____
___ Cautery, type/site _____
_____
___ Destruction of lesion(s), extensive, site: ___
_____
___ Destruction of lesion(s), simple, site: ___
_____
___ Emergency surgery (list above), reason: ___
_____
___ Excision, type/site _____
___ I & D abscess, type/site: _____
_____
___ Insertion/Removal of IUD, type _____
___ Major surgery, type/site _____
_____
___ Minor surgery, type/site _____
_____
___ Sonogram _____
___ Other _____

Miscellaneous

___ Immunization _____
___ Injection _____
_X_ Supplies _Soft wrist splint_
___ Surgical tray

___ Patient Teaching (Preventive medicine)
_____
_X_ Other _Xray (L) wrist—2 views_
         _$35.00   73100_
_____
_____

Outside Lab

___ Beta HCG, Serum
___ Biopsy/Pathology
___ Biopsy, Mult./Pathology
_X_ CBC _$15.00 85025_
___ Cholesterol   _$15.00_
___ Culture, throat
_X_ Cultures (source) _Urine 87088_
___ Glucose, ___1hr glucose, ___3hr glucose
___ Estrogen
___ Herpes simplex, AB
___ Mononucleosis
___ Pap Smear
___ PT___PTT
___ Sed rate
___ SMAC
_X_ Urinalysis, w/micro _$20.00 81001_
___ HIV
___ Other _____
_____
_____
_____

Diagnosis Codes

1. _842.00_
2. _590.00_
3. _E 849.0_
4. _E 885.9_

Appointment in __2__ Weeks
Procedure in _____ Weeks
Sent Labs to_____
Call in _____ Mos./Weeks

Previous Balance $ ___0___
Co-Pay $ _Medigap_
Paid Today Cash/Check $ _____
Yes-No All Diagnosis, Procedures, & VS above are documented in Record
Doctor's Signature _Aaron Rubin MD_

New Charges $ _260.00_
New Balance $ _260.00_
Check Number _____

FIGURE C-10, E

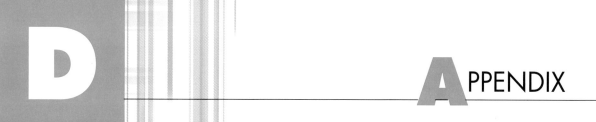

Quick Guide to HIPAA for the Physician's Office

*Brenda K. Burton**

Health Insurance Portability and Accountability Act (HIPAA)

The U.S. health care system has undergone rapid change with regard to the separate issues of privacy, security, and claims processing over the past decade. Any business that is involved with the health care industry must conform its practices to follow the principles and practices as identified by state and federal agencies. These efforts are generally identified as *compliance*. The professional elements include regulations and recommendations to protect individuals, streamline processes, and increase system-wide stability. A compliance strategy provides a standardized process for handling business functions, leading to consistent and effective management and staff performance. Failure to comply with mandates leads to sanctions and fines from state and federal agencies; failure to follow guidelines potentially results in more fraud and abuse in the claims reimbursement cycle.

The Health Insurance Portability and Accountability Act of 1996 (HIPAA), Public Law 104-191, will have significant impact on both individuals and health care providers over the next several years. There are two provisions of HIPAA, *Title I: Insurance Reform* and *Title II: Administrative Simplification*. HIPAA projects long-term benefits that include lowered administrative costs, increased accuracy of data, increased patient and customer satisfaction, and reduced revenue cycle time, ultimately improving financial management.

*Brenda K. Burton, Director, MEDEXTEND, Fayetteville, GA 30215, http://medextend.com.

This paper is intended to promote awareness. It is not all encompassing in regard to HIPAA and OIG compliance. It is not intended to replace policy and procedures manuals and similar policy documents.

Definitions from the *Federal Register* are excerpts, used for ease of understanding.

Title I: Health Insurance Reform

The primary purpose of HIPAA Title I, *Insurance Reform* is to provide continuous insurance coverage for workers and their insured dependents when they change or lose jobs. This aspect of HIPAA affects individuals as consumers, not particularly as patients. Previously, when an employee left or lost a job and changed insurance coverage, a "preexisting" clause prevented or limited coverage for certain medical conditions. HIPAA now limits the use of preexisting condition exclusions, prohibits discrimination for past or present poor health, and guarantees certain employees and individuals the right to purchase new health insurance coverage after losing a job. Additionally, HIPAA allows renewal of health insurance coverage regardless of an individual's health condition that is covered under the particular policy.

Title II: Administrative Simplification

The goals of HIPAA Title II, *Administrative Simplification,* focus on the health care practice setting and are intended to reduce administrative costs and burdens. This will be accomplished by standardizing the exchange of health care data, which will, in itself, increase the use and efficiency of computer-to-computer methods transactions. Additional provisions are meant to ensure the privacy and security of an individual's health data. Standardizing electronic transmissions of administrative and financial information will reduce the number of forms and methods used in the claims processing cycle and reduce the nonproductive effort that goes into processing paper or nonstandard electronic claims.

The two parts of the Administrative Simplification provisions are as follows:

1. Development and implementation of standardized electronic transactions using common sets of descriptors (i.e., Standard Code Sets). These must be used to represent health care concepts and procedures when performing health-related financial and administrative activities electronically (i.e., Standard Transactions).
   - ❏ Electronic Health Transaction Standards (specific format information transmitted using Electronic Data Interchange)
   - ❏ Standard Code Sets (identify diagnosis, procedures, services, drugs, and supplies)
   - ❏ Unique Identifiers for Providers, Employers, Health Plans, and Patients (numeric and alphanumeric strings attached to identify a particular provider, employer, etc.)
2. Implementation of privacy and security procedures to prevent the misuse of health information by ensuring confidentiality.
   - ❏ Privacy and confidentiality
   - ❏ Security of health information

Administrative simplification has created uniform sets of standards that protect and place limits on how confidential health information can be used. For years, health care providers have locked medical records in file cabinets and refused to share patient health information. Patients now have specific rights regarding how their health information is used and disclosed because federal and state laws regulate the protection of an individual's privacy. Knowledge and attention to the rights of patients are important to the compliance endeavor in a health care practice. Providers are entrusted with health information and are expected to recognize when certain health information can be used or disclosed. Patients have the legal right to request (1) access and amendments to their health records, (2) an accounting of those who have received their health information, and (3) restrictions on who can access their health records. Understanding the parameters concerning these rights is crucial to complying with HIPAA.

Health care providers and their employer can be held accountable for using or disclosing patient health information inappropriately. HIPAA regulations

Examples of Administrative Information	Examples of Financial Information
Referral Certification and Authorization for Services	Healthcare Claim Submission for Services
Enrollment/Disenrollment of Individual into Health Plan	Process Health Plan Premium Payment
Health Plan Eligibility	Check Status of a Previously Submitted Claim
	Healthcare Payment and Remittance Advice
	Coordination of Benefits

will be enforced, as clearly stated by the U.S. government. The revolution of HIPAA will take time to understand and implement correctly, but once the standards are in place both within the practice setting and across the sector, greater benefits will be appreciated by the health care provider, staff, and patients.

COMPLIANCE DEADLINES

Before a rule (or law) becomes final, a preliminary draft is published in the *Federal Register* (FR) as a Notice of Proposed Rule Making (NPRM). As defined by the U.S. Government Printing Office, "The *Federal Register* is the official daily publication for Rules, Proposed Rules, and Notices of Federal agencies and organizations, as well as Executive Orders and other Presidential Documents." After the comment period, the NPRM is usually modified to reflect the consensus of the comments and the best judgment of the staff. Generally, once final rules are published, there is a 2 year plus 60 day period before the rule becomes effective. Upcoming legislation with further mandates from HIPAA will bring more changes. Specific rules and their deadlines at this time are as follows:

- ❏ Transactions and Code Set Standards: October 16, 2003
- ❏ Medicare Requirement to Submit Electronic Claims: October 16, 2003
- ❏ Privacy: April 14, 2003
- ❏ Standard Unique Employer Identifier: July 30, 2004
- ❏ Security Standards: April 21, 2005
- ❏ Standard Unique Health Care Provider Identifier: final rule not yet published, estimate of September 2003
- ❏ Standard Unique Health Plan Identifier: proposed rule estimated to publish September 2003
- ❏ Standard Unique Individual Identifier: halted due to privacy concerns
- ❏ Standard for Claims Attachments: proposed rule to adopt standards for claims attachments

DEFINING ROLES AND RELATIONSHIPS: KEY TERMS

HIPAA legislation required the U.S. Department of Health and Human Services (HHS) to establish national standards and identifiers for electronic transactions as well as implement privacy and security standards. In regard to HIPAA, *Secretary* refers to the HHS Secretary or any officer or employee of HHS to whom the authority involved has been delegated.

The Centers for Medicare and Medicaid Services (CMS) will enforce the insurance portability and transaction and code set requirements of HIPAA. This federal organization was known as the Health Care Financing Administration (HCFA) until June 2001.

The Office of Civil Rights (OCR) will enforce privacy standards.

A covered entity transmits health information in electronic form in connection with a transaction covered by HIPAA. The covered entity may be (1) a health plan such as Blue Cross Blue Shield, (2) a health care clearinghouse through which claims are submitted, or (3) a health care provider such as the primary care physician.

A business associate is a person who, on behalf of the covered entity, performs or assists in the performance of a function or activity involving the use or disclosure of individually identifiable health information, including claims processing or administration, data analysis, processing or administration, utilization review, quality assurance, billing, benefit management, practice management, and repricing. For example, if a provider practice contracts with an outside billing company to manage its claims and accounts receivable, the billing company would be a business associate of the provider (the covered entity).

Electronic media refers to the mode of electronic transmission, including the following:

- ❏ Internet (wide open)
- ❏ Extranet or private network using Internet technology to link business parties
- ❏ Leased phone or dial-up phone lines, including fax modems (speaking over phone not considered an electronic transmission)
- ❏ Transmissions that are physically moved from one location to another using magnetic tape, disk, or compact disk media

A health care provider is a provider of medical or health services and any other person or organization who furnishes, bills, or is paid for health care in the normal course of business.

Privacy and security officers oversee the HIPAA-related functions. These individuals may or may not be employees of a particular health care practice. A privacy officer or privacy official (PO) is designated to help the provider remain in compliance by setting policies and procedures in place, training and managing the staff regarding HIPAA and patient rights, and generally functioning as the contact person for questions and complaints. A security officer protects the computer and networking systems within the practice and implements protocols such as password assignment, back-up procedures, firewalls, virus protection, and contingency planning for emergencies.

A *transaction* refers to the transmission of information between two parties to carry out financial or administrative activities related to health care. These information transmissions include the following:

1. Health care claims or equivalent encounter information
2. Health care payment and remittance advice
3. Coordination of benefits
4. Health care claim status
5. Enrollment and disenrollment in a health plan
6. Eligibility for a health plan
7. Health plan premium payments
8. Referral certification and authorization
9. First report of injury
10. Health claim attachments
11. Other transactions that the Secretary may prescribe by regulation

TPO refers to treatment, payment, and health care operations.

Application to Practice Setting

The previous "roles" create relationships that guide the health care provider and the practice. A health care provider can include a nurse practitioner, social worker, chiropractor, radiologist, or dentist; HIPAA does not affect only medical physicians. The health care provider is designated as a HIPAA-mandated Covered Entity under certain conditions. It is important to remember that health care providers who transmit any health information in electronic form in connection with a HIPAA transaction are covered entities. Electronic form or media can include floppy disk, compact disk (CD), or file transfer protocol (FTP) over the Internet. Voice-over-modem faxes, meaning a phone line, are not considered electronic media, although a fax from a computer (e.g., WinFax program) is considered an electronic medium.

HIPAA Focus

Simply put, if a health care provider either transmits directly or utilizes a "business associate" (e.g., billing company or clearinghouse) to transmit information electronically for any of the transactions listed, the health care provider is a "covered entity" and must comply with HIPAA.

HIPAA requires the designation of a PO to develop and implement the organization's policies and procedures. The PO for an organization may hold another position within the practice or may not be an employee of the practice at all. Often, the PO is a contracted professional and available to the practice through established means of contact.

The business associate often is considered an extension of the provider practice. If an office function is outsourced with use or disclosure of individually identifiable health information, the organization that is acting on behalf of the health care provider is considered a business associate. For example, if the office's medical transcription is performed by an outside service, the transcription service is a Business Associate of the Covered Entity (the health care provider/practice).

HIPAA privacy regulations as a federal mandate will apply unless the state laws are contrary or more stringent with regard to privacy. State preemption, a complex technical issue not within the scope of the health care provider's role, refers to instances when state law takes precedence over federal law. The PO will determine when the need for preemption arises.

PRIVACY RULE: CONFIDENTIALITY AND PROTECTED HEALTH INFORMATION

What I may see or hear in the course of the treatment or even outside of the treatment in regard to the life of men, which on no account one must spread abroad, I will keep to myself holding such things shameful to be spoken about.

Hippocrates, 400 BC

The Hippocratic Oath, federal and state regulations, professional standards, and ethics all address patient privacy. Because current technology allows easy access to health care information, HIPAA imposes new requirements for health care providers. Since computers have become indispensable for the health care office, confidential health data have been sent across networks, e-mailed over the Internet, and even exposed by hackers, with few safeguards taken to protect data and prevent information from being intercepted or lost. With the implementation of standardizing electronic transactions of health care information, the use of technologies will pose new risks for privacy and security. These concerns were addressed under HIPAA, and regulations now closely govern how the industry handles its electronic activities.

Privacy is the condition of being secluded from the presence or view of others. Confidentiality is using discretion in keeping information secret.

Integrity plays an important part in the health care setting. Staff members of a health care organization need a good understanding of HIPAA's basic requirements and must be committed to protecting the privacy and rights of the practice's patients.

Disclosure means the release, transfer, provision of access to, or divulging in any other manner of information outside the entity holding the information. An example of a "disclosure" would be if you give information to the hospital's outpatient surgery center about a patient you are scheduling for a procedure.

Individually identifiable health information (IIHI) is any part of an individual's health information, including demographic information (e.g., address, date of birth) collected from the individual that is created or received by a covered entity. This information relates to the individual's past, present, or future physical or mental health or condition; the provision of health care to the individual; or the past, present, or future payment for the provision of health care. IIHI data identify the individual or establish a reasonable basis to believe the information can be used to identify the individual. For example, if you as health care provider are talking to an insurance representative, you will likely give information such as the patient's date of birth and last name. These pieces of information would make it reasonably easy to identify the patient. If you are talking to a pharmaceutical representative about a drug assistance program that covers a new pill for heartburn, and you only say that your practice has a patient living in your town who is indigent and has stomach problems, you are not divulging information that would identify the patient.

Protected health information (PHI) refers to IIHI that is transmitted by electronic media, maintained in electronic form, or transmitted or maintained in any other form or medium. PHI does not include IIHI in education records covered by the Family Educational Right and Privacy Act.

Traditionally, there has been focus on protecting paper medical records and documentation that held patient's health information, such as laboratory results and radiology reports. HIPAA Privacy Regulation expands these protections to apply to PHI. The individual's health information is protected regardless of the type of medium in which it is maintained. This includes paper, the health care provider's computerized practice management and billing system, spoken words, and x-ray films.

Use means the sharing, employment, application, utilization, examination, or analysis of IIHI within an organization that holds such information. When a patient's billing record is accessed to review the claim submission history, the individual's health information is in "use."

HIPAA imposes requirements to protect not only disclosure of PHI outside of the organization but also for internal uses of health information. PHI may not be used or disclosed without permission of the patient or someone authorized to act on behalf of the patient, unless the use or disclosure is specifically required or permitted by the regulation (e.g., TPO). The two types of disclosure required by HIPAA Privacy Rule are to the individual who is the subject of the PHI and to the Secretary or DHHS to investigate compliance with the rule.

PRIVACY RULE: PATIENT RIGHTS UNDER HIPAA

Patients are granted the following federal rights that allow them to be informed about PHI and to control how their PHI is used and disclosed:

1. Right to Notice of Privacy Practices
2. Right to request restrictions on certain uses and disclosures of PHI
3. Right to request confidential communications
4. Right to access (inspect and obtain a copy of) PHI
5. Right to request an amendment of PHI
6. Right to receive an accounting of disclosures of PHI

Right to Notice of Privacy Practices

Under HIPAA, patients are entitled to receive the written Notice of Privacy Practices (NPP) of their provider at the first appointment. The NPP outlines the individual's rights and covered entity's legal duties in regard to PHI. The NPP must be provided and written in "plain language" and the staff must make a reasonable "best effort" to obtain a signature from the patient acknowledging receipt. This can be recorded simply as signing a label on the inside cover of the chart. The front desk reception area is an ideal location for distribution of the NPP to the patient with the registration sheet and other required forms. If the patient cannot or will not sign, a staff member can sign and date the receipt for them. An NPP will be tailored to each organization and must explain the following:

- ❑ How PHI may be used and disclosed by the organization
- ❑ Health provider duties to protect PHI
- ❑ Patient rights regarding PHI
- ❑ How complaints may be filed with the office and HHS if the patient believes his or her privacy rights have been violated
- ❑ Whom to contact for further information (usually the PO)
- ❑ Effective date of the NPP

As a health care provider, you may have already seen these notices posted at your pharmacy or had to sign an acknowledgment that you read a copy of the NPP at your personal physician's office. Your patients must have ready access to your organization's NPP. This Notice must be posted prominently in the office (e.g., on the wall by the reception desk) and must be available in paper form for patients who request it. If your office has a website, the Notice must be posted prominently there as well. HIPAA states that covered entities may not require individuals to waive their rights "as a condition of the provision of treatment or payment."

Right to Request Restrictions on Certain Uses and Disclosures of PHI

Patients do have the right to ask for restrictions on how your office uses and discloses PHI for TPO. Patients may have items in their previous medical history that are not applicable to the current disclosure and may even cause the patient embarrassment; patients may request that this PHI not be disclosed (e.g., a patient had a successfully treated STD many years before and requests that, whenever possible, this material not be disclosed). The covered entity is not required to agree to these requests but must have a process to review the requests, accept and review any appeal, and give a sound reason for not agreeing to the request. If agreed upon, however, the restrictions must be documented and followed. Such restrictions may be tracked by flagging the patient's medical chart that a restriction applies or by using a pop-up note in the practice management software. There must be an implemented procedure in place to check for any restrictions before PHI is disclosed.

A practice may disclose confidential information in certain situations *without* a written authorization from the patient (e.g., reporting communicable diseases, reporting about victims of abuse, and for law enforcement purposes). You can ask your PO or refer to the *Policy and Procedure Manual* for clarification when disclosures are permissible.

In addition, unless a patient has requested that such disclosures not occur and the provider has agreed, health information may be disclosed to a family member, relative, close friend, or any other person identified by the patient.

Right to Request Confidential Communications

A patient can request to receive confidential communications by alternative means or at an alternative location. For example, a patient may ask that the health care provider call the patient at work rather than at the residence or patients may request that their test results be sent to them in writing rather than by phone. It is the patient's right to request such alternative methods of communication, and the health care office must accommodate *reasonable* requests. This can become a serious issue, especially in cases of domestic violence when the individual is at risk for physical harm within the home environment. The patient does not need to explain the reason for the request. The health care office must have a process in place both to evaluate requests and appeals and to respond to the patient.

Patients may be required by the office to make their request in writing. Documenting such requests in writing with the patient's signature is an effective way to protect the practice's compliance endeavors. The office may even condition the agreement by arranging for payment of any additional costs from the patient that the request has created. For example, the patient asks that all correspondence be sent by registered mail; this request may be able to be honored without significant additional staff time but the patient should expect to incur the actual additional mailing costs.

Right to Access PHI (Inspect and Obtain a Copy)

A patient has the right to access, inspect, and obtain a copy of his or her confidential health information. Privacy regulations allow the provider to require the patient make the request for access in writing. Generally, a request must be acted on within 30 days. A reasonable, cost-based fee for copies of PHI may only include the costs for the following:

- ❏ Supplies and labor for copying
- ❏ Postage when mailed
- ❏ Preparing a summary of the PHI if the patient has agreed to this instead of complete access

This "fee" for copying varies widely by state and each provider should be aware of the state allowances and conform their fee to that which gives most relief to the patient. The HIPAA-determined fee applies *only* to fees for copies to patients and not copies for other required or allowed disclosures, e.g. subpoenas. The fee structures for other disclosures are often set by state law. If you are a staff member involved in applying fees for copying, you should seek guidance from your privacy officer.

Under HIPAA Privacy Regulation, patients do not have the right to access the following:

- ❏ Psychotherapy notes
- ❏ Information compiled in reasonable anticipation of, or for use in, legal proceedings
- ❏ Information exempted from disclosure under the Clinical Laboratory Improvements Amendment (CLIA)

In regard to the patient's right to request restrictions on certain uses and disclosures of PHI, you will find key terms addressed in the NPP that apply to this right.

❑ **Minimum Necessary.** Privacy regulations require that use or disclosure of only the minimum amount of information necessary to fulfill the intended purpose be permitted. There are some exceptions to this rule. You do not need to limit PHI for disclosures in regard to health care providers for treatment, the patient, HHS for investigations of compliance with HIPAA, or as required by law.

Minimum necessary determinations for uses of PHI must be determined within each organization, and reasonable efforts must be made to limit access to only the minimum amount of information needed by identified staff members. In smaller offices, employees may have multiple job functions. If a medical assistant helps with the patient exam, documents vital signs, and then collects the patient's co-pay at the reception area, the assistant will likely access clinical and billing records. Simple policy and procedure (P&P) about appropriate access to PHI may be sufficient to satisfy the minimum necessary requirement. Larger organizations may have specific restrictions on who should have access to different types of PHI, because staff members tend to have a more targeted job role. Remain knowledgeable about your office's policy regarding minimum necessary. If you are strictly scheduling appointments, you may not need access to the clinical record. An x-ray technician will likely not need to access the patient billing records.

Minimum necessary determinations for disclosures of PHI are distinguished by two categories within the Privacy Rule:

1. For disclosures made on a routine and recurring basis, you may implement policies and procedures, or standard protocols, for what will be disclosed. These disclosures would be common in your practice. Examples may include disclosures for workers' compensation claims or school physical forms.
2. For other disclosures that would be considered nonroutine, criteria should be established for determining the minimum necessary amount of PHI and to review each request for disclosure on an individual basis. There will be a staff member (e.g., PO, medical records supervisor) likely assigned to determine this situation when need arises.

As a general rule, remember that you must limit your requests to access PHI to the minimum necessary to accomplish the task for which you will need the information.

❑ **De-identification of Confidential Information.** Other requirements relating to uses and disclosures of PHI include health information that does not identify an individual or leaves no reasonable basis to believe that the information can be used to identify an individual. This "de-identified" information is no longer individually identifiable health information (IIHI). Most providers will never have the need to de-identify patient information, and the requirements for de-identifying PHI are lengthy. The regulations give specific directions on how to ensure all pieces of necessary information are removed to fit the definition. De-identified information is not subject to the privacy regulations because it does not specifically identify an individual.

❑ **Marketing** refers to communicating about a product or service where the goal is to encourage patients to purchase or use the product or service. For instance, a dermatologist may advertise for a discount on facial cream when you schedule a dermabrasion treatment. You will likely not be involved in marketing, but keep in mind the general rule that PHI (including names and addresses) cannot be used for marketing purposes without specific authorization of the patient. Sending appointment reminders and general news updates about your organization and the services you provide would not be considered marketing and would not require patient authorization.

❑ **Fundraising.** Again, you will likely not be involved in fundraising activities, but HIPAA allows demographic information and dates of care to be used for fundraising purposes without patient authorization. The disclosure of any additional information requires patient authorization. Your organization's NPP will state that patients may receive fundraising materials and are given the opportunity to opt out of receiving future solicitations.

The office may deny patient access for the above reasons without giving the patient the right to review the denial. Also, if the PHI was obtained from an individual other than a health care provider under a promise of confidentiality, access may be denied if such access would likely reveal the identity of the source. Other circumstances in which an individual may be denied access will be detailed in the practice's policy manual.

If the health care provider has determined that the patient would be endangered (or cause danger to another person) from accessing the confidential health information, access may be denied. In this case the patient has the right to have the denial reviewed by another licensed professional who did not participate in the initial denial decision.

HIPAA specifically excludes from psychotherapy notes information about medication management, start and stop times of sessions, frequency and type of treatment provided, results of testing, and summaries of diagnosis, treatment plan, symptoms, prognosis, and progress to date. These are, however, PHI. Psychotherapy notes are not stored in the general client record, nor are personal notes.

HIPAA affords psychotherapy notes more protection—most notably from third-party payers—than they had been given in the past. Under HIPAA, disclosure of psychotherapy notes requires more than just generalized consent; it requires patient authorization—or specific permission—to release this sensitive information (e.g., to a third party).

Though the privacy rule does afford patients the right to access and inspect their health records, psychotherapy notes are treated differently: Patients do not have the right to obtain a copy of these under HIPAA. Under the new law, psychologists can decide whether to release their psychotherapy notes to patients, unless patients would have access to their psychotherapy notes under state law. If a psychologist denies a patient access to these notes, the denial isn't subject to a review process, as it is with other records.

There is a catch in the psychotherapy notes provision. HIPAA's definition of psychotherapy notes explicitly states that these notes are kept separate from the rest of an individual's record. So, if a psychologist keeps this type of information in a patient's general chart, or if it is not distinguishable as separate from the rest of the record, access to the information does not require specific patient authorization.

State law must be considered since, in all cases where state law is more strict or gives the patient more access to information, state law takes precedence.

Right to Request Amendment of PHI

Patients have the right to request that their PHI be amended. As with the other requests, the provider may require the request be in writing. The provider must have a process to accept and review both the request and any appeal in a timely fashion. The health care provider may deny this request in the following circumstances:

- ❑ The provider who is being requested to change the PHI is not the creator of the information (e.g., office has records sent by referring physician).
- ❑ The PHI is believed to be accurate and complete as it stands in the provider's records.
- ❑ The information is not required to be accessible to the patient (see Right to Access PHI).

Generally, the office must respond to a patient's request for amendment within 60 days. If a request is denied, the patient must be informed in writing of the reason for the denial. The patient must also be given the opportunity to file a statement of disagreement. These rules are complex in regard to steps of appeal, rebuttal, and documentation that must be provided if a request for amendment is denied. The PO will instruct providers on additional responsibilities if they are directly involved in this process.

Right to Receive an Accounting of Disclosures of PHI

Providers should maintain a log of disclosures of PHI, either paper or within the organization's computer system, of all disclosures other than those made for TPO, facility directories, and some national security and law enforcement agencies. The process for providing an accounting should be outlined in

---

HIPAA Focus

HIPAA regulations recognize that certain kinds of mental health information need to be protected more than other types of information. Under HIPAA, psychotherapy notes are defined as "notes recorded in any medium by a mental health professional documenting or analyzing the contents of conversation during a private counseling session." These notes, which capture the psychologist's impressions about the patient and can contain information that is inappropriate for a medical record, are similar to what psychologists have historically referred to as "process notes."

the practice's policy manual. Patients may request an accounting (or tracking) of disclosures of their confidential information and are granted the right to receive this accounting once a year without charge. Additional accountings may be assessed a cost-based fee.

These accountings are only required to start on April 14, 2003, when privacy regulations became enforceable. Items to be documented must include the following:

❑ Date of disclosure
❑ Name of the entity or person who received the PHI, including their address if known
❑ Brief description of the PHI disclosed
❑ Brief statement of the purpose of the disclosure

The patients cannot keep their confidential health information from being used for treatment, payment or health care operations (TPO) nor may they force amendments to their health record. As you become more acclimated to your organization's policies and procedures regarding the handling of PHI, you will be better able to recognize how your position is an important part in HIPAA compliance.

ORGANIZATION AND STAFF RESPONSIBILITIES IN PROTECTING PATIENT RIGHTS

The covered entity must implement written policies and procedures (P&P) that comply with HIPAA standards. P&P are tailored guidelines established to accommodate each health care practice and designed to address PHI. HIPAA requires each practice to implement P&P that comply with privacy and security rules. The office should have a *Policy and Procedure Manual* to train providers and to serve as a resource for situations that need clarification. Revisions in P&P must be made as necessary and appropriate to comply with laws as they change. Documentation must be maintained in written or

HIPAA Focus

In summary, patients have the right to:

❑ Be informed of the organization's privacy practices by receiving a Notice of Privacy Practices (NPP).
❑ Have their information kept confidential and secure.
❑ Obtain a copy of their health record.
❑ Request to have their health records amended.
❑ Request special considerations in communication.

HIPAA Focus

Health care providers and staff will likely not be reading the *Federal Register* and thus will want to familiarize themselves with the general forms used in their practice setting. They should be aware of the following:

❑ **Written acknowledgment.** After providing the patient with the NPP, a "good faith" effort must be made to obtain written acknowledgment of the patient receiving the document. If the patient refuses to sign or is unable to sign, this must be documented in the patient record.
❑ **Authorization forms.** Use and disclosure of PHI is permissible for TPO because the NPP describes how PHI is used for these purposes. The health care provider is required to obtain signed authorization to use or disclose health information for situations beyond the TPO. This is a protection for the practice. Providers must learn about the particular "authorization" forms used in their office. Psychotherapy notes are handled separately under HIPAA. Such notes have additional protection, specifically, that an authorization for any use of disclosure of psychotherapy notes must be obtained.

Your organization will be expected to handle requests made by patients to exercise their rights. You must know your office's process for dealing with each specific request. With your understanding of HIPAA and your organization's policy manual, you will be guided in procedures specific to your health care practice.

electronic form and retained for 6 years of its creation or when it was last in effect, whichever is later.

Verification of Identity and Authority

Before any disclosure, you must verify the identity of persons requesting PHI if they are unknown to you. You may request identifying information such as date of birth, Social Security number, or even a code word stored in your practice management system that is unique to each patient. Public officials may show you badges, credentials, official letterheads, and other legal documents of authority for identification purposes. Additionally, you must verify that the requestor has the right and the need to have the PHI.

Exercising professional judgment will fulfill your verification requirements for most disclosures because you are acting on "good faith" in believing the identity of the individual requesting PHI. It is good practice, when making any disclosure, to note the "authority" of the person receiving the PHI and how this was determined. This evidence of due diligence on your part would enforce a needed structure on your staff and dampen any complaints that might arise.

Validating Patient Permission

Before making any uses or disclosures of confidential health information other than for the purposes of TPO, your office must have appropriate patient permission. Always check for conflicts between various permissions your office may have on file for a given patient. This information should be maintained either in your practice management system or in the medical chart, where it can be easily identified and retrieved.

For example, if a covered entity has agreed to a patient's request to limit how much of the PHI is sent to a consulting physician for treatment, but then received the patient's authorization to disclose the entire medical record to that physician, this would be a conflict. In general, the more restrictive permission would be the deciding factor. Privacy regulations allow resolving conflicting permissions by either obtaining new permission from the patient or by communicating orally or in writing with the patient to determine the patient's preference. Be sure to document any form of communication in writing.

Training

Under HIPAA regulations, a covered entity must train all members of its workforce. This training must include the practice's policies and procedures with respect to PHI as "necessary and appropriate for the members of the workforce to carry out their function within the covered entity." This training will address how your role relates to PHI in your office, and you will be instructed on how to handle confidential information. The PO for your health care practice will likely be the instructor for this type of training. HIPAA training focuses on how to handle confidential information securely in the office, as discussed later.

Safeguards: Ensuring That Confidential Information Is Secure

Every covered entity must have appropriate safeguards to ensure the protection of an individual's confidential health information. Such safeguards include administrative, technical, and physical measures that will "reasonably safeguard" PHI from any use or disclosure that violates HIPAA, whether intentional or unintentional.

Complaints to Health Care Practice and Workforce Sanctions

Individuals, both patients and staff, must be provided with a process to make a complaint concerning the P&P of the covered entity. If a violation involves the misuse of PHI, this incident should be reported to the practice's PO. Should there be further cause, the OCR may also be contacted.

Workforce members are subject to appropriate sanctions for failure to comply with the P&P regarding PHI set forth in the office. Types of sanctions applied will vary depending on factors involved with the violation. Sanctions can range from a warning to suspension to termination. This information should be covered in the P&P manual. Written documentation of complaints and sanctions must be prepared with any disposition.

Mitigation

Mitigation means to "alleviate the severity" or "make mild." In reference to HIPAA, the covered entity has an affirmative duty to take reasonable steps in response to breaches. If a breach is discovered, the health care provider is required to mitigate, to the extent possible, any harmful effects of the breach. For example, if you learn you have erroneously sent medical records by fax to an incorrect party, steps should be taken to have the recipient destroy the PHI. Mitigation procedures also include activities of the practice's business associates. Being proactive and responsible by mitigating will reduce the potential for a more disastrous outcome from the breach or violation.

Refraining from Intimidating or Retaliatory Acts

HIPAA privacy regulations prohibit a covered entity from intimidating, threatening, coercing, discriminating against, or otherwise taking retaliatory action against:

- ❑ Individuals for exercising HIPAA privacy rights
- ❑ Individuals for filing a complaint with HHS or testifying, assisting, or participating in an investigation about the covered entity's privacy practices or reasonably opposing any practice prohibited by the regulation

Example Administrative Safeguard	Example Technical Safeguard	Example Physical Safeguard
Verifying the identity of an individual picking up health records	User name/password required to access patient records from computer	Locked, fireproof filing cabinets for storing paper records

TRANSACTION AND CODE SET REGULATIONS: STREAMLINING ELECTRONIC DATA INTERCHANGE

HIPAA Transaction and Code Set (TCS) regulation was developed to introduce efficiencies into the health care system. The objectives are to achieve a higher quality of care and to reduce administrative costs by streamlining the processing of routine administrative and financial transactions. HHS has estimated that by implementing TCS, almost $30 billion over 10 years would be saved.

Technology and the use of electronic data interchange (EDI) has made the processing of transactions more efficient and reduced administrative overhead costs in other industries. EDI is the exchange of data in a standardized format through computer systems. Standardizing transactions and code sets is required to use EDI effectively, with the implementation of standard formats, procedures, and data content.

TCS regulation requires the implementation of specific standards for transactions and code sets by October 16, 2003. The intent of TCS requirements is to achieve a single standard. As an example in the pre-HIPAA environment, when submitting claims for payment, health care providers have been doing business with insurance payers who require the use of their own version of local code sets (e.g., state Medicaid programs) or identifiers and paper forms. More than 400 versions of a National Standard Format (NSF) exist to submit a claim for payment. HIPAA will streamline the standards and enable greater administrative efficiencies throughout the health care system. Health care provider offices will benefit from less paperwork, and standardizing data will result in more accurate information and a more efficient organization.

HIPAA standardization actions are similar to using a bank's automatic teller machine (ATM) or the grocery store's self-checkout. A magnetic strip on a bankcard or the bar code on a grocery item can be swiped across a reading mechanism, allowing customers to process a transaction more quickly than with traditional methods. As these methods are adapted, there are benefits to both the end user and the business providing the technology (Table D-1).

A provider is *considered a covered entity* under HIPAA in the following circumstances:

❏ If the provider submits electronic transactions to any payer.
❏ If the provider submits paper claims to Medicare and has 10 or more employees, the provider is required to convert to electronic transactions (no later than October 16, 2003), and therefore HIPAA compliance is required.

According to the CMS, "After October 16, 2003, Electronic Claims will not be processed if they are in a format other than in the HIPAA format. Providers who are not small providers (institutional organizations with fewer than 25 full-time employees or physicians with fewer than 10 full-time employees) must send all claims electronically in the HIPAA format."

A provider is *not considered a covered entity* under HIPAA in the following circumstances:

❏ If the provider has fewer than 10 employees and submits claims only on paper to Medicare (not electronic). The provider may continue to submit on paper and therefore is not required to comply with any part of HIPAA (i.e., not required to submit electronically).
❏ If the provider submits only paper claims until and after April 14, 2003, and does not send claims to Medicare, the provider is not required to comply with sending electronic claims.

TABLE D-1
Recognized Benefits of TCS and EDI

Benefit	Result
More reliable and timely processing	Fast eligibility evaluation; reduced accounts receivable cycle; industry averages for claim turnarounds are 9-15 days for electronic vs. 30-45 days for paper claims.
Quicker reimbursement from payor	Improves cash flow for the health care organization.
Improved accuracy of data	Decreases processing time, increases data quality, and leads to better reporting.
Easier and more efficient access to information	Improves patient support.
Better tracking of transactions	Facilitates tracking of transactions (i.e., when sent and received), allowing for monitoring (e.g., prompt payments).
Reduction of data entry/manual labor	Electronic transactions facilitate automated processes (e.g., auto payment posting).
Reduction in office expenses	Reduces office supplies, postage, and telephone charges.

Data from HIPAA docs Corporation.

Transaction and Code Set Standards

TCS standards by the American National Standards Institute (ANSI) have been adopted for medical transactions. HIPAA transactions are the electronic files in which medical data are compiled to produce a given format. This is *electronic* and not a paper form. The provider cannot print out a "HIPAA claim form" to submit for reimbursement.

In general, code sets are the allowable set of codes that anyone could use to enter into a specific space on a form. All health care organizations using electronic transactions will have to use and accept (either directly or through a clearinghouse) the code set systems required under HIPAA that document specific health care data elements, including medical diagnoses and procedures, drugs, physician services, and medical suppliers. These codes have already been in common use (required in Medicare and Medicaid claims), which should help ease the transition to the new transaction requirements. What has been a standard in the health care industry and recognized by most payers now is simply mandated under HIPAA.

HIPAA standard codes are used in conjunction with the standard electronic transactions. The health care industry will recognize a standard that will eliminate ambiguity when processing transactions. In turn, this will ultimately improve the quality of data and result in improved decision making and reporting in administrative and clinical processes.

Medical code sets are data elements used uniformly to document why patients are seen (diagnosis, ICD-9-CM) and what is done to them during their encounter (procedure, CPT-4, and HCPCS). Each covered entity organization is responsible for implementing the updated codes in a timely manner, using the new HIPAA-mandated TCS codes and deleting old or obsolete ones (Table D-2).

HIPAA also provides standards for the complete cycle of administrative transactions and electronic standard formats (Table D-3).

"Out with the Old, In with the 837": Understanding Data Requirements

The health care provider practice and staff will learn about the 837. The role of the billing specialist in the health care organization will likely not change drastically because the HIPAA-enabled practice management software system will produce the required HIPAA standard electronic formats. Additionally, the continued use of clearinghouses will eliminate much of the confusion for the organization. However, if you are directly involved in the claims processing procedures, you will need to know the most important items to look for in regard to HIPAA requirements and situational data and how to successfully construct a compliant and payable

TABLE D-2
HIPAA Medical Code Sets and Elements

Standard Code Sets	Medical Data Elements
International Classification of Diseases, Ninth Revision, Clinical Modification (ICD-9-CM), Vols. 1 and 2	Diseases Injuries Impairments
ICD-9-CM replaces DSM-IV.	Other health-related problems and their manifestations Causes of injury, disease, impairment, or other health-related problems
ICD-9-CM, Vol. 3	Procedures or other actions taken for diseases, injuries, and impairments on hospital inpatients reported by hospitals, including prevention, diagnosis, treatment, and management
Current Procedural Terminology, Fourth Edition (CPT-4)	Physician services Physician and occupational therapy services Radiologic procedures Clinical laboratory tests Other medical diagnostic procedures Hearing and vision services Transportation services (e.g., helicopter, ambulance) Other services
Code on Dental Procedures and Nomenclature (CDT)	Dental services
National Drug Codes (NDC) for Retail Pharmacy transactions	Pharmaceuticals Biologics
International Classification of Diseases, Tenth Revision, Clinical Modification (ICD-10-CM) (diagnosis) ICD-10-PCS (to replace ICD-9-CM, Vol. 3 procedural coding system)	Expected to replace ICD-9-CM, but no date has been set

DSM-IV, Diagnostic and Statistical Manual of Mental Disorders, Fourth Edition.

TABLE D-3
HIPAA Transaction Functions and Formats

Standard Transaction Function	Industry Format Name
Eligibility Verification/Response	ASC X12N 270/271 Version 4010
Referral Certification and Authorization	ASC X12N 278 Version 4010
Claims or Equivalent Encounters and Coordination of Benefits	ASC X12N 837 Version 4010. You will become very familiar with this format. The 837P (Professional) will take over the paper CMS-1500 form and the electronic National Standard Format (NSF). The 837I (Institutional) will replace the paper UB-92. 837D (Dental) will be used for dentistry. The encounter for Retail Drug NCPCP v. 32.
Functional Acknowledgment	ASC X12N 997 Version 4010
Health Claim Status Inquiry/Response	ASC X12N 276/277 Version 4010
First Report of Injury (pending)	ASC X12N 148
Payment and Remittance Advice	ASC X12N 835
Health Claims Attachment (pending)	ASC X12 275 & HL7 TBD (No more copying paper attachments and stapling to a CMS-1500)

HIPAA Focus

When a patient comes into your office and is treated, his or her confidential health information is collected and put into the computerized practice management system. The services rendered are assigned a standard code from the HIPAA-required code sets (e.g., CPT), and the diagnosis is selected from another code set (e.g., ICD-9-CM); much the same as before HIPAA.

When claims are generated for electronic submission, all data collected are compiled and constructed into a HIPAA standard transaction. This EDI is recognized across the health care sector in computer systems maintained by providers, the clearinghouses, and insurance payers. The harmony among the covered entities results in a more efficient claim lifecycle.

insurance claim. You will be trained on the practice management software system on where to put additionally captured data that have not been collected on the CMS-1500 form or electronic NSF.

In addition to the major code sets (ICD-9 and CPT/HCPCS), several supporting code sets encompass both medical and nonmedical data (Table D-4). When constructing a claim, the *supporting code sets are made up of "Required" and "Situational" data elements, similar to those on the CMS-1500 paper form.* These supporting code sets are embedded in the data elements identified by the HIPAA standard electronic formats. You will not need to know all these specific codes, but it will be helpful to know they do exist, especially if you are active in the claims-processing procedures. When reviewing reports from the clearinghouse or the insurance payer, you may have to correct claims that were rejected for not having correct data elements.

Required refers to data elements that must be used to be in compliance with a HIPAA standard transaction. Conversely, *situational* means that the item depends on the data content or context. For example, a baby's birth weight is obviously "situational" when submitting a claim for the delivery of the infant. Another situational data element would be the last menstrual period (LMP) when a female is pregnant. Determining the required and situational data elements not currently collected for the CMS-1500 claim or NSF electronic format can be quite complex; you will learn this process when you are in the office performing claims-processing duties. In addition to other data elements required under HIPAA TCS, examples include the following:

❏ *Taxonomy codes.* Provider specialty codes assigned to each health care provider. Common taxonomy codes include "general practice 203BG0000Y," "family practice 203BF10100Y," and "nurse practitioner 363L00000N."
❏ *Patient account number.* To be assigned to every claim.
❏ *Relationship to patient.* Expanded to 25 different relationships, including indicators such as "grandson," "adopted child," "mother," and "life partner."
❏ *Facility code value.* Facility-related element that identifies the place of service, with at least 29 to choose from, including "office," "ambulance air or water," and "end-stage renal disease treatment facility."
❏ *Patient signature source code.* Indicates how the patient or subscriber signatures were obtained for authorization and how signatures are retained by the provider. Codes include letters such as *B* for "signed signature authorization form or forms for both CMS-1500—claim

TABLE D-4
HIPAA Supporting Code Sets

Adjustment Reason Code	Exception Code	Provider Code
Agency Qualifier Code	Facility Type Code	Provider Organization Code
Ambulatory Patient Group Code	Functional Status Code	Provider Specialty Certification
Amount Qualifier Code	Hierarchical Child Code	Code
Attachment Report Type Code	Hierarchical Level Code	Provider Specialty Code
Attachment Transmission Code	Hierarchical Structure Code	Record Format Code
Claim Adjustment Group Code	Immunization Status Code	Reject Reason Code
Claim Filing Indicator Code	Immunization Type Code	Related-Causes Code
Claim Frequency Code	Individual Relationship Code	Service Type Code
Claim Payment Remark Code	Information Release Code	Ship/Delivery or Calendar Pattern
Claim Submission Reason Code	Insurance Type Code	Code
Code List Qualifier Code	Measurement Reference ID Code	Ship/Delivery Pattern Time Code
Condition Codes	Medicare Assignment Code	Student Status Code
Contact Function Code	Nature of Condition Code	Supporting Document Response
Contract Code	Non-Visit Code	Code
Contract Type Code	Note Reference Code	Surgical Procedure Code
Credit/Debit Flag Code	Nutrient Admin Method Code	Transaction Set Identifier Code
Currency Code	Nutrient Admin Technique Code	Transaction Set Purpose Code
Disability Type Code	Place of Service Code	Unit or Basis Measurement Code
Discipline Type Code	Policy Compliance Code	Version Identification Code
Employment Status Code	Product/Service Procedure Code	X-Ray Availability Indicator Code
Entity Identifier Code	Prognosis Code	

TABLE D-5
Data Grouping in 837P Standard Transaction Format

Level	Information
High-Level Information: Applies to the entire claim and reflects data pertaining to the billing provider, subscriber, and patient.	Billing/Pay to Provider Information Subscriber/Patient Information Payer Information
Claim-Level Information: Applies to the entire claim and all service lines and is applicable to most claims.	Claim Information
Specialty Claim–Level Information: Applies to specific claim types.	Specialty
Service Line–Level Information: Applies to specific procedure or service that is rendered and is applicable to most claims.	Service Line Information
Specialty Service Line–Level Information: Applies to specific claim types. Required data are required only for the specific claim type.	Specialty Service Line Information
Other Information	Coordination of Benefits (COB) Repriced Claim/Line Credit/Debit Information Clearinghouse/VAN Tracking

form block 12 and block 13 are on file" and *P* for "signature generated by provider because the patient was not physically present for services."

Grouping of Information for 837P

Because the 837P is an electronic format and not a paper form, data collected to construct and submit a claim are grouped by levels. Again, it is important for claims-processing staff to know the language when following up on claims. You will likely not need to know exactly how these are grouped. However, if the clearinghouse or payer states that you have an invalid item at the "High Level," you will need to

understand that it could be incomplete or erroneous information pertaining to the provider, subscriber, or payer (Table D-5).

A "friendlier" way to understand this new stream-of-data format is to address a "crosswalk" between the legacy CMS-1500 (Figure D-1) and the 837P (Table D-6; note that dates on HIPAA transactions will be in the format YYYYMMDD [20030806]). Refer to the sample Health Insurance Claim Form.

Standard Unique Identifiers

The use of standard unique identifiers will improve efficiency in the management of health care by simplifying administration systems. This will enable

PLEASE
DO NOT
STAPLE
IN THIS
AREA

FIGURE D-1

CMS-1500 Health Insurance Claim Form, also known as the "universal claim form," used by outpatient facilities for claims submission. (Courtesy U.S. Department of Health and Human Services, Centers for Medicare and Medicaid Services.)

CPT only © 2005. Current Procedural Terminology, 2006, Professional Edition, American Medical Association. All Rights Reserved.

TABLE D-6
Comparison of CMS-1500 and 837P

Ref. No. on CMS	CMS-1500 Box No.	CMS-1500 Box Name	837P Data Element No.	837P Data Element Name
1	1	Government Program	66	Identification Code Qualifier
2	1a	Insured ID number	67	Subscriber Primary Identifier
3-4-5-6	2	Patients Name L, F, MI	1035	Patient Last Name
			1036	Patient First Name
			1037	Patient Middle Name
			1039	Patient Name Suffix
7	3	Patient Date of Birth	1251	Patient Date of Birth
8	3	Sex	1068	Patient Gender Code
9-10-11-12	4	Insured Name L, F, MI	1035	Patient Last Name
			1036	Patient First Name
			1037	Patient Middle Name
			1039	Patient Name Suffix
13-14	5	Patient Address	166	Patient Address Line
			166	Patient Address Line
15	5	City	19	Patient City Name
16	5	State	156	Patient State Code
17	5	Zip		Patient Postal Zone or Zip Code
18	5	Telephone		NOT USED in 837P
19-20	6	Patient relationship to Insured, Self, Spouse	1069	Individual Relationship Code
21-22	7	Insured Address	166	Subscriber Address Line
			166	Subscriber Address Line
23	7	City	19	Subscriber City Name
24	7	State	156	State Code
25	7	Zip Code	116	Subscriber Postal Zone or Zip Code
26	7	Telephone		NOT USED in 837P
27-28-29-30-31		Patient Status Single, Married	1069	Individual Relationship Code
	8	Other	1069	Individual Relationship Code
	8	Employed		NOT USED in 837P
	8	Full-time Student		NOT USED in 837P
	8	Part-time Student		NOT USED in 837P
32-33-34-35	9	Other Insured's Name L, F, MI	1035	Other Insured First Name
			1036	Other Insured Middle Name
			1037	Other Insured Name Suffix
			1039	Other Insured Group Name
36	9a	Other insured Policy or Group Number	93	
37	9b	Other insured date of birth	1251	
38	9b	Sex	1068	
39	9c	Employer's name or school name		NOT USED in 837P
40	9d	Insurance plan name or program name	93	Other Insured group name
41	10	Is patient's condition related to:		Related causes information:
42	10a	Employment (current or previous)	1362	Related causes code
43	10b	Auto Accident	1362	Related causes code
44	10b	Place (state)	156	Auto accident state or province code
45	10c	Other Accident	1362	Related causes code
46	11	Insured's Policy Group or FECA number		
47	11a	Insured's Date of Birth	1251	Subscriber's birth date
48	11a	Sex	1068	Subscriber gender code
49	11b	Employer's name or school name		NOT USED in 837P
50	11c	Insurance plan name or program name	93	Other insured group name
51	11d	Is there another health benefit plan	98	Entity identifier code
52-53	12	Patient's or authorized person's signature (and date)	1363	Release of information code
			1351	Patient Signature source code
54	13	Insured's or authorized person's signature		Benefits assignment certification indicator

TABLE D-6
Comparison of CMS-1500 and 837P—cont'd

Ref. No. on CMS	CMS-1500 Box No.	CMS-1500 Box Name	837P Data Element No.	837P Data Element Name
55-56-57	14	Date of current: Illness, Injury, Pregnancy (LMP)	1251	Initial treatment date
			1251	Accident date
			1251	LMP
58	15	If patient has had same or similar illness, give first date	1251	Similar illness or symptom date
59	16	Dates patient unable to work in current occupation: From		Last worked date
60	16	To	1251	Work return date
61	17	Name of Referring Physician or other source		
62	17a	ID number of referring physician		
63	18	Hospitalization dates related to current services: From	1251	Related hospitalization
64	18	To		Related hospitalization discharge date
65	19	Reserved for local use		
66	20	Outside Lab?		
67	20	$ Charges		
68	21	Diagnosis or nature of illness or injury, 1	1271	Diagnosis code
69	21	2	1271	Diagnosis code
70	21	3	1271	Diagnosis code
71	21	4	1271	Diagnosis code
72	22	Medicaid Resubmission code		NOT USED in 837P
73	22	Original ref. No.	127	Claim original reference number
74	22	Prior authorization number	127	Prior Authorization number
75	24A	Dates of service: From MM DD YY	1251	Order Date
76	24A	To MM DD YY	1331	Order Date
77	24B	Place of Service		Place of Service Code
78	24C	Type of Service		NOT REQUIRED in 837P
79	24D	Procedures, services, or supplies CPT/HCPCS	234	Procedure code
80-81	24D	Modifier	1339	Procedure Modifier
			1339	Procedure Modifier
			1339	Procedure Modifier
82-83-84-85	24E	Diagnosis Code	1328	Diagnosis code pointer
				Diagnosis code pointer
				Diagnosis code pointer
				Diagnosis code pointer
86	24F	$ Charges	782	Line item charge amount
87	24G	Days or units	380	Service unit count
88	24H	EPSDT Family Plan	1366	Special program indicator
89	24I	EMG	1073	Emergency indicator
90	24J	COB		
91	24K	Reserved for local use	127	Rendering provider Secondary Identifier
92	25	Federal Tax ID Number	67	Rendering provider Identifier
93	25	SSN, EIN	66	Identification code qualifier
94	26	Patient's Account No.	1028	Patient account number
95	27	Accept Assignment	1359	Medicare assignment code
96	28	Total charge	782	Total claim charge amount
97	29	Amount Paid	782	Patient amount paid
98	30	Balance Due		
99-100	31	Signature of Physician or supplier (and date)	1073	Provider or supplier signature indicator
101-106; 108-115	32	Name and address of facility where services were rendered	1035	Laboratory or facility name
			166	Laboratory or facility address line
			19	Laboratory or facility city
			156	Laboratory facility state or province code
			116	Laboratory or facility postal zone or zip code

Continued.

TABLE D-6
Comparison of CMS-1500 and 837P—cont'd

Ref. No. on CMS	CMS-1500 Box No.	CMS-1500 Box Name	837P Data Element No.	837P Data Element Name
			OR	
			1036	Submitter first name
			1035	Billing provider last or organizational name
			1036	Billing provider first name
			166	Billing provider address line
			166	Billing provider address line
			19	Billing provider city name
			156	Billing provider state or province code
			116	Billing provider postal zone or zip code
116-122	33	Physicians' suppliers billing name, address, zip code, & phone number	1035	Billing provider last or organization name
			1036	Billing provider first name
			166	Billing provider address line
			166	Billing provider address line
			19	Billing provider city name
			156	Billing provider state or province code
			116	Billing provider postal zone or zip code
123	33	Pin #	127	Billing provider additional identifier
124	33	GRP#	67	Billing provider identifier

Data from MEDEXTEND.

the efficient electronic transmission of certain health information used across the industry.

❑ *Standard Unique Employer Identifier* (use EIN to identify employers; compliance by July 30, 2004). The EIN will be used to identify employers rather than inputting the actual name of the company. Employers can use their EINs to identify themselves in transactions involving premium payments to health plans on behalf of their employees or to identify themselves or other employers as the source or receiver of information about eligibility. Employers can also use EINs to identify themselves in transactions when enrolling or disenrolling employees in a health plan.

❑ *Standard Unique Health Care Provider Identifier.* Final rule estimated to publish September 2003. This is proposed to be an eight-position alphanumeric identifier for the health care provider.

❑ *Standard Unique Health Plan Identifier.* Proposed rule estimated to publish September 2003.

❑ *Standard Unique Patient Identifier.* The intention to create a standard for a uniform patient identifier prompted protest among public interest groups, who saw a universal identifier as a civil liberties threat. Therefore the issue of a universal Patient Identifier is on hold indefinitely.

Corrective Action Plan

The CMS has implemented a Corrective Action Plan to address issues of noncompliance in regard to TCS. Details at this time are forthcoming and will be available at the CMS website: http://www.cms.gov.

SECURITY RULE: ADMINISTRATIVE, PHYSICAL, AND TECHNICAL SAFEGUARDS

Security measures encompass all the administrative, physical, and technical safeguards in an information system. The Security Rule addresses only *electronic* protected health information (ePHI), but the concept of protecting PHI that will become ePHI makes attention to security for the entire office important. The Security Rule is divided into three main sections: administrative safeguards, technical safeguards, and physical safeguards.

Administrative safeguards prevent unauthorized use or disclosure of PHI through administrative actions and P&P to manage the selection, development, implementation, and maintenance of security measures to protect ePHI. These management controls guard data integrity, confidentiality, and availability and include the following:

❑ Information access controls authorize each employee's physical access to PHI. This is management of password and access for separate employees that restricts their access to records in accordance with their responsibility in the health care organization. For example, the medical records clerk who has authorization to retrieve medical records will likely not have access to billing records located on the computer.

❑ Internal audits allow the ability to review who has had access to PHI to ensure that there is no intentional or accidental inappropriate access, in both the practice management software system and the paper records or charges.

❑ Risk analysis and management is a process that assesses the privacy and security risks of various safeguards and the cost in losses if those safeguards are not in place. This process is newly introduced into healthcare compliance and each organization must evaluate their vulnerabilities and the associated risks and decide how to mitigate those risks. Reasonable safeguards must be implemented to protect against known risks.

❑ Termination procedures should be formally documented in the P&P manual and include terminating the employee's access to PHI. Other procedures would likely include changing office security pass codes, deleting user access to computer systems, deleting terminated employee's e-mail account, collecting any access cards or keys.

Technical safeguards are technological controls in place to protect and control access to information on computers in the health care organization and include the following:

❑ Access controls consist of user-based access (system set up to place limitations on access to data tailored to each staff member) and role-based access (limitations created for each job category, e.g., scheduling, billing, clinical).

❑ Audit controls keep track of log-ins to the computer system, administrative activity, and changes to data. This includes changing passwords, deleting user accounts, or creating a new user.

❑ Automatic log-offs prevent unauthorized users from accessing a computer when it is left unattended. The computer system or software program should automatically log off after a predetermined period of inactivity. Your office's practice management software may have this useful feature; if not, the feature may be temporarily mimicked using a screen-saver and password.

❑ Each user should have a unique identifier or "username" and an unshared, undisclosed password to log into any computer with access

to PHI. Identifying each unique user allows the functions of auditing and access controls to be implemented. Other authentication techniques involve more sophisticated devices, such as a magnetic card or fingerprints. You likely will be dealing only with a password in your organization. Passwords for all users should be changed on a regular basis and should never be common names or words.

❑ *Physical safeguards* also prevent unauthorized access to PHI. These physical measures and P&P protect a covered entity's electronic information systems and related buildings and equipment from natural and environmental hazards and unauthorized intrusion. Appropriate and reasonable physical safeguards should include the following:

❑ Media and equipment controls are documented P&P regarding the management of media and equipment containing the PHI. Typical safeguard policies include how the organization handles the retention, removal, and disposal of paper records, as well as the recycling of computers and destruction of obsolete data disks or software programs containing PHI.

❑ Physical access controls limit unauthorized access to areas where equipment is stored as well as medical charts. Locks on doors are the most common type of control.

❑ Secure workstation locations minimize the possibility of unauthorized viewing of PHI. This includes making sure that password-protected screensavers are in use on computers when unattended and that desk drawers are locked.

APPLICATION TO PRACTICE SETTING

HIPAA affects all areas of the health care office, from the reception area to the provider. In conjunction with being educated and trained in job responsibilities, every staff member must be educated about HIPAA and trained in the P&P pertinent to the organization.

Best practices are strategies for constantly improving productivity and service. Best practices are deployed and produce demonstrable results that meet federal and state mandates and the practice's objectives. Results and benefits are documented and measured periodically to assess for efficiency in terms of dollars, time, and other resource costs. "Best" does not mean "most," as in "most organizations do things this way" or "the most expensive solution."

Best practice is a way to perform in the most efficient and effective manner for your particular organizational environment. In the revenue or claims cycle, for example, your office may have all charges for services posted by Thursday afternoon and may not see patients on Fridays. Your organization may employ a "best practice" of generating and transmitting claims every Friday afternoon. This is efficient because there are no distractions with patient appointments, and the routine of every Friday keeps claims filed in a timely manner. This leads to a positive cash flow.

Reasonable safeguards are measurable solutions based on accepted standards that are implemented and periodically monitored to demonstrate that the office is in compliance. Reasonable efforts must be made to limit the use or disclosure of PHI. If you are the front desk receptionist and you close the privacy glass between your desk and the waiting area when you are making a call to a patient, this is a reasonable safeguard to prevent others in the waiting room from overhearing.

Incidental uses and disclosures are permissible under HIPAA only when reasonable safeguards or precautions have been implemented to prevent misuse or inappropriate disclosure of PHI. When incidental uses and disclosures result from failure to apply reasonable safeguards or adhere to the minimum necessary standard, the Privacy Rule has been violated. If you are in the reception area and you close the privacy glass when having a confidential conversation, and you are still overheard by an individual in the waiting room, this would be "incidental." You have applied a reasonable safeguard to prevent this from happening.

Guidelines for HIPAA Privacy Compliance
As a health care provider, you will likely answer the telephone and speak during the course of your business, and there will be questions about what you can and cannot say. Reasonable and appropriate safeguards must be taken to ensure that all confidential health information in your office is protected from unauthorized and inappropriate access, including both verbal and written forms.

1. Consider that conversations occurring throughout the office could be overheard. The reception area and waiting room are often linked, and it is easy to hear the scheduling of appointments and exchange of confidential information. It is necessary to observe areas and maximize efforts to avoid unauthorized disclosures. Simple and affordable precautions include using privacy glass at the front desk and having conversations away from settings where other patients or visitors are present. Health care providers can move their dictation stations away from patient areas or wait until no patients are present before dictating. Phone conversations by providers in front of patients, even in emergency situations, should be avoided. Providers and staff must use their best professional judgment.

2. Be sure to check in the patient medical record and in your computer system to see if there are any special instructions for contacting the patient regarding scheduling or reporting test results. Follow these requests as agreed by the office.

3. Patient sign-in sheets *are* permissible, but limit the information you request when a patient signs in, and change it periodically during the day. A sign-in sheet must not contain information such as reason for visit because some providers specialize in treating patients with sensitive issues. Showing that a particular individual has an appointment with your practice may pose a breach of patient confidentiality.

4. Make sure you have patients sign a form acknowledging receipt of the NPP. The NPP allows you to release the patient's confidential information for billing and other purposes. If your practice has other confidentiality statements and policies besides HIPAA mandates, these must be reviewed to ensure they meet HIPAA requirements.

5. Formal policies for transferring and accepting outside PHI must address how your office keeps this information confidential. When using courier services, billing services, transcription services, or e-mail, you must ensure that transferring PHI is done in a secure and compliant manner.

6. Computers are used for a variety of administrative functions, including scheduling, billing, and managing medical records. Computers typically are present at the reception area. Keep the computer screen turned so that viewing is restricted to authorized staff. Screensavers should be used to prevent unauthorized viewing or access. The computer should automatically log off the user after a period of being idle, requiring the staff member to reenter their password.

7. Keep your username and password confidential, and change it often. Do not share this information. An authorized staff member such as the PO will have administrative access to reset your password if you lose it or if someone discovers it. Also, practice manage-

ment software can track users and follow their activity. Do not set yourself up by giving out your password. Safeguards include password protection for electronic data and storing paper records securely.

8. Safeguard your work area; do not place notes with confidential information in areas that are easy to view by nonstaff. Cleaning services will access your building, usually after business hours; ensure that you safeguard PHI.

9. Place medical record charts face down at reception areas so the patient's name is not exposed to other patients or visitors to your office. Also, when placing medical records on the door of an examination room, turn the chart so that identifying information faces the door. If you keep medical charts in the office on countertops or in receptacles, it is your duty to ensure that nonstaff persons will not access the records. Handling and storing medical records will certainly change because of HIPAA guidelines.

10. Do not post the health care provider's schedule in areas viewable by nonstaff individuals. The schedules are often posted for professional staff convenience, but this may be a breach in patient confidentiality.

11. Fax machines should not be placed in patient examination rooms or in any reception area where nonstaff persons may view incoming or sent documents. Only staff members should have access to the faxes.

12. If you open your office mail or take phone calls pertaining to medical record requests, direct these issues to the appropriate staff member.

13. If you are involved in coding and billing, be sure to recognize, learn, and use HIPAA TCS.

14. Send all privacy-related questions or concerns to the appropriate staff member.

15. Immediately report any suspected or known improper behavior to your supervisor or the PO so that the issue may be documented and investigated.

16. If you have questions, contact your supervisor or the PO.

Health care organizations face challenges in implementing the HIPAA requirements; do not let these overwhelm you. Your office is required to take reasonable steps to build protections specific to your health care organization. Compliance is an ongoing endeavor involving teamwork. Understand your office's established P&P. Monitor your own activities to ensure you are following the required procedures. Do not take shortcuts when your actions involve patient privacy and security.

Be alert to other activities in your office. Help your co-workers change work habits that do not comply with HIPAA. Do not ignore unauthorized uses and disclosures of PHI, and do not allow unauthorized persons to access data. You have an obligation to your employer and the patients you serve.

CONSEQUENCES OF NONCOMPLIANCE WITH HIPAA

The prosecution of HIPAA crimes is handled by different governing bodies. HHS handles issues regarding TCS and security. Complaints can be filed against a covered entity for not complying with these rules. The OCR oversees privacy issues and complaints, referring criminal issues to the Office of Inspector General (OIG). The OIG provides the workup for referral cases, which may involve the FBI and other agencies.

Serious civil and criminal penalties apply for HIPAA noncompliance. General noncompliance with the privacy, security and transaction regulations result in a $100 fine per violation and up to $25,000 per person for identical violations in a given calendar year. Specific to the Privacy Rule is a $50,000 fine and imprisonment for 1 year if one knowingly obtains or discloses IIHI. The person who obtains or discloses such health information under false pretenses is subject to a $100,000 fine. If one obtains or discloses PHI with the intent to sell, transfer, or use it for commercial advantage, personal gain, or malicious harm, a maximum fine of $250,000 and up to 10 years' imprisonment may be applied.

Office of Inspector General

The mission of the OIG is to safeguard the health and welfare of the beneficiaries of HHS programs and to protect the integrity of HHS programs (Medicare and Medicaid). The OIG was established to identify and eliminate fraud, abuse, and waste and

"to promote efficiency and economy in departmental operations." HIPAA legislation has radically changed the focus and mission within the OIG. HIPAA pushed the OIG into a new era, guaranteeing funding for OIG programs and mandating initiatives to protect the integrity of all health care programs. The OIG undertakes nationwide audits, as well as investigations and inspections to review the claim submission processes of providers and reimbursement patterns of the programs. Recommendations are made to the HHS Secretary and the U.S. Congress on correcting problematic areas addressed in the federal programs. According to the OIG:

> Efforts to combat fraud were consolidated and strengthened under Public Law 104-191, the Health Insurance Portability and Accountability Act of 1996 (HIPAA). The Act established a comprehensive program to combat fraud committed against all health plans, both public and private. The legislation required the establishment of a national Health Care Fraud and Abuse Control Program (HCFAC), under the joint direction of the Attorney General and the Secretary of the Department of Health and Human Services (HHS) acting through the Department's Inspector General (HHS/OIG). The HCFAC program is designed to coordinate Federal, State, and local law enforcement activities with respect to health care fraud and abuse. The Act requires HHS and DOJ [Department of Justice] to detail in an Annual Report the amounts deposited and appropriated to the Medicare Trust Fund, and the source of such deposits.

Health care providers must be aware of the potential liabilities when submitting claims for payment that are deemed to be "fraudulent" or inappropriate by the government. The government may impose significant financial and administrative penalties when health care claims are not appropriately submitted, including criminal prosecution against the offending party. Fraud, according to the OIG, can result from deliberate unethical behavior or simply from mistakes and miscues that cause excessive reimbursement. The OIG is the professional health care provider's (and their agents') "partner" in fighting fraud and abuse.

Compliance Program Guidance recommendations from the OIG must be the guiding principle of a health care practice in regard to the potential for unethical behavior or the mistakes that may occur within the organization. The *Individual and Small Group Physician Practices* and *Compliance Program Guidance for Third-Party Medical Billing Companies* are two publications in a series for the health care industry that provides guidance and acceptable principles for business operations.

If you are involved in the claims-processing procedures in your organization, note the importance and urgency in following the legal and ethical path when performing your duties. Your "honest mistake" could lead to a situation that puts the health care provider at risk for investigation of fraud, waste, or abuse.

FRAUD AND ABUSE LAWS

Fraud can occur when deception is used in a claim submission to obtain payment from the payer. Individuals who knowingly, willfully, and intentionally submit false information to benefit themselves or others commit fraud. Fraud can also be interpreted from mistakes that result in excessive reimbursement. No proof of "specific intent to defraud" is required for fraud to be considered.

Abuse occurs when a health care organization practices behavior that is not indicative of sound medical or fiscal activity.

Federal False Claims Act (31 US Code §3729-33)

"A false claim is a claim for payment for services or supplies that were not provided specifically as presented or for which the provider is otherwise not entitled to payment." Presenting a claim for an item or service based on a code known to result in greater payment or submitting a claim for services not medically necessary is also a violation of the False Claims Act (FCA). The government uses the FCA as a primary enforcement tool.

Although no proof of specific intent to defraud is required, liability can occur when a person knowingly presents or causes to present such a claim or makes, uses, or causes a false record or statement to have a false or fraudulent claim paid or approved by the federal government.

Qui Tam "Whistleblower"

Qui Tam in the FCA provisions allows a private citizen to bring a civil action suit for a violation on behalf of the federal government. This involves fraud by government contractors and other entities who receive or use government funds. The Qui Tam "whistleblower" shares in any money recovered.

Civil Monetary Penalties Law (42 US Code §320a-27a)

The U.S. Congress enacted the Civil Monetary Penalty (CMP) statute to provide administrative remediation to combat health care fraud and abuse. HIPAA's final rule includes civil monetary penalties when there is a pattern of upcoded claims or billing for medically unnecessary services. The CMP imposes civil money penalties and assessments against a person or organization for making false or improper claims against any federal health care program.

Criminal False Claims Act (18 US Code)

The Criminal False Claims Act did not apply specifically to the health care industry before HIPAA. HIPAA amendments to the criminal code include the following:

❏ **Theft or Embezzlement (18 US Code §669).** This law brings fines and imprisonment against any individual who "knowingly and willfully embezzles, steals, or otherwise without authority converts to the use of any person other than the rightful owner, or intentionally misapplies any of the moneys, funds, securities, premiums, credits, property, or other assets of a health care benefit program." This law does not just affect Medicare and Medicaid programs.

❏ **False Statement Relating to Health Care Matters (18 US Code §1035).** Any individual who knowingly and willfully "falsifies, conceals, or covers up by any trick, scheme, or device a material fact; or makes any materially false, fictitious, or fraudulent statements or representations, or makes or uses any materially false writing or document knowing the same to contain any materially false, fictitious, or fraudulent statement or entry, in connection with the delivery of or payment for health care benefits, items, or services" is subject to fines and imprisonment.

❏ **Health Care Fraud (18 US Code §1347).** Any individual who knowingly and willfully "executes, or attempts to execute, a scheme or artifice to defraud any health care benefit program; or to obtain, by means of false or fraudulent pretenses, representations, or promises, any of the money or property owned by, or under the custody or control of, any health care benefit program, in connection with the delivery of or payment for health care benefits, items, or services" is subject to fines and imprisonment. If seriously bodily injury or even death occurs, the person may face life imprisonment.

❏ **Obstruction of Criminal Investigations of Health Care Offenses (18 US Code §1518).** An individual is subject to fines and imprisonment when the person "willfully prevents, obstructs, misleads, delays or attempts to prevent, obstruct, mislead, or delay the communication of information or records relating to a violation of a Federal health care offense to a criminal investigator."

Stark Laws (42 US Code §1395)

Stark laws prohibit the submission of claims for "designated services" or referral of patients if the referring physician has a "financial relationship" with the entity that provides the services. Originally named "Stark I," this law pertained only to clinical laboratories. Stark laws carry exceptions, so it is important to understand the referral processes and in-office ancillary services used by your health care organization.

Antikickback Statute

According to the CMS, discounts, rebates, or other reductions in price may violate the Antikickback Statute because such arrangements induce the purchase of items or services payable by Medicare or Medicaid. However, some arrangements are clearly permissible if they fall within a "safe harbor." One safe harbor protects certain discounting practices. For purposes of this safe harbor, a "discount" is the reduction in the amount a seller charges a buyer for a good or service based on an "arms-length" transaction. In addition, to be protected under the discount safe harbor, the discount must apply to the original item or service purchased or furnished; that is, a discount cannot be applied to the purchase of a different good or service than the one on which the discount was earned. A "rebate" is defined as a discount that is not given at the time of sale. A "buyer" is the individual or entity responsible for submitting a claim for the item or service that is payable by the Medicare or Medicaid programs. A "seller" is the individual or entity who offers the discount.

Safe Harbors

Safe harbors specify various business and service arrangements that are protected from prosecution under the Antikickback Statute. These include certain investments, care in underserved areas, and other arrangements.

Additional Laws and Compliance

Other laws pertaining to fraud and abuse include the Federal Deposit Insurance Corporation (FDIC) Mail and Wire Fraud provisions, as follows:

❏ **§1341. Frauds and swindles.** An individual is subject to both fines and imprisonment when having "devised or intending to devise any scheme or artifice to defraud, or for obtaining money or property by means of false or fraudulent pretenses" by use of the U.S. Postal Service, whether sent by or delivered to the Postal Service.

❏ **§1343. Fraud by wire, radio, or television.** An individual will be fined and/or imprisoned "for obtaining money or property by means of false or fraudulent pretenses, representations, or promises, transmits or causes to be transmitted by means of wire, radio, or television communication."

The U.S. government is clearly committed to the investigation and prosecution of health care fraud.

As with HIPAA policies and procedures, it is imperative that health care entities develop their own compliance program to identify and prevent fraud.

GOVERNMENT STRATEGIES TO REDUCE HEALTH CARE FRAUD

Health Care Fraud and Abuse Program

HCFAP has created a national fraud and abuse program by coordinating efforts of enforcement agencies at local, state, and federal levels.

Operation Restore Trust

Launched in 1995, Operation Restore Trust (ORT) was designed to coordinate the activities of the OIG along with the CMS and other HHS entities in identifying and preventing fraud. An established hotline (1-800-HHS-TIPS) for the public allows reporting issues that might indicate fraud, abuse, or waste. ORT has been successful due to planning with the Department of Justice (DOJ) and other law enforcement agencies, training state and local organizations to detect fraud and abuse, and implementing statistical methods to identify providers for audits and investigations.

Medicare Integrity Program

The goal of the Medicare Integrity Program (MIP) is to identify and reduce Medicare overpayments through a series of audits and reviews of provider claims and cost report data. Initiatives of the MIP include identifying plan beneficiaries with additional insurance and educating health care providers. Program integrity contractors help expand the scope of the MIP. This endeavor has recovered several billions of dollars in the fight against fraud waste and abuse in the Medicare program.

Correct Coding Initiative

The Correct Coding Initiative (CCI) was developed to detect improperly coded claims through the use of computer edits. Services that should be grouped together and paid as one item rather than billed separately to obtain higher reimbursement are identified with the computer system.

Increased Staffing and Expanded Penalties for Violations

A significant increase in staffing among the OIG, DOJ, and FBI over the past decade has included prosecutors (400% increase since 1993) and FBI agents (300% since 1993). With additional employees, the industry has seen the promotion of compliance endeavors across the health care sector. Penalties for violations have increased.

Special Alerts, Bulletins, and Guidance Documents

Special Fraud Alerts are published by the OIG to alert the industry concerning specific patterns or trends related to fraudulent or abusive activities regarding the Medicare and Medicaid programs. Special Advisory Bulletins report industry practices and arrangements that may implicate fraud and abuse. Other guidance documents include updates, response letters, and alerts important to more specifically targeted matters. All notices are available at the OIG website, and you can sign up for their mailing list.

Exclusion Program

According to the OIG:

> No program payment will be made for anything that an excluded person furnishes, orders, or prescribes. This payment prohibition applies to the excluded person, anyone who employs or contracts with the excluded person, any hospital or other provider where the excluded person provides services, and anyone else. The exclusion applies regardless of who submits the claims and applies to all administrative and management services furnished by the excluded person.

Excluded persons/facilities are convicted for program-related fraud and patient abuse, actions from licensing boards, and defaulting on Health Education Assistance Loans.

Your health care organization must not conduct business with any health care provider or subcontract with any agent who has been listed as an Excluded Individual. Be sure to check the updated listings at the OIG website.

COMPLIANCE PROGRAM GUIDANCE FOR INDIVIDUAL AND SMALL GROUP PHYSICIAN PRACTICES

The OIG published the *Individual and Small Group Physician Practices* in September 2000. This guidance recommended by the OIG is voluntary; however, an effective plan reduces the risk of legal action and creates a "good faith" effort in combating fraud, waste, and abuse. A compliance plan requires that a health care practice review all billing processes through audits and establish controls that will correct weaknesses and prevent errors.

A well-designed compliance program can speed the claims-processing cycle; optimize proper payment or claims; minimize billing mistakes; reduce the likelihood of a government audit; avoid conflict with Stark laws and the Antikickback Statute; show a "good faith" effort that claims will be submitted appropriately; and relay to staff that there is a duty to report mistakes and suspected or known misconduct.

If you are a claims-processing staff member, your organization's claims-processing supervisor should research industry sector program guidance to help with specific concerns regarding the specialty/facility setting. Check the OIG website to view addendums, comments, and drafts of additional compliance guidance subjects. Other program guidance includes the following:

- ❏ April 2003: Guidance for Pharmaceutical Industry
- ❏ March 2003: Ambulance Suppliers
- ❏ September 2000: Individual and Small Group Physician Practices
- ❏ February 2000: Nursing Facilities
- ❏ November 1999: Medicare + Choice Organizations
- ❏ September 1999: Hospices
- ❏ June 1999: Durable Medical Equipment Prosthetics, Orthotics, and Supply Industry
- ❏ November 1998: Third-Party Medical Billing Companies
- ❏ August 1998: Home Health Agencies
- ❏ August 1998: Clinical Laboratories
- ❏ February 1998: Hospitals

Increased Productivity and Decreased Penalties with Compliance Plan

The presence of an OIG compliance program can significantly mitigate imposed penalties in the event of an OIG audit or other discovery of fraudulent billing activities. These P&P can be found in the provider's P&P manual. For those not currently in the role of a privacy/security/compliance officer, knowledge about P&P as they pertain to both HIPAA and the OIG will be invaluable throughout their career.

Because health care providers rely on the expertise of their billing and coding staff to process claims accurately and promptly, they also look to these staff members for advice and guidance. If you are directly involved in this area of your organization, you will likely be expected to understand the complexities of the various laws and regulations governing the medical claims process.

Compliance plans effectively become a "meeting of the minds" among the players; providers, claims-processing staff, and payers when all are agreeing to process claims in accordance with shared values. Consider your organization's OIG compliance program as a way to integrate regulatory requirements directly into your claims-processing procedures. The OIG views the experienced claims-processing staff as the critical screen for the health care provider's

claims. The common denominators in the key benefits identified by the OIG are efficiency, consistency, and integrity.

SEVEN BASIC COMPONENTS OF A COMPLIANCE PLAN

The OIG outlines the following seven components of an effective program guidance plan specifically for the individual and small group physician practices:

1. Conducting internal monitoring and auditing
2. Implementing compliance and practice standards
3. Designating a compliance officer or contact
4. Conducting appropriate training and education
5. Responding appropriately to detected offenses and developing corrective action
6. Developing open lines of communication
7. Enforcing disciplinary standards through well-publicized guidelines

Conducting Internal Monitoring and Auditing

A comprehensive auditing and monitoring program will not eliminate misconduct within an organization but will minimize the risk of fraud and abuse by identifying the risk areas. The OIG does not provide a specific set of guidelines on conducting audits or ongoing monitoring. The compliance officer, with the committee's assistance, should identify problem areas and should have established auditing priorities and procedures as part of the organization's compliance program.

Special attention should be made to the risk areas associated with claims submission and processing. Also, a thorough review of the organization's standards and written P&P should be conducted to ensure proper guidelines for complying with state and federal laws and insurance payer requirements.

Implementing Compliance and Practice Standards

Written standards and procedures will address risk areas that an office needs to monitor and follow. Specific risk areas identified by the OIG include the following:

- ❏ Billing for items or services not rendered or not provided as claimed
- ❏ Submitting claims for equipment, medical supplies, and services that are not reasonable and necessary
- ❏ Double billing resulting in duplicate payment
- ❏ Billing for noncovered services as if covered
- ❏ Knowing misuse of provider identification numbers, which results in improper billing

- ❑ Unbundling, or billing for each component of the service instead of billing or using an all-inclusive code
- ❑ Failure to use coding modifiers properly
- ❑ Clustering
- ❑ Upcoding the level of service provided

In addition to these risk areas, policies should be developed that address the following:

- ❑ Reasonable and necessary
- ❑ Proper medical documentation
- ❑ Federal sentencing guidelines
- ❑ Record retention

You should be able to access your organization's P&P manual to review the standards and protocol for these issues involving your practice.

Designating a Compliance Officer or Contact

As with the HIPAA privacy officer (PO), the compliance officer is the key individual overseeing your organization's compliance program monitoring with the support of the Compliance Committee. Again, as with HIPAA, policies and procedures (P&P) need to be drafted. These established guidelines identify and prevent fraud and abuse activities as described by the OIG.

The number of members on your Compliance Committee is not important, and prospective staff members from human resources, claims auditing, billing, legal, and medicine can ensure a comprehensive mix. You may currently participate on your office's Compliance Committee or may be asked to do so in the future. The Compliance Committee acts as a review board. Some committees consist of provider-client office staff and billing company staff. Some committees are simply the provider-client and the billing company staff, or a combination of the provider-client, their practice manager, and the billing company staff. The Committee, empowered by management, legitimizes the compliance strategy within your organization. In addition to possessing professional experience in claims processing and auditing, Committee members will be expected to use good judgment and high integrity to fulfill committee obligations.

Conducting Appropriate Training and Education

Because OIG compliance program guidelines are based on Federal Sentencing Guidelines, significant elements of an effective compliance program involve proper education and training of staff. Every employee and individual who interacts with your health care organization and may be accountable for potential misconduct should be considered in the organization's training sessions.

You should be required to attend training in a "general" compliance training session at least annually. For staff members involved in claims processing (coding and billing), a separate training session should be held to cover internal procedures, federal and state laws regarding fraud and abuse, and specific government and other payer reimbursement policies. Periodic professional courses in continuing education should be available. Coding and billing personnel should receive training at least annually to remain updated on CPT/HCPCS and ICD-9-CM codes for each year. You will attend training either on site, at a remote location, or both.

Effective training can reduce potential errors, penalties, and fines. An educated staff makes fewer errors, reduces your organization's risks, and requires less micromanagement.

Responding Appropriately to Detected Offenses and Developing Corrective Action

When faced with the discovery of an offense or an error, inaction may be interpreted as indifference. This could impose a potential jeopardy to the reputation of the health care provider's practice. Your office should have a process for investigating problems and taking necessary corrective action. Issues that would raise concern include significant change in claims that are rejected; software edits that show pattern of misuse of codes or fees; unusually high volume of charges, payments, or rejections; and notices from insurance payers regarding claims submitted by your office.

You and your fellow staff members should be encouraged to report concerns for any suspected or known misconduct, with an established chain of command in the reporting path. Some incidences of misconduct may violate criminal, civil, or administrative law. Should the situation warrant, the Compliance Officer should report the misconduct promptly to the appropriate government authority.

Report fraud and abuse. Contact the OIG/HHS as follows:

- ❑ PHONE HOTLINE 800-HHS-TIPS (800-447-8477)
- ❑ TTY 800-377-4950
- ❑ FAX 800-223-8164
- ❑ http://oig.hhs.gov/hotline.html

Developing Open Lines of Communication

Effective lines of communication provide a channel for employees to report suspected or known misconduct without immediately resorting to an external agency. In this way your health care organization can resolve issues internally. "Open door" policies ensure an environment where staff members feel secure to ask about the organization's existing P&P and to report questionable activities. Your role as a conscientious employee will allow you to know the steps to take in reporting any suspicious business activity.

You will learn your office's procedure for reporting misconduct. It is important to follow these guidelines to protect your reputation and credibility within the workplace. Depending on the size of the practice, the methods for contacting managerial staff may include anonymous telephone calls through a "hotline" or written report forms.

Enforcing Disciplinary Standards through Well-Publicized Guidelines

The unfortunate downside to compliance is that misconduct does occur. For this reason, health care organizations must have established disciplinary guidelines and must make these well known to employees and other agents who contract with the organization. We all want to know what will happen if we "make a mistake" and what progressive forms of discipline await situations involving misconduct. Disciplinary standards include the following:

- ❑ Verbal warning
- ❑ Written warning
- ❑ Written reprimand
- ❑ Suspension or probation
- ❑ Demotion
- ❑ Termination of employment
- ❑ Restitution of any damages
- ❑ Referral to federal agencies for criminal prosecution

Whether the misconduct was intentional or negligent, all levels of employees need to know what is expected of them. Your office must publish this information and disseminate it to all employees.

WHAT TO EXPECT FROM YOUR HEALTH CARE PRACTICE

Although every health care organization or practice is different in regard to policies and procedures, you now know what to expect in the workplace, as follows:

- ❑ Practice Adherence to HIPAA and OIG Mandates and Recommendations

- ❑ Privacy/Security/Compliance Officer (even if one person)
- ❑ Policy and Procedure Manual
- ❑ Employee Training and Education (at least annually and whenever there are changes in business operations that affect staff members directly)
- ❑ Complaint and Sanctions Process

COMPLIANCE LESSONS LEARNED

You must strongly consider the lessons learned from the privacy, transaction, and security rules in conjunction with OIG compliance recommendations. The most important points are to read your organization's P&P manual and to ask questions about the many aspects of HIPAA or the general operations of your organization. Always use your ethical and "best practice" approach to be an informed and effective employee.

DATA SOURCES AND REFERENCES

American Health Information Management Association
http://www.ahima.org

Centers for Medicare and Medicaid Services
http://www.cms.gov

HIPAAdocs Corporation
http://www.hipaadocs.com

MEDEXTEND
http://www.medextend.com

Office of Civil Rights
http://www.hhs.gov/ocr/hipaa

Office of Inspector General
http://www.oig.hhs.gov

OIG Compliance Program Guidance for Third-Party Medical Billing Companies, *Federal Register* 63(243):70141, 1998.

OIG Compliance Program for Individual and Small Group Physician Practices, *Federal Register* 65(194):59439, 2000.

Phoenix Health Systems: HIPAA Advisory
http://www.hipaadvisory.com

Workgroup for Electronic Data Interchange
http://www.wedi.org

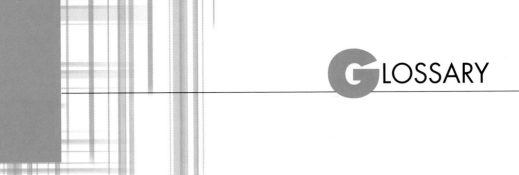

GLOSSARY

ABN Advance Beneficiary Notice; a Medicare waiver that notifies the patient that Medicare might not pay for a service either because it is a noncovered service or because medical necessity, as defined by Medicare, might not be met, even though the physician feels the service is medically necessary. The patient may then choose to pay for the service if Medicare does not or may choose to decline the service. This form must be signed by the patient before the service is provided or you cannot bill the patient if Medicare does not pay.

actuaries mathematicians who study trends and set insurance premiums, deductibles, and copays.

add-on codes codes used to expand the scope of a basic procedure code. Add-on codes are never used alone, and they are never listed first.

adjustment codes codes used by payors to explain why a claim or a service is paid differently than it was billed.

AFDC Aid to Families with Dependent Children; a government assistance program for those with qualifying low incomes.

aging reports reports used to report the status of claims to the physician and identify individual transactions that require follow-up.

alphabetical index an alphabetical listing of diagnoses, located in Section 1 of Volume 2 of the ICD-9-CM codebook.

alphabetical index to external causes of injury and poisoning an alphabetical listing of causes and places of injuries and poisoning, located in Section 3 of Volume 2 of the ICD-9-CM codebook, right after the table of drugs and chemicals.

ambulatory payment classification (APC) the prospective payment system used by Medicare to determine payment for hospital outpatient services. It is based on the procedure codes billed. Also called OPPS.

amount and/or complexity of data to be reviewed documentation of the review of (1) results of diagnostic tests; (2) personal review of films or slides to confirm or augment reported results; (3) collaboration with other health professionals regarding test results or prior history; (4) review of old records or history from other sources.

anatomic modifiers Level II HCPCS modifiers that identify specific anatomical parts of the body; they are used when the procedure code does not include that information.

ancillary medical providers professionals with a limited license to practice medicine and medical therapists who perform billable services.

ANSII format a complex format used to send electronic claims. It is very versatile; the electronic medical records may be attached to the claim.

appeal a formal request submitted to an insurance plan to have a payment decision changed or a penalty reversed.

assignment of benefits instructs the insurance company to send payment directly to the medical practice or provider. (The patient will pay copayments and deductibles at the time of service.)

associated signs and symptoms details that are included in the definition of a medical problem, or details that are used to narrow the choices when a diagnosis has not yet been established. An element of HPI.

authorization number proof that prior approval was obtained for a specific service: treatment, test, or procedure. It does not guarantee coverage if the claim does not establish medical necessity.

bad debt write-off a write-off that records payments owed, but not collectable. It does not represent a discount.

balance billing billing the patient for the balance remaining after the insurance payment has been posted.

beneficiary a person entitled to benefits under an insurance policy.

benefit period the time period in which an additional hospitalization for a Medicare patient is considered to be part of a previous hospitalization for the purpose of calculating the Medicare Part A patient financial responsibility. Readmission within 60 days of discharge is considered to extend an existing benefit period. When there have been 60 consecutive days without inpatient status, a new benefit period begins. There is no limit on how many benefit periods a person may have.

billing address the mailing address for the patient or the mailing address for the payor.

billing manager the supervisor in charge of medical billing and collections; may or may not include medical coding.

birthday rule when a dependent child is covered by insurance plans from both parents' employers, the policy for the parent whose birthday falls earliest in the calendar year is the primary payor and is billed first.

Blue Cross and Blue Shield (BCBS) medical plans organized during the Great Depression as nonprofit, low-cost medical plans operating under special laws with less government red tape. Blue Cross covered hospital costs and Blue Shield covered physician costs. The plans have since merged, and many states dropped the nonprofit status to compete. They are no longer low cost.

brief HPI a brief history of present illness; the medical record documentation should describe one to three elements of the present illness.

business office personnel employees in the medical business office: office manager, billing manager, schedulers, receptionists, billers, collections employees, medical records employees, and professional medical coders.

capitation a method to pay physicians based on the number of patients assigned by the medical plan rather than actual costs incurred. The physician controls the expense of rendering care.

carrier the insurer or medical plan chosen to administer the portions of a government medical plan specific to one state. For Medicare, the private insurer chosen to administer Part B claims. Also refers to a payor or medical plan chosen to administer or underwrite a range of health benefit programs.

case number a payor-assigned number that must appear on each page of each document sent with an appeal.

categorically needy the state is *required* to give these people Medicaid coverage if the state is to be eligible for federal funds.

category three-digit related codes within each section of a chapter in the Volume 1 tabular list of codes in the ICD-9-CM codebook.

CC (1) chief complaint; a concise statement describing the reason for an outpatient visit; (2) complications and comorbidities; those additional conditions that increase the length of an inpatient stay by at least 1 day in at least 75% of patients.

certified coding professional someone who has met the educational and experience prerequisites and who has passed a medical coding certification test administered by a professional coding organization.

CHAMPUS Civilian Health and Medical Program of the Uniformed Services; the law that established an entitlement program to provide medical coverage for families of military service members.

CHAMPVA Civilian Health and Medical Program of Veterans Affairs; the law that established an entitlement program to provide medical coverage for dependents of veterans totally disabled with a service-connected disability and dependents of veterans who died while on active duty and in the line of duty.

chapter the first major division in the tabular list in Volume 1 of the ICD-9-CM codebook. Chapters represent body systems or types of conditions.

circulatory system uses the heart, blood, and blood vessels in a complex delivery system for the body. The heart pumps the blood and keeps it flowing through the blood vessels. Arteries carry blood away from the heart and veins carry blood back to the heart.

claim audits check for duplication of services or billing that is in excess of normal.

claim edits check for completeness and accuracy of claim form.

clean claim a claim that passes payor claim edits and claim audits.

clinical staff the production employees in the medical practice: physicians, NPs, PAs, ancillary medical providers, nursing personnel, and technicians.

clinical support staff the members of the clinical staff who do not practice medicine, although some do practice nursing: RNs, LPNs, technicians, CMAs, and RMAs.

CMA certified medical assistant; an employee whose education places an emphasis on the outpatient medical office and encompasses both clinical and business office functions and who has passed a certification examination administered by the American Association of Medical Assistants (AAMA), a professional association.

CMS-1500 claim form the claim form used by physicians and other nonfacility providers to bill payors for medical charges incurred by someone covered by the medical plan.

coinsurance the portion of covered medical care costs for which the patient has a financial responsibility. Often a deductible must be met first. *Copay* refers to either coinsurance or copayment.

collections agency an outside resource option to collect delinquent payments from patients.

collections employee an employee with responsibility for collecting payments from insurance companies and patients.

combining vowel a vowel inserted to link word parts together to make them easier to read.

comment period the time during which everyone may review proposed rules and requirements developed by the Secretary of Health and Human Services to meet a specific law. Anyone may submit comments and suggestions during this time.

comorbidity secondary diagnoses and conditions that influence treatment; diagnoses that coexist.

complete PFSH complete past, family, and/or social history; a documented review of two or all three PFSH areas, depending on the category of E/M service. All three areas are required for comprehensive assessments.

complete ROS complete review of systems; the documented report of an inquiry about the body system(s) directly related to the problem(s) identified in the history of present illness (HPI) plus all additional body systems (at least 10).

compliance deadline the date when a "final rule" developed by the Secretary of Health and Human Services to meet a specific law becomes mandatory and is strictly enforced.

complications and comorbidities (CC) Those additional conditions that increase the length of stay by at least one day in at least 75% of patients.

comprehensive code a code that includes all the services essential to accomplishing a service or procedure; also called a bundle or a package.

comprehensive exam (1) *1995 guidelines*: a general multi-system examination or a complete examination of a single organ system or body area; (2) *1997 guidelines for multi-system exam*: should include at least nine organ systems or body areas. For each system/area selected, all elements of the examination identified in a table by a bullet (●) should be performed, unless specific directions limit the content of the examination. For each area/system, documentation of at least two elements identified in a table by a bullet (●) is expected; (3) *1997 guidelines for single organ system exam*: should include performance of all elements identified in a table by a bullet (●), whether in a shaded or unshaded box. Documentation of every element in each shaded box and at least one element in each unshaded box is expected.

comprehensive history documentation must include the chief complaint, an extended history of presenting illness (HPI), a complete review of systems (ROS), and complete past, family, and/or social history (PFSH).

concurrent payment audit an audit that occurs at the time payments are posted to evaluate the correctness of payments received on the day of the audit.

constitutional signs and symptoms includes vital signs and an assessment of a person's general well being.

consultation used when only an opinion or treatment advice is requested from the consulting physician. The consultant must send a written report to the requesting physician, or both physicians must document a telephone discussion.

context details that relate a medical problem to other factors (not timing) about other specific events (e.g., right upper quadrant abdominal pain or right shoulder pain that occurs after eating when only fatty foods are eaten). An element of HPI.

contributory elements the elements of documentation that confirm or augment the selection of codes for E/M services but that usually do not play a large enough role to make a difference in code choice. The exception is when counseling or coordination of care takes more than half the intraservice time for the encounter; then time is used to determine code selection.

conversion number the dollar value assigned to each RVU (relative value unit) to find the allowed fee in an RBRVS (resource-based relative value system) fee schedule.

coordination of benefits allows payors to reduce payments by the amount of coverage provided elsewhere so reimbursement is never greater than the actual charge.

copayment a cost-sharing agreement in which the patient pays a specified fee for specified services, and the medical plan pays the remainder of the cost. *Copay* can refer to either copayment or coinsurance.

Correct Coding Initiative (CCI) a Medicare editing system designed to control improper coding.

CPT *Current Procedural Terminology;* the Level I HCPCS procedure codebook updated and maintained by the American Medical Association.

credentialing the process of verifying credentials to establish that a person has not misrepresented accomplishments, that licensure remains current, and that the person has not been excluded from participation in federal medical plans.

curriculum vitae an expansive résumé that documents credentials, education, work history, and specific accomplishments, such as research projects, speaking engagements, and published works.

custodian of records the employee who is legally responsible for the care and handling of medical records for the medical practice.

DC doctor of chiropractic medicine; schooling focuses on medical health in relation to spinal alignment; fully licensed to practice chiropractic medicine.

deductible a specified amount of expense the patient must pay before the medical plan pays anything.

DEERS Defense Enrollment Eligibility Reporting System; the military organization that determines eligibility and issues military ID cards for CHAMPUS.

delinquent payment or account a payment or account that is overdue.

demographics statistics about a person or a population, such as name, age, gender, race, address, zip code, telephone number, and area code.

detailed exam (1) *1995 guidelines*: an extended examination of the affected body areas or other symptomatic or related organ systems; (2) *1997 guidelines for multi-system exam*: should include at least six organ systems or body areas. For each system/area selected, performance and documentation of at least two elements identified in a table by a bullet (●) is expected. Alternatively, a detailed examination may include performance and documentation of at least 12 elements identified in a table by a bullet (•) in two or more organ systems or body areas; (3) *1997 guidelines for single organ system exam*: examinations other than eye or psychiatric examinations should include performance and documentation of at least 12 elements identified in a table by a bullet (•), whether in a shaded or unshaded box. Eye and psychiatric examinations should include the performance and documentation of at least nine elements identified in a table by a bullet (•), whether in a shaded or unshaded box.

detailed history documentation must include the chief complaint, an extended history of present illness (HPI), an extended review of systems (ROS), and a pertinent past, family, and/or social history (PFSH).

diagnosis related group (DRG) the prospective payment system used by Medicare to determine payment for hospital inpatient services. It is based on the diagnosis codes billed.

digestive system processes food to provide nutrients to the body and processes solid waste that is expelled by the body.

disability income policies policies to replace lost wages during an extended illness or injury.

DO doctor of osteopathy; similar to an MD, but schooling places a larger emphasis on the role of the musculoskeletal system in overall health; a graduate from an osteopathic school of medicine who is fully licensed by the state to practice medicine.

documentation guidelines official guidelines developed by the CMS and published in the *Federal Register*; a method of evaluating physician performance by defining services and counting the items documented. All physicians are required by law to follow either the 1995 or the 1997 guidelines, or the most current guidelines once another set of guidelines is released.

downcoding a code is chosen for a less severe condition than is recorded in the patient's medical record, or for a lesser procedure than was actually performed; undercoding.

duplicate claim resubmission of an identical claim—mirror image—with no changes. Also called double billing; duplicate claims are considered fraud.

duration the length of time involved for each episode or occurrence of a medical problem or symptom. An element of the history of present illness (HPI).

E-code an explanatory code that lists the external causes and places of occurrence for injuries and poisonings.

EDI electronic data interchange; the process used to send claims electronically.

electronic payment posting the payor automatically posts a payment to your practice management system after making an automatic deposit into the practice bank account.

electronic remittance voucher an electronic EOB (explanation of benefits) that is sent when the payor sends an electronic payment that is automatically deposited in the practice bank account.

encounter form a fee ticket or superbill that ties reimbursement to specific encounters for line item billing.

endocrine system uses ductless glands to produce hormones. Hormones regulate many body functions.

end-stage renal disease (ESRD) end-stage renal disease is kidney failure.

EOB explanation of benefits; a notification of the payor's decision regarding a claim, accompanied by payment when payment is due.

EOMB explanation of Medicare benefits; a notice sent from Medicare to a beneficiary informing the beneficiary of Medicare's payment decisions and bills paid or not paid for the beneficiary.

eponym a word, such as a medical diagnosis or procedure, that is named after a person or a place.

EPSDT Medicaid's early periodic screening and diagnostic testing program; a preventive medicine program for certain children covered by Medicaid.

established patient one who has been seen within the last 3 years by the practice or by the specialty group within a multi-specialty practice.

evaluation and management (E/M) the process of evaluating a patient for suspected, known, or potential problems or conditions; assessing the findings; rendering an opinion; and developing and initiating a plan of action.

examination the process of obtaining and recording the physician's or other health care provider's medically significant observations and findings.

expanded problem-focused exam (1) *1995 guidelines*: a limited examination of the affected body area or organ system and other symptomatic or related organ systems; (2) *1997 guidelines for multi-system exam*: performance and documentation of at least six elements identified in a table by a bullet (•) in one or more organ system(s) or body area(s); (3) *1997 guidelines for single organ system exam*: performance and documentation of at least six elements identified in a table by a bullet (•), whether in a shaded or unshaded box.

expanded problem-focused history documentation must include the chief complaint, a brief history of present illness (HPI), and a problem-pertinent review of systems (ROS).

explanatory notes these give additional information about items referenced by footnotes or symbols on an EOB.

extended HPI the medical record documentation describes at least four elements of the present illness or describes the status of at least three chronic and/or inactive conditions.

extended ROS extended review of systems; the documented report of an inquiry about the body system(s) directly related to the problem(s) identified in the history of present illness (HPI) and a limited number (two to nine) of additional body systems.

face-to-face time documented time spent face-to-face with a patient or a patient's family in an office or other outpatient setting; outpatient intraservice time.

facility fee a charge representing the expenses incurred by a facility when providing a service.

False Claims Act a law that makes it illegal to submit a false or an inaccurate claim to the government for payment. This law covers all types of government payments, not just medical claims.

family history a documented review of the history of medical events in the patient's family, including hereditary diseases, contagious diseases, and any other diseases or conditions that place the patient at risk.

FBI Federal Bureau of Investigation; they investigate and prosecute federal offenses and criminal activity.

fee for service (FFS) the physician is paid a fee for each service provided; private fee-for-service medical plans are an option under Medicare Part C.

fee ticket a record of the day's charges for a patient.

FEIN Federal Employer Identification Number; a tax ID number issued to a business.

final rule the official release of new rules or standards developed by the Secretary of Health and Human Services to meet a specific law. Once a final rule is officially released, you may begin using the rule. After an implementation period, a compliance deadline is established.

financial class a person's income or ability to pay a debt.

financial hardship discount a discount given when a patient is in financial difficulty and cannot meet the patient financial obligation. A hardship waiver must be on file before this discount is given. The physician collects the payor's portion of the charge and writes off the patient portion of the charge.

financial policy statement a patient-signed document that protects the physician's right to collect money earned.

financial record documentation of a patient's financial transactions, i.e., billing and collections.

fiscal intermediary (FI) the insurer or medical plan chosen to administer Medicare Part A and some Medicare Part B claims for the government, or the insurer or medical plan chosen to administer other government programs (e.g., Medicaid, CHAMPUS, TRICARE).

floor/unit time documented time spent working directly on behalf of an inpatient while physically present on the patient's floor or unit; inpatient intraservice time. It includes but is not limited to face-to-face time.

FPL federal poverty line.

fragmentation occurs when a service that is normally completed in one visit is broken apart to require two or more visits.

gag clause prohibits a physician from discussing with a patient treatment options the payor does not cover, such as experimental treatments or treatments that are expensive, even when one of these treatments represents the best course of action for the patient.

genitourinary system the reproductive and urinary systems. The male and female reproductive systems work together to create a baby. The urinary system processes and expels liquid waste from the body.

global period the time period during which all care related to a procedure is considered to be part of the code that reports the procedure, and it may not be billed separately.

greatest level of specificity the code with the greatest level of detail that matches the patient's medical record with the greatest accuracy.

group medical plans medical insurance plans offered to groups, usually at a discounted rate or with special provisions. Employers are offered guarantee-issued coverage—employees cannot be excluded from the plan, and preexisting conditions are covered in accordance with the Health Insurance Portability and Accountability Act of 1996 (HIPAA) and subsequent related laws.

HCPCS *HCFA Common Procedure Coding System*; the Level II HCPCS procedure codebook updated and maintained by the CMS.

health insurance portability allows individuals to keep employer-group medical insurance plans when changing jobs.

high-complexity medical decision-making documentation of (1) an extensive number of diagnoses or management options; (2) an extensive amount of data or complexity of data to be reviewed; and (3) a high risk of complications and/or morbidity or mortality.

high-severity presenting problem a medical problem in which the risk of morbidity without treatment is high to extreme; there is moderate to high risk of mortality without treatment *or* high probability of severe, prolonged functional impairment.

HIPAA Health Insurance Portability and Accountability Act of 1996; a federal law that governs many aspects of health care.

history of present illness (HPI) a chronologic description of (1) the development of the patient's present illness or problem from the first sign or symptom; *or* (2) the development of the patient's present illness or problem from the previous encounter to the present. It includes the following elements: location, quality, severity, duration, timing, context, associated signs and symptoms, and modifying factors.

HMO health maintenance organization; a managed care medical plan.

hypertension table a table to assist with code choices for hypertension; part of the alphabetical index in Section 1 of Volume 2 of the ICD-9-CM codebook.

ICD-9-CM *International Classification of Diseases, Ninth Revision, Clinical Modification*; the version of the diagnosis codebook used in the United States for diagnosis coding until the date ICD-10-CM is implemented.

ICD-10-CM *International Classification of Diseases, Tenth Revision, Clinical Modification*; the next version of the diagnosis codebook that will be used in the United States. It might be used for diagnosis coding as early as October 2007, but implementation could be delayed until a later year.

IME independent medical exam; a second opinion requested and paid for by a third party. There must be a valid reason for conducting the exam. Valid reasons include but are not limited to confirmation of level of impairment or injury or confirmation of medical condition for workers' compensation, disability insurance, liability lawsuit, other legal proceedings, etc.

immune system uses the lymphatic system and the spleen to fight infection and regulate immune responses. Also regulates the amount of fluid in and around body cells.

indemnity the purest form of commercial medical insurance. The patient directs his or her own care and pays a deductible as well as a percentage of the costs.

indicators CCI indicators designate which codes can be pulled out of a bundle and which cannot.

individual medical plans insurance policies offered to individuals rather than groups. Individuals can be denied coverage. Under HIPAA, insurance portability is tied to employer-group plans in which an employee changes jobs.

insurance write-off the insurance discount given to a payor in a contract.

insured the person entitled to benefits under an insurance policy. The *insured* is the policyholder, the person whose name is listed in the medical plan's files as the owner of the policy. Some medical plans call the insured a "subscriber," and Medicare calls the insured a "beneficiary."

integumentary system consists of skin, hair, nails, sebaceous glands, and sweat glands. It is the body's largest organ system and the first line of defense against infection.

intraservice time documented face-to-face time or floor/unit time used to calculate the level of E/M code when time is the determining factor.

key components the elements of documentation that best describe the amount of work performed and that are used to determine the code choice for E/M services.

Kyle provision legislation included in the 1997 Balanced Budget Act that allows providers who opt out of the Medicare program (minimum 2 year opt-out) to enter into private contracts with Medicare recipients for services that would normally be covered by Medicare. Special rules apply.

LCSW licensed clinical social worker; a limited-license mental health professional with a minimum of a bachelor's degree and who has passed a state licensure examination.

ledger card an old-fashioned patient accounting method that does not allow you to track payments by transaction.

length of stay (LOS) the actual length of time a patient spends as an inpatient in the hospital.

lifetime reserve an extra 60 days of hospital coverage that a Medicare recipient may use only once. When the days are gone, Medicare coverage for hospitalization beyond 90 days ceases.

limited license the scope of medical practice has limitations; the number and the type of services are less than for a full license to practice medicine: often limited to a particular specialty and to specific services within that specialty.

line item posting an accounting method by which every payment is posted to the exact transaction for which the payment is received.

living will a legal document that communicates a patient's decision regarding life support measures in the event the patient is unconscious or otherwise unable to make that decision.

location the anatomical location of a medical problem. An element of history of present illness (HPI).

low-complexity medical decision-making documentation of (1) a limited number or diagnoses or management options; (2) a limited amount of data or complexity of data to be reviewed; and (3) a low risk of complications and/or morbidity or mortality.

low-severity presenting problem a medical problem where the risk of morbidity without treatment is low; there is little to no risk of mortality without treatment; full recovery without functional impairment is expected.

LPN licensed practical nurse; a limited-license nursing professional whose education places an emphasis on the clinical aspects of nursing and who has passed a state licensure examination.

main term the word to look up in an alphabetical index; in ICD-9-CM, a condition, disease, or injury.

major diagnostic category (MDC) each category groups patients who are medically related by diagnosis, treatment similarity, and statistically similar length of hospital stay. The more than 10,000 available ICD-9-CM diagnosis codes are divided into 25 major diagnostic categories.

MD medical doctor; a graduate from medical school who is fully licensed by the state to practice medicine.

MedCHAMP a program for CHAMPUS-eligible persons younger than age 65 who qualify for both Medicare and CHAMPUS. Medicare is the primary payor and CHAMPUS is the secondary payor.

Medicaid a government medical program developed to provide coverage for qualified low-income applicants.

medical biller a medical business office employee who prepares and submits medical claim forms.

Medical Care Cost Recovery Program (MCCRP) a program developed to enable the Department of Veterans Affairs (VA) to bill third-party payors for non–service-connected care rendered by the VA to veterans, and to collect copayments from veterans with less than a 50% service-connected disability rating for non–service-connected care rendered, based on ability to pay.

medical decision-making (MDM) documentation of the thought processes required to evaluate medical findings, documentation of the amount of work performed when evaluating medical data, and documentation of the conclusions drawn and the resulting plan of care. The amount of risk involved also is factored into the level of MDM chosen.

medical necessity a medically sound reason for ordering a specific service.

medical record documentation of a patient's medical visits and care rendered.

medical records employee a medical business office employee who is responsible for handling and safeguarding patient medical records.

medically needy this option allows states to extend Medicaid eligibility to additional people as defined by the state—usually people who can meet ordinary expenses but cannot afford medical care.

Medicare the federal medical program that provides hospital and medical expense protection for the elderly (age 65 or older), anyone who suffers from chronic kidney disease (any age), and those who receive Social Security disability benefits.

Medicare Advantage the current name for Medicare Part C, formerly Medicare + Choice; options Medicare beneficiaries may choose instead of traditional Medicare. Enrollees must have Medicare Part A and Part B, and they cannot have end-stage renal disease (kidney failure).

Medicare Part A a Medicare program that provides coverage for hospital and hospitalization-related expenses.

Medicare Part B a Medicare program that provides coverage for physician services, ambulances, diagnostic tests, medical equipment and supplies, and ancillary services.

Medicare Part C also called Medicare + Choice and Medicare Advantage; a Medicare program that gives Medicare recipients the option of replacing traditional Medicare with a plan that covers Part A and Part B services in one plan. In order to qualify, the enrollee must have both Part A and Part B coverage, and the enrollee cannot have end-stage renal disease (kidney failure).

Medicare Part D was created by the Medicare Modernization Act of 2003. It is a voluntary program designed to provide a prescription drug benefit.

Medicare provider number a Medicare-assigned number that identifies the exact physician in a practice who provided the service reported on line 24 of the CMS-1500 claim form. This number is placed in block No. 24K for a group practice and for a single- physician practice that is incorporated. It is placed in block No. 33 for a single-physician practice not incorporated. This will be replaced by the National Provider Identifier (NPI) when the NPI becomes available. Providers began obtaining NPIs in June 2005, but the implementation date to begin using the NPI is expected to be at least 1 year later.

Medicare Select Medicare supplemental policies similar to Medigap, except they only provide coverage when preferred providers are used, and they cost less than unrestricted Medigap plans.

Medicare UPIN a unique provider identification number issued by Medicare to identify each individual physician who is authorized to give referrals for Medicare patients. On a claim form, the UPIN distinguishes between the referring physician and the rendering physician. This number will be replaced with the National Provider Identifier (NPI) when the NPI becomes available.

Medigap Medicare supplemental policies designed to cover some or all the costs not covered by traditional Medicare. Enrollees must have both Medicare Part A and Medicare Part B.

MIB Medical Information Bureau; an organization formed by insurance companies in 1902 to share or pool subscriber information related to health and lifestyle in order to prevent fraud.

minimal presenting problem a medical problem that may not require the presence of a physician, but the service is provided under the physician's supervision.

MMI maximum medical improvement and impairment rating; measures long-term impairment, often as a percentage of total body function.

moderate-complexity medical decision-making documentation of (1) multiple diagnoses or management options; (2) a moderate amount of data or complexity of data to be reviewed; and (3) a moderate risk of complications and/or morbidity or mortality.

moderate severity presenting problem a medical problem in which the risk of morbidity without treatment is moderate; there is a moderate risk of mortality without treatment; uncertain prognosis or increased probability of prolonged functional impairment.

modifiers used with a procedure code to report that a service or procedure has been altered by a specific circumstance.

modifying factors details that alter the definition or scope of a medical problem (e.g., the fact that a patient smokes must be considered and it changes the scope of many medical problems). An element of history of present illness (HPI).

morbidity sickness or statistical incidence of disease.

mortality death or statistical incidence of death.

MRN Medicare remittance notice; also called remittance advice (RA); this notice is sent from Medicare to the physician (or other medical provider) giving notification of Medicare's payment decision regarding a claim, accompanied by payment when payment is due.

MSA medical savings account; a medical plan option under Medicare Part C.

musculoskeletal system muscles and bones provide the framework that gives the body shape, form, and movement.

mutually exclusive code pairs service or procedure combinations that would not or could not reasonably be performed at the same session, by the same provider, on the same patient.

neoplasm table a table to assist with code selection for neoplasms; located in the alphabetical index in Section 1 of Volume 2 of the ICD-9-CM codebook.

nervous system the electronic computer system for the body. It gathers, stores, and interprets information, and it initiates responses. It includes the central nervous system, the peripheral nervous system, and the autonomic nervous system.

new patient a patient who is new to the practice or who has not been seen by a physician in the practice (or the specialty in a multi-specialty group) within the past 3 years.

nonparticipating provider a provider who signs a Medicare contract but does not accept assignment of benefits.

non–service-connected a medical problem that did not develop during military service and is not related to or caused by military service.

no-show a patient who fails to arrive for a scheduled appointment and who has not called to cancel the appointment.

NP nurse practitioner; a registered nurse who has received advanced education and has passed a state certification examination to obtain a limited license to practice medicine in addition to practicing nursing.

NPI National Provider Identifier; a number that Medicare began issuing in June 2005 to replace the unique provider identification number (UPIN), practice (or physician) identification number (PIN), and provider number systems used historically before that time. A physician will have just one number to use in every location and every state to identify who he or she is. This number may be used in blocks 17B, 24K, and sometimes 33 on the CMS-1500 claim form for physician billing and in FL 82 and FL 83 on the UB-92 claim form for hospital and facility billing.

NSF National Standard Format; a simpler format used to send electronic claims. New versions are issued periodically. Only the data on the claim form are transmitted electronically. Supporting documentation is sent under separate cover.

number of diagnosis or management options documentation of (1) every diagnosis and every diagnosis option the physician thought about and considered, including new diagnoses, the status of previously established diagnoses, and rule-out of possible diagnoses; and (2) every treatment and every treatment option the physician thought about and considered, including the initiation of or changes actually made in treatment and alternative treatment options discussed with the patient.

OCR optical character recognition; a process by which a computer "reads" information that is scanned into the computer.

office manager the top-level supervisor in a medical practice whose responsibilities encompass both business office and clinical duties.

OIG/HHS Office of Inspector General, Department of Health and Human Services.

OT occupational therapist or occupational therapy; requires a minimum of a bachelor's degree and passing a state licensure examination to obtain a license in occupational therapy.

outlier payors use software programs to determine patterns of code use. They know the usual patterns for every region and every physician who submits claims. Those who fall outside the normal statistical patterns for a specialty or for a region are called outliers. Claims from outliers are scrutinized more carefully.

out-of-plan services rendered by providers or hospitals that do not have a contract agreement with the patient's medical plan.

outpatient prospective payment system (OPPS) the prospective payment system used by Medicare to determine payment for hospital outpatient services. It is based on the procedure codes billed. Also called APC.

outside lab a lab that bills the physician for tests the physician purchased on behalf of a patient. The physician then bills the patient's medical plan. When an outside lab is used, the lab is identified in block No. 32 on the CMS-1500 claim form.

PA physician's assistant; a medical provider who has completed the required education and passed a state licensure examination to obtain a limited license to practice medicine.

participating physician (1) a physician who signed a contract with a medical plan and agreed to provide services to plan members; (2) a physician who signed a Medicare contract and agreed to provide services and accept the Medicare fee schedule for Medicare patients.

participating provider a provider who signs a Medicare contract and accepts assignment of benefits. Also, a provider who signs a Medicaid or an HMO managed care contract.

past, family, and/or social history (PFSH) a documented review of the patient's past history, family history, and/or age-appropriate social history and activities.

past history documentation of the patient's past experience with illness, operations, injuries, and/or treatments.

patient account number a number assigned by the practice for internal identification of the patient's financial record.

patient discount often offered to self-pay patients if they pay their bills on time. It must not cause the total fee to become lower than the Medicare fee schedule for the service.

patient eligibility the process of contacting each payor and verifying that the patient is covered by the policy, the policy information is correct, and the policy has not expired. Sometimes additional information is needed to determine the primary payor for the claim.

patient financial responsibility the portion of the bill that the patient legally is required to pay.

patient-supplied information the billing information for the top half of the medical claim form.

payor the insurance company responsible for paying the medical claim.

peer review organization (PRO) PROs consist of physicians and other health care professionals (nurses, data technicians, etc.) who review the care given to Medicare patients. Hospitals must enter into a contract with a PRO in order to receive DRG payments. The federal government pays PROs, but they are separate from Medicare and have their own functions. The newest title for this organization is quality improvement organization, or QIO.

penalized claim a claim that did not pass the payor's claim edits or claim audits and a penalty was applied, reducing the payment.

pertinent PFSH a documented review of past, family, and/or social history (PFSH) that is directly related to the history of present illness (HPI). At least one item from any of the three PFSH areas must be documented.

physical address the actual location of a building or the actual location where a person lives—not a post office box.

physician a person who is fully licensed to practice medicine: MD or DO.

pigeonholing the practice of using a short list of diagnosis codes and using those codes for all patients, regardless of whether the codes match actual diagnoses and conditions.

PIN (Medicare) a practice identification number assigned to a group practice or a solo physician who has incorporated the practice. It is used in block No. 33 on the CMS-1500 claim form.

place of service codes codes used to identify where a service is rendered.

policyholder the primary person entitled to benefits under an insurance policy, and the person whose name is listed as the owner of the policy. Some medical plans call the policyholder a "subscriber," and Medicare calls the policyholder a "beneficiary." On the CMS-1500 claim form, the policyholder is the "insured."

POS point of service; an option that allows HMO patients limited coverage for out-of-plan providers.

PP/PM per patient per month; the amount of money a physician receives each month for each assigned patient under a capitation payment system. Some payors call it per member, per month.

PPO preferred provider organization; a managed care medical plan.

preauthorization the process of obtaining prior approval before a service: treatment, test, or procedure. It does not guarantee coverage if the claim form does not establish medical necessity.

preexisting condition any condition with which a person has ever been diagnosed or for which a person has ever received medical treatment.

preferred provider a physician who has signed a contract with a PPO-type of medical plan (similar to an HMO participating provider).

prefix a word part attached at the beginning of a word to add to or alter the meaning of the word.

prescription an order for a drug, treatment, or device, written or given by a properly licensed professional.

preventive medicine treatment rendered to prevent medical problems and reduce the incidence of costly medical care.

primary diagnosis the condition that prompted an outpatient visit or treatment or the underlying cause for a hospital visit.

primary payor the insurance company that legally should be billed first when more than one insurance company can be billed.

principal diagnosis the condition that is found after study to be chiefly responsible for a hospitalization.

problem-focused exam (1) *1995 guidelines*: a limited examination of the affected body area or organ system; (2) *1997 guidelines for multi-system exam*: performance and documentation of one to five elements identified in a table by a bullet (•) in one or more organ system(s) or body area(s); (3) *1997 guidelines for single organ system exam*: performance and documentation of one to five elements identified in a table by a bullet (•), whether in a shaded or unshaded box.

problem-focused history documentation must include the chief complaint and a brief history of present illness (HPI).

problem-pertinent ROS problem-pertinent review of systems; the documented report of an inquiry about the body system(s) directly related to the problem(s) identified in the history of present illness (HPI).

professional courtesy the physician sees a patient at no charge.

profit the money remaining from a payment after all expenses for the service, including employee expenses, have been paid.

proposed standard the first draft of new rules or standards developed by the Secretary of Health and Human Services to meet a specific law. After a public comment period, a final rule is developed.

provider number (Medicare) a number assigned by Medicare to identify individual providers in a group and to identify solo physicians who are not incorporated. For Medicare, the National Provider Identifier (NPI) will replace this number. Medicare began issuing NPIs in June 2005.

provider-supplied information the billing information for the bottom half of the medical claim form.

PSO provider-sponsored organization; a new medical plan created by Medicare Part C.

PT physical therapist, or physical therapy; requires a minimum of a bachelor's degree and passing a state licensure examination to obtain a license in physical therapy.

quality the details used to distinguish differences between similar problems (e.g., pain may be sharp, stabbing, cramping, dull, heavy, burning). An element of history of present illness (HPI).

quality improvement organization (QIO) The new title for peer review organization, or PRO. QIOs consist of physicians and other health care professionals (nurses, data technicians, etc.) who review the care given to Medicare patients. Hospitals must enter into a contract with a QIO in order to receive DRG payments. The federal government pays QIOs, but they are separate from Medicare and have their own functions.

Qui Tam a provision of the False Claims Act designed to allow ordinary citizens to report violations without repercussions.

RBRVS resource-based relative value system; the prospective payment system used by Medicare to pay physicians. It considers the *Current Procedural Terminology* (CPT) code in relation to work, overhead expenses, and malpractice (risk). A geographical adjustment is then made to account for cost-of-living differences throughout the nation.

rebill the process of resubmitting a corrected claim.

receptionist the business office employee who greets patients and obtains or verifies the patient-supplied information for the medical claim form.

referral used whenever partial or total care of the patient is transferred to another physician.

reimbursement decision tree a tool to help you decide what your next action is when you receive an EOB from a payor.

rejected claim a claim that did not pass payor claim edits and claim audits, and no payment was sent.

relative value unit (RVU) a numeric value assigned to each procedure code in the RBRVS. This number represents the total of each of three parts (work, overhead, and malpractice). Each part is multiplied by the geographic practice site indicator (GPSI) and then added together to get a total adjusted RVU. The total adjusted RVU is multiplied by the conversion factor (the assigned per-RVU dollar value) to arrive at the RBRVS fee allowed for the service.

relator the person who reports a violation under the False Claims Act. A whistleblower.

release of information the patient authorizes the medical practice to send specific records, such as billing information, to a payor or to a specific person or place.

repeat claims corrected claims that have been resubmitted with information that has changed; not the same as duplicate claims.

resource-based relative value system (RBRVS) the prospective payment system used by Medicare to pay physicians. It considers the *Current Procedural Terminology* (CPT) code in relation to work, overhead expenses, and malpractice (risk). A geographical adjustment is then made to account for cost-of-living differences throughout the nation.

respiratory system uses breathing to bring oxygen into the body and to expel carbon dioxide from the body.

retrospective payment audit an audit that tracks and evaluates patient financial records for a specific number of completed transactions. It verifies the correctness of payments received from every source and the correctness and appropriateness of the write-offs for each transaction.

review of systems (ROS) a documented inventory of normal and abnormal subjective findings and/or symptoms reported by the patient or others.

right of subrogation allows physicians to be reimbursed by medical plan payors for some or all of the patient charges until payor responsibility can be determined. This is considered a good faith payment. If a different payor is later found to be responsible, the medical plan that paid first is reimbursed for those expenses.

risk of significant complications, morbidity, and/or mortality risks are based on documentation of the presenting problem(s), the procedure(s) performed, treatments ordered, and other possible management options.

RMA registered medical assistant; an employee whose education places an emphasis on the outpatient medical office and encompasses both clinical and business office functions and who has passed a certification examination administered by the American Medical Technologists (AMT), a professional association.

RN registered nurse; a fully licensed nursing professional. Must complete required education and pass a state licensure examination to obtain a license as a registered nurse.

root word the word part that gives the basic meaning of the word.

RVU relative value unit; a numeric value assigned to each procedure code in the RBRVS. This number represents the total of each of three parts (work, overhead, and malpractice). Each part is multiplied by the geographic practice site indicator (GPSI) and then added together to get a total adjusted RVU. The total adjusted RVU is multiplied by the conversion factor (the assigned per-RVU dollar value) to arrive at the RBRVS fee allowed for the service.

scheduler a business office employee who schedules patient appointments.

scope of practice the legal limits of licensure or certification; the number and type of services that can be performed with a given set of credentials.

secondary diagnosis a diagnosis that contributes to a condition for an outpatient visit; it may include the underlying cause.

secondary payor the insurance company that legally should be billed second for any remaining unpaid bills after the primary payor has sent payment.

section related groups of codes within a chapter in the tabular list in Volume 1 of ICD-9-CM; the major divisions within each chapter.

Security Standards for Health Information a law that governs the security of electronic patient records.

self-limited or minor presenting problem a medical problem that runs a definite and prescribed course, is transient in nature, and is not likely to permanently alter heath status *or* has a good prognosis when treatment is given as ordered.

service connected a medical problem that arose while the person was serving on active duty or that was caused by active duty military service, or a problem that was incurred during reserve duty with a military unit.

severity the details used to distinguish levels of seriousness for a medical problem. An element of history of present illness (HPI).

sign a change from normal noted or observed by the examiner.

significant finding a change from normal (a sign or a symptom) or a significant normal finding that narrows the options and leads to a diagnosis.

single component codes codes used to bill services when only one component of a comprehensive procedure is performed.

social history a documented, age-appropriate review of the patient's past and current activities.

special report a report that explains or clarifies an unusual, variable, or infrequently performed service or procedure.

SSI Supplemental Security Income; a Social Security program that provides additional income to qualified beneficiaries.

SSN Social Security number; a tax ID number issued to an individual.

ST speech therapist or speech therapy. Requires a minimum of a bachelor's degree and passing a state licensure examination to obtain a license in speech therapy.

standards of care protocols tests and procedures are only considered covered services for specific predetermined diagnoses that are not usually disclosed to the physician because they are considered trade secrets. These are commonly called black-box edits.

Stark laws laws that regulate many activities relating to consultations and referrals. They prevent physicians and other providers from profiting from the consultations and referrals they give out. They are often called the antikickback laws.

starred procedures deleted in 2004, starred procedures were relatively minor surgical procedures that were not bundled and did not have a global period. All preprocedure and postprocedure work was reported separately.

straightforward medical decision-making documentation of a minimal number or diagnoses or management options, zero to minimal data or complexity of data to be reviewed, and a minimal risk of complications and/or morbidity or mortality.

subcategory the fourth digit in an ICD-9-CM code; further defines the codes within a category in the Volume 1 tabular list of codes.

subclassification the fifth digit in an ICD-9-CM code; adds more specificity to distinguish between codes within a subcategory in the Volume 1 tabular list of codes.

subscriber the primary person entitled to benefits under an insurance policy. The subscriber is the policyholder—the person whose name is listed in the medical plan's files as the owner of the policy. The subscriber is the "insured" for purposes of completing a medical claim form.

suffix a word part attached at the end of a word that adds to or alters the meaning of the word.

superbill a tool to report chart documentation for billing purposes; part of the financial record.

symptom a change or suspected change from normal noted or observed by the patient.

table of drugs and chemicals a table to assist with code selections that identify drugs and other chemicals. It is located in Section 2 of Volume 2 in ICD-9-CM, right after the alphabetical index.

tabular list a numerical list of diagnosis codes presented in a format similar to a table; it is located in Volume 1 of ICD-9-CM and is arranged by body system or types of conditions.

TANF Temporary Assistance for Needy Families.

timing the details that relate a medical problem to when other specific events occur, or that identify a pattern of occurrences. An element of history of present illness (HPI).

TRICARE a program with three levels of coverage established to administer CHAMPUS.

type of service codes codes used to categorize the type of service and give a clearer picture of what occurred.

UCR usual, customary, and reasonable; often the average payment rate that same-specialty providers have accepted in a given region.

unbundling when a group of procedures covered by a single comprehensive code are each reported separately instead of using the comprehensive code.

Uniform Bill 1992 (UB-92) the claim form used in facility billing.

unlisted procedure codes used when *Current Procedural Terminology* (CPT) does not contain an appropriate entry. They end in -9 or -99. Each section of CPT has unlisted procedure codes.

unprocessable claim a claim that could not be processed by a payor because of missing key information.

upcoding a code is chosen for a more severe condition or for a more extensive procedure than is documented in the patient's medical record; overcoding.

UPIN (Medicare) unique physician identifier number; used by Medicare to identify a referring physician. Medicare began replacing this number with the National Provider Identifier (NPI) in June 2005.

V-code a supplemental code that describes reasons other than illness for which a person might encounter the health care system; many V-codes cannot be used as a principal or primary diagnosis.

vendor a representative from another company that wishes to sell a product or a service to the medical practice.

vital signs a minimum of 3 of 10 possible examination items identified by the American Medical Association considered critical to assess body function.

whistleblower a relator in a Qui Tam action; the person who reports a violation of the False Claims Act.

workers' compensation employer-owned combination medical insurance and disability income policy that covers employees' work-related illnesses, injuries, and deaths.

working aged any person age 65 or older who continues to work.

write-off a discount the physician has given a patient or has authorized in a payor contract.

Page numbers followed by f indicate figures; t, tables; b, boxes.